Clinical Cardiac MRI With Interactive CD-ROM

J. Bogaert · S. Dymarkowski · A. M. Taylor (Eds.)

Softcover Edition

Originally published in:

Medical Radiology – Diagnostic Imaging

Editors:
A. L. Baert, Leuven · K. Sartor, Heidelberg

J. Bogaert · S. Dymarkowski · A. M. Taylor (Eds.)

Clinical
Cardiac MRI

With Interactive CD-ROM

With Contributions by

N. Al-Saadi · J. Bogaert · H. Bosmans · S. Dymarkowsi · P. Hamaekers · S. R. Hegde
V. Muthurangu · Y. Ni · R. Razavi · A. M. Taylor

Foreword by
A. L. Baert

With 437 Figures in 1218 Separate Illustrations, 92 in Color and 52 Tables

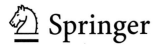 Springer

JAN BOGAERT, MD, PhD
Professor of Medicine
Department of Radiology
Gasthuisberg University Hospital
Catholic University of Leuven
Herestraat 49
3000 Leuven
Belgium

STEVEN DYMARKOWSKI, MD, PhD
Department of Radiology
Gasthuisberg University Hospital
Catholic University of Leuven
Herestraat 49
3000 Leuven
Belgium

ANDREW M. TAYLOR, MD, MRCP, FRCR
Senior Clinical Lecturer and
Honorary Consultant in Cardiovascular MR
Cardiothoracic Unit
Institute of Child Health and
Great Ormond Street Hospital for Children
London WC1N 3JH
UK

Originally published in:

MEDICAL RADIOLOGY · Diagnostic Imaging and Radiation Oncology
Series Editors: A. L. Baert · L. W. Brady · H.-P. Heilmann · M. Molls · K. Sartor
ISBN 3-540-40170-9 Springer Berlin Heidelberg New York
Continuation of Handbuch der medizinischen Radiologie · Encyclopedia of Medical Radiology

Library of Congress Control Number: 2004094688

ISBN 3-540-26217-2 Springer Berlin Heidelberg New York
ISBN 978-3-540-26217-6 Springer Berlin Heidelberg New York

Springer is part of Springer Science+Business Media

http//www.springeronline.com
© Springer-Verlag Berlin Heidelberg 2005
Printed in Germany

Medical Editor: Dr. Ute Heilmann, Heidelberg
Desk Editor: Ursula N. Davis, Heidelberg
Production Editor: Kurt Teichmann, Mauer
Cover-Design and Typesetting: Verlagsservice Teichmann, Mauer

Printed on acid-free paper – 21/3150xq – 5 4 3 2 1 0

This book is dedicated to

Brigitte, Christophe, Sébastien and Julie Jan Bogaert

Ursula, Karen and Steven Jr. Steven Dymarkowski

Nazneen and Haroon Andrew Taylor

Foreword

Few areas in radiology attract so much attention as cardiac MRI, because of its unique ability to study cardiac function – more specifically cardiac contraction, myocardial perfusion and valvular function – in a non-invasive way.

The editors and contributing authors have prepared this book on the basis of their personal long-standing involvement with clinical cardiac MRI. It is, however, their aim to provide the readers not only with the fruits of their personal experience but also with current opinions and the latest developments in the field. The fascinating possibilities of clinical cardiac MRI in children and adults are covered comprehensively and the full range of clinical cardiac diseases is discussed, but the limitations of the method are also clearly outlined.

One of the strengths of this volume is its extensive and superb illustrations, complemented by a wonderful CD-ROM to better demonstrate the specific dynamic information provided by cardiac MRI.

I would like to thank the editors and the authors and congratulate them sincerely for their superb efforts in producing this excellent volume, a comprehensive update of our knowledge of cardiac MRI. This book will be a daily reference for radiologists involved in cardiac imaging, cardiologists and cardiac surgeons.

I am confident that it will meet the same success with readers as the previous volumes published in this series.

Leuven   ALBERT L. BAERT

Preface

We have compiled and written this textbook to highlight the clinical indications and applications of cardiac magnetic resonance imaging (MRI). Over the past few decades, MRI has become an essential element of decision making for many medical specialties. However, though cardiovascular diseases are a major cause of morbidity and mortality throughout the world, MRI of the heart and great vessels has experienced relatively slow acceptance. In part this is due to the technical difficulties of imaging a structure that is affected by both its own motion and that of respiration, and the effects of flowing blood. Although the first publications on cardiac MRI coincided with those on applications in other organs of the human body, the radiology and cardiology communities have always considered cardiac MRI promising, but not yet ready for clinical use.

It has taken nearly two decades, and the perseverance of several small groups of advocates, to establish cardiac MRI more broadly. Nowadays, the initial skepticism has been replaced by increasing optimism from imagers, clinicians and manufacturers alike. In recent years, not only has cardiac MRI benefited from technical MRI advances, but several publications have demonstrated unequivocally the advantages of MRI over other cardiac imaging modalities. Furthermore, several dedicated cardiac MRI societies have acted to promote cardiac MRI throughout the medical community. As a result, there is now a rapid growth in interest in cardiac MRI. This sudden change in mentality must be treated with some caution. Cardiac MRI is not a panacea for imaging the heart and great vessels, and over-promotion of promising pre-clinical research may lead to expectations that cannot be fulfilled, with potentially disastrous consequences for the long-term future of cardiac MRI.

The main incentive for writing this textbook was the desire to pass on our own experience of cardiac MRI, and in particular to provide guidance to those who are new to this field. Understanding cardiovascular MRI physics, and developing the skills to adjust and optimize sequence parameters in individual patients, is a major key to success. This book is edited and written by people who are active in clinical cardiac MRI, on routine MR scanners, on a daily basis. They contribute their personal experience, fueled with current state-of-the-art opinions on their subjects. They are well aware of what is, and what is not, currently achievable with cardiac MRI. The clinical indications for cardiac MRI are widely discussed, while potentially interesting but clinically premature applications are highlighted. Moreover, for some applications where the role of cardiac MRI has not yet been defined, the pros and cons of performing cardiac MRI are discussed.

The first part of this textbook deals with the more technical aspects of cardiac MRI – cardiovascular MRI physics, contrast agents, and the practical aspects of performing a cardiac MRI study. The second part of the book deals with cardiovascular anatomy, image positioning for the heart and great vessels, and the assessment of ventricular function and myocardial perfusion. In the third and largest part of the book, the role of cardiac MRI in different cardiovascular diseases is extensively covered. Finally, the current and future role of interventional cardiac MRI is discussed.

It is hoped that this book will serve as a useful reference to guide the daily interpretation of cardiac MRI studies. To achieve this goal, the textbook is extensively illustrated and includes tables with normal values and practical schemes, with a series of summary statements for each chapter. A CD-ROM is also included, containing 50 clinical teaching cases covering the widest possible range of cardiovascular pathologies. This new medium enables depiction of some of the major strengths of cardiac MRI, such as the study of cardiac contraction, myocardial perfusion, and valvular function, that are difficult to represent in static images. These cases illustrate well the comprehensive approach of current clinical cardiac MRI. The authors hope that this book will help you to understand and appreciate the exciting world of cardiac MRI.

Leuven

JAN BOGAERT
STEVEN DYMARKOWSKI

London

ANDREW TAYLOR

Contents

1 Cardiac MRI Physics

Steven Dymarkowski and Hilde Bosmans

CONTENTS

S. Dymarkowski, MD, PhD; H. Bosmans, PhD
Department of Radiology, Gasthuisberg University Hospital,
Catholic University of Leuven, Herestraat 49, 3000 Leuven,
Belgium

1.1
Basic Principles of Cardiac MRI

1.1.1
Introduction

The basic principles of cardiac MRI are essentially the same as for MRI techniques in other parts of the human body. During an examination, the patient is brought into a high-strength static magnetic field that aligns the spins of the human body (Hendrick 1994). These spins can be excited and subsequently detected with coils. The signal arising from the tissues is influenced by two relaxation times (T1 and T2), proton density, flow and motion, changes in susceptibility, molecular diffusion, magnetization transfer, etc. The timing of the excitation pulses and the successive magnetic field gradients determine the image contrast (Smith and McCarthy 1992).

The purpose of this chapter is to provide insight into the essentials of MR image formation and to discuss specific features of cardiac MRI, rather than to elaborate with a detailed mathematical description of every physical phenomenon associated with cardiac MRI.

1.1.2
The Nuclear-Spin Phenomenon,
T1 and T2 Relaxation

The asymmetric nucleus of a proton is sensitive to the presence of an external magnetic field. The interaction of a nucleus with this field can be described via a property that has been called a "spin." This spin or "magnetic moment" revolves or precesses with a specific frequency, the Larmor frequency, around the magnetic field. The larger the field strength, the higher will be the precessional frequency.

In a large group of spins, such as present in any tissue, the net effect is an alignment of these spins parallel to the long axis of the external magnetic field. A radiofrequency (RF) pulse whose frequency matches the Larmor frequency can perturb this alignment, resulting in a magnetic moment that is no longer aligned with the field. This magnetic moment of the tissue can now be deconstructed in a vector that is still aligned with the field, the so-called longitudinal magnetization, and a component perpendicular to the field, the transverse magnetization.

After excitation, the spins gradually return to their resting state, i.e., aligned with the field, as this is energetically the most favorable situation. Therefore, their magnetic component along the magnetic field will increase; and the component in the transverse plane will gradually disappear. The first process is described as the T1-relaxation time (Fig. 1.1). A tissue with a long T1 recovers slowly after an RF pulse; the spins of tissues with short T1 align very quickly with the magnetic field. The gradual disappearance of magnetization in the transverse plane after the excitation pulse is called T2 relaxation (Fig. 1.2). Tissues in which the transverse magnetization is rapidly lost are said to have a short T2. These T1- and T2-relaxation processes have a major influence on the image contrast in most MR images (van Geuns et al. 1999).

1.1.3
Slice Encoding, Phase Encoding, and Frequency Encoding

Measurement of T1 and T2 relaxation in itself is not enough to construct an image of the patient. The coil has in itself no way of determining where in the patient the signals are arising from. This is achieved through spatial encoding. A detailed discussion on how the spatial encoding is performed is beyond the scope of this text, but can be found in any basic MR textbook. The procedure is based on the Larmor equation, namely that the precessional frequency of the spins is proportional to the magnetic field at the location of the spin (Duerk 1999). In practice, this means that magnetic field gradients are applied over the volume of interest. Let us assume the example of reconstructing a transverse slice. To acquire the signal from only this slice, a first magnetic gradient is applied. Along the direction of this gradient (caudal to cranial), the magnetic field, thus also the precessional frequency of the spins, becomes slightly different. As an RF pulse with one

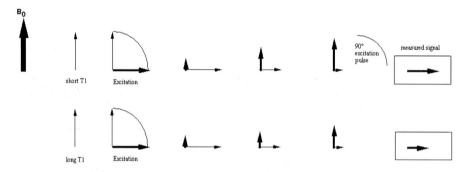

Fig. 1.1. Schematic of T1 relaxation. After the excitation pulse, magnetization is flipped in the transverse plane. During relaxation, longitudinal relaxation (*T1*) recovers, faster for tissue with short T1 than for tissues with long T1. A second 90° pulse flips the recovered signal again in the transverse plane, where it can be measured.

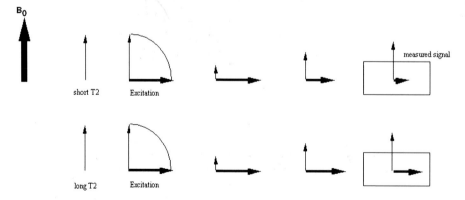

Fig. 1.2. Schematic of T2 relaxation. After the excitation pulse, magnetization is flipped in the transverse plane. During relaxation, transverse magnetization (*T2*) gradually decreases, faster for tissues with short T2 that for tissues with long T2. A second 90° pulse flips the recovered signal again in the transverse plane, where it can be measured.

specific RF frequency will excite only the spins with the corresponding precessional frequency, the use of this first magnetic field gradient results in selective excitation of a single transverse slice (slice encoding; Fig. 1.3a).

During the measurement of the signal from this slice, a second magnetic field gradient is applied along another direction (left to right). This is defined as the readout direction. As a consequence, spins of different columns in the excited slice precess with a different frequency, and the measured signal consists of the sum of magnetic moments with different frequencies (frequency encoding; Fig. 1.3b). For example, if this particular signal is measured during 256 successive time points, it is possible to redistribute the signals afterwards over 256 different columns. The necessary mathematical technique to perform this "column reconstruction" technique is the well-known Fourier transformation.

In order to create differences between the different rows in an image, an encoding scheme has to be used for this direction too. A third magnetic field gradient is applied between RF excitation pulse and signal readout. It forces the spins of different rows onto a different frequency during a certain time. The result of this magnetic field gradient will be a different phase for spins from different rows (phase encoding; Fig. 1.3c).

From the above example, it is clear that a basic acquisition scheme is a complex process. For an image with a given resolution of 256^2, 256 different phase-encoding gradients have to be applied on the same group of spins, and 256 frequency encodings are performed to encode for the horizontal resolution. A series of successive measurements is therefore necessary. The time in between successive RF excitation pulses is called the repetition time (TR). All the measurements are written in the raw data plane and two-dimensional (2D) Fourier transformation of these data is performed. Because of the common mathematical use of the parameter "κ" in Fourier calculations, the raw data space is often called the "κ-space" (PETERSSON et al. 1993).

The κ-space has a central role in MRI. The total amount of data in the κ-space determines the image matrix. The direction of filling (bottom-to-top, cen-

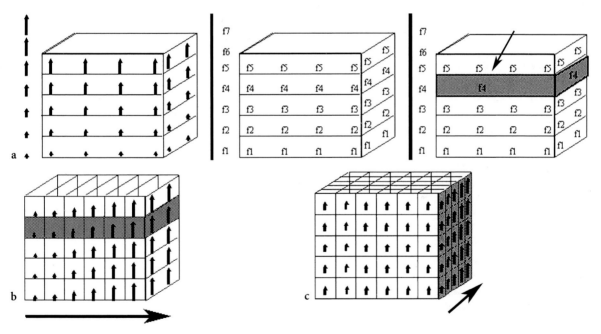

Fig. 1.3. a For slice encoding, a magnetic gradient is applied in the *Z* direction (*left*). Along the direction of this gradient (caudal to cranial), the magnetic field, thus also the precessional frequency of the spins, becomes slightly different (*f1–f6, middle*). A radiofrequency (RF) pulse with one specific RF frequency (*arrow, right*) will excite only the spins with the corresponding precessional frequency, resulting in selective excitation of a single transverse slice. **b** For frequency encoding, a second magnetic field gradient is applied along a secondary direction (*large arrow*). Spins of different columns in the excited slice will precess with a different frequency. To reconstruct the image from this encoded measurement, a Fourier reconstruction needs to be performed. **c** For phase encoding, a third magnetic field gradient is applied between RF excitation pulse and signal readout (*large arrow*). It forces the spins of different rows onto a different frequency during a certain time. The result of this magnetic field gradient will be a different phase for spins from different rows.

tric reordered, spiral, etc.) and the sparseness of data sampling (e.g., half-Fourier techniques) have consequences on contrast and image resolution (DUERK 1999). Since each line in κ-space has experienced different phase-encoding and readout gradients, the information derived from each line is different. Lines which have experienced the strongest gradients are written near the periphery of the κ-space; it is these which make the greatest contribution to the final image resolution. The data samples acquired with the weakest gradients are saved in the center of κ-space. They have a major influence on the image contrast.

The different geometries and acquisition schemes using these specific κ-space properties is explained in the following section and outlined with detail in relevance to cardiac MRI examinations.

1.1.4
κ-space Geometry

The coordinates of κ-space are spatial frequencies with units of reciprocal distance, such as millimeter^{-1}. These spatial frequencies describe how image features change as a function of position in the image (PASCHAL and MORRIS 2004). For example: the MRI signal from a large object does not change while passing through its spatial configuration. Otherwise stated: the signal from this object is reflected in low-spatial frequencies. It is only at the border of this object that the transition, e.g., to air or the interface with another object produces a change in signal. Edges in the images produce high spatial frequencies. The low spatial-frequency information (signal from the object, contrast information) is placed in the center of κ-space. The high spatial-frequency information (edges of the object, resolution information) is put outward in the periphery of κ-space. This theory is illustrated in Fig. 1.4. When an image is reconstructed only using the low spatial-frequency information from the center of κ-space, the result is a low-resolution image (Fig. 1.4a), while an image reconstructed from only the peripheral κ-space lines reveals the borders of the organ with very little contrast (Fig. 1.4b). By gradually adding more peripheral information to the image (Fig. 1.4c), the spatial resolution in the image improves without changing the image contrast. The important elements to remember from this difficult theory are that the center of the κ-space contains image contrast and that the resolution of the image is governed by the extent of peripheral κ-space lines (HENNIG 1999).

The ways in which κ-space can be filled are almost infinite. The classic filling scheme or "trajectory" is sequential bottom-to-top, i.e., the bottom peripheral line is sampled first, continuing in a linear trajectory through the center of κ-space toward the top line. Other schemes include centric-reordered (centrally outward), reversed linear (peripherally inward), radial and spiral. The choice of a particular κ-space filling scheme is directed by the information which is to be obtained from the image, e.g., high T2-weighted contrast, first pass of a contrast agent bolus, etc. The different κ-space trajectories relevant for cardiac MRI are summarized in Table 1.1.

1.1.5
Spin Echoes and Gradient Echoes

Within the range of sequences used for cardiac MRI, two large families exist. The first commonly used pulse sequence is the spin-echo pulse sequence. In a spin-echo sequence, a 90° pulse is first applied to the spin system. The 90° degree pulse rotates the magnetization into the XY plane. The transverse magnetization begins to dephase. At some point in time after the 90° pulse (usually half of the echo time or TE), a 180° pulse is applied. This pulse rotates the magnetization by 180° about the axis. The 180° pulse causes the magnetization to at least partially rephase and to produce a signal called an echo (HADDAD et al. 1995; Fig. 1.5a).

In cardiac MRI, conventional spin-echo techniques suffer from disturbing motion artifacts, even when performed with many signal averages (WINTERER et al. 1999). This technique has therefore been largely abandoned. Developments in MRI have gone in the direction of techniques that can be acquired during a single breath-hold. Most frequently, a fast spin-echo technique (FSE/TSE) is used with the TR adjusted to the cardiac frequency. For T1-weighting, the TE is kept short (5–15 ms) and TR is chosen to coincide with one single R–R interval of the patient's ECG (STEHLING et al. 1996; BOGAERT et al. 2000). Images are formed by acquiring a number of κ-space lines (typically 9–15, named "turbofactor" or "echo train") during diastole, in order to minimize motion artifacts. Since the number of κ-space lines per excitation pulse determines the total acquisition window per heart cycle, in practice the number of lines has to be adapted inversely proportional to the heart rate of the patient (Fig. 1.5b).

Spin-echo imaging has a major disadvantage. For maximum signal, the transverse magnetization

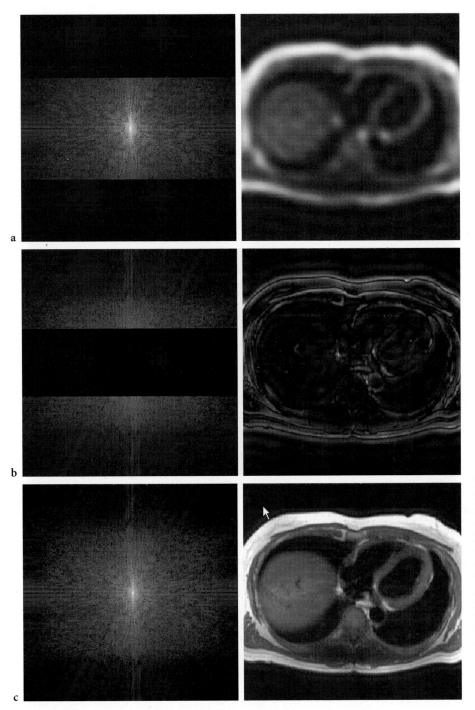

Fig. 1.4a-c. Influence of κ-space filling on image properties. **a** When only the low spatial-frequency information (center of κ-space) is acquired, a low resolution image is obtained. **b** An image reconstructed from only the peripheral κ-space lines reveals the contours of the body and organs with very little contrast. **c** When the entire κ-space is filled, the image has maximal resolution and contrast.

needs to recover to its equilibrium position before TR is repeated. When T1 is long, this can significantly lengthen the imaging sequence.

In a gradient-echo (GE) imaging sequence, first a slice-selective RF pulse is applied to the imaged object. This RF pulse typically produces a rotation angle of between 10° and 90°. A slice-selection gradient is applied with the RF pulse.

A phase-encoding gradient is applied next. A dephasing frequency-encoding gradient is applied at the same time as the phase-encoding gradient so as to cause the spins to be in phase at the center of the acquisition period. This gradient is negative in sign from that of the frequency-encoding gradient turned on during the acquisition of the signal. An echo is produced when the frequency-encoding gra-

Table 1.1. Different κ-space trajectories

κ-space trajectory	Variant	Mechanism	Application in cardiac MRI
Rectilinear	Sequential	Single line acquired in a separate readout, from top to bottom of κ-space	Spin-echo anatomical imaging (older technique)
	Turbosequential	Multiple lines of κ-space per excitation are acquired, each line preceded by a 180° pulse	TSE or FSE anatomical imaging
	Centric-reordered	κ-space lines are acquired starting at the center line of κ-space and alternating up and down on successive excitations	Intended to acquire image contrast in the beginning of the sequence, e.g., first-pass imaging in contrast-enhanced MR angiography
	Reversed centric	κ-space lines are acquired starting with the outer lines of κ-space and working inward from either edge in successive excitations	Intended for high-resolution images with long TE (avoids T2-blurring), e.g., T2-weighted TSE for myocardial edema
	Half-Fourier	Lines are acquired, usually bottom-to-top up to ±67–75% of κ-space. The missing data is replaced by a copy of the bottom part	Faster scanning for which resolution is less important, e.g., fast T2-TSE or HASTE for short-axis determination
	Zero filling	Usually in a centric reordered sequence, κ-space line acquisition is stopped after 50–66% and missing data is replaced by zeros. Equivalent to interpolating a low resolution image to make a higher resolution image	Mainly used in MR angiography to reduce scan time. For example a 144×256 matrix is acquired and reconstructed to 256×256
Radial or propeller		κ-space is not traversed line-by-line but rotate around the centerpoint like the spoke of a wheel or a fan blade	Used for sequences requiring high SNR (frequent sampling of the center of κ-space) Used in coronary MRA and post contrast T1-weighted 3D imaging (scar imaging)
Spiral		κ-space is usually covered using with multiple, interleaved spiral trajectories, each after a separate excitations. Known to have complicated reconstruction algorithms	Used for fast acquisitions requiring high spatial resolution. Currently under investigation for coronary MRA

dient is turned on, because this gradient refocuses the dephasing which occurred from the dephasing gradient (Fig. 1.6).

A period called the echo time (TE) is defined as the time between the start of the RF pulse and the maximum in the signal. The sequence is repeated every TR seconds. The TR period can be as short as tens of milliseconds (Frahm et al. 1990).

1.1.6
Parallel Imaging

Imaging speed is a key factor in most cardiovascular MRI applications of MRI. As a means of enhancing scan speed in MRI, alternative signal acquisition strategies have been developed. These techniques make use of spatial information related to the spatially varying sensitivity of different receiver coils.

Parallel imaging using multiple RF coils has considerably enhanced the performance of cardiac MRI. For example, SMASH and SENSE, acronyms for simultaneous acquisition of spatial harmonics and sensitivity encoding, respectively, are two widely used imaging techniques where imaging time has been reduced with a limited sacrifice in signal-to-noise ratio (SNR) (Pruessmann et al. 1999; Sodickson and Manning 1997; Kyriakos et al. 2000). Both techniques rely on the use of coils with different elements (phased arrays). As the sensitivity of each separate coil element for the geometry of a given object is different, this information can be used to reconstruct information from this sensitivity without actively measuring it, thus saving imaging time. In the SMASH method proposed by Sodickson, the sensitivity profiles of the coils is calculated in one direction. These profiles are then weighted appropriately and combined linearly in

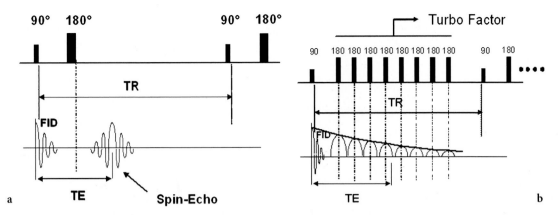

Fig. 1.5. a Schematic of the spin-echo principle. After an initial 90° pulse, the magnetization is rotated into the *XY* plane. At *TE*/2, a 180° pulse is applied, which initiates rephasing. At the echo time (*TE*), a spin-echo is produced. *FID*, free induction decay or initial signal after excitation; *TR*, repetition time. **b** Schematic of a fast spin-echo (TSE) technique. After the 90° excitation pulse, multiple 180° pulses (called "echo train" or "turbo factor") produce a spin-echo signal at TE.

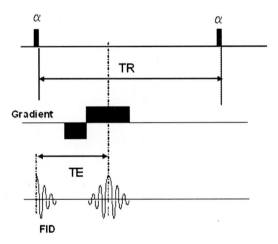

Fig. 1.6 Schematic of the gradient-echo principle. After the excitation pulse, a phase-encoding gradient and simultaneously a dephasing frequency-encoding gradient are applied to produce a rephasing signal at the center of the acquisition period (*TE*).

order to form sinusoidal harmonics which are used to generate the κ-space lines that are missing due to undersampling. SMASH has some inflexibility in the choice of imaging planes due its restriction on the placement of receiver coils along one direction, slice geometry, and reduction factor.

The SENSE method proposed by Pruessmann is another parallel-imaging technique which relies on the use of sensitivity profile information in order to reduce image acquisition times in MRI. In SENSE, substantial reductions of scan time are obtained by increasing the distance between the lines in κ-space (this reduces the field of view in the image domain).

In doing so, κ-space is basically undersampled, resulting in aliasing. Each pixel of an aliased single-coil image reflects the sum of signal components of multiple origins, with each component individually weighted according to local coil sensitivity. The sensitivity-profile information is then used to remove the infolding from the image (Fig. 1.7).

Each method is characterized by a tradeoff in SNR. This is dependent on the data-reduction factor, the configuration and placement of receiver coils, and the accuracy of determination of coil-sensitivity profiles.

Theoretically, the acceleration factor of a parallel-imaging scan is equal to the amount of coils used. In practice however, the degree of scan acceleration is limited by the SNR of the images. In parallel imaging, the SNR is inversely proportional to the square root of the acceleration factor. Furthermore, in image reconstruction from sensitivity-encoded data, noise enhancement occurs in regions where the geometric relations of coil sensitivities are not optimal. Therefore, when parallel imaging is used in cardiac MRI, generally acceleration factors are limited to 2–3.

Parallel imaging is often used to accelerate common breath-hold imaging sequences and to increase the temporal resolution of cine MRI sequences, up to 75 frames/s. Cardiac real-time scanning is one of the greatest achievements of parallel imaging, which will be discussed in Sect. 1.2.1.5 (WEIGER et al. 2000). Other applications of parallel imaging in cardiac MRI include decreasing the duration of 3D sequences to fit in a single breath-hold period for assessment of myocardial contrast enhancement (CE-

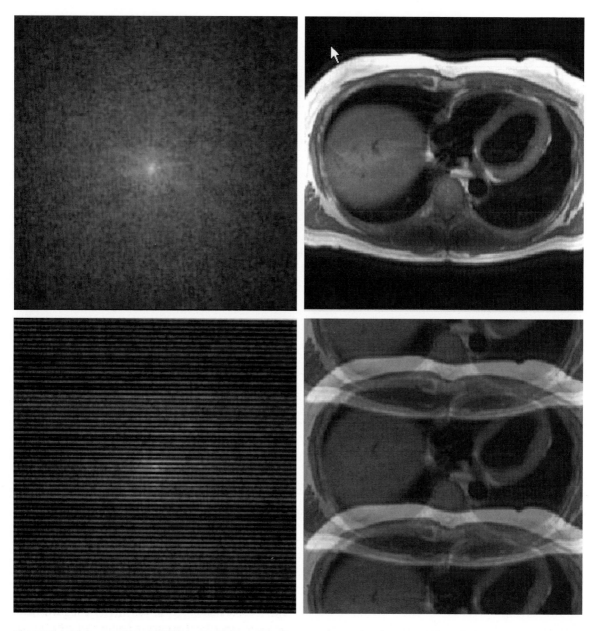

Fig. 1.7 Sensitivity encoding (SENSE) – parallel imaging. *Top row:* conventional κ-space filling (*left*) with resulting image reconstruction. By reducing the sampling density (increasing the distance between sampling lines in κ-space, *bottom left*), SENSE allows substantial reduction of scan time. Because κ-space is undersampled, an aliased image is produced (*bottom right*). In SENSE reconstruction using phased-array coils, the encoding effect of the different coil sensitivities is taken into account to enable separation of aliased pixels by means of linear algebra.

IR MRI; see Sect. 1.3.4.5) and multislice perfusion imaging.

The most recent advance in this field is to use parallel imaging in the time domain (Tsao et al. 2003). Due to the intrinsic process of excitation and spatial encoding, in most cardiac MRI sequences, the duration of acquisition of a single time frame is long,

if seen relative to the actual motion of the heart. Therefore, it can be assumed that there is a certain degree of redundancy in the acquired data. This redundancy is found in the specific spatiotemporal relationship of each individual time frame. Based on this approach, two methods were developed to significantly improve the performance of dynamic imaging, named κ-t BLAST (broad-use linear acquisition speed-up technique) and κ-t SENSE (sensitivity encoding). In this method, signal correlations are learned from a set of training data and the missing data is recovered afterwards. By using this method, it is possible to increase temporal resolutions of ungated imaging beyond current capabilities during the acquisition stage. It should, however, be remarked that the precise process of temporal parallel imaging is currently not clinically available on most MRI machines.

1.2
Specific Measures in Cardiac MRI Sequences

Compared with other anatomical regions, MRI of the heart faces specific difficulties to overcome, such as cardiac and respiratory motion, flow phenomena, etc. Therefore MRI sequences have been adjusted or are acquired differently for use in cardiac MRI.

1.2.1
Cardiac Motion

1.2.1.1
Synchronization with ECG

The contraction of the heart muscle is a major determining factor in the image quality of cardiac MR images. The application of a conventional MRI protocol would result in unreadable images due to overwhelming motion artifacts (LANZER et al. 1984). Using the electrical activity of the heart, MRI data acquisition can be synchronized to the corresponding mechanical events. In this way, cardiac motion can be "frozen". Different methods and systems are currently available to perform ECG gating in an MRI environment. The user should, however, be aware that the surface electrodes also measure other electrical currents, such as those induced by the magnetic field on the blood flow in the cardiac chambers and vessels. A principal source of artifacts in the ECG due to the magnetic field itself is the magnetohydrodynamic effect. This effect consists of a voltage induced by ions flowing within blood vessels that are exposed to the magnetic field. This voltage artifact is mainly superimposed on the ST segment of the ECG during the ejection of blood in systole. The increase in amplitude of the ST segment

can thus cause a false QRS detection in certain R-wave detection algorithms.

Since accurate peak detecting in the ECG is critically important for good-quality scans, several systems have been designed to provide superior detection. These systems use the spatial information in a vector cardiogram (VCG) to improve R-wave detection in the MRI environment. With a three-dimensional and orthogonal lead system, the electrical activity of the heart is deconstructed in dipolar elements, which allows the R–R interval to be registered as a 3D spatial vector that varies in magnitude and direction throughout the cardiac cycle. Since it has been shown that the average electrical moment of the heart and the average moment of the magnetohydrodynamic artifact manifest significantly different spatial orientations, separation of the QRS loop and the blood flow-induced artifact can be obtained (FISCHER et al. 1999).

Other sources of noise in the ECG include that from the RF pulses and the switching of the gradient fields. This has been largely overcome by the introduction of fiber optics in the ECG-detection systems, replacing the formerly used carbon leads. The use of low-power semiconductor optic or laser technology for optimal signal transduction has further improved ECG triggering in the MRI environment.

1.2.1.2
Prospective Triggering and Retrospective Gating

There are different ways in which ECG is used to guide acquisition. One technique is to use a preceding R-wave to act as a trigger to acquire information during the following R–R interval or cardiac cycle. This is called "prospective triggering." Another strategy is to acquire data continuously and to retrospectively match this to the ECG tracing which is recorded into the memory buffer of the acquisition computer, this is called "retrospective gating." Both techniques have different applications and will be further elaborated.

Prospective triggering is the more traditional approach: an R-wave serves as a trigger pulse. Instead of acquiring a traditional phase-encoding scheme in which the measurements are performed continuously, by using triggering in cardiac MRI, κ-space is segmented into individual lines or groups of lines. Every group of lines requires another phase-encoding such that they can be saved in the appropriate row of the κ-space. An individual group of lines acquired per R–R interval pulse is called a κ-space segment. After each excitation pulse, phase-encoding tables are incremented and acquisition of a segment is performed (Fig. 1.8a). Depending on the sequence, this can mean that a single segment is acquired for static morphological imaging or a series of segments for multiphase imaging. The key issue to prospective triggering is that the length of the acquisition itself must be shorter that the average R–R interval. If the acquisition length should supersede this period, the next R-wave would be ignored, resulting in unnecessary prolongation of the total acquisition time or breath-hold period, if applicable. For some acquisitions, the changes in effective TR due to changes in R–R interval in case of missed R-wave could also lead to artifacts.

A limitation of prospective triggering is that, due to this constraint, the end of diastole and the early atrial contraction is missed. This can result in poor visualization of physiological phenomena during relaxation and inaccurate readings in flow measurements through the atrioventricular valves. In the clinical setting of diastolic heart failure, restrictive heart disease, or constrictive pericarditis, these are elements that must certainly not be missed. Therefore, preference is given to retrospective gating techniques, which acquire the full R-R interval.

In retrospective gating a continuous succession of excitation and data readout is performed and phase-encoding tables are incremented after a fixed time, calculated a priori from an estimated averaged R–R interval. The ECG is recorded during the measurement and, after this measurement, signals are redistributed over the κ-space according to their timing over the cardiac cycle. In older sequences, the total acquisition time is usually longer, because in these sequences the actual R–R interval is overestimated to ensure the complete coverage of the heartbeat for each phase-encoding increment. Newer sequences use real-time rescaling of the acquired κ-space information to an average R–R interval, and overestimation is no longer necessary (Fig. 1.8b).

1.2.1.3
Single-phase Imaging:
Timing Of Acquisition During Diastasis

In morphological imaging such as T1-weighted imaging of the myocardium and coronary MR angiography, cardiac contraction induces severe motion artifacts related to the length of acquisition if the placement of the acquisition shot is not planned accurately, i.e., during systole or early diastole, when motion of the heart muscle is maximal. Using a time delay, imaging is fixed during the period of diastasis, which is a relative rest period during the mid-to-late diastole. In this period, the heart motion is minimal (HOFMAN et al. 1998).

The exact timing for diastasis is inversely related to the cardiac frequency of the patient. The length of diastasis decreases as the heart rate goes up. This has implications for artifact-free imaging. In patients with low heart rates, this leaves some margin for error but, in higher heart rates, the length of the

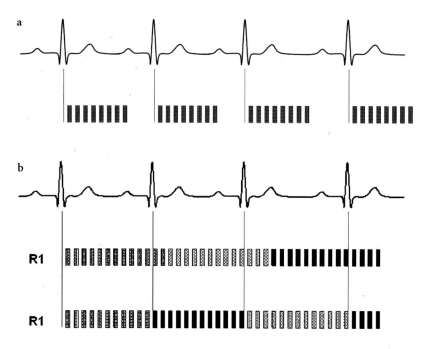

Fig. 1.8a,b Prospective triggering. In this example of a multiphase acquisition, after each R-wave, a number of κ-space lines is acquired. Note that the acquisition length is shorter than the R-R interval and, at this sampling rate, the end of the cardiac cycle is missed. **b** Using conventional retrospective gating schemes (*R1*), the acquisition interval supersedes the R-R interval. This ensures effective acquisition of the complete cardiac cycle, but lengthens the total acquisition duration. In optimized retrospective schemes (*R2*) real-time rescaling of the acquisition interval to the R-R interval eliminates the need for overestimation.

acquisition should be decreased to avoid motion artifacts.

There are different ways to calculate the precise timing for diastasis. A first strategy is to calculate the time delay using the empirical Weissler formula. In this formula, trigger delay = [(R–R interval – 350)×0.3]+350.

A much easier method is to perform a cine MRI scan with very high temporal resolution, e.g., 10 ms and to review this in loop mode. Hence the period of diastasis can be assessed as the period of least motion of the ventricle or the coronary artery. The time after the trigger pulse can usually be read in the image information on the scanner and be used as a trigger delay in single-phase imaging sequences.

1.2.1.4
Multiphase Acquisitions

The most common method to acquire dynamic information (e.g., cine MRI or flow measurements) is the single-slice multiphase approach. This approach is typically performed with GE acquisitions, as these can be performed with short TRs in between successive excitations. These sequences are used to study dynamic phenomena of the heart such as the myocardial contractility and valvular function. The number of phases that can be acquired over the heart cycle are calculated from the acquisition time per phase and the averaged R–R interval. The entire set of images can be loaded into an endless cine loop, providing information on dynamic cardiac processes similarly to other cardiac imaging techniques such as echocardiography, but taking into account the fact that the MR images acquired with this particular scheme are usually not real-time images but are acquired over several heartbeats. Real-time dynamic MRI will be discussed in Sect. 1.2.1.5.

In most acquisition schemes, several κ-space lines are acquired per image and per cardiac cycle. The κ-space corresponding to one particular image is then filled with a fixed number of κ-lines per heartbeat (Fig. 1.9). This part of κ-space is defined as a "segment," and the corresponding technique is a "segmented acquisition." Multiphase measurements of successive images can even share κ-space data (echo- or view-sharing; Fig. 1.10), which further increases temporal resolution without length-

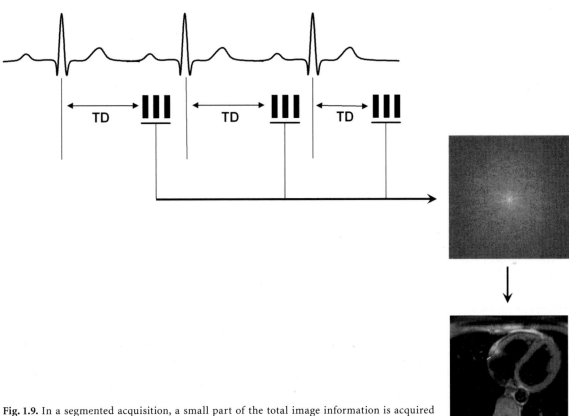

Fig. 1.9. In a segmented acquisition, a small part of the total image information is acquired after every heartbeat and arranged in κ-space. After complete acquisition, the definitive image is obtained by Fourier transformation.

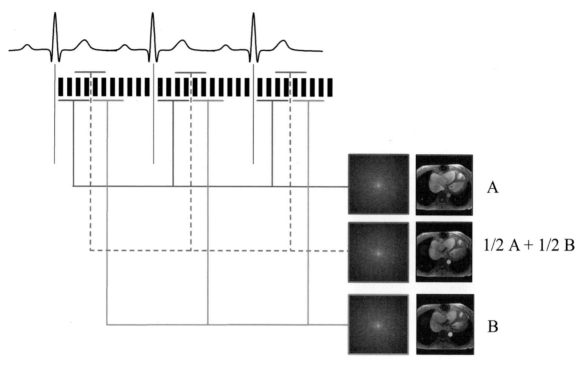

Fig. 1.10. View sharing. Each individual cine MR image is formed from different κ-space segments. Virtual images are formed from the half of each preceding and following segment through κ-space interpolation.

ening the duration of acquisition. These techniques are usually run during breath-hold.

1.2.1.5
Real-Time Dynamic MRI

With current modern MRI systems and the newest scanning techniques, high temporal and spatial resolution can be achieved in cine MRI sequences. Using a SSFP protocol (Sect. 1.3.3) and parallel imaging, a complete set of cine MR images can be obtained in 5–10 breath-hold periods of 10 s. Nevertheless, this procedure can be complicated by arrhythmias and patient difficulty with long or multiple breath-holds, especially in a group with cardiac illness.

For cine MRI, sequences have been adapted allowing for imaging in real time. In a conventional κ-space sampling strategy, each image is composed of κ-space segments acquired over several R–R intervals during cardiac triggering or gating. In real-time sequences, κ-space is generally filled in a single shot. The imaging matrix is reduced. e.g., 128^2, no cardiac triggering is used, and parallel imaging is used to increase the data sampling rate. A single image can thus be acquired in less than 100 ms. Since the acquisition duration is short, breath-holding is optional, so it can be used even in critically ill pa-

tients. Studies have shown this technique to produce comparable results with standard multiple breath-hold examinations (Fig. 1.11; SPUENTRUP et al. 2003; HORI et al. 2003).

A further evolution of this technique tackles another potential source of errors both in segmented breath-hold and free-breathing scans, namely slice misregistration between multiple successive slices. Depending on the imaging plane, diaphragmatic shifts between breath-holds of unequal depth or during free breathing can cause cardiac shifts of up to 1 cm. This could result in over- or underestimation of cardiac volumes during quantification.

The abovementioned real-time scans can be combined with retrospective gating to produce a real-time, retrospectively gated, multislice scan with retrospective reordering of the acquired real-time images into the R–R interval over which they were acquired. A further advantage over nontriggered scans is that these images can be accepted by postprocessing software as triggered cardiac studies and can be quantitatively analyzed.

Similar evolutions exist for myocardial perfusion sequences, which visualize the first pass of contrast agents in the myocardium (see also Chap. 7). High spatial resolution is not a basic requirement for perfusion studies. The major prerequisites for perfu-

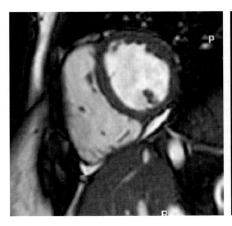
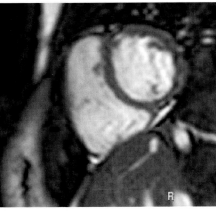

Fig. 1.11. Comparison of retrospective cine MRI (*left*) and real-time ungated cine MRI (*right*). The ungated image has lower spatial resolution, since priority during the acquisition is given to temporal resolution.

sion acquisitions are a short acquisition time and an adequate T1 weighting. In practice, single-shot T1-weighted gradient-echo sequences are used. These sequences use a saturation-recovery prepulse, a 90° pulse which guarantees the nulling of the entire signal prior to the effective acquisition, allowing clear visualization of the first-pass effects.

1.2.2
Respiratory Motion

Respiration and the associated motion of the organs in the thorax and the abdomen are well-known problems in MRI. This kind of motion superimposes on the signal acquisition during cardiac contraction and is of approximately equal importance for image quality.

From early experience with MRI, increasing the number of signal averages decreased motion artifacts in the images. However, as the total acquisition time is proportional to this number, this approach was very time-consuming. In addition, even for properly adjusted T1-weighted spin-echo techniques, good results could never be guaranteed. Since in the present era most imaging techniques used in cardiac MRI use accelerated acquisition schemes (fast spin-echo, turbo-gradient echo) other strategies are maintained to keep images clear of respiratory artifacts (PETTIGREW et al. 1999).

1.2.2.1
Respiratory Gating

Similar to cardiac triggering, acquisitions can be triggered by the respiratory cycle. By use of a respiratory belt, excitation and signal readout is guided to the period of end-expiration. In cardiac MRI,

this technique presumes that cardiac and respiratory gating are combined. The disadvantage of this approach is that acquisitions become very long. As one respiratory cycle can easily take 5 s or longer, the minimal effective TR for an acquisition would be 5 s. In practice, this technique is rarely used.

1.2.2.2
Breath-Hold Cardiac MRI

The developments in MRI tending toward fast-acquisition schemes make imaging during a single breath-hold possible. Generally speaking, a random patient can hold his or her breath for about 10–15 s. The goal is to use an acquisition that can be performed in this time frame. Clear patient instructions before the examination can aid in improving the efficiency of this approach. It can also be useful to provide patients short of breath with an oxygen mask or nasal cannula during the examination to alleviate the often frequent breath-holds.

For morphological imaging in breath-hold, usually a FSE or TSE sequence is used, in which the number of lines per heartbeat can be tailored to coincide with the period of diastasis in diastole, as described in Sect. 1.2.3. If T2-weighting is required, one should consider that, in view of the long echo times, there is a linear relationship between the length of the acquisition shot and the amount of blurring in the image due to dephasing. A compromise should be found between the length of breath-holding and the length of the acquisition. If necessary, parallel-imaging technology can be used to shorten the total acquisition duration. Similar acquisition schemes in GE protocols allow for cine MRI and flow measurements to be captured in a single slice per breath-hold.

1.2.2.3
Free-Breathing Navigator-Echo Acquisitions

In longer imaging sequences such as high-resolution flow measurements and especially in coronary MR angiography, abovementioned strategies have little chance of success. The long acquisitions need a different approach to filter the respiratory motion out of the acquisition. This is performed by navigator-gated scans. This technique will be briefly described here, since it is elaborated in Chap. 14. A navigator is usually a 2D RF pulse, representing a single signal readout of a sagittal slice, positioned over the right diaphragmatic dome. It is positioned there in order not to pick up any signal from the heart. The signal readout of this RF pulse allows determination of the position of the diaphragm, since there is high contrast between the liver and the lungs. During the acquisition of the imaging sequence, this signal or position is read out every heartbeat, thus providing a real-time measurement of the diaphragmatic excursion. By use of a threshold value within which range to accept data, the MRI system can be directed only to include information into the κ-space of the given protocol, for instance at end expiration. All other data are rejected (Fig. 1.12). The length of the total acquisition depends on the efficiency of the navigator and thus on the regularity of the breathing pattern of the patient. If respiratory drift occurs, for instance when the patient falls asleep, or there is bulk motion, the efficiency is limited. It is therefore important to carefully instruct the patient to breathe regularly and consistently.

There are many variations in navigator gating. Some tracking algorithms exist to compensate for drifts in respiratory excursion, and many investigators have works with navigator beams positioned on the heart itself. Additional information about coronary MR angiography can be read in Chap. 14.

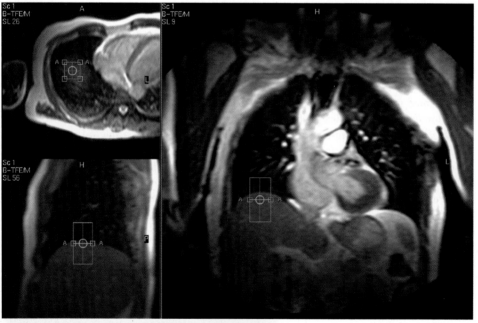

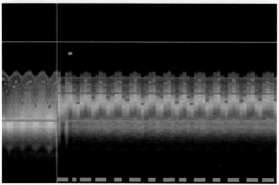

Fig. 1.12 Principle of navigator echo acquisitions. A navigator pencil beam is placed on the right diaphragmatic dome as shown on the *top part*. The navigator registers the motion of the diaphragm during respiration and determines end-expiration as the top of the excursion curve. All data points of the acquired sequence within a certain acceptance window (indicated by the *blue lines*) are kept for image formation, while other points are rejected.

1.3
Contrast Mechanisms in Cardiac MRI

1.3.1
T1- and T2-Weighted Techniques

Static images in cardiac MRI are often used for anatomical evaluation. These images require high image contrast and a sufficient spatial resolution. The required weighting is in practice application-dependent. For instance, the visualization of myocardial edema is optimal with a T2-weighted acquisition, whereas other indications such as evaluation of the right ventricular (RV) wall, LV wall thickness, and pericardial thickening benefit from T1-weighted measurements. The visualization of enhancing structures after an intravenous injection of contrast agents (infarction, mass, fibrosis) also requires a T1-weighted approach (Fig. 1.13a,b).

Conventional spin-echo techniques suffer from disturbing motion artifacts, even when performed with many signal averages and a long TE. This technique has therefore been largely abandoned. Developments in MRI have gone in the direction of techniques that can be acquired during a single breath-hold. Most frequently, a fast spin-echo technique (FSE/TSE) is used with the TR adjusted to the cardiac frequency. For T1-weighting, the TE is kept short (5–15 ms) and TR is chosen to coincide with one single R–R interval of the patient's ECG. Images

are formed by acquiring a number of κ-space lines (typically 9–15) every diastole, in order to minimize motion artifacts. Since the number of κ-space lines per excitation pulse determines the total acquisition window per heart cycle, in practice the number of lines has to be adapted inversely proportionate to the heart rate of the patient.

GE acquisitions can be used as an alternative to T1-weighted TSE acquisitions. A GE or turbo-FLASH (fast low-angle shot technique) acquisition can be used as a single-shot or multishot technique, with TR/TE minimal and an inversion-recovery (IR) preparation pulse to improve the image contrast (FRAHM et al. 1990).

T2-weighted acquisitions can also be performed with fast acquisition schemes. Both fast spin-echo (TSE/FSE) and echoplanar imaging (EPI)-based techniques have been explored. The turbo-factor or number of κ-space lines that can be accepted for T2-weighted imaging is subject to the same type of compromise as T1-weighted acquisitions. For T2-weighted TSE, the turbo factor in TSE imaging is usually higher (21–33) and TR is longer (2 or 3 heartbeats), which is beneficial for T2-weighted contrast. These measurements are often combined with fat-suppression techniques to increase image contrast (STEHLING et al. 1996) To increase the contrast in T1- and T2-weighted images, these sequences can be fitted with a double inversion or "black-blood" pulse to increase image contrast between cardiac structures and the blood. This functionality is discussed in Sect. 1.3.4.4.

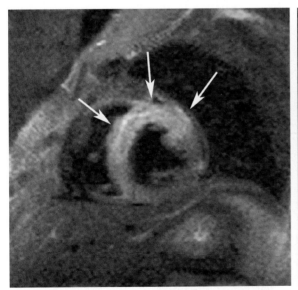 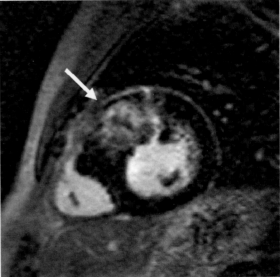

Fig. 1.13 T1- and T2-weighted techniques. *Left:* T2-weighted TSE image with fat suppression acquired in a patient with acute myocardial infarction. The tissue edema due to the infarction is expressed as elevated signal intensity in the anterior wall. *Right:* T1-weighted gradient-echo acquisition after injection of contrast in a patient with asymmetric septal hypertrophy. Disarray of myocardial fibers and increase in interstitial fibrosis is shown as a contrast-enhancing wall segment.

Postcontrast T1-weighted MRI, for instance in the setting of ischemic heart disease, is used to distinguish between myocardial infarction and normal myocardium. Different authors have shown that visualization of contrast enhancement can be best performed using GRE acquisitions. Newer MR sequences, such as inversion-recovery fast GE (e.g., IR-FLASH, IR-FFE, CE-IR MRI) sequences can be used to obtain T1-weighting, while the inversion-recovery prepulse (inversion time, TI, variable between 200 and 300 ms, depending on contrast dose and time after injection) suppresses the normal myocardium and thus improves the contrast difference between normal and pathological myocardium (Fig. 1.14) (SANDSTEDE 2003). This technique will be further elaborated in Chap. 8, Ischemic Heart Disease.

1.3.2
Intracardiac Flow and Gradient-Echo Acquisitions

Most conventional MRI sequences presume that the spins in the tissues do not move during the procedure. For flowing spins, such as those in the ventricular cavity, the great vessels, or in the coronary arteries, this assumption is not valid. Spins moving along the direction of a magnetic field gradient acquire a phase angle that depends on the magnetic field and on their flow. A paradoxical signal enhancement of flowing blood is observed in GE acquisitions whenever the spins experience only a restricted number of RF excitation pulses and then disappear from the imaged volume. Hence, the continuous refreshment or inflow of the spins ensures a maximal alignment of spins with the external field prior to the excitation

pulses. Compared with the partially relaxed signals in the stationary tissues, subjected to a long series of RF pulses, the signal in the vessel or cardiac chamber can therefore be very strong. Apart from being the basis for time-of-flight (TOF) MR angiography acquisitions, this principle is used for GE cine MRI sequences (Fig. 1.15; SEMELKA et al. 1990). Usually single-slice, segmented multiphase GRE protocols or hybrid variations (GRE-EPI) with small flip angles are used for this purpose. The myocardium can be delineated due to hyperintense signals in the cavity, and these sequences possess a sufficiently high temporal resolution to acquire 15–20 frames per cardiac cycle. Sharing of the measured raw data (echo- or view-sharing) increases the temporal resolution further (BOGAERT et al. 1995).

There have been a number of alternative acquisition schemes proposed over the last 5–10 years, such as multishot echo planar MRI (EPI), IR single-shot turbo-FLASH and biphasic spin-echo sequences as compared to the well-validated conventional GRE technique. Although these techniques all provided accurate measurements of global LV function and mass in a time-efficient manner, they are now largely abandoned for balanced steady-state free precession (b-SSFP) sequences, which are discussed in Sect. 1.3.3.

The flow-induced phase effects caused by extra bipolar pulses in GRE sequences can be exploited to study intracardiac or valvular flow. Due to a bipolar pulse, flowing spins acquire a phase angle that is, in a first approach, proportional to the amplitude of the gradients, the time between the onset of the first and the second pulse, and, most importantly, the velocity of the spins (whenever their motion can be described by a constant velocity flow during the application of the gradients). Under well-controlled

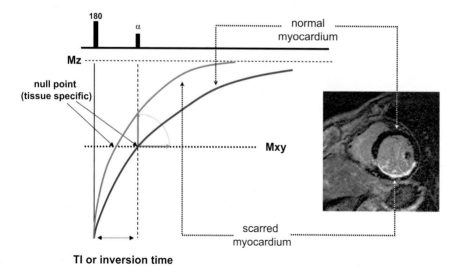

Fig. 1.14 Contrast-enhanced inversion-recovery (CE-IR MRI) technique. Since longitudinal relaxation is tissue-specific, a 180° (inversion) prepulse can be used to enhance the contrast between normal (dark) and scarred (bright) myocardium as shown in a patient with an old inferior myocardial infarctation. Midventricular short-axis view, obtained 20 minutes following injection of 0.2 mmol Gd-DTPA/kg body weight, using an inversion time of 270 ms.

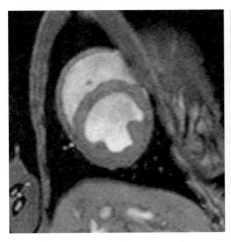 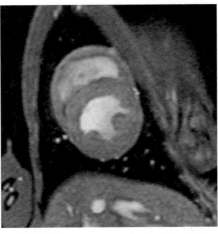

Fig. 1.15 Gradient-echo cine MR image in cardiac short-axis. There is moderate blood-to-myocardium contrast, mainly due to intracavitary flow.

conditions, the velocity of the spins can thus be measured from the phase angles (HIGGINS et al. 1991). A typical flow-encoded phase image is shown in Fig. 1.16a. Measuring the phase angle over the cardiac cycle permits the calculation of the mean flow over, for example, the descending aorta, as shown in Fig. 1.16b. The range of velocities that can be measured is determined by the gradients and generally described by the strength of the VElocity-ENCoding bipolar pulse (VENC).

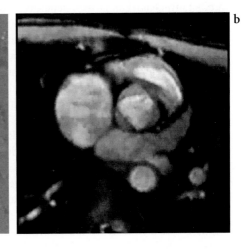

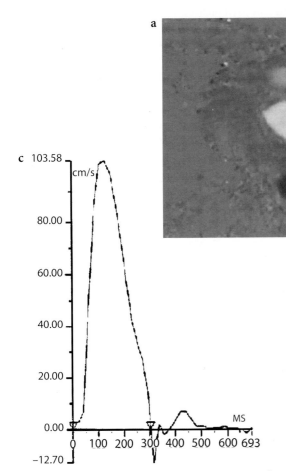

Peak Velocity: 103.58 cm/s Vascular Area: 4.79 cm^2
Mean Velocity: 54.30 cm/s Mean Flow: 259.84 cm/s

Fig. 1.16a–c Gradient-echo phase-contrast flow measurement of the aortic valve. **a** Phase-encoded image. Flow in cranial direction is displayed as white pixels, while flow in the caudal direction as black pixels. Stationary tissues appear as intermediate gray-scale image points. **b** corresponding magnitude image. **c** flow velocity curve obtained by measuring the flow profile over time.

1.3.3
Balanced Steady-State Free Precession Sequences

Since the introduction of powerful gradient MRI systems into clinical practice, great interest has re-emerged for b-SSFP techniques. These sequences have many monikers, such as TrueFISP (Siemens), balanced FFE (Philips), and FIESTA (GE). As very shrewdly described by Scheffler et al., many authors unify these sequences under the name "steady-state free precession techniques" (SSFP) and emphasize that the unique feature of this sequence is the acquisition of magnetization during steady state. Scheffler accurately remarks that is very confusing and wrong, since all rapid GE sequences are SSFP sequences (SCHEFFLER and LEHNHARDT 2003). The remarkable features and contrast mechanisms of the b-SSFP sequence do not originate from the steady state but from the unique gradient-switching pattern through which it generates contrast.

As previously described, a GE is made up of a number of excitation pulses, separated by a given time interval (TR). The acquisition and the spatial encoding of the GE is performed between consecutive excitation pulses by means of switched gradient pulses along read, phase, and slice direction. The amount of signal dephasing within TR depends on the spatial position and on the gradient strength. In addition the spatial specific dephasing, T1 and T2 relaxation unavoidably occurs during TR, resulting in further signal decay. The next excitation pulse is superimposed on the altered magnetization, and the process of excitation and relaxation is repeated every TR. After several TR periods – providing this is a constant period – a steady state of the magnetization is established (Fig. 1.17). This situation is called "steady-state free precession" (SSFP). All types of fast GE sequences are SSFP techniques. The difference between the various types of GE sequences is a different gradient-switching pattern between the consecutive excitation pulses. Different gradient-switching patterns produce different dephasings within TR, which finally result in different types of steady states and, more importantly, in different image contrasts.

b-SSFP is a special type of SSFP sequence where the gradient-induced dephasing within TR is exactly zero. In other words, within TR each applied gradient pulse is compensated by a gradient pulse with opposite polarity, which ensures maximum recovery of transverse magnetization. The overall magnetization consists of a single vector that is not spatially dephased, as for non-balanced SSFP

sequences. Absence of this linear dephasing of the magnetization as seen in conventional excitation schemes results in much higher signal gain in the image (Fig. 1.18).

Besides a favorable SNR, the most important feature of an imaging sequence is its contrast. While the classic spin-echo sequence shows either a T1- or a T2-weighted contrast, rapid GE sequences, including b-SSFP, exhibit a relatively complicated contrast that is composed of T1 and T2 contributions (HENNIG et al. 2002). In cardiac MRI, due to the transient signal of inflowing blood and the steady-state signal of muscle (which is low due to a low T2/T1 ratio) can be observed, which makes b-SSFP very useful for cardiac imaging. The high contrast of b-SSFP is produced both by the different ratio of T2 and T1 of blood and myocardium and by inflow effects. A second advantage of b-SSFP is its high SNR even for very short TR. A GRE sequence with comparable TR and optimized flip angle exhibits a much lower SNR and contrast-to-noise ratio.

The new b-SSFP technique is presently the preferred cine MRI technique to study ventricular function, since it yields a better contrast between blood and myocardium, thus providing better visualization of small anatomical structures such as endocardial trabeculations, papillary muscles, and valve leaflets (THIELE et al. 2001). Combined with parallel imaging (SMASH, SENSE), the temporal resolution can be increased by a factor of 2–4 (i.e., temporal resolution <10 ms), albeit at the expense of SNR.

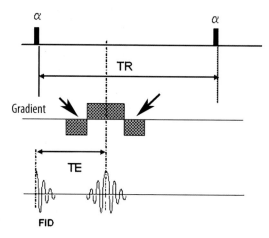

Fig. 1.17 Schematic of a balanced steady-state free precession (b-SSFP) sequence. In this acquisition scheme, all three gradient axes are refocused or balanced. If compared with non-balanced SSFP (**Fig. 1.6**), in b-SSFP the readout gradient is perfectly symmetrical (*arrows*), resulting in completely rephased magnetization after one TR period.

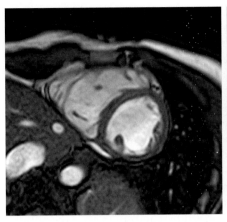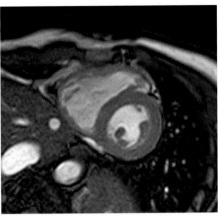

Fig. 1.18 Balanced steady-state free precession (b-SSFP) cine MR image in cardiac short-axis. In comparison with standard gradient-echo cine MRI, the blood-to-myocardium contrast is higher. This technique allows better delineation of intracardiac structures such as papillary muscles and trabeculations.

b-SSFP requires short TRs (3–6 ms) to minimize artifact behavior. This is the main reason why b-SSFP has only become feasible (and popular) during the past 3–5 years. With the design of very fast gradient amplifiers, it was possible to reduce the time to switch all relevant gradients needed for echo encoding to a few milliseconds. The b-SSFP also requires relatively high flip angles, between 50 and 80°, to generate the highest possible signal. This can easily exceed the SAR limits, which may limit its use in ultrahigh field systems, such as recently introduced 3 T MRI units.

1.3.4
Use of Preparation Pulses

Preparation pulses create a preexisting condition in the spin population prior to the applications of RF pulses destined for signal readout. Typical examples are fat-suppression pulses, inversion pulses, and saturation pulses. Other types of preparation pulses have applications in other parts of the body, such as magnetization transfer pulses, vessel tracking pulses, spin-labeling pulses, but are beyond the scope of this chapter.

1.3.4.1
Fat-Suppression Techniques

Fat suppression in cardiac MR images may be desirable for a variety of reasons. An examination aimed at the diagnosis of right ventricular pathology may require fat-suppressed TSE images to distinguish the fine anterior wall from the pericardial fat. Fat suppression is commonly used in coronary MR an-

giography and in contrast-enhanced sequences used for myocardial viability assessment.

A robust way to perform fat suppression is to use sequences with an IR prepulse. These sequences are called STIR sequences, which is an acronym for short-tau inversion recovery. This sequence starts with a 180° RF pulse that inverts the magnetization (SIMONETTI et al. 1996). After this pulse, the spin population relaxes: it realigns its magnetization with the external magnetic field. This relaxation behavior is, by definition, described by the T1 relaxation time. A time constant "TI" is associated with the use of this pulse: it defines the time in between the IR pulse and the actual measuring process. This sequence parameter could be set to optimize the T1-weighted contrast. Fat suppression is achieved with a TI of about 120 ms. At this TI, the signal of the fat crosses the zero point. STIR is most commonly explained with reference to an inversion-recovery spin-echo (IRSE) sequence, but the approach is also applicable to TSE, GRE, and EPI acquisitions.

IR prepulses can also be added to a T2-weighted sequence, for instance to visualize myocardial edema in the setting of an acute myocardial infarction (DYMARKOWSKI et al. 2002). The combination of T2-weighting, usually in the form of a TSE sequence and fat suppression causes high contrast between the edematous myocardium and the surrounding tissues. Beware, however, that overall SNR decreases as TE is increased. For adequate SNR, an echo time of 60 ms can be chosen (Fig. 1.19).

In spectral fat suppression, or SPIR, a spectrally selective "fat-pulse" is used to flip fat spins and, after the time interval that lets the longitudinal magnetization of fat reach zero, the excitation pulse is applied which causes the signal of the water spins to contribute to most of the signal. The best fat suppression is achieved with a 180 spectral inversion pulse and a time delay equal to that used in normal STIR imaging (Fig. 1.20).

1.3.4.2
Saturation Bands

Saturation bands are normal 90° RF excitation pulses that are applied on tissues prior to the measurement, thereby avoiding interference of their signal with the images. This is an efficient way to suppress image artifacts originating from a traceable source that does not have to be visualized in the image. A commonly used application of saturation bands is slabs positioned over the chest wall to avoid high signal from subcutaneous fat in T1-weighted imaging or to avoid motion-related artifacts in coronary MR angiography (Fig. 1.21). Another very interesting application of these saturation bands is the selective saturation of parts of the myocardium, as first de-

scribed by Zerhouni et al. The saturated tissues can be used as noninvasive markers or "tags" to study the myocardial deformation and motion during the heart cycle (ZERHOUNI et al. 1988; see Chap. 6).

1.3.4.3
Saturation Recovery Pulses

The saturation recovery (SR) sequences are only rarely used for imaging. Their primary use at this time is as a technique to measure T1 times more quickly than an IR pulse sequence. SR sequences consist of multiple 90° RF pulses at relatively short TRs. Longitudinal magnetization after the first 90° RF pulse is dephased by a spoiling gradient (in this case with the slice select gradient). Longitudinal magnetization that develops during the TR period after the dephasing gradient is rotated into the transverse plane by another 90° pulse. A GE is acquired immediately after this. The signal will reflect T1

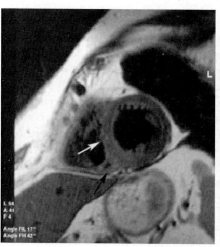 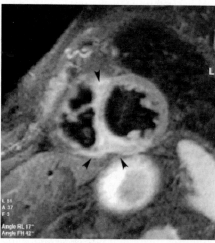

Fig. 1.19 Use of fat suppression in T2-weighted MRI. *Left:* T2-weighted TSE image in the cardiac short-axis in a 64-year-old patient with acute myocardial infarction. In this image without fat suppression, the tissue edema is only marginally visible (*arrow*). *Right:* corresponding fat-suppressed image shows increased contrast between the edematous and normal myocardium (*arrowheads*).

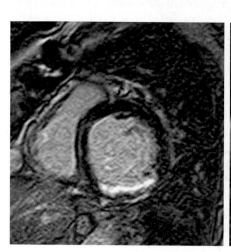 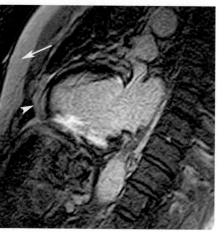

Fig. 1.20 In CE-IR-MRI, spectral fat suppression is used to suppress the signal of chest wall (*arrow*) and pericardial (*arrowhead*) tissue to increase contrast between the myocardium and surrounding fat.

differences in tissues because of different amounts of longitudinal recovery during the TR period. The primary use of these prepulses is in myocardial perfusion sequences (HUNOLD et al. 2004; Fig. 1.22).

1.3.4.4
Dark-Blood or PRESTO Inversion Prepulses

Dark-blood pulses consists of a 180° inversion pulse applied over a large part of the heart, including the slice to be imaged. A slice-selective 180° pulse im-

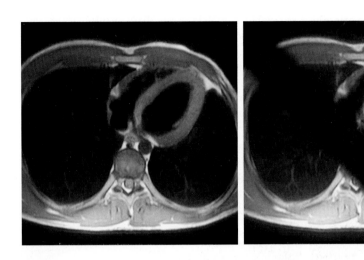

Fig. 1.21 Right: transverse T1-weighted TSE image. *Left:* Identical image with saturation band positioned over the atria. The signal covered by the saturation band is selectively destroyed before the actual image acquisition.

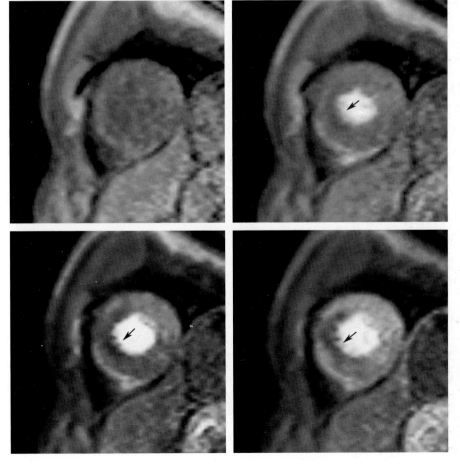

Fig. 1.22 Short-axis perfusion MR images acquired during injection of contrast agent. Before the gadolinium agent enters circulation, there is no contrast between the blood pool and the myocardium. During the perfusion phase of the myocardium, signal of blood and myocardium increases, revealing a perfusion defect in the anteroseptal wall (*arrows*).

mediately follows this pulse. This pulse is called preceding IR preparing pulse pair (PRESTO) and the sequences that have such a pulse are also known as double IR sequences (STEHLING et al. 1996).The dark-blood pulse cancels the effects of the first pulse in the stationary tissues in the particular slice. In the ideal situation, there is no net effect for the spins in the myocardium. Most spins in the blood pool and especially those with high velocity experience only parts of the two pulses. Their signal is significantly reduced and/or partly inverted. A black signal in the cavity will occur with the image acquisition process starting at the time when the spins in the cavity have no net magnetization (Fig. 1.23). The optimal TI between the preparation pulses and image acquisition is patient- and flow-dependent. Usually a TI of about 600 ms is a good compromise. In practice, the pulse is used prior to single-shot techniques or acquisitions with a long echo train length, in which it is a very helpful and robust technique, not only

to suppress the artifacts from the cavity but also to better delineate the myocardium (GREENMAN et al. 2003). A third IR pulse may be added to null the signal from fat to produce a triple IR sequence.

Disadvantages of these pulses are that slowly flowing blood near the myocardium can be incompletely suppressed and may appear hyperintense. Furthermore, parts of the myocardium can be partially suppressed, which would result in hypointense regions.

1.3.4.5
Contrast-Enhanced Inversion-Recovery MRI of the Myocardium

Several studies have shown that myocardial infarction tissue can be best imaged after injection of paramagnetic contrast agents using GE acquisitions with a 180° IR prepulse, called contrast-enhanced inversion recovery MRI (CE-IR MRI;

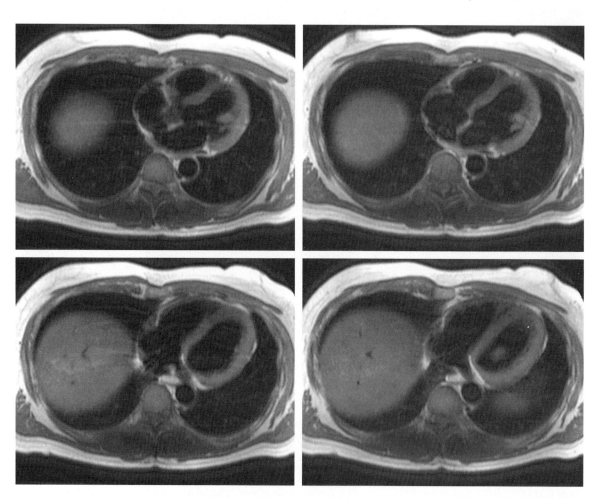

Fig. 1.23 Example of black-blood T1-weighted TSE MRI. The signal from the blood flow is negated by the double inversion prepulse during the acquisition.

Kim et al. 2000; Wagner et al. 2003). In these sequences, the IR pulse is not used to suppress the signal of fat as is done in STIR sequences (Sect. 1.3.4.1), but from normal myocardial tissue (Fig. 1.14). The TI or inversion time for this sequence in not predefined, but variable, and is dependent on many factors such as patient weight, contrast dose, renal function, and timepoint after injection. After the inversion pulse, tissues recover magnetization, and the issue is to acquire image data exactly when normal myocardium crosses the zero line. The resulting image will show normal myocardium as dark, and hyperenhanced myocardium as bright. It can also be used to suppress other tissues than fat. Because the TI in these sequences is used for myocardial suppression, additional fat suppression is achieved with another technique, namely spectral fat-suppression (Fig. 1.24; Bornert et al. 2002).

Both 2D and 3D sequences for CE-IR MRI exist. The definite advantage of 3D sequences is the ability to cover the entire ventricle in a single breath-hold period. Nevertheless, to achieve a 3D acquisition in a single breath-hold, the echo train length has to be quite long, which can lead to motion blurring in patients with higher heart rates (Kuhl et al. 2004). This functionality will be further elaborated in Sect. 1.4.4 and in Chap. 8.

1.4
Specific Protocols

1.4.1
Cardiac Morphology

Breath-hold prospective-triggered TSE images with dark-blood pulses provide excellent delineation of cardiac anatomy with minimal respiratory artifacts. These sequences are widely used for the visualization of ventricles, atria, and great vessels. When good blood suppression can be obtained, visualization of valve leaflets is also possible. The relative ease in application make them extremely useful in the evaluation of postoperative congenital heart disease, since these sequences are relatively insensitive to susceptibility artifacts arising from prosthetic valves and sternotomy wires. The fact that they are available in both T1- and T2-weighted version with or without fat suppression makes this technique especially appealing in characterization of cardiac masses and the detection of fat in right ventricular dysplasia.

For T1-weighting, the TE is kept short, usually ranging from 5 to 15 ms, and TR is kept constant at 1 R–R interval. A turbo factor of 9–15 is used with minimal echo spacing to keep the acquisition duration short. A linear profile order is preferred. Useful slice thickness ranges from 5 to 8 mm.

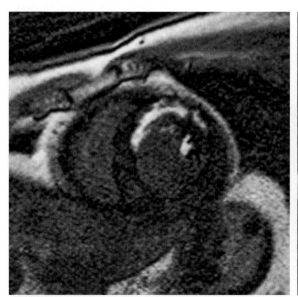
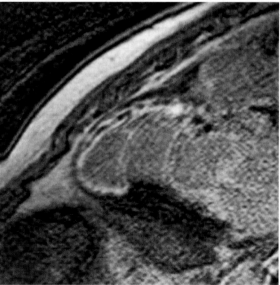

Fig. 1.24 CE-IR MRI, cardiac short–axis (left) and vertical long–axis (right) acquired 25 min after contrast injection. The larger part of the left ventricle appears hypointense, due to the inversion pulse which is adapted to the exact zero crossover of normal myocardium. The blood is slightly more intense, and infarcted myocardium appears most intense due to the shorter T1 value (higher gadolinium content).

For T2-weighting, TE is longer. Beware, however, that overall SNR decreases as TE is increased, due to dephasing. Useful TEs range from 60 to 88 ms, and TR is longer (2 heartbeats). Since a long TE in cardiac MRI causes the breath-hold duration to increase, turbo factors are usually higher (23–33). Fat suppression may be added to increase contrast in the image. This technique has also proved very effective in imaging acute myocardial infarction, highlighting the edema associated with this pathology.

1.4.2
Cardiac Function

Routine cine MR Imaging is most commonly done during brief periods of breath-holding.

The basic approach uses the segmented GE sequence, with very short TE and TR. Multiple lines in κ-space are acquired per heartbeat for each phase in the cine sequence. In these sequences there is a trade-off in the temporal resolution versus the duration of the breath-hold period. If greater temporal resolution is needed, the number of image resolution lines acquired per heartbeat should be reduced with a proportionate increase in scan time (Fig. 1.25).

Despite the obvious virtues of this technique, traditional GRE sequences are rapidly losing ground to the newer generation of b-SSFP techniques, due to their inherent higher contrast. The high contrast of b-SSFP is produced both by the different ratio of T2 and T1 of blood and myocardium and by inflow effects. A second advantage of b-SSFP is its high SNR despite very short TRs and TEs. High flip angles between 50° and 80° are preferred to generate the high-

est possible signal. The b-SSFP technique is presently the preferred cine MRI technique to study global and regional ventricular function, since it yields a better contrast between blood and myocardium, thus providing better visualization of small anatomical structures such as endocardial trabeculations, papillary muscles, and valve leaflets (Fig. 1.26). Parallel imaging (SMASH, SENSE) can furthermore be used to increase the temporal resolution without lengthening breath-hold durations, albeit at the expense of SNR.

The traditional GRE cine MRI sequences are still used in the evaluation of regional myocardial deformation analysis, i.e., cardiac tagging (ZERHOUNI et al. 1988; AXEL and DOUGHERTY 1989). In cardiac tagging, thin saturation pulses are applied immediately after the R-wave and prior to the multiphase acquisition scheme. This RF excitation pulse suppresses specific parts of the myocardium by nulling the magnetization. The so-called tagged tissue will produce markedly decreased signal intensity during a certain period after the application of the saturation pulse. In a multiphase acquisition, the position of this tag can be traced.

Different types of tagged sequences have been developed. The first uses normal saturation pulses, applying one RF pulse per tagging line (Fig. 1.27). Tagging in the short-axis plane is then performed with a series of radial tagging lines through the center of the myocardium. Parallel lines can be used on long-axis views of the heart. It is possible to merge the information of two such data sets to calculate the true 3D positions of the myocardium over the cardiac cycle. In a next step, it is possible to track the contraction of the left ventricle to calculate the

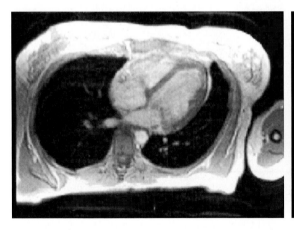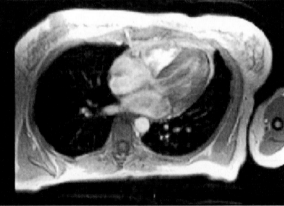

Fig. 1.25 End-diastolic (*left*) and end-systolic (right gradient-echo cine MR image in horizontal long-axis orientation. Because the through-plane flow component is smaller in orientations other than short axis, using this flow-dependent technique, intracavitary contrast can be severely compromised, resulting in difficult detection of the endocardial border (*arrow*).

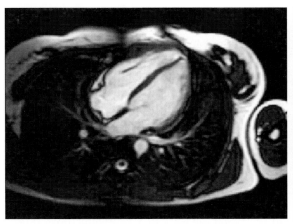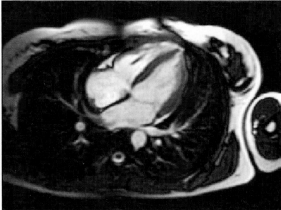

Fig. 1.26 End-diastolic (*left*) and end-systolic (right b-SSFP cine MR image in horizontal long-axis orientation. The complete rephasing in all three gradient directions renders the technique relatively independent of flow effects. There is higher contrast between blood and myocardium than in standard gradient-echo cine MRI.

strains in the ventricle and to estimate the related wall stress in particular regions.

Other centers apply a grid of tag lines on the image. Saturation is typically achieved with a series of flip angles, e.g., +30°, –60°, +60°, and –30°. A magnetic gradient modulates the phases of the spins, such that spins in a first series of lines end up with a 0° flip angle and others, in other lines, experience effectively 90°. The latter are saturated. This technique is known as "SPAMM" (spatial modulation of magnetization). The acquisitions are straightforward, but postprocessing (and in particular the 3D analysis) is more difficult (Fig. 1.28).

1.4.3
Myocardial Perfusion

The goal of myocardial-perfusion MR images is to assess the relative perfusion of the myocardium by monitoring the first transit of a bolus of a contrast agent (ISHIDA et al. 2003) This requires an ultrafast acquisition scheme, since it is the goal to acquire multiple slices through the heart, preferably within a single heartbeat. A second goal is to minimize the signal contribution in the image from the previous image to increase the conspicuousness of the contrast agent and its passage. Myocardial contrast uptake (T1 decrease) is achieved by using a 90° satu-

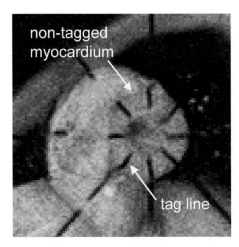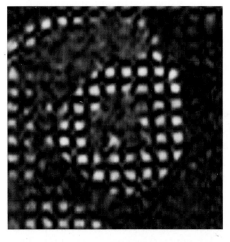

Fig. 1.27 Radial tagging. Applying very thin saturation bands centered around a rotation point in the center of the left ventricular cavity, part of the tissue is saturated before image acquisition.

Fig. 1.28 Spatial modulation of magnetization (SPAMM) tagging. A grid of intersecting thin saturation bands superimposes a pattern on the left ventricular wall contour, used for deformation analysis.

ration recovery prepulse before acquisition of the image data.

Current imaging protocols allow 3–5 slices to be imaged per heartbeat. This permits whole-heart first-pass perfusion imaging to be qualitatively assessed and quantitative indexes of relative myocardial perfusion to be measured.

Preferred sequences are T1-weighted, hybrid turbo GE (TGE) sequences with EPI readouts to acquire 5–9 lines of data for each RF excitation. This permits ultrashort image acquisition times, often less than 100 ms. The use of parallel imaging has also allowed for TGE sequences without EPI acceleration to be acquired within the same time frame. There is still some controversy in the literature about which technique is preferred. The TGE-EPI strategy has lower SNR, but is more sensitive to changes in T1, thus theoretically more sensitive to assess perfusion.

Absolute quantification of contrast uptake also remains difficult. First, using extracellular contrast agents, there is a significant leakage of the agent to the extracellular tissues during the first pass through the myocardium. As a result, the amount of contrast agent in the tissue is not proportional to the blood flow into the tissue. A second restriction results from the MR acquisition technique itself. Signal intensities are not necessarily proportional to the local concentrations of the contrast agent (PRAKASH et al. 2004). Trials with intravascular contrast agents are currently underway to investigate the potential of these agents for determination of absolute myocardial blood flow.

T2- or T2*-weighted, single-shot techniques are rarely used for cardiac perfusion measurements. In the literature, evidence is provided that the EPI approach is feasible for perfusion measurements. Quantification of the tissue perfusion using these techniques is difficult for the same reasons as in the case of T1-weighted measurements.

1.4.4
Myocardial Viability Assessment

It has been known for many years that regions of acute and chronic myocardial necrosis such as myocardial infarction exhibit higher signal intensity on T1-weighted MR images following administration of extracellular contrast agents (KIM et al. 2001; SANDSTEDE 2003). In the chronic patient populations, this technique has been shown to have a close agreement with FDG positron-emission tomogra-

phy (-PET) studies in detecting transmural myocardial scars, PET still being considered to be the gold standard in myocardial viability assessment. Numerous studies of myocardial infarction have been performed using a variety of pulse sequences to differentiate injured from normal myocardium. Delayed-contrast enhanced MRI allows assessment of myocardial viability in patients with acute and chronic ischemic heart disease. Typically, the heart is imaged at 15–30 min after administration of a contrast agent. In myocardium with increased extravascular space or abnormal contrast wash-in and washout characteristics, this results in increase in the signal intensity in a T1-weighted MR image. Sequences formerly used for this purpose include T1-weighted spin-echo and TSE, IR TSE and IR GRE. The role of the IR prepulse is to increase T1 weighting, which results in improved contrast between enhanced and nonenhanced tissues. It was shown by SIMONETTI et al. that a segmented GRE pulse sequence (turbo-FLASH) with a TI set to null normal myocardial signal intensity after contrast-material administration produced the greatest differences in regional myocardial MR image signal intensity compared with other MRI techniques (Fig. 1.29).

The initial described technique advocated a 2D MR imaging sequence with high spatial resolution images. However, this necessitates multiple, successive breath-holds to generate a set of MR images that cover the entire heart, which is time-consuming and proves difficult for patients.

Therefore 3D acquisition sequences have been developed with which a complete volume can be acquired within one breath-hold. In a recent comparative study by Kühl, both 2D and 3D techniques are compared for the accuracy of presence of delayed enhancement and the degree of transmurality (KÜHL et al. 2004). The total myocardial area and contrast-enhanced area agree well between the two sequences. A high level of agreement has also been found for the presence of hyperenhancement, while agreement is poor for the transmural extent of hyperenhancement, which is attributed to the blurred appearance of the 3D MR images. In fact this makes sense, since the number of κ-space lines is much larger in the 3D sequence than in a 2D sequence (in the abovementioned study, 77 versus 25, respectively). Long acquisition durations lead to blurring due to motion superposition and T2-dephasing effects (Fig. 1.30).

From our experience, we recommend starting 3D measurements shortly after injection to visualize no-reflow areas, which appear initially dark. After 15–30 min, the ideal period to perform accurate de-

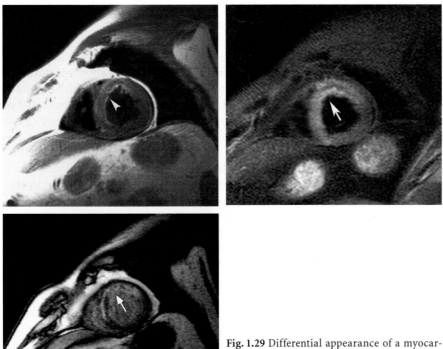

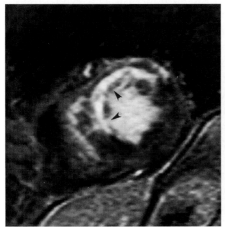

Fig. 1.29 Differential appearance of a myocardial infarction on different sequences. *Left:* T1-weighted contrast-enhanced TSE image (*white arrowhead*); *middle:* T2-weighted T2 short-tau inversion-recovery (STIR) image (*white arrow*); *right:* CE-IR MR image (*black arrow*).

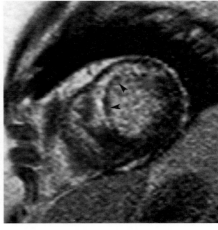

Fig. 1.30 Most commonly, 3D CE-IR MRI sequences are used to image the entire ventricle in one single breath-hold (*left*). These sequences have higher signal-to-noise than 2D sequences (*right*) but may suffer form more motion blurring and slightly less sharp delineation of infarction tissue (*arrowheads*).

layed-enhancement imaging, we perform a single 3D volume for a general presence of delayed enhancement and multiple 2D breath-hold slices in different orientations though the areas that exhibit abnormal contrast enhancement. The higher spatial resolution of the 2D sequences allow detailed mapping of the pathological area.

The importance of spatial resolution has been stressed by a study by HUNOLD et al. which shows that, due to the superior spatial resolution, contrast-enhanced MRI is able to detect and quantify subendocardial scarring better than nuclear medicine techniques. Currently, several large studies using functional recovery after revascularization as an endpoint are investigating whether MRI might replace PET as the standard of reference in the assessment of myocardial viability.

It should also be stressed that contrast enhancement of the myocardium is not a specific sign for myocardial infarction (BOGAERT et al. 2003). The presence of hyperenhancement on postcontrast T1-weighted images merely suggests that the normal fluid homeostasis within the heart has been altered due to rupture of cell membranes or ultrastructural changes in myocyte organization. Many authors have described delayed hyperenhancement in myocarditis, infiltrative cardiomyopathy, pericardial inflammation, hypertrophic cardiomyopathy, and cardiac masses (BOGAERT et al. 2004).

Other studies in myocardial infarction which have focused on T2-weighted MRI have suggested that, although T2-weighted MRI may be able to detect the presence of myocardial damage, the areas that exhibit increased signal intensity are probably related to the presence of myocardial edema, rather than the myocardial infarction, especially in the acute phase (DYMARKOWSKI et al. 2002; MILLER et al. 2003).

Many authors have focused on comparisons between contrast-enhanced T1-weighted MRI and functional deficits measured with cine MRI The main finding of these studies is that T2-weighted images overestimate the size of the infarct area and correlate well with the dysfunctional myocardial region. This region has been called "the peri-infarction zone" in recent literature and has been defined as both the necrotic and the viable tissue after myocardial infarction. If T2-weighted images of myocardium are obtained in the context of acute myocardial infarction, they can serve as a means to quantify the amount of myocardial edema occurring early after myocardial infarction. T2-weighted MRI might therefore be considered as a valuable technique for sizing the peri-infarction area. Until evidence of the contrary is presented, we need to assume that this area represents stunned but viable myocardium, in which recovery can be gained after revascularization.

1.4.5
MR Coronary Angiography

Since the early 1990s, several groups have investigated the use of MRI for depiction of the coronary artery anatomy and stenoses. The traditional 2D MR techniques have been replaced for the most part by 3D MR coronary angiography techniques, which are performed during either breath-holding or free breathing with navigator echoes (KIM et al. 2001; DIRKSEN et al. 2003).

This technique will be only briefly described in this section, since it is elaborated in Chap. 14.

3D sequences for visualization of the coronary arteries are complex and consist of many subparts, which all have a separate function. A prototype of a coronary MR angiography scan is a 3D submillimeter turbo-field-echo (TFE) sequence. This sequence starts with a flow-insensitive, T2-weighted prepulse for myocardial suppression followed by the navigator prepulse, which allows image acquisition during the period of diastasis during diastole. The navigator pulse is again followed by a spectrally selective fat-saturation pulse, and finally the TFE image acquisition (Fig. 1.31).

Using a field of view of 360 mm and a matrix of 360×512 results in an in-plane acquisition spatial resolution of 1.0×0.7 mm². The TFE factor, or number of κ-space lines acquired per cardiac cycle, is usually adapted to the patient's heart rate.

The real-time navigator gating window, or allowance window, is usually set at 5 mm. Thus, shots are only accepted when the diaphragm is within the gating window at end-expiration.

In analogy to the good clinical results of b-SSFP techniques in cine MRI, 3D b-SSFP protocols have also been developed for coronary MR angiography (WEBER et al. 2003). The results of these studies show a significant shortening of acquisition times and improved image quality, supplying images with less flow-dependent contrast between the ventricu-

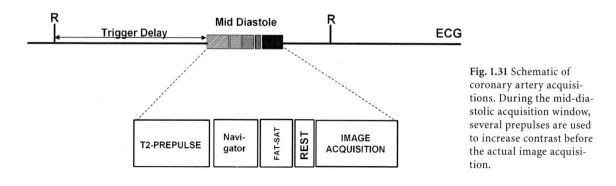

Fig. 1.31 Schematic of coronary artery acquisitions. During the mid-diastolic acquisition window, several prepulses are used to increase contrast before the actual image acquisition.

lar lumen and the surrounding myocardium, as well as sharper delineation. In a comparative study by GIORGI et al. (2002), the b-SSFP technique yielded a higher blood-to-myocardium and blood-to-pericardial fluid contrast ratio, resulting in a significantly longer segment of the three major coronary arteries visualized (Fig. 1.32).

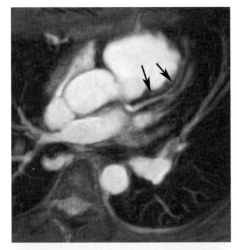

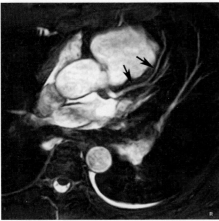

Fig. 1.32 *Top:* Gradient-echo coronary MR angiography image of the left anterior descending (LAD) coronary artery. *Bottom:* Corresponding b-SSFP image shows sharper delineation and longer depiction of the coronary artery.

1.4.6
MR Angiography of Thoracic Vessels

Flow-dependent and phase-contrast techniques for thoracic MR angiography have largely been abandoned, due to long acquisition duration and artifact-prone behavior. The availability of stronger gradients on modern MRI systems allows for ultra-

fast gradient switching, resulting in 3D techniques with extremely short TR and TE. The T1-weighting of these sequences is in fact limited: only with a highly concentrated contrast agent in the vessels is a high signal intensity observed. It can thus be stated that these sequences provide a morphological rather than a physiological image of the blood vessel, since the technique does not rely on intrinsic inflow effects. In theory, the appearance of the blood vessels is closer to the classic angiographic image than is the time-of-flight or phase-contrast angiogram (Fig. 1.33).

In practice, contrast-enhanced MR angiography has to be performed during the first pass of the contrast bolus. There are a couple of practical problems to be solved for this condition to be fulfilled (HANY et al. 1997). Indeed, the majority of the (3D) GE acquisitions takes longer than the passage of a contrast bolus. A typical high-resolution MRA acquisition may use parameters in the following range: TR 2.5 ms, matrix 192×256 or 192×512, 32 partitions, FOV 300×400 mm, and partition thickness of 1–2 mm. This leads to a total acquisition time of 17 s. Contrast boluses can be made much shorter. Next, it may be difficult to predict the exact arrival time of the bolus. To obtain a positive blood vessel contrast, the T1 of the blood has to be sufficiently short during the measurement of the central κ-space lines. For most conventional acquisition schemes, this occurs halfway through the measurement. Centric-reordered or elliptically reordered acquisitions typically acquire the center of κ-space during another

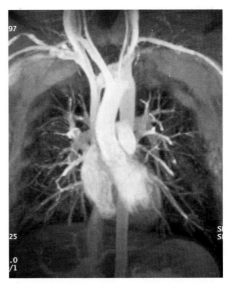

Fig. 1.33 Typical example of coronal contrast-enhanced MR angiography of the thoracic aorta.

period of the measurement. Finally, due to a rapid
venous return, it is difficult to exactly time the acquisition such that there is, on the one hand, a lot of
contrast material in the arteries, while the veins, on
the other hand, are not yet filled. Several strategies
have been worked out to match the acquisitions and
the passage of the contrast bolus for the particular
applications. In the optimal case, the center of κ-
space is scanned during the first pass of the bolus.
The following two approaches can be used to reach
this target: (1) to calculate the bolus arrival time, (2)
to track the arrival of the contrast bolus and scan the
κ-space center at the appropriate time (PRINCE et al.
1997), (3) to acquire a series of ultrashort acquisitions, such that at least one acquisition lines up with
the bolus arrival (time-resolved MRA, KOROSEC et
al. 1996). These techniques will be further discussed
in Chap. 16, Great Vessels.

Key Points

- A wide variety of prepulses, segmentation algorithms, and triggering techniques are used to
adapt MRI sequences to the specific requirements for cardiac studies.
- Parallel imaging and real-time MRI are recent
evolutions that contribute significantly to the
interactive nature of a cardiac MRI examination
- Careful choice of sequences and the knowledge
of the tissue properties they reveal allow comprehensive studies of cardiac pathology.

References

Axel L, Dougherty L (1989) Heart wall motion: improved
method for spatial modulation of magnetization for MR
imaging. Radiology 172:349-350
Bogaert JG, Bosmans HT, Rademakers FE et al (1995) Left
ventricular quantification with breath-hold MR imaging:
comparison with echocardiography. MAGMA 3:5-12
Bogaert J, Kuzo R, Dymarkowski S et al (2000) Follow-up of
patients with previous treatment for coarctation of the
thoracic aorta: comparison between contrast-enhanced
MR angiography and fast spin-echo MR imaging. Eur
Radiol 10:1847-1854
Bogaert J, Goldstein M, Tannouri F et al (2003) Late myocardial enhancement in hypertrophic cardiomyopathy
with contrast-enhanced MR imaging. Am J Roentgenol
180:981-985
Bogaert J, Taylor AM, Kerkhove F van, Dymarkowski S
(2004) Use of inversion recovery contrast-enhanced MRI
for cardiac imaging: spectrum of applications. Am J
Roentgenol 182:609-615

Bornert P, Stuber M, Botnar RM et al (2002) Comparison of
fat suppression strategies in 3D spiral coronary magnetic
resonance angiography. J Magn Reson Imaging 15:462-
466
Dirksen MS, Lamb HJ, Doornbos J et al (2003) Coronary
magnetic resonance angiography: technical developments and clinical applications. J Cardiovasc Magn
Reson 5:365-386
Duerk JL (1999) Principles of MR image formation and
reconstruction. Magn Reson Imaging Clin North Am
7:629-659
Dymarkowski S, Ni Y, Miao Y et al (2002) Value of T2-
weighted magnetic resonance imaging early after myocardial infarction in dogs: comparison with bis-gadolinium-mesoporphyrin enhanced T1-weighted magnetic
resonance imaging and functional data from cine magnetic resonance imaging. Invest Radiol 37:77-85
Fischer SE, Wickline SA, Lorenz CH (1999) Novel real-time
R-wave detection algorithm based on the vector cardiogram for accurate gated magnetic resonance acquisitions.
Magn Reson Med 42:361-370
Frahm J, Merboldt KD, Bruhn H et al (1990) 0.3-second
FLASH MRI of the human heart. Magn Reson Med
13:150-157
Giorgi B, Dymarkowski S, Maes F et al (2002) Improved visualization of coronary arteries using a new three-dimensional submillimeter MR coronary angiography sequence
with balanced gradients. Am J Roentgenol 179:901-910
Greenman RL, Shirosky JE, Mulkern RV, Rofsky NM (2003)
Double inversion black-blood fast spin-echo imaging of
the human heart: a comparison between 1.5 T and 3.0 T.
J Magn Reson Imaging 17:648-655
Haddad JL, Rofsky NM, Ambrosino MM et al (1995) T2-
weighted MR imaging of the chest: comparison of electro-
cardiograph-triggered conventional and turbo spin-echo
and nontriggered turbo spin-echo sequences. J Magn
Reson Imaging 5:325-329
Hany TF, McKinnon GC, Pfammatter T, Debatin JF (1997)
Optimization of contrast timing for breath-hold, contrast
enhanced three-dimensional MR angiography. J Magn
reson Imaging 7:551-556
Hendrick RE (1994) The AAPM/RSNA physics tutorial for
residents. Basic physics of MR imaging: an introduction.
Radiographics 14:829-846
Hennig J (1999) κ-space sampling strategies. Eur Radiol
9:1020-1031
Hennig J, Speck O, Scheffler K (2002) Optimization of
signal behavior in the transition to driven equilibrium
in steady-state free precession sequences. Magn Reson
Med 48:801-809
Higgins CB, Wagner S, Kondo C et al (1991) Evaluation of
valvular heart disease with cine gradient echo magnetic
resonance imaging. Circulation 84:I198-I207
Hofman MB, Wickline SA, Lorenz CH (1998) Quantification
of in-plane motion of the coronary arteries during the
cardiac cycle: implications for acquisition window duration for MR flow quantification. J Magn Reson Imaging
8:568-576
Hori Y, Yamada N, Higashi M et al (2003) Rapid evaluation
of right and left ventricular function and mass using real-
time true-FISP cine MR imaging without breath-hold:
comparison with segmented true-FISP cine MR imaging
with breath-hold. J Cardiovasc Magn Reson 5:439-450

Hunold P, Maderwald S, Eggebrecht H et al (2004) Steady-state free precession sequences in myocardial first-pass perfusion MR imaging: comparison with TurboFLASH imaging. Eur Radiol 14:409-416

Ishida N, Sakuma H, Motoyasu M et al (2003) Noninfarcted myocardium: correlation between dynamic first-pass contrast-enhanced myocardial MR imaging and quantitative coronary angiography. Radiology 229:209-216

Kim RJ, Wu E, Rafael A et al (2000) The use of contrast-enhanced magnetic resonance imaging to identify reversible myocardial dysfunction. N Engl J Med 343:1445-1453

Kim WY, Danias PG, Stuber M et al (2001) Coronary magnetic resonance angiography for the detection of coronary stenoses. N Engl J Med 345:1863-1869

Korosec FR, Frayne R, Grist TM, Mistretta CA (1996) Time resolved contrast-enhanced 3D MR angiography. Magn Reson Med 36:345-351

Kuhl HP, Papavasiliu TS, Beek AM et al (2004) Myocardial viability: rapid assessment with delayed contrast-enhanced MR imaging with three-dimensional inversion-recovery prepared pulse sequence. Radiology 230:576-582

Kyriakos WE, Panych LP, Kacher DF et al (2000) Sensitivity profiles from an array of coils for encoding and reconstruction in parallel (SPACE RIP). Magn Reson Med 44:301-308

Lanzer P, Botvinick EH, Schiller NB et al (1984) Cardiac imaging using gated magnetic resonance. Radiology 150:121-127

Miller S, Helber U, Brechtel K et al (2003) MR imaging at rest early after myocardial infarction: detection of preserved function in regions with evidence for ischemic injury and non-transmural myocardial infarction. Eur Radiol 13:498-506

Paschal CB, Morris HD (2004) κ-space in the clinic. J Magn Reson Imaging 19:145-159

Petersson JS, Christoffersson JO, Golman K (1993) MRI simulation using the κ-space formalism. Magn Reson Imaging 11:557-568

Pettigrew RI, Oshinski JN, Chatzimavroudis G et al (1999) MRI techniques for cardiovascular imaging. J Magn Reson Imaging 10:590-601

Prakash A, Powell AJ, Krishnamurthy R, Geva T (2004) Magnetic resonance imaging evaluation of myocardial perfusion and viability in congenital and acquired pediatric heart disease. Am J Cardiol 93:657-661

Prince MR, Chevenert TL, Foo TK et al (1997) Contrast-enhanced abdominal MR angiography: optimization of imaging delay time by automating the detection of contrast material arrival in the aorta. Radiology 203:109-114

Pruessmann KP, Weiger M, Scheidegger MB, Boesiger P (1999) SENSE: sensitivity encoding for fast MRI. Magn Reson Med 42:952-962

Sandstede JJ (2003) Assessment of myocardial viability by MR imaging. Eur Radiol 13:52-61

Scheffler K, Lehnhardt S (2003) Principles and applications of balanced SSFP techniques. Eur Radiol 13:2409-2418

Semelka RC, Tomei E, Wagner S et al (1990) Normal left ventricular dimensions and function: interstudy reproducibility of measurements with cine MR imaging. Radiology 174:763-768

Simonetti OP, Finn JP, White RD et al (1996) "Black blood" T2-weighted inversion-recovery MR imaging of the heart. Radiology 199:49-57

Smith RC, McCarthy S (1992) Physics of magnetic resonance. J Reprod Med 37:19-26

Sodickson DK, Manning WJ (1997) Simultaneous acquisition of spatial harmonics (SMASH) : fast imaging with radiofrequency coil arrays. Magn Reson Med 38:591-603

Spuentrup E, Mahnken AH, Kuhl HP et al (2003) Fast interactive real-time magnetic resonance imaging of cardiac masses using spiral gradient echo and radial steady-state free precession sequences. Invest Radiol 38:288-292

Stehling MK, Holzknecht NG, Laub G et al (1996) Single-shot T1- and T2-weighted magnetic resonance imaging of the heart with black blood: preliminary experience. MAGMA 4:231-240

Thiele H, Nagel E, Paetsch I et al (2001) Functional cardiac MR imaging with steady-state free precession (SSFP) significantly improves endocardial border delineation without contrast agents. J Magn Reson Imaging 14:362-367

Tsao J, Boesiger P, Pruessmann KP (2003) k-t BLAST and k-t SENSE: dynamic MRI with high frame rate exploiting spatiotemporal correlations. Magn Reson Med 50:1031-1042

Van Geuns RJ, Wielopolski PA, Bruin HG deet al (1999) Basic principles of magnetic resonance imaging. Prog Cardiovasc Dis 42:149-156

Wagner A, Mahrholdt H, Holly TA (2003) Contrast-enhanced MRI and routine single photon emission computed tomography (SPECT) perfusion imaging for detection of subendocardial myocardial infarcts: an imaging study. Lancet 361:374-379

Weber OM, Martin AJ, Higgins CB (2003) Whole-heart steady-state free precession coronary artery magnetic resonance angiography. Magn Reson Med 50:1223-1228

Weiger M, Pruessmann KP, Boesiger P (2000) Cardiac real-time imaging using SENSE. SENSitivity Encoding scheme. Magn Reson Med 43:177-184

Winterer JT, Lehnhardt S, Schneider B et al (1999) MRI of heart morphology. Comparison of nongradient echo sequences with single- and multislice acquisition. Invest Radiol 34:516-522

Zerhouni EA, Parish DM, Rogers WJ et al (1988) Human heart: tagging with MR imaging – a method for noninvasive assessment of myocardial motion. Radiology 169:59-63

2 Contrast Agents for Cardiac MRI

Yicheng Ni and Steven Dymarkowski

CONTENTS

2.1 Introduction

Magnetic resonance imaging (MRI) has rapidly evolved into a major player in the armamentarium of clinical diagnostic imaging. This development is a great symbol of contemporary medicine. Acknowledging its significance, the 2003 Nobel Prize in Physiology or Medicine was awarded jointly to Lauterbur and Mansfield for their pivotal contributions in the discovery and utility of MRI (Gore 2003).

Compared with any other body structures, the ever-pumping heart in the respiratory-tided thorax represents the most difficult organ to image. Nonetheless cardiac MRI is now entirely feasible thanks to the implemented techniques such as ECG

Y. Ni MD, PhD; S. Dymarkowski MD, PhD
Department of Radiology, Gasthuisberg University Hospital, Catholic University of Leuven, Herestraat 49, 3000 Leuven, Belgium

triggering, respiration gating, ultrafast or even real-time imaging methods that have efficiently minimized cardiac and breathing motion artifacts (Kuhl et al. 2004). Over the last decade, there has been tremendous progress in MRI of both cardiac morphology and function. Further advances toward faster acquisition with real-time imaging, higher resolution for plaque imaging, and quantitative analysis are taking place at a rapid pace.

Thus, for cardiac imaging, MRI has become advantageous over other modalities owing to its versatile strengths, including noninvasiveness; nonionizing safety; superb spatial and temporal resolution; inherent 3D data acquisition with unlimited orientation; intrinsic contrast, exploitable for tissue characterization; sensitivity to blood flow and cardiac wall motion; and potential for in vivo measurement of myocardial metabolism, using MR spectroscopy or MRS; as well as for any further technical breakthroughs (van der Wall et al. 1996).

Despite all these strengths, it is of no doubt that only when complemented with the use of contrast agents can cardiac MRI fully play its pivotal role in clinical diagnosis and therapeutic decision-making. In fact, the potential and necessity of using contrast materials to promote MRI capacity was recognized soon after the invention of this imaging technology (Lauterbur et al. 1978). In particular, MR coronary angiography (MRCA), perfusion mapping, and cellular membrane integrity or myocardial viability assessment rely more on the use of appropriate contrast agents for eased imaging acquisition, enhanced image quality, and/or improved diagnostic sensitivity and specificity. In addition, contrast agents may be useful for MRI-guided interventional procedures such as angioplasty and localized delivery in gene or other advanced therapies in the future. Further research and development of more targeted MRI contrast agents at the cellular and molecular levels will help to more specifically identify different cardiovascular pathologies, including ischemia, atherosclerosis, inflammation, necrosis, and angiogenesis. Only by joining together all these indispensable elements can the comprehensive "one-stop shop" cardiac MRI examination become the reality of clinical cardiology (Ni 1998).

The current chapter aims to provide an overview on the main topics related to MRI contrast agents, including the mechanisms of MRI contrast and contrast agents, classification of both commercially available and preclinically investigational contrast agents useful for cardiac MRI, as well as the general scope of contrast agent applications in relevant clinical and experimental research.

2.2
Basic Principle of MRI Contrast Agents

2.2.1
Origins of Imaging Signals for Current Clinical MR

About two-thirds of the human body consists of water, which exists either freely or confined within the life-maintaining molecules. Water is formed by one atom of oxygen bound to two atoms of hydrogen (^1H). Another, more "MRI-discernible" body constituent is fat, which is chemically composed of fatty acids such as stearic, palmitic, and oleic acids, covalently bound in various proportions with glyceryl, all are enriched with ^1H.

The imaging signals in the clinically applied MRI at present stem from the abundant ^1H in the human body, which is inherent in magnetic property due to its single positively charged proton. A similar property is also found in other less abundantly occurring isotopic nuclei such as ^{13}C, ^{19}F, ^{23}Na, and ^{31}P, with only odd numbers of protons, but not in ^{12}C, ^{14}N, and ^{16}O, with even numbers of protons and neutrons.

When the body is exposed to a strong magnetic field, the ^1H nuclei in the tissue orient themselves within this magnetic field. While sending in a pulse of radio waves at a certain frequency, the energy content as well as the orientation of the nuclei changes, and, as they relax to their previous states, a resonance radio wave or an MRI signal is emitted. In 1971, Lauterbur pioneered spatial information encoding principles that made image formation possible by utilizing such emitted MRI signals. The further studies of Mansfield on the concept of echoplanar imaging dramatically decreased acquisition time and allowed functional and dynamic imaging (Gore 2003).

The frequencies of electromagnetic waves or radiations used for MRI are from 10^6 to 10^9 Hz approximately, i.e., within radiofrequency range,

which are much lower than that of ionizing X-rays (10^{16}–10^{20} Hz) and γ-rays (10^{21}–10^{24} Hz) used for radiography and nuclear medicine, respectively, and are therefore considered biologically safe.

Besides ^1H, other magnetic nuclei such as ^{23}Na, ^{13}C, ^{19}F, and ^{31}P in the human body can also generate MRI signals, though normally with much less intensity, but under much more technically demanding conditions and/or at much higher costs (Ardenkjaer-Larsen et al. 2003; Cannon et al. 1986; Fishman et al. 1987; Friedrich et al. 1995; Golman et al. 2003; Kim et al. 1997, 1999; Svensson et al. 2003). Some of these techniques are of particular cardiovascular relevance. The feasibility of obtaining cardiac ^{23}Na MRI at both 4.7-T animal and 1.5-T human scanners has been recently demonstrated using double-resonant ^{23}Na-^1H surface radiofrequency coils for myocardial viability determination (Cannon et al. 1986; Kim et al. 1997). In this context, the dramatic alteration of extra- versus intracellular ^{23}Na concentration during acute myocardial ischemia was exploited as an intrinsic source of contrast to identify irreversibly damaged myocytes due to disruption of sodium concentration gradient across cellular membranes. However, as the authors admitted, clinical feasibility does not imply clinical utility. Further efforts have to be made before cardiac ^{23}Na MRI can be incorporated as part of the clinical routine (Kim et al. 1999). On the other hand, ^{31}P chemical shift imaging may provide a profile of regional adenosine triphosphate (ATP) and phosphocreatine (PCr) contents, hence an estimation of energy status and viability of the myocardium (Friedrich et al. 1995). Recently a new revolutionary technology that utilizes biomolecules bearing certain prepared hyperpolarized (HP) nuclei such as HP ^{13}C-urea has shown the promise in ultrafast, high-resolution MR angiography with unprecedented signal-to-noise (SNR) and contrast-to-noise (CNR) ratios even at very low magnetic field (e.g., 0.01 T). This may also open new horizons for molecular imaging with MRI (Ardenkjaer-Larsen et al. 2003; Golman et al. 2003; Svensson et al. 2003). Despite the high performance of such novel approaches, it is likely that conventional ^1H MRI will still serve as the mainstream method for providing the basic morphological and functional information of normal and diseased cardiovascular tissues.

2.2.2
Unique Mechanisms of MRI Contrast Agents

Image contrast is the basis for human visual perception to differentiate between regions on the object. Contrast media or agents denote extrinsic or intrinsic substances that are intended to improve the image contrast of the target tissues by means of increasing or decreasing the attenuation of X-rays in radiography, the signal intensity (SI) in MRI, and the echo amplitude in ultrasonography. The radiopharmaceuticals can also be considered as contrast media to a certain extent. Since there is virtually no native radioactivity in the human body, introduction of a radiopharmaceutical into the body always increases positively the contrast of the target tissue over the background. Acceptable biotolerance remains one of the basic requirements for any potential contrast agents.

The main contrast determinants in MRI are ^{1}H proton density, longitudinal (T1) or transverse (T2) relaxation times of ^{1}H protons, and magnetic susceptibility. Since water content or ^{1}H proton density in the tissue is virtually unchangeable, magnetic properties of T1, T2, and susceptibility have therefore been the major parameters dominating the development of MRI contrast agents. Although T1 and T2 are generally prolonged in injured myocardium, there is considerable overlap of relaxation times between normal, reversibly injured and irreversibly damaged myocardium on native MRI, a fact stressing the need of contrast agents for cardiac MRI.

Some paramagnetic transition metal elements such as gadolinium (Gd^{3+}), manganese (Mn^{2+}), dysprosium (Dy^{3+}), and iron (Fe^{3+}) contain in their outer shells of the electron orbit a number of unpaired electron spins, which have relatively long electron-spin relaxation time. The magnetic field produced by an electron is much stronger than that by a ^{1}H proton, and therefore these paramagnetic elements are ideal candidates for producing MRI contrast agents that affect T1 and T2 of tissue ^{1}H protons, hence the tissue SI and/or contrast. Contrast enhancement is achieved by either increasing or decreasing the SI of a tissue; thus its signal over background noise ratio (SNR), its contrast relative to another tissue (contrast ratio or CR) and/or to the background noise (CNR), can be enhanced.

Differing from the direct and linear principles of contrast formation with the high-density contrast media for radiography or the gamma ray emitting-isotopes for nuclear scintigraphy, the mechanisms of the current MRI contrast agents are basically indirect and nonlinear, and much more complicated. They rest on the distinct magnetic properties and interactions of native ^{1}H protons toward introduced MRI contrast agents. Depending on influential factors, including the dose of the contrast agent and

MRI sequence applied, either T1-shortening (positive) or T2-shortening (negative) contrast effects can be predominant.

The positive contrast agents are typically Gd- or Mn-containing paramagnetic chelates. They shorten both T1 and T2 of the tissue, but, since T1 is much longer than T2, their predominant effect at low doses is T1 shortening. Therefore the tissue taking up such contrast agents becomes bright or hyperintense on T1-weighted MR images. However, when the local concentration of a T1 or positive contrast agent becomes very high, its T2-shortening effect appears or becomes even predominant, as often seen in the renal pelvis shortly after an intravenous dosage or as exemplified in the case of experimental acute myocardial infarction (AMI) enhanced with a necrosis-avid contrast agent (NACA; Fig. 2.1).

The negative contrast agents are often termed "superparamagnetic or susceptibility contrast agents" that can be created as small Fe_3O_4 particulate aggregates consisting of ferromagnetic or superparamagnetic crystals or particles smaller than 300 nm. They generate local magnetic field gradients that disrupt the homogeneity of the primary magnetic field over the tissue. Besides a T2-shortening effect due to the diffusion of water through these field gradients, their more prominent effect is a T2*-shortening or -susceptibility effect; both effects darken the region of interest or produce hypointense signals on T2, T2*, and even T1-weighted MR images. However, depending on their particle size and coating, they can also produce substantial T1-shortening effect and function as positive contrast agents used, for example, for MR angiography (MRA).

There are also intrinsic MRI contrast substances such as hemoglobin. The paramagnetic property of deoxyhemoglobin to cause local magnetic field distortion and susceptibility has been exploited as the source of blood oxygen level-dependent (BOLD) contrast for functional MRI of the brain (TURNER 1997).

In principle, it is their magnetic impact on the ^{1}H proton relaxation rather than the MRI contrast agents themselves that creates enhanced contrast on MR images. In other words, MRI contrast agents do not generate signals but only modify the amplitude of the signals generated by ^{1}H protons in the presence of a magnetic field.

Because of such an indirect mechanism of action, a lack of linear relation between the SI and the local concentration represents a drawback for accurate quantification of studied MRI contrast agents. Nevertheless, similar to radiopharmaceuticals or radiographic con-

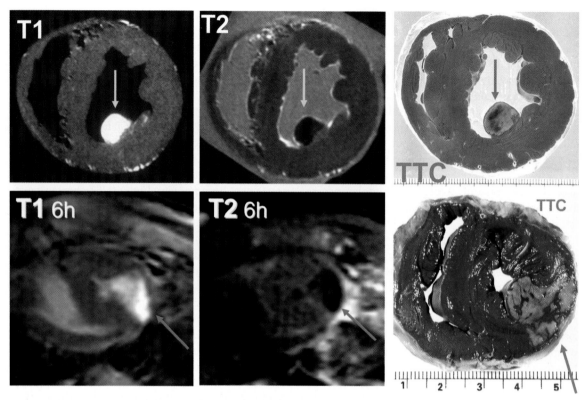

Fig. 2.1. Nonporphyrin necrosis-avid contrast agents (NACAs) at the same intravenous dose of 0.05 mmol/kg induced both T1 and T2 contrast enhancement (CE) with relevant MRI sequences in reperfused MI (*arrow*) on postmortem images of a dog overnight after injection of *bis*-Gd-DTPA-pamoic acid derivative (ECIII-60; *upper row*) and on in vivo images of a pig 6 h after injection of *bis*-Gd-DTPA-bis-indole derivative (ECIV-7; *lower row*), suggesting the chemotactic accumulation of NACAs in the necrotic myocardium as proven by the corresponding TTC-stained specimen

trast media, in unconventional MRI, when the scanner is tuned to the resonant frequencies for nuclei of ^{23}Na, ^{13}C, ^{19}F, and ^{31}P, the generated images will only show regions where these nuclei are present, hence feasible for quantitative data analysis with a direct SI and nucleus concentration relationship.

2.2.3
Dosage in Relation to Contrast-Enhancing Efficacy

Normally MRI contrast agents are chemically formulated in a manner similar to that for producing radiopharmaceuticals. Due to the fact that the sensitivity of ^{1}H MRI to detect contrast agent-induced effects visible on the image is higher than that of radiography but much lower than that of nuclear scintigraphy, the MRI contrast agents can be given with doses of micromoles per kilogram (about 5–300 µmol/kg), i.e., about 10^2–10^3 times lower than that for radiographic contrast media at a millimoles-per-kilogram level, but 10^4–10^6 times higher than that for radiopharmaceuticals at a nanomole- or even picomole-per-kilogram level. Usually, the physicians' knowledge and experience with CT contrast media can be extended to the use of clinically available MRI extracellular fluid (ECF) space contrast agents. However, as illustrated in Fig. 2.1, MRI contrast agents possess both T1- and T2-shortening effects, and their positive or negative effects of contrast enhancement (CE) depend on not only the total dosage administered, but also the local concentration of the accumulated agent in a given target tissue, as well as interaction between the contrast agent and the tissue components. Such a unique phenomenon differing from that with CT and nuclear imaging should be taken into account when contrast-enhanced MRI is interpreted.

Based on the diagnostic purpose as well as safety considerations, the exact doses and manners of contrast agent administration vary among different cardiac MRI protocols. For a first-pass myocardial-perfusion MRI, a bolus of a contrast agent at a relatively low dose of 0.005–0.05 mmol/kg is intravenously injected at a high speed (e.g., 3–5 ml/s) and flushed with a certain volume of 9% saline by using a power injector. This is usually followed by another normal dose of contrast agent for delayed CE for estimation of MI or viability (Chiu et al. 2003). To compensate the unstable CE in the AMI due to the use of ECF contrast agents, a constant infusion of Gd-DTPA is recommended for more accurate determination of myocardial necrosis in a clinical setting (Pereira et al. 2000). Diversely, slow intravenous infusion is also a common practice for administration of Mn-based intracellular contrast agents, but to avoid acute side-effects caused by calcium disturbance in myocardium (Bremerich et al. 2000; Flacke et al. 2003).

2.3
Classifications of Contrast Agents for Cardiac MRI

2.3.1
Extracellular Fluid Space Contrast Agents

The first generation MRI contrast agents, including Gd-DTPA and Gd-DOTA (Table 2.1, Fig. 2.2), are created by chelating the lanthanide metal element gadolinium with linear or cyclic multidentate ligands (DTPA or DOTA) to form thermodynamically stable and biologically inert complex or coordination compounds so that the paramagnetic properties of gadolinium can be utilized for enhancing MRI contrast, whereas the toxicity of both gadolinium and the ligands, if each applied alone, can thus be avoided. After intravenous injection, these contrast agents randomly distribute in intravascular and interstitial ECF spaces, and are eliminated rapidly in their unchanged forms through glomerular filtration in the kidney (Fig. 2.2), which makes the "renal-specific" property exploitable for evaluation of renal function. These contrast agents also allow possible diagnosis of certain pathological conditions with altered distribution space at vascular level, such as hemangioma and blood–brain barrier (BBB) breakdown, at interstitial level, such as inflammatory edema and regenerative fibrosis, and at cellular membrane integral level, such as tissue necrosis or infarction, e.g., AMI. However, normally they do not allow definite histological diagnoses owing to the intrinsic feature of nonselective distribution over all the abovementioned pathologies. Alternatively, analyses of enhancement kinetics have been elaborated for differential diagnosis between malignant and benign lesions (Heywang et al. 1989; Kaiser and Zeitler 1989), for quantitative assessment of tumor angiogenesis and microvascular density (Hawighorst et al. 1999), and for determination of cerebral blood flow and volume (Villringer et al. 1988). Lack of real tissue and/or disease specificity of these contrast agents has prompted further research and development of more specific MRI contrast agents. One noteworthy issue is that other, more advanced specific or targeting contrast agents always share more or less the nonspecific properties of the ECF contrast agents especially in their early systemic distribution phase, which has been explored for multipurpose applications of certain organ- or tissue-specific contrast agents such as the hepatobiliary Gd-BOPTA (Cavagna et al. 1997) and necrosis-avid contrast agents (NACAs; Ni et al. 2002a, 2002b; Table 2.1).

2.3.2
Blood-Pool Contrast Agents

This unique type refers to a variety of contrast agents that are confined by purpose to the intravascular space and dedicated exclusively to cardiovascular applications. Such blood-pool property can be realized by controlling the distribution and elimination of the contrast agents, which in turn is determined by their size relative to the permeability of the capillary endothelium in different organs. Although BPCAs are partially or completely limited in passing through the endothelial membrane elsewhere, they can still be excreted by the kidneys (Fig. 2.2). Usually, the higher the molecular weight of macromolecular compounds, the slower the blood elimination half-life and total blood clearance. In tissues such as myocardium, the lumen of the continuous capillaries is lined with an uninterrupted endothelial layer, which only allows diffusion of drugs with small molecular weight such as Gd-DTPA (590 Da); whereas, in the kidneys, glomerular capillaries are fenestrated with pores of 60–70 nm in diameter, which facilitate passage of any drug molecules weighted approximately below 20,000 Da. Above this molecular weight, renal excretion then depends on the lipophilicity and polarity of the agent as well as the pH of the environment. Molecules larger than 70,000 Da cannot pass the glomerular filter but are metabolized before excretion (Brasch 1991).

Relative to the ECF contrast agents with a short period of peak vascular enhancement, BPCAs pos-

Table 2.1. Contrast agents that could be used for cardiac MRI[a]

Category	Short Name	Generic Name	Trade Name	Feature
Extracellular Fluid Space Contrast Agents[b]	Gd-DTPA	Gadopentetate dimeglumine	Magnevist	Positive[c]
	Gd-DOTA	Gadoterate meglumine	Dotarem	Positive
	Gd-DTPA-BMA	Gadodiamide injection	Omniscan	Positive
	Gd-HP-DO3A	Gadoteridol injection	ProHance	Positive
	Gd-DTPA-BMEA	Gadoversetamide	Optimark	Positive
	Gd-DO3A-butriol	Gadobutrol	Gadovist	Positive
	Gd-BOPTA	Gadobenate dimeglumine	Multi-Hance	Positive
	Porphyrin and Nonporphyrin NACAs			Positive
Blood Pool Contrast Agents	NC-100150	PEG-feron (USPIO)	Clariscan	Positive
	SH U 555 C	ferucarbotran (USPIO)	Supravist	Positive
	MS-325		Angiomark	Positive
	B-22956	Gadocoletic Acid		Positive
	Gadomer-17			Positive
	P792	Macromolecular Gd-DOTA derivate	Vistarem	Positive
	AMI-227	ferumoxtran (USPIO)	Sinerem / Combidex	positive or negative
	Gd-BOPTA	Gadobenate dimeglumine	Multi-Hance	Positive
	Porphyrin and Nonporphyrin NACAs			Positive
Intracellular Contrast Agents	Mn-DPDP	Mangafodipir Trisodium	Teslascan	Intramyocytic uptake, positive
	MnCl2, MP-680, CVP 1001-1			Experimental, positive
Necrosis-Avid Contrast Agents (NACAs)	Bis Gd-DTPA meso-porphyrin		Gadophrin-2 Gadophrin-3*	Experimental, positive; *Central chelation of Cu
	ECIII-60	Gd-DTPA pamoic acid derivative	Nonporphyrin NACA	Experimental, positive
	ECIV-7	Gd-DTPA bisindole derivative	Nonporphyrin NACA	Experimental, positive
	Gadofluorine-M			Experimental, positive
Plaque-Specific Contrast Agents	Gadofluorine-M			Experimental, positive
	Porphyrin and Nonporphyrin NACAs			Experimental, positive

[a]Approved or in development
[b]All ECF space contrast agents are excreted via urine
[c]With high local concentration, negative contrast can be observed, e.g., first-pass perfusion

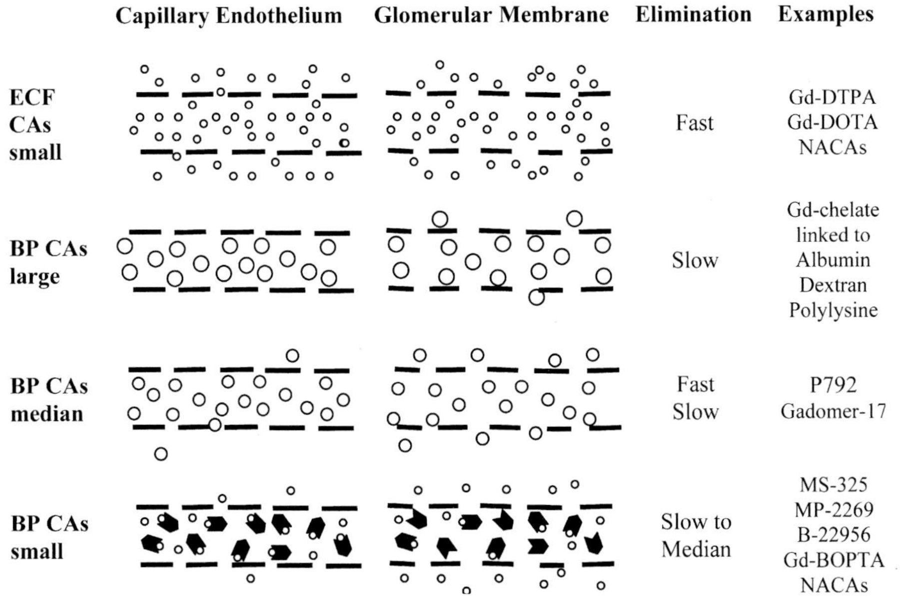

	Capillary Endothelium	Glomerular Membrane	Elimination	Examples
ECF CAs small			Fast	Gd-DTPA Gd-DOTA NACAs
BP CAs large			Slow	Gd-chelate linked to Albumin Dextran Polylysine
BP CAs median			Fast Slow	P792 Gadomer-17
BP CAs small			Slow to Median	MS-325 MP-2269 B-22956 Gd-BOPTA NACAs

Fig. 2.2. Extracellular fluid (*ECF*) space versus blood-pool (*BP*) contrast agents (*CAs*)

sess longer plasma half-life and render a higher intravascular signal, and therefore facilitate MRA with improved flexibility, accuracy, and versatility. With the use of BPCAs, the time interval between contrast injection and imaging acquisition becomes less crucial due to the resultant optimal imaging window in tens of minutes instead of seconds with the use of ECF contrast agents.

An adequate and uniform particulate size, a high ratio of T1 over T2 relaxivity, an initial intravascular space distribution, a sufficient eventual body clearance, and a lack of toxicity and/or immunogenecity are the basic requirements for an ideal BPCA. Several concepts dominate the development of BPCAs (Fig. 2.2). One approach is to synthesize large and median molecules of Gd-containing polymer for prolonged intravascular retention and slower extravasation during renal elimination, as represented by Gd-polylysine (BOGDANOV et al. 1993), Gadomer-17 (MISSELWITZ et al. 2001) and P792 (PORT et al. 2001; TAUPITZ et al. 2001), which may feature rapid urinary clearance kinetics. Another approach utilizes the reversible protein-binding property of certain small molecular Gd-chelates to form a type of "semi-endogenous" blood-pool markers, as represented by gadofosveset trisodium (formerly identified as MS-325 or Angiomark; LAUFFER et al. 1998), MP-2269 (WALLACE et al. 1998) and B-22956 (LA NOCE et al. 2002), as well as other protein-binding (though perhaps somewhat weaker) agents such as Gd-BOPTA (CAVAGNA et al. 1997) and NACAs (NI 1998; NI et al. 2002). MS-325 has been the most clinically advanced agent of this class (LAUFFER et al. 1998). While all above BPCAs are based on paramagnetic gadolinium, the third class is based on small or ultrasmall superparamagnetic iron oxides (USPIO) optimized for blood retention and minimized for susceptibility effects (CHAMBON et al. 1993; MAYO-SMITH et al. 1996; STILLMAN et al. 1996). Furthermore, clinical trials with starch-coated and stabilized iron oxide particles code-named NC 100150 (Clariscan) have been performed (AHLSTROM et al. 1999). These particulate contrast agents are slowly cleared up from the circulation and recycled through the mononuclear phagacytotic or reticuloendothelial system (MPS or RES), a metabolic route completely different from that used by gadolinium-based contrast agents. The potential cardiovascular applications of BPCAs include MRCA, assessment of myocardial perfusion, pulmonary and peripheral MRA, as well as evaluation of microvascular permeability in different pathological conditions. While a slower bolus of BPCAs is administered for dynamic arterial-phase MRA, higher injection speed as a very fast bolus often necessary for myocardial first-pass perfusion MRI remains one of the safety concerns that have to be taken into account before BPCAs can be applied in a clinical routine. The speed of injection appears to be crucial in acute toxicity effects of any contrast agents. However, the injection rate at about 1 ml/min used in laboratories to determine LD_{50} values in experimental animals is probably too slow to detect early deaths (within a few minutes after administration), which are mainly caused by osmotic expansion of the plasma volume and failure of the cardiovascular circulation (DE HAEN et al. 1994).

Other factors that are responsible for adverse reactions to contrast agents are chemotoxicity, osmotoxicity, ion toxicity, allergy, and dose (ALMEN 1994).

2.3.3
Intracellular Contrast Agents

In nuclear scintigraphic tomography, active uptake of radioactive thallium-201 (^{201}Tl) as a potassium analog (SCHOEDER et al. 1993), and manganese-52m (^{52m}Mn) and manganese-54 (^{54}Mn) as calcium antagonists (ATKINS et al. 1979; CHAUNCEY et al. 1977) by viable myocytes has been applied for assessment of myocardial viability (MV). A similar approach has been adopted in cardiac MRI using cold cation Mn^{2+} preparations as intracellular contrast agents for infarct imaging, since Mn^{2+} is potent for T1 shortening and is taken up only in cells capable of active calcium (Ca^{2+}) transport, and thereby provides an analog to ^{201}Tl imaging in cardiac scintigraphy (BREMERICH et al. 2000; FLACKE et al. 2003; KARLSSON et al. 2001; KROMBACH et al. 2004; STOREY et al. 2003). Mn^{2+} has an ionic radius similar to that of Ca^{2+} and is known to enter myocytes via voltage-facilitated calcium channels. These agents feature bifacial functions, i.e., for myocardial perfusion imaging with the initial blood-pool effect and as viability markers for functional myocytes at the equilibrium phase. Among these preparations, manganese chloride salt ($MnCl_2$) has shown the highest contrast-enhancing efficacy with the ability even to identify stunned myocardium (FLACKE et al. 2003; KROMBACH et al. 2004). However, because Mn^{2+} functions as a potent antagonist at the voltage-dependent Ca^{2+} channel across cellular membrane and competes with Ca^{2+} uptake of myocardium, concerns about the potential cardiac toxicity for negative inotropic effects or reduction of myocardial contractility have led to various formulations, all intended to lower cardiac toxicity, such as injection solution of $MnCl_2$ dissolved in calcium gluconate (FLACKE et al. 2003) and chelated preparations as slower Mn^{2+} releasers, including MP-680 or Mn[EDTA-bis(aminopropanediol)] (FLACKE et al. 2003), EVP 1001-1 (STOREY et al. 2003), and mangafodipir trisodium (manganese dipyridoxyl diphosphate, Mn-DPDP, or Teslascan; BREMERICH et al. 2000; FLACKE et al. 2003). The latter is already marketed for liver imaging with a plasma half-life less than 25 min (HUSTVEDT et al. 1997) and LD$_{50}$ about 5.4 mmol/kg in mice (ELIZONDO et al. 1991).

Interestingly, recent experimental studies in pigs have revealed that the metabolite from Mn-DPDP, namely manganese dipyridoxyl ethyldiamine (MnPLED), could reduce postischemic reperfusion-induced cardiac dysfunction and infarct size (KARLSSON et al. 2001). Therefore, the use of a Mn^{2+}-releasing contrast agents such as Mn-DPDP may be a promising multipurpose approach. In addition to the suggested therapeutic effects of antioxidative myocardial protection (BRUROK et al. 1999; KARLSSON et al. 2001), with noninvasive MRI, more functional information about myocardial metabolism and MV might be acquired by depicting differential patterns of T1 relaxation changes in relation to regional coronary flow, cellular cation uptake and retention, ion channel function, and metabolism in patients with coronary heart disease. However, all these encouraging outcomes are still experimental. Before clinical cardiac MRI might enjoy the CE with an intracellular contrast agent, its formulation, dosage, imaging protocol, and especially biotolerance have to be optimized through further strenuous preclinical and clinical research.

2.3.4
Necrosis-Avid or Multipurpose Contrast Agents?

The ECF contrast agents such as Gd-DTPA have been applied widely to enhance cardiac MRI in both clinical practice and experimental research owing to their immediate availability and excellent safety. Despite the considerable consensus to regard them as viability markers with "necrosis-specific" property to discriminate between viable and nonviable myocardium at delayed-phase contrast-enhanced MRI (KIM et al. 2000; PEREIRA et al. 2001; RAMANI et al. 1998; WEINMANN et al. 2003), inaccuracy, uncertainty, and dependency of using them on multiple influential factors for imaging interpretation have also been evidenced (CHOI et al. 2002; JUDD and KIM 2002; NI et al. 2001b; OSHINSKI et al. 2001; SAEED et al. 2001). Particularly, they are still incapable of making explicit distinctions between reversibly and irreversibly injured myocardium, between acute and chronic infarction, and between ischemic and inflammatory lesions. Therefore there has been a continuing strategy for searching more specific contrast agents that can offer unambiguous and indisputable imaging diagnosis.

Phosphonate-modified Gd-DTPA complexes could produce a persistent and strong CE in diffuse and occlusive MI owing to their affinity for calcium-rich tissues and subsequent formation of insoluble calcium phosphate precipitates in the damaged myocardium. However, they may cause disordered calcium-homeostasis and consequently impaired ventricular contractility (ADZAMLI et al. 1993). Besides, studies with technetium-99m pyrophosphate, a scintigraphic analog of this type, shows a lack of specificity between ischemic and necrotic myocardium (BIANCO et al. 1983), leading to a significant overestimation of the infarct (KHAW et al. 1987).

Anti-myosin antibody-labeled magnetopharmaceuticals denote an appealing approach. However, possible immunogenic side-effects, insufficient expression of antigens or MRI sensitivity to the currently available relaxation enhancers, and complexity in preparation and handling of the agents challenge their clinical applicability (WEISSLEDER et al. 1992).

What do X-rays, nylon, and vaccination have in common? They were discovered by accident or serendipitously. The word "serendipity" was first introduced in the middle of eighteenth century to express the phenomenon of discovery "by accident and sagacity" (ROBERTS 1989). What probably also belongs to this type is the discovery of another category of necrosis-targeting contrast agents, which represents an ongoing multiepisode story. To distinguish them from other antibody- or receptor mediated-specific contrast agents with better-defined molecular targets, we propose to nominate these newly discovered porphyrin and nonporphyrin species "necrosis-avid contrast agents" (NACAs) because of their remarkable affinity for necrotic and/or infarcted tissues (CRESENS et al. 2001; NI 1998; NI et al. 1999, 2001; PISLARU et al. 1999).

Porphyrin derivatives have been investigated for decades in diagnosis and treatment of malignant tumors (GOMER 1989; KESSEL 1984; NELSON et al. 1990; PASS 1993). The rationales governing porphyrin-mediated cancer photodynamic therapy are based on "tumor-localizing" and photosensitizing properties of the agents. By analogy, the tumor "preferential uptake" of porphyrins has also been exploited for developing paramagnetic metalloporphyrins as "tumor-seeking" MRI contrast agents (BOCKHORST et al. 1990; CHEN et al. 1984; EBERT et al. 1992; FIEL et al. 1990; FURMANSKI and LONGLEY 1988; HINDRE et al. 1993; NELSON and SCHMIEDL 1991; OGAN et al. 1987; PLACE et al. 1992; SAINI et al. 1995; VAN ZIJL et al. 1990; YOUNG et al. 1994).

However, the research activities in this laboratory have dramatically converted metalloporphyrins from being used as tumor-seeking contrast agents into magnetic markers of MI (NI et al. 1996). During the early 1990s, in helping the former Institut für Diagnostikforschung, Berlin, Germany, to screen and confirm a few potentially tumor-specific porphyrin contrast agents, including bis-Gd-DTPA-mesoporphyrin (later named Gadophrin-2) and Mn-tetraphenylporphyrin (Mn-TPP), we conducted experiments on our well-established animal models of primary and secondary liver tumors (NI et al. 1992). By using the methodologies dissimilar to those in the previous studies, we found that the notified "specific" CE could be attributed only to nonviable (typically necrotic) instead of viable tumor components (NI et al. 1995), an observation contrary to the assumption raised by an earlier study (EBERT et al. 1992). To support our findings and to convince people of porphyrins' tumor-nonspecificity, more metalloporphyrins were assessed in rats with various induced "benign" necroses and the so-called tumor-localizing phenomenon could be reproduced without exceptions (NI et al. 1997b). Although, unfortunately, these contrast agents can no longer be considered tumor-specific, their superb necrosis targetability has elicited even more exciting, novel applications for MRI visualization of acute MI (HERIJGERS et al. 1997; MARCHAL et al. 1996; MARCHAL and NI 2000; NI et al. 1994, 1998, 2001; PISLARU et al. 1999) and brain infarction (SCHNEIDER et al. 1995). The local concentration of Gd is frequently more than 10s of times higher in infarcted compared with normal myocardium. Finally, the potent effects of Gadophrin-2 for labeling spontaneous and therapeutic necroses, including MI and lesions of radiofrequency ablation (RFA), on MRI were widely recognized a few years later, after multi-institutional reproducibility studies (BARKHAUSEN et al. 2002; CHOI et al. 2000; JEONG et al. 2001; LIM and CHOI 1999; SAEED et al. 1999, 2001; STILLMAN et al. 1999; WENDLAND et al. 1999).

Besides a normal intravenous dose at 0.05–0.1 mmol/kg for cardiac MRI to visualize MI with an extended imaging window of 3–48 h (HERIJGERS et al. 1997; MARCHAL et al. 1996; MARCHAL and NI 2000; NI et al. 1994; NI 1998; PISLARU et al. 1999; BARKHAUSEN et al. 2002; CHOI et al. 2000; JEONG et al. 2001; LIM and CHOI 1999; SAEED et al. 1999; STILLMAN et al. 1999; WENDLAND et al. 1999), intracoronary delivery of a tiny dose at 0.005 mmol/kg in combination with the percutaneous transcatheter coronary angioplasty (PTCA) procedure serves as a diagnostic adjuvant for MV determination and therapeutic assessment (NI et al. 1998, 2001).

So far, triphenyltetrazolium chloride (TTC) staining has been used as the only gold standard for mac-

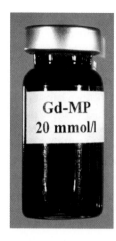
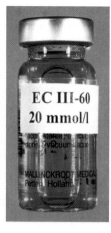
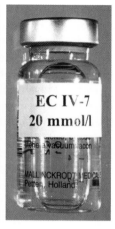

Fig. 2.3. Vials contain the porphyrin-derived NACA Gadophrin-2 on the left, the nonporphyrin NACA *bis*-Gd-DTPA-pamoic acid derivative (*ECIII-60*) in the middle and the nonporphyrin NACA *bis*-Gd-DTPA-bis-indole derivative (*ECIV-7*) on the right at the same concentration of 20 mmol/l. In contrast to the nontransparent, dark-colored pigment-like Gadophrin-2, nonporphyrin NACAs appear as either a transparent light-yellowish (ECIII-60) or completely colorless (ECIV-7) water solutions

roscopic identification or quantification of acute MI. However, it is a postmortem technique and not clinically applicable. Studies with both intravenous and intracoronary NACA injections have revealed that what is specifically enhanced on cardiac MRI corresponds exactly to what TTC dye does not stain on the excised heart, resulting in the same accuracy for MI delineation (CHOI et al. 2000; HERIJGERS et al. 1997; JEONG et al. 2001; LIM and CHOI 1999; MARCHAL et al. 1996; MARCHAL and NI 2000; NI et al. 1994, 1998, 2001a, 2001b; NI 1998; PISLARU et al. 1999; SAEED et al. 1999; STILLMAN et al. 1999; WENDLAND et al. 1999; Fig. 2.1). Experimentally, NACA-enhanced MRI has been used as a surrogate of TTC histochemical staining or an in vivo viability gold standard for evaluation of medicinal myocardial protection (LUND et al. 2001) and interventional RFA (NI et al. 1997a, 2004b). By chelating a copper ion in the center of the cyclic tetrapyrrole ring, Gadophrin-3 has been introduced to improve its structural stability and safety yet still retain its targeting efficacy (BARKHAUSEN et al. 2002; SCHALLA et al. 2004). Except for slight discoloration that fades considerably over 24 h, during animal experiments no detectable side-effects have been reported with porphyrin agents at a 0.05–0.1 mmol/kg dose range (CHOI et al. 2000; HERIJGERS et al. 1997; JEONG et al. 2001; LIM and CHOI 1999; MARCHAL et al. 1996; MARCHAL and NI 2000; NI 1998; NI et al. 1994, 1997a, 1997b, 1998, 2001a, 2001b; PISLARU et al. 1999; SAEED et al. 1999, 2001; SCHNEIDER et al. 1995; STILLMAN et al. 1999; WENDLAND et al. 1999). Nevertheless, despite optimistic expectations (KROMBACH et al. 2002), further commercial development of these colored porphyrin complexes has unfortunately been abandoned by the industry (Weinmann, Schering AG, personal communication), most likely due to the predicted unsatisfactory clinical tolerance resulting from the unchangeable nature of dark-colored pigments of this type of chemical (Fig. 2.3).

In order to overcome the discoloration, phototoxicity, and other side-effects related to the use of porphyrin derivatives, we have made continuing efforts to search for more effective, less toxic and less colored compounds. First, to verify whether the cyclic tetrapyrrole structure characteristic of all porphyrins is essential or not for the observed necrosis targeting, we checked more metalloporphyrins and found that four out of nine metalloporphyrins did not prove necrosis-avid (NI et al. 1999). Such unequal performances among different porphyrins, also occurring in cancer photodynamic therapy (KESSEL 1984; PASS 1993) and tumor imaging (EBERT et al. 1992), suggest that the tetrapyrrole ring does not appear to be a common structural requirement for the specific targetability. Furthermore, other Gd chelates conjugated to either open-chain tetrapyrroles such as bilirubin and biliverdin or smaller constituents such as mono-, bis- and tri-pyrrole derivatives also failed to reveal a necrosis-specificity (NI et al. 2002a, 2002b). These findings not only disprove an inevitable link between porphyrin-related structures and the affinity for necrosis but also imply the possibility of generating totally different nonporphyrin molecules that could be more effective and less colored or even colorless and, therefore, deprived of any unwanted effects associated with porphyrins. Along this line, we have been able to successfully synthesize a few promising leading compounds such as the light-yellowish ECIII-60 (bis-Gd-DTPA-pamoic acid) and the colorless ECIV-7 (bis-Gd-DTPA-bisindole; CRESENS et al. 2001; MARCHAL et al. 1999; NI et al. 2002a, 2002b), with both featuring extraordinary necrosis avidity (Figs. 2.1, 2.3). All studied NACAs, whether porphyrin or nonporphyrin species, allow differential diagnoses between reversible ischemic injury and irreversible infarct, acute and healing MI, and occlusive and reperfused MI (CHOI et al. 2000; JEONG et al. 2001; NI et al. 2002; SAEED et al. 1999, 2002). Even negative findings after CE with NACAs help to reliably exclude the presence of necrosis, which would also be of high significance for differential diagnosis (MARCHAL et al. 1996; NI 1998).

In a recently proposed "one-stop shop" comprehensive package of cardiac MR for MV assessment, the NACA serves as the only key factor that can provide a clear-cut distinction between viable and necrotic myocardium (NI 1998). In addition to the necrosis-targeting property, NACAs also share some exploitable features commonly seen with other existing contrast agents, for instance their relatively long plasma half-life due to protein-binding facilitates their utility as BPCAs for MR angiography (Fig. 2.4) especially of coronary arteries; their amphiphilicity, as well as hepatobiliary and renal pathways, may render applications for liver- and kidney-specific CE. Therefore, with combined specific and nonspecific capacities, NACAs may serve well as versatile or multipurpose contrast-enhancing agents (NI et al. 2002a, 2002b, 2002c). A similar example can be found with Gd-BOPTA or trade-named MultiHance (CAVAGNA et al. 1997), which is albeit void of necrosis acidity. (Table 2.1). Indeed, it appears that both porphyrin and nonporphyrin NACAs exert their necrosis-targeting function only when there exists denatured nonviable tissue debris in a living being, otherwise they just behave like other, less specific contrast agents such as ECF contrast agents used, e.g., for the first-pass myocardial perfusion, BPCAs used for MRCA, and hepatobiliary and urinary contrast agents for liver and kidney CE (NI et al. 2005a).

Nobel Prize laureate Arthur Kornberg (1918) once thus said: "You cannot prove a mechanism; you can only disprove a mechanism," which is exactly reflected by the current status of the mechanism research on NACAs. Hofmann et al. have attributed the accumulation mechanism of Gadophrin-2 to its binding to albumin in the plasma and interstitium and subsequent trapping in intratumoral necrotic regions (HOFMANN et al. 1999). However, this conclusion was disproved in another study in which only Gadophrin-2, but not the strong albumin-binding BPCA MP2269 revealed in vivo necrosis avidity

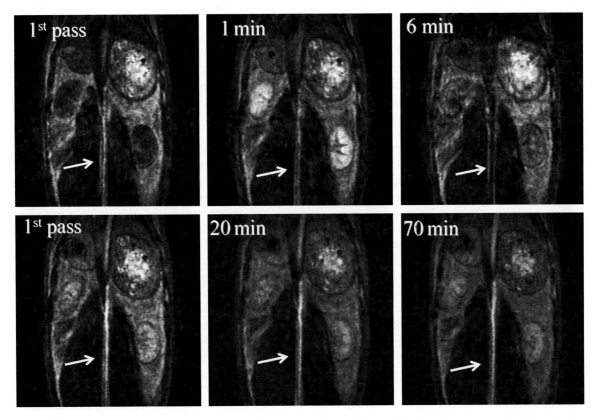

Fig. 2.4. MR angiography of rabbit aorta (*arrow*) comparing Gd-DTPA at 0.1 mmol/kg (*upper row*) and the nonporphyrin NACA ECIV-7 at 0.05 mmol/kg (*lower row*) display rapid clearance of Gd-DTPA from the circulation and blood-pool (BP) effect of ECIV-7 over 70 min

(NI et al. 2001a, 2001b). This finding suggests that only few albumin-binding contrast agents possess the NACA property, although to some extent most of the NACAs tend to bind plasma proteins (typically albumin); in other words, the necrosis avidity is an outstanding feature beyond the general pharmacological process of albumin binding-mediated drug transportation (NI et al. 2005a, 2005b).

Hypothetically, NACA-induced necrosis targeting may arise in a seemingly chemotactic fashion as follows. While circulating in the blood pool after administration, the agents approach the necrotic region by a time-consuming process of perfusion through residual vessels, extravasation, and interstitial diffusion, wherein a reperfused infarction is more favorable than an occlusive one for NACA accumulation due to the ampler access. The disintegrated cell-membrane after autolysis facilitates contact and communication of NACAs with the tissue debris, which in turn may further augment the relaxivity due to macromolecular interactions leading always to a striking CE of the infarct (LAUFFER 1991). Our recent studies suggest that such local interaction and retention seems strictly chemo-structure dependent rather than a simple trapping or sluggish wash-in and washout, because either a slight modification or even an isomer transformation may drastically switch off the necrosis-targeting effect of certain NACA molecules (NI et al. 2005a, 2005b). With respect to target tissues, the size and site of infarcted areas as well as the presence or absence of postischemic reperfusion determine what the NACA-induced necrosis-specific CE looks like (i.e., patchy or bulky, subendocardial or transmural, and complete or rim-like) and how long it may persist. Unlike the "detrapping" process of nonspecific contrast agents in a few hours, the eventual clearance of NACAs from necrotic foci typically takes a few days after administration and parallels the natural healing process, during which the necrotic tissues are progressively infiltrated and phagocytozed by inflammatory cells (mainly neutrophils, monocytes, and/or macrophages) and replaced by the granulation tissue. Therefore the retained NACAs in necrosis are most likely removed together with necrotic materials by phagocytosis. Questions remain as to whether the Gd complex of NACAs is still stable after being taken up by macrophages and what the fate and consequence are of this small necrosis-binding fraction of NACAs in the human body (NI 1998; NI et al. 2001, 2002a, 2002b, 2005a). These have to be further elucidated. Alternatively, to substitute the bioincompatible lanthanide element Gd^{3+} with the physiological trace metal element Mn^{2+} in the complex of NACAs may eliminate the concerns about any potential side-effects due to gadolinium body retention.

In addition to the above-identified porphyrin and nonporphyrin NACAs, there appears to be a large variety of synthetic or natural, endogenous or exogenous substances such as the organic dye Evans blue used for intravital staining (HAMER et al. 2002), the botanical extract hypericin derived from St. Johns Wort (NI et al. 2004, 2005), the heme-related cofactor hematoporphyrin for oxygen transportation (GOMER 1989; KESSEL 1984; NELSON et al. 1990; NELSON and SCHMIEDL 1991; PASS 1993), and the urinary-excretable glucarate catabolized from UDP (uridine diphosphate)-glucose (ORLANDI et al. 1991), which all seem to share a common necrosis avidity. They may firmly bind to the denatured, nonviable tissue components such as positively charged histone, collagen, and other reduced subcellular organelle proteins found in necrotic debris (NI et al. 2004, 2005a, 2005b). However, unless they are inherently colored or fluorescent, their existence can hardly be discerned prior to their labeling with detectable markers as to form radiopharmaceuticals (NI et al. 2004, 2005a, 2005b) and magnetopharmaceuticals (CHOI et al. 2000; HERIJGERS et al. 1997; JEONG et al. 2001; LIM and CHOI 1999; MARCHAL et al. 1996; MARCHAL and NI 2000; NI 1998; NI et al. 1994, 1998, 2001; PISLARU et al. 1999; SAEED et al. 1999, 2001; SCHNEIDER et al. 1995; STILLMAN et al. 1999; WENDLAND et al. 1999).

Furthermore, such generally perceived structural diversity versus functional similarity supports our hypothesis that the avidity of certain chemicals to necrotic debris in the living body is an ever-existing phenomenon as part of the natural wound-healing process, which has never been well recognized yet deserves to be wisely exploited for medical purposes (NI et al. 2002a, 2002b, 2004, 2005a, 2005b). The key steps to realize this more close-to-nature strategy include understanding the underlying mechanisms of necrosis avidity and identifying the exact local structural configuration responsible for such a strong physicochemical reaction through careful analyses on the structure–function relationship among all available NACA-like substances. Then, it might be possible to create dedicated, all-in-one, multifunctional contrast agents by purposely tailoring the chemical structures. In contrast to more aggressive and sophisticated approaches such as transgenic or cloning techniques that are prone to potential ecological hazards, such more-biocompatible molecular engineering may render additional NACA targetability onto any known nontoxic substances that could be the more physiological life molecules such as vitamins, simple carbohydrates and amino acids, and/or even existing medications already in use such as anti-ischemic and thrombolytic drugs. Development in this promising direction may open a new horizon certainly for the diagnosis and treatment of diseases in clinical cardiology, wherein interdisciplinary collaborations from both academics and industry are warranted. The ultimate beneficiary would be the entire human society.

2.3.5
Potential Plaque- and Thrombus-Specific Contrast Agents

Atherosclerosis and thrombosis are two sequential, interdependent processes causative for acute coronary syndrome (ACS) in patients with chronic cardiovascular disease. Noninvasive, high-resolution MRI may depict 3D microanatomy of the lumen and the vascular wall, characterize the composition of the atherosclerotic plaque, identify lesions vulnerable to rupture or erosion, and therefore provide information about not only the individual high-risk plaques but also overall plaque burden in each patient. These diagnostic messages are critical for making decisions in emergent therapeutic interventions and monitoring progression and regression of atherosclerosis during preventive treatment with, e.g., lipid-lowering drug regimes. It is believed that the high resolution of MRI in combination with sophisticated contrast agents under development may offer the promise of in vivo molecular imaging of the plaque (FAYAD 2003).

There have been some developments in favor of plaque- and thrombus-specific contrast agents that can target either matrices or cellular compositions of the lesion (Table 2.1).

Fibrin-specific paramagnetic nanoparticles formulated with Gd-DTPA-bis-oleate (BOA) or Gd-DTPA-phosphatidylethanolamine (PE) are reported to have high affinity for fibrin-rich thrombus and the potential to sensitively detect active vulnerable plaques on T1-weighted MRI (FLACKE et al. 2001).

Macrocyclic gadolinium-based Gadofluorines prone to form nanomicelles were originally intended for intravenous lymphography but have been found also to be able to accumulate in the deeper-layer intima (rich in foam cells and cellular debris) of the atherosclerotic aorta, leading to a strong positive CE in a genetically hyperlipidemic rabbit model 1 day after intravenous injection (BARKHAUSEN et al.

2003). Gadofluorine B can also be regarded as another nonporphyrin NACA because of characteristic pharmacodynamic behaviors similar to those commonly seen with other NACAs (Misselwitz, Schering AG, personal communication).

Interestingly, porphyrins and an expanded porphyrin target atherosclerotic plaques too (SPOKOJNY et al. 1986; VEVER-BIZET et al. 1989; WOODBURN et al. 1996; YOUNG et al. 1994). Given the clues collected in the studies on porphyrin and nonporphyrin species of NACAs as described in detail above, their multiple pyrrole ring structures are unlikely to be essential for their preferential accumulation in the nonviable matrices of the plaques. A secondary macrophage uptake following NACA-necrosis binding may also count for their local enrichment. Further studies may reveal that plaque-targeting could well be one of the NACAs' versatile functions.

Besides functioning as positive BPCAs for MR angiography and negative contrast agents for lesion delineation in the lymph node, liver, and spleen, long-circulating USPIOs also accumulate in atherosclerotic plaques due to active uptake by localized monocytes and macrophages. At a relatively high intravenous dose (e.g., 1 mmol/kg), persistent, hypointense signals could be detected over a few days in the wall of atherosclerotic arteries from the same rabbit atherosclerotic models (KOOI et al. 2003; RUEHM et al. 2001; SCHMITZ et al. 2000). Nonetheless, from the viewpoints of dose efficacy and safety, so far none of these agents have convincingly shown their even remote clinical feasibility.

2.3.6
Emerging Molecular Imaging Contrast Agents

Molecular imaging can be defined typically as the technology that is established for developing targeted and activatable imaging agents to exploit specific molecular targets, pathways, or cellular processes to generate image contrast with appropriate imaging modalities (JAFFER and WEISSLEDER 2004). Strictly speaking, what also fall well into this plausible definition would be many already existing MRI contrast agents, including albumin-targeting BPCAs, Mn-based intracellular contrast agents, and even NACAs that are involved in several pathophysiological processes such as protein-binding, chemotactic interaction with necrotic tissues, and hepatobiliary and renal pathways.

The underpinning hypothesis of this newer approach to imaging is that most disease processes have a molecular basis that can be exploited to (1) detect disease earlier, (2) stratify disease subsets (e.g., active versus inactive), (3) objectively monitor novel therapies by imaging molecular biomarkers, and (4) to prognosticate disease (JAFFER and WEISSLEDER 2004).

Although still far from the clinical reality in cardiac MRI, the research in this discipline is rapidly advancing, with a few leading molecular probes already emerging from laboratory experiments for MRI monitoring of cardiovascular pathological processes or consequences such as atherosclerosis (WINTER et al. 2003), thrombosis (JOHANSSON et al. 2001), and heart failure (SCHELLENBERGER et al. 2002), as well as therapeutic intervention (KRAITCHMAN et al. 2003). It has been predicted that in the ensuing years fundamental aspects of cardiovascular biology will be detectable in vivo and that promising molecular imaging agents will be translated into the clinical arena to guide diagnosis and therapy of human cardiovascular illness (JAFFER and WEISSLEDER 2004). This would again offer opportunities for people to witness whether such anticipations could bring about the breakthroughs that are really beneficial to patients suffering from, and to clinicians fighting against, cardiovascular diseases.

2.4
Application Scopes of Contrast Agents for Cardiac MRI

As demonstrated in the many chapters throughout the contents in this handbook, the use of contrast agents has undoubtedly become an integral part of the daily practice of cardiac MRI because of their efficacy and their excellent tolerance profile. Their application scope cover almost all aspects of cardiac MRI, including noninvasive depiction of cardiac anatomy (Chap. 4) and real-time monitor of cardiac function (Chap. 6), in particular myocardial perfusion (Chap. 7) and cardiac output quantification. The indispensable role of contrast agents is exemplified in comprehensive diagnoses of ischemic (Chap. 8) and nonischemic (Chap. 9) heart diseases, as well as heart failure (Chap. 10) and neoplasms (Chap. 12). More delicate evaluations with CE MRI on pericardial diseases and valvular heart diseases are addressed in Chaps. 11 and 13, respectively. The state-of-the-art techniques for MR coronary artery imaging is introduced in Chap. 14. The images by courtesy of Dr. Debiao Li illustrate well the crucial added value of contrast agents by comparing MRCA in a swine without contrast agent with an ECF contrast agent and with a BPCA injection (Fig. 2.5). In addition, the usefulness of contrast agents has also been proven for clinical diagnoses of congenital heart diseases (Chap. 15) and abnormalities in great vessels (Chap. 16).

2.5
Conclusion

Despite the appreciable maturity with continuing excellence at 30 years of age, it is encouragingly evident that MRI would still have its best years to come toward a one-stop shop final solution of noninvasive, 3D, high-resolution real time imaging of the cardiovascular system particularly boosted by the new inventions and applications of MRI contrast agents.

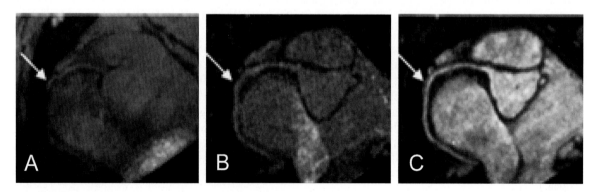

Fig. 2.5a-c. Comparison of MR angiography of the right coronary artery (*arrow*) in the same pig without contrast agent injection (**a**), with an ECF agent Gd-DTPA at 0.2 mmol/kg (**b**) and with a blood-pool contrast agent Gadomer-17 at 0.1 mmol/kg (**c**) demonstrate the indispensable role of contrast agents, especially the blood-pool agent, in MR coronary angiography. The images are displayed after multiplanar reconstruction. (*By courtesy of Debiao Li, Biomedical Engineering Department, Northwestern University, Evanston, Ill., USA*)

References

Adzamli IK, Blau M, Pfeffer MA, Davis MA (1993) Phosphonate-modified Gd-DTPA complexes. III. The detection of myocardial infarction by MRI. Magn Reson Med 29:505-511

Ahlstrom KH, Johansson LO, Rodenburg JB, Ragnarsson AS, Akeson P, Borseth A (1999) Pulmonary MR angiography with ultrasmall superparamagnetic iron oxide particles as a blood pool agent and a navigator echo for respiratory gating: pilot study. Radiology 211:865-869

Almen T (1994) The etiology of contrast medium reactions. Invest Radiol 29 [Suppl 1]:S37-S45

Ardenkjaer-Larsen JH, Fridlund B, Gram A, Hansson G, Hansson L, Lerche MH, Servin R, Thaning M, Golman K, Petersson JS, Mansson S, Leunbach I (2003) Increase in signal-to-noise ratio of >10,000 times in liquid-state NMR molecular imaging with endogenous substances. Proc Natl Acad Sci USA 100:10158-10163

Atkins HL, Som P, Fairchild RG, Hui J, Schachner E, Goldman A, Ku T (1979) Myocardial positron tomography with manganese-52m. Radiology 133:769-774

Barkhausen J, Ebert W, Debatin JF, Weinmann HJ (2002) Imaging of myocardial infarction: comparison of magnevist and gadophrin-3 in rabbits. J Am Coll Cardiol 39:1392-1398

Barkhausen J, Ebert W, Heyer C, Debatin JF, Weinmann HJ (2003) Detection of atherosclerotic plaque with Gadofluorine-enhanced magnetic resonance imaging. Circulation 108:605-609

Bianco JA, Kemper AJ, Taylor A, Lazewatsky J, Tow DE, Khuri SF (1983) Technetium-99m(Sn^{2+})pyrophosphate in ischemic and infarcted dog myocardium in early stages of acute coronary occlusion: histochemical and tissue-counting comparisons. J Nucl Med 24:485-491

Bockhorst K, Hohn-Berlage M, Kocher M, Hossmann KA (1990) Proton relaxation enhancement in experimental brain tumors – in vivo NMR study of manganese(III)TPPS in rat brain gliomas. Magn Reson Imaging 8:499-504

Bogdanov AA Jr, Weissleder R, Frank HW, Bogdanova AV, Nossif N, Schaffer BK, Tsai E, Papisov MI, Brady TJ (1993) A new macromolecule as a contrast agent for MR angiography: preparation, properties, and animal studies. Radiology 187:701-706

Brasch RC (1991) Rationale and applications for macromolecular Gd-based contrast agents. Magn Reson Med 22:282-287, 300-303

Bremerich J, Saeed M, Arheden H, Higgins CB, Wendland MF (2000) Normal and infarcted myocardium: differentiation with cellular uptake of manganese at MR imaging in a rat model. Radiology 216:524-530

Brurok H, Ardenkjaer-Larsen JH, Hansson G, Skarra S, Berg K, Karlsson JO, Laursen I, Jynge P (1999) Manganese dipyridoxyl diphosphate: MRI contrast agent with antioxidative and cardioprotective properties? Biochem Biophys Res Commun 254:768-772

Cannon PJ, Maudsley AA, Hilal SK, Simon HE, Cassidy F (1986) Sodium nuclear magnetic resonance imaging of myocardial tissue of dogs after coronary artery occlusion and reperfusion. J Am Coll Cardiol 7:573-579

Cavagna FM, Maggioni F, Castelli PM, Dapra M, Imperatori LG, Lorusso V, Jenkins BG (1997) Gadolinium chelates with weak binding to serum proteins. A new class of high-efficiency, general purpose contrast agents for magnetic resonance imaging. Invest Radiol 32:780-796

Chambon C, Clement O, Le Blanche A, Schouman-Claeys E, Frija G (1993) Superparamagnetic iron oxides as positive MR contrast agents: in vitro and in vivo evidence. Magn Reson Imaging 11:509-519

Chauncey DM, Jr., Schelbert HR, Halpern SE, Delano F, McKegney ML, Ashburn WL, Hagan PL (1977) Tissue distribution studies with radioactive manganese: a potential agent for myocardial imaging. J Nucl Med 18:933-936

Chen CW, Cohen JS, Myers CE, Sohn M (1984) Paramagnetic metalloporphyrins as potential contrast agents in NMR imaging. FEBS Lett 168:70-74

Chiu CW, So NM, Lam WW, Chan KY, Sanderson JE (2003) Combined first-pass perfusion and viability study at MR imaging in patients with non-ST segment-elevation acute coronary syndromes: feasibility study. Radiology 226:717-722

Choi C, Haji-Momenian S, Dimaria J et al (2002) Contrast washout by MRI identifies stunned myocardium in patients after reperfused myocardial infarction (abstract). J Cardiovasc Mag Res 4:19

Choi SI, Choi SH, Kim ST, Lim KH, Lim CH, Gong GY, Kim HY, Weinmann HJ, Lim TH (2000) Irreversibly damaged myocardium at MR imaging with a necrotic tissue-specific contrast agent in a cat model. Radiology 215:863-868

Cresens E, Ni Y, Adriaens P, Verbruggen A, Marchal G (2001) Substituted bis-indole derivatives useful as contrast agents, pharmaceutical compositions containing them and intermediates for producing them, Belgium, International patent, Application number PCT/BE01/00192, Application date November 7, 2001

De Haen C, Morisetti A, Bertani F, Tirone P (1994) The factor time in acute intravenous toxicity studies of contrast media. Invest Radiol 29 [Suppl 2]:108-110

Ebert E, Hofmann S, Swiderski U et al (1992) Metallopophyrins: tumor-specific contrast agents? European Magnetic Resonance Forum Foundation, Hamburg, Germany

Elizondo G, Fretz CJ, Stark DD, Rocklage SM, Quay SC, Worah D, Tsang YM, Chen MC, Ferrucci JT (1991) Preclinical evaluation of MnDPDP: new paramagnetic hepatobiliary contrast agent for MR imaging. Radiology 178:73-78

Fayad ZA (2003) MR imaging for the noninvasive assessment of atherothrombotic plaques. Magn Reson Imaging Clin North Am 11:101-113

Fiel RJ, Musser DA, Mark EH, Mazurchuk R, Alletto JJ (1990) A comparative study of manganese meso-sulfonatophenyl porphyrins: contrast-enhancing agents for tumors. Magn Reson Imaging 8:255-259

Fishman JE, Joseph PM, Floyd TF, Mukherji B, Sloviter HA (1987) Oxygen-sensitive 19F NMR imaging of the vascular system in vivo. Magn Reson Imaging 5:279-285

Flacke S, Fischer S, Scott MJ, Fuhrhop RJ, Allen JS, McLean M, Winter P, Sicard GA, Gaffney PJ, Wickline SA, Lanza GM (2001) Novel MRI contrast agent for molecular imaging of fibrin: implications for detecting vulnerable plaques. Circulation 104:1280-1285

Flacke S, Allen JS, Chia JM, Wible JH, Periasamy MP, Adams MD, Adzamli IK, Lorenz CH (2003) Characterization of viable and nonviable myocardium at MR imaging: comparison of gadolinium-based extracellular and blood pool contrast materials versus manganese-based contrast materials in a rat myocardial infarction model. Radiology 226:731-738

Friedrich J, Apstein CS, Ingwall JS (1995) 31P nuclear magnetic resonance spectroscopic imaging of regions of remodeled myocardium in the infarcted rat heart. Circulation 92:3527-3538

Furmanski P, Longley C (1988) Metalloporphyrin enhancement of magnetic resonance imaging of human tumor xenografts in nude mice. Cancer Res 48:4604-4610

Golman K, Ardenkjaer-Larsen JH, Petersson JS, Mansson S, Leunbach I (2003) Molecular imaging with endogenous substances. Proc Natl Acad Sci USA 100:10435-10439

Gomer CJ (1989) Photodynamic therapy in the treatment of malignancies. Semin Hematol 26:27-34

Gore J (2003) Out of the shadows – MRI and the Nobel Prize. N Engl J Med 349:2290-2292

Hamer PW, McGeachie JM, Davies MJ, Grounds MD (2002) Evans Blue Dye as an in vivo marker of myofibre damage: optimising parameters for detecting initial myofibre membrane permeability. J Anat 200:69-79

Hawighorst H, Knapstein PG, Knopp MV, Vaupel P, van Kaick G (1999) Cervical carcinoma: standard and pharmacokinetic analysis of time-intensity curves for assessment of tumor angiogenesis and patient survival. Magma 8:55-62

Herijgers P, Laycock SK, Ni Y, Marchal G, Bogaert J, Bosmans H, Petre C, Flameng W (1997) Localization and determination of infarct size by Gd-Mesoporphyrin enhanced MRI in dogs. Int J Card Imaging 13:499-507

Heywang SH, Wolf A, Pruss E, Hilbertz T, Eiermann W, Permanetter W (1989) MR imaging of the breast with Gd-DTPA: use and limitations. Radiology 171:95-103

Hindre F, Le Plouzennec M, de Certaines JD, Foultier MT, Patrice T, Simonneaux G (1993) Tetra-p-aminophenylporphyrin conjugated with Gd-DTPA: tumor-specific contrast agent for MR imaging. J Magn Reson Imaging 3:59-65

Hofmann B, Bogdanov A Jr, Marecos E, Ebert W, Semmler W, Weissleder R (1999) Mechanism of gadophrin-2 accumulation in tumor necrosis. J Magn Reson Imaging 9:336-341

Hustvedt SO, Grant D, Southon TE, Zech K (1997) Plasma pharmacokinetics, tissue distribution and excretion of MnDPDP in the rat and dog after intravenous administration. Acta Radiol 38:690-699

Jaffer FA, Weissleder R (2004) Seeing within: molecular imaging of the cardiovascular system. Circ Res 94:433-445

Jeong AK, Choi SI, Kim DH, Park SB, Lee SS, Choi SH, Lim TH (2001) Evaluation by contrast-enhanced MR imaging of the lateral border zone in reperfused myocardial infarction in a cat model. Korean J Radiol 2:21-27

Johansson LO, Bjornerud A, Ahlstrom HK, Ladd DL, Fujii DK (2001) A targeted contrast agent for magnetic resonance imaging of thrombus: implications of spatial resolution. J Magn Reson Imaging 13:615-618

Judd RM, Kim RJ (2002) Imaging time after Gd-DTPA injection is critical in using delayed enhancement to determine infarct size accurately with magnetic resonance imaging (author reply). Circulation 106:e6

Kaiser WA, Zeitler E (1989) MR imaging of the breast: fast imaging sequences with and without Gd-DTPA. Preliminary observations. Radiology 170:681-686

Karlsson JO, Brurok H, Eriksen M, Towart R, Toft KG, Moen O, Engebretsen B, Jynge P, Refsum H (2001) Cardioprotective effects of the MR contrast agent MnDPDP and its metabolite MnPLED upon reperfusion of the ischemic porcine myocardium. Acta Radiol 42:540-547

Kessel D (1984) Porphyrin localization: a new modality for detection and therapy of tumors. Biochem Pharmacol 33:1389-1393

Khaw BA, Strauss HW, Moore R, Fallon JT, Yasuda T, Gold HK, Haber E (1987) Myocardial damage delineated by indium-111 antimyosin Fab and technetium-99m pyrophosphate. J Nucl Med 28:76-82

Kim RJ, Lima JA, Chen EL, Reeder SB, Klocke FJ, Zerhouni EA, Judd RM (1997) Fast 23Na magnetic resonance imaging of acute reperfused myocardial infarction. Potential to assess myocardial viability. Circulation 95:1877-1885

Kim RJ, Judd RM, Chen EL, Fieno DS, Parrish TB, Lima JA (1999) Relationship of elevated ^{23}Na magnetic resonance image intensity to infarct size after acute reperfused myocardial infarction. Circulation 100:185-192

Kim RJ, Wu E, Rafael A, Chen EL, Parker MA, Simonetti O, Klocke FJ, Bonow RO, Judd RM (2000) The use of contrast-enhanced magnetic resonance imaging to identify reversible myocardial dysfunction. N Engl J Med 343:1445-1453

Kooi ME, Cappendijk VC, Cleutjens KB, Kessels AG, Kitslaar PJ, Borgers M, Frederik PM, Daemen MJ, van Engelshoven JM (2003) Accumulation of ultrasmall superparamagnetic particles of iron oxide in human atherosclerotic plaques can be detected by in vivo magnetic resonance imaging. Circulation 107:2453-2458

Kraitchman DL, Heldman AW, Atalar E, Amado LC, Martin BJ, Pittenger MF, Hare JM, Bulte JW (2003) In vivo magnetic resonance imaging of mesenchymal stem cells in myocardial infarction. Circulation 107:2290-2293

Krombach GA, Higgins CB, Gunther RW, Kuhne T, Saeed M (2002) MR contrast media for cardiovascular imaging. Rofo Fortschr Geb Rontgenstr Neuen Bildgeb Verfahr 174:819-829

Krombach GA, Saeed M, Higgins CB, Novikov V, Wendland MF (2004) Contrast-enhanced MR delineation of stunned myocardium with administration of MnCl(2) in rats. Radiology 230:183-190

Kuhl HP, Spuentrup E, Wall A, Franke A, Schroder J, Heussen N, Hanrath P, Gunther RW, Buecker A (2004) Assessment of myocardial function with interactive non-breath-hold real-time MR imaging: comparison with echocardiography and breath-hold Cine MR imaging. Radiology 231:198-207

La Noce A, Stoelben S, Scheffler K, Hennig J, Lenz HM, La Ferla R, Lorusso V, Maggioni F, Cavagna F (2002) B22956/1, a new intravascular contrast agent for MRI: first administration to humans-preliminary results. Acad Radiol 9 [Suppl 2]:404-406

Lauffer RB (1991) Targeted relaxation enhancement agents for MRI. Magn Reson Med 22:339-342, 343-346

Lauffer RB, Parmelee DJ, Dunham SU, Ouellet HS, Dolan RP, Witte S, McMurry TJ, Walovitch RC (1998) MS-325: albumin-targeted contrast agent for MR angiography. Radiology 207:529-538

Lauterbur P, Mendonca Dias H, Rudin A (1978) Augmentation of tissue proton spin-lattice relaxation rates by in vivo addition of paramagnetic ions. In: Dutton PO LJ, Scarpa A (eds) Frontiers of biological energetics. Academic Press, New York, pp 752-759

Lim TH, Choi SI (1999) MRI of myocardial infarction. J Magn Reson Imaging 10:686-693

Lund GK, Higgins CB, Wendland MF, Watzinger N, Weinmann HJ, Saeed M (2001) Assessment of nicorandil therapy in ischemic myocardial injury by using contrast-enhanced and functional MR imaging. Radiology 221:676-682

Marchal G, Ni Y (2000) Use of porphyrin-complex or expanded porphyrin-complex as an infarction localization diagnosticum. USA Patent Office, USA

Marchal G, Ni Y, Herijgers P, Flameng W, Petre C, Bosmans H, Yu J, Ebert W, Hilger CS, Pfefferer D, Semmler W, Baert AL (1996) Paramagnetic metalloporphyrins: infarct avid contrast agents for diagnosis of acute myocardial infarction by MRI. Eur Radiol 6:2-8

Marchal G, Verbruggen A, Ni Y, Adriaens P, Cresens E (1999) Non-porphyrin compounds for use as a diagnosticum and/or pharmaceutical, Belgium, International application No. PTC (Patent Cooperation Treaty)/BE99/00104; Priority date: August 14, 1998. Filing date: 5 August, 1999

Mayo-Smith WW, Saini S, Slater G, Kaufman JA, Sharma P, Hahn PF (1996) MR contrast material for vascular enhancement: value of superparamagnetic iron oxide. AJR Am J Roentgenol 166:73-77

Misselwitz B, Schmitt-Willich H, Ebert W, Frenzel T, Weinmann HJ (2001) Pharmacokinetics of Gadomer-17, a new dendritic magnetic resonance contrast agent. Magma 12:128-134

Nelson JA, Schmiedl U (1991) Porphyrins as contrast media. Magn Reson Med 22:366-371; discussion 378

Nelson JA, Schmiedl U, Shankland EG (1990) Metalloporphyrins as tumor-seeking MRI contrast media and as potential selective treatment sensitizers. Invest Radiol 25 [Suppl 1]:71-73

Ni Y (1998) Myocardial viability. In: Bogaert JDA, Rademakers FE (eds) Magnetic resonance of the heart and great vessels: clinical applications. Medical radiology - diagnostic imaging and radiation oncology. Springer, Berlin Heidelberg New York, pp 113-132

Ni Y, Marchal G, van Damme B, van Hecke P, Michiels J, Zhang X, Yu J, Baert AL (1992) Magnetic resonance imaging, microangiography, and histology in a rat model of primary liver cancer. Invest Radiol 27:689-697

Ni Y, Marchal G, Petré C, Lukito G, Herijgers P, Flameng W, Yu J, Hilger C, Ebert W, Maier F, Semmler W (1994) Metalloporphyrin enhanced magnetic resonance imaging of acute myocardial infarction (abstract). Circulation 90 [Suppl]: I-468

Ni Y, Marchal G, Yu J, Lukito G, Petre C, Wevers M, Baert AL, Ebert W, Hilger CS, Maier FK et al (1995) Localization of metalloporphyrin-induced «specific» enhancement in experimental liver tumors: comparison of magnetic resonance imaging, microangiographic, and histologic findings. Acad Radiol 2:687-699

Ni Y, Marchal G, Herijgers P, Flameng W, Petre C, Ebert W, Hilger CS, Pfefferer D, Semmler W, Baert AL (1996) Paramagnetic metalloporphyrins: from enhancers of malignant tumors to markers of myocardial infarcts. Acad Radiol 3 [Suppl 2]:395-397

Ni Y, Miao Y, Bosmans H, Yu J, Semmler W, Baert A, Marchal G (1997a) Evaluation of interventional liver tumor ablation with Gd-mesoporphyrin enhanced magnetic resonance imaging (abstract). Radiology 205:319

Ni Y, Petre C, Miao Y, Yu J, Cresens E, Adriaens P, Bosmans H, Semmler W, Baert AL, Marchal G (1997b) Magnetic resonance imaging-histomorphologic correlation studies on paramagnetic metalloporphyrins in rat models of necrosis. Invest Radiol 32:770-779

Ni Y, Pislaru C, Bosmans H, Pislaru S, Miao Y, van de Werf F, Semmler W, Marchal G (1998) Validation of intracoronary delivery of metalloporphyrin as an in vivo «histochemical staining» for myocardial infarction with MR imaging. Acad Radiol 5 [Suppl 1]:S37-S41; discussion 45-46

Ni Y, Miao Y, Cresens E, Adriaens P, Yu J, Semmler W, Marchal

G (1999) Paramagnetic metalloporphyrins: there exist necrosis-avid and non-avid species. 7th annual scientific meeting for ISMRM, Philadelphia, Pennsylvania, USA

Ni Y, Adzamli K, Miao Y, Cresens E, Yu J, Periasamy MP, Adams MD, Marchal G (2001a) MRI contrast enhancement of necrosis by MP-2269 and Gadophrin-2 in a rat model of liver infarction. Invest Radiol 36:97-103

Ni Y, Pislaru C, Bosmans H, Pislaru S, Miao Y, Bogaert J, Dymarkowski S, Yu J, Semmler W, van de Werf F, Baert AL, Marchal G (2001b) Intracoronary delivery of Gd-DTPA and Gadophrin-2 for determination of myocardial viability with MR imaging. Eur Radiol 11:876-883

Ni Y, Cresens E, Adriaens P, Dymarkowski S, Bogaert J, Zhang H, Bosmans H, Verbruggen A, Marchal G (2002a) Exploring multifunctional features of necrosis avid contrast agents. Acad Radiol 9 [Suppl 2]:488-490

Ni Y, Cresens E, Adriaens P, Miao Y, Verbeke K, Dymarkowski S, Verbruggen A, Marchall G (2002b) Necrosis-avid contrast agents: introducing nonporphyrin species. Acad Radiol 9 [Suppl 1]:S98-S101

Ni Y, Dymarkowski S, Chen F, Bogaert J, Marchal G (2002c) Occlusive myocardial infarction enhanced or not enhanced with necrosis-avid contrast agents at MR imaging. Radiology 225:603-605

Ni Y, Huyghe D, Chen F, Bormans G, Verbruggen A, Marchal G (2004a) Research on necrosis avid contrast agents: further expansion of scope. Acad Radiol 11 [Suppl] (in press)

Ni Y, Mulier S, Miao Y, Michel L, Marchal G (2004b) A review of the general aspects of radiofrequency ablation (invited review). Abdominal Imaging 29 (in press)

Ni Y, Bormans G, Chen F, Verbruggen A, Marchal G (2005a) Necrosis avid contrast agents: functional similarity vs structural diversity. Magma (in press)

Ni Y, Huyghe D, Verbeke K, de Witte P, Nuyts J, Mortelmans L, Chen F, Marchal G, Verbruggen A, Bormans G (2005b) First evaluation of mono-[123I]iodohypericin as a necrosis avid tracer agent. J Nucl Med (in press)

Ogan MD, Revel D, Brasch RC (1987) Metalloporphyrin contrast enhancement of tumors in magnetic resonance imaging. A study of human carcinoma, lymphoma, and fibrosarcoma in mice. Invest Radiol 22:822-828

Orlandi C, Crane PD, Edwards DS, Platts SH, Bernard L, Lazewatsky J, Thoolen MJ (1991) Early scintigraphic detection of experimental myocardial infarction in dogs with technetium-99m-glucaric acid. J Nucl Med 32:263-268

Oshinski JN, Yang Z, Jones JR, Mata JF, French BA (2001) Imaging time after Gd-DTPA injection is critical in using delayed enhancement to determine infarct size accurately with magnetic resonance imaging. Circulation 104:2838-2842

Pass HI (1993) Photodynamic therapy in oncology: mechanisms and clinical use. J Natl Cancer Inst 85:443-456

Pereira RS, Wisenberg G, Prato FS, Yvorchuk K (2000) Clinical assessment of myocardial viability using MRI during a constant infusion of Gd-DTPA. Magma 11:104-113

Pereira RS, Prato FS, Wisenberg G, Sykes J, Yvorchuk KJ (2001) The use of Gd-DTPA as a marker of myocardial viability in reperfused acute myocardial infarction. Int J Cardiovasc Imaging 17:395-404

Pislaru SV, Ni Y, Pislaru C, Bosmans H, Miao Y, Bogaert J, Dymarkowski S, Semmler W, Marchal G, van de Werf FJ (1999) Noninvasive measurements of infarct size after thrombolysis with a necrosis-avid MRI contrast agent. Circulation 99:690-696

Place DA, Faustino PJ, Berghmans KK, van Zijl PC, Chesnick AS, Cohen JS (1992) MRI contrast-dose relationship of manganese(III)tetra(4-sulfonatophenyl) porphyrin with human xenograft tumors in nude mice at 2.0 T. Magn Reson Imaging 10:919-928

Port M, Corot C, Rousseaux O, Raynal I, Devoldere L, Idee JM, Dencausse A, Le Greneur S, Simonot C, Meyer D (2001) P792: a rapid clearance blood pool agent for magnetic resonance imaging: preliminary results. Magma 12:121-127

Ramani K, Judd RM, Holly TA, Parrish TB, Rigolin VH, Parker MA, Callahan C, Fitzgerald SW, Bonow RO, Klocke FJ (1998) Contrast magnetic resonance imaging in the assessment of myocardial viability in patients with stable coronary artery disease and left ventricular dysfunction. Circulation 98:2687-2694

Roberts R (1989) Serendipity: accidental discoveries in science. Wiley, New York

Ruehm SG, Corot C, Vogt P, Kolb S, Debatin JF (2001) Magnetic resonance imaging of atherosclerotic plaque with ultrasmall superparamagnetic particles of iron oxide in hyperlipidemic rabbits. Circulation 103:415-422

Saeed M, Bremerich J, Wendland MF, Wyttenbach R, Weinmann HJ, Higgins CB (1999) Reperfused myocardial infarction as seen with use of necrosis-specific versus standard extracellular MR contrast media in rats. Radiology 213:247-257

Saeed M, Lund G, Wendland MF, Bremerich J, Weinmann H, Higgins CB (2001) Magnetic resonance characterization of the peri-infarction zone of reperfused myocardial infarction with necrosis-specific and extracellular nonspecific contrast media. Circulation 103:871-876

Saeed M, Wendland MF, Bremerich GL, Weinmann HJ, Higgins CB (2002) Assessment of myocardial viability using standard extracellular and necrosis specific MR contrast media. Acad Radiol 9 [Suppl 1]:84-87

Saini SK, Jena A, Dey J, Sharma AK, Singh R (1995) MnPcS4: a new MRI contrast enhancing agent for tumor localisation in mice. Magn Reson Imaging 13:985-990

Schalla S, Wendland MF, Higgins CB, Ebert W, Saeed M (2004) Accentuation of high susceptibility of hypertrophied myocardium to ischemia: complementary assessment of Gadophrin-enhancement and left ventricular function with MRI. Magn Reson Med 51:552-558

Schellenberger EA, Bogdanov A, Jr., Hogemann D, Tait J, Weissleder R, Josephson L (2002) Annexin V-CLIO: a nanoparticle for detecting apoptosis by MRI. Mol Imaging 1:102-107

Schmitz SA, Coupland SE, Gust R, Winterhalter S, Wagner S, Kresse M, Semmler W, Wolf KJ (2000) Superparamagnetic iron oxide-enhanced MRI of atherosclerotic plaques in Watanabe hereditable hyperlipidemic rabbits. Invest Radiol 35:460-471

Schneider G, Hayd C, Mühler A et al (1995) Contrast enhanced MRI of experimentally induced brain infarctions in rabbits using Bis-Gd-MP as MR contrast agent. 3rd annual scientific meeting, Society of Magnetic Resonance, Nice, France. Society of Magnetic Resonance, p 1144

Schoeder H, Friedrich M, Topp H (1993) Myocardial viability: what do we need? Eur J Nucl Med 20:792-803

Spokojny AM, Serur JR, Skillman J, Spears JR (1986) Uptake of hematoporphyrin derivative by atheromatous plaques: studies in human in vitro and rabbit in vivo. J Am Coll Cardiol 8:1387-1392

Stillman AE, Wilke N, Li D, Haacke M, McLachlan S (1996) Ultrasmall superparamagnetic iron oxide to enhance MRA of the renal and coronary arteries: studies in human patients. J Comput Assist Tomogr 20:51-55

Stillman AE, Wilke N, Jerosch-Herold M (1999) Myocardial viability. Radiol Clin North Am 37:361-378, vi

Storey P, Danias PG, Post M, Li W, Seoane PR, Harnish PP, Edelman RR, Prasad PV (2003) Preliminary evaluation of EVP 1001-1: a new cardiac-specific magnetic resonance contrast agent with kinetics suitable for steady-state imaging of the ischemic heart. Invest Radiol 38:642-652

Svensson J, Mansson S, Johansson E, Petersson JS, Olsson LE (2003) Hyperpolarized 13C MR angiography using true-FISP. Magn Reson Med 50:256-262

Taupitz M, Schnorr J, Wagner S, Kivelitz D, Rogalla P, Claassen G, Dewey M, Robert P, Corot C, Hamm B (2001) Coronary magnetic resonance angiography: experimental evaluation of the new rapid clearance blood pool contrast medium P792. Magn Reson Med 46:932-938

Turner R (1997) Signal sources in bold contrast fMRI. Adv Exp Med Biol 413:19-25

Van der Wall EE, Vliegen HW, de Roos A, Bruschke AV (1996) Magnetic resonance techniques for assessment of myocardial viability. J Cardiovasc Pharmacol 28 [Suppl 1]:37-44

Van Zijl PC, Place DA, Cohen JS, Faustino PJ, Lyon RC, Patronas NJ (1990) Metalloporphyrin magnetic resonance contrast agents. Feasibility of tumor-specific magnetic resonance imaging. Acta Radiol [Suppl] 374:75-9

Vever-Bizet C, L'Epine Y, Delettre E, Dellinger M, Peronneau P, Gaux JC, Brault D (1989) Photofrin II uptake by atheroma in atherosclerotic rabbits. Fluorescence and high performance liquid chromatographic analysis on post-mortem aorta. Photochem Photobiol 49:731-737

Villringer A, Rosen BR, Belliveau JW, Ackerman JL, Lauffer RB, Buxton RB, Chao YS, Wedeen VJ, Brady TJ (1988) Dynamic imaging with lanthanide chelates in normal brain: contrast due to magnetic susceptibility effects. Magn Reson Med 6:164-174

Wallace RA, Haar JP Jr, Miller DB, Woulfe SR, Polta JA, Galen KP, Hynes MR, Adzamli K, Adams MD (1998) Synthesis and preliminary evaluation of MP-2269: a novel, non-aromatic small-molecule blood-pool MR contrast agent development of a novel nonaromatic small-molecule MR contrast agent for the blood pool. Magn Reson Med 40:733-739

Weinmann HJ, Ebert W, Misselwitz B, Schmitt Willich H (2003) Tissue-specific MR contrast agents. Eur J Radiol 46:33-44

Weissleder R, Lee AS, Khaw BA, Shen T, Brady TJ (1992) Anti-myosin-labeled monocrystalline iron oxide allows detection of myocardial infarct: MR antibody imaging. Radiology 182:381-385

Wendland MF, Saeed M, Lund G, Higgins CB (1999) Contrast-enhanced MRI for quantification of myocardial viability. J Magn Reson Imaging 10:694-702

Winter PM, Morawski AM, Caruthers SD, Fuhrhop RW, Zhang H, Williams TA, Allen JS, Lacy EK, Robertson JD, Lanza GM, Wickline SA (2003) Molecular imaging of angiogenesis in early-stage atherosclerosis with alpha(v)beta3-integrin-targeted nanoparticles. Circulation 108:2270-2274

Woodburn KW, Fan Q, Kessel D, Wright M, Mody TD, Hemmi G, Magda D, Sessler JL, Dow WC, Miller RA, Young SW (1996) Phototherapy of cancer and atheromatous plaque with texaphyrins. J Clin Laser Med Surg 14:343-348

Young SW, Sidhu MK, Qing F, Muller HH, Neuder M, Zanassi G, Mody TD, Hemmi G, Dow W, Mutch JD et al (1994) Preclinical evaluation of gadolinium (III) texaphyrin complex. A new paramagnetic contrast agent for magnetic resonance imaging. Invest Radiol 29:330-338

3 Practical Setup

Steven Dymarkowski and Pascal Hamaekers

CONTENTS

3.1 Introduction

There are many practical aspects that need to be taken into consideration when performing a cardiovascular MRI examination. Although seemingly trivial, successful image acquisition and interpretation requires a working knowledge of adequate patient preparation, ECG lead placement, breath-hold instructions, and contrast injection. This expertise should be accompanied by knowledge of safety issues and precautions in the MRI environment, relating to the use of strong magnetic fields, radio frequency (RF) energy, magnetic field gradients, and cryogenic liquids.

S. Dymarkowski, MD, PhD
Department of Radiology, Gasthuisberg University Hospital, Herestraat 49, 3000 Leuven, Belgium
P. Hamaekers, RN
Radiological Technician, Department of Radiology, Gasthuisberg University Hospital, Herestraat 49, 3000 Leuven, Belgium

The purpose of this chapter is to provide MRI users, in particular those who aim to perform cardiovascular MRI studies in daily clinical practice, with a practical introduction to setting up and performing an MR scan.

3.2 The Physical MRI Environment and Safety Issues

As with other imaging techniques, MRI has its risks, and precautions need to be taken to ensure that potentially hazardous situations do not occur. Attraction of ferromagnetic objects due to the static magnetic field is the most important consideration, but the potential unwanted effects of RF-induced heating and peripheral nerve stimulation in the MR environment should also be considered, in particular in patients with permanent pacemakers, automatic implantable cardiac defibrillators (AICDs), long lengths of temporary cardiac pacing wires, metallic stents, and prosthetic valves.

Monitoring physiological parameters within the MR scanners can also be problematic. For example, use of MRI-incompatible ECG electrodes may be associated with third-degree burns, and distortion of the ECG by the magnetic field may interfere with monitoring of ischemic changes during MR examinations. Specifically designed hardware to reduce this distortion is under development.

Thus, appropriate knowledge of the MR environment is essential to eliminate the risks that can be associated with the specific physical properties of MRI.

3.2.1 Static Magnetic Field

MRI personnel are expected to be familiar with the dangers associated with the presence of ferromagnetic objects in the vicinity of the strong static magnetic field of MR scanners. However, other medical professionals, insufficiently experienced with MRI, and patients themselves may not be aware, and the trained MR staff should remain vigilant about MR safety.

Magnetic fields from large bore magnets may pull large ferromagnetic items into the bore of the magnet. In practice, all ferromagnetic objects should be removed from the MR suite. Such objects can become fast-moving projectiles within the magnetic field, which can cause severe injury to an individual inside the magnet or can seriously damage the magnet itself. The force exerted on a large metal object of sufficient size induces enough kinetic energy to destroy and injure anything in its path.

Despite numerous safety warnings issued by the manufacturers and the medical profession, sad but true stories of objects being pulled into MR scanners circulate, with, in extreme cases, fatal outcomes. Special consideration should be given to objects that are associated with patient management, for example oxygen cylinders, monitors, injection systems, and drip stands (Fig. 3.1).

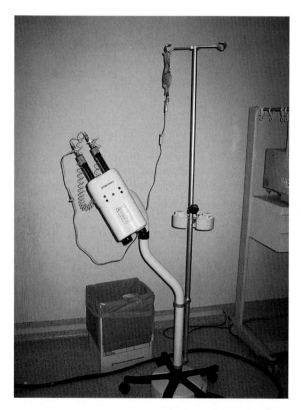

Fig. 3.1. Typical example of MRI-compatible power injection with dual injection system (contrast agent and saline), equipped with a nonferromagnetic (aluminum) infusion stand

Similar forces are at work on ferromagnetic metal implants or foreign matter inside those being imaged. These forces can pull on these objects, cutting and compressing healthy tissue. For these reasons individuals with foreign metal objects such as shrapnel or older ferromagnetic implants are not imaged.

The physical boundary up to which ferromagnetic objects can be safely manipulated is indicated as the 5-gauss line (Fig. 3.2). In some MR suites, this is visually indicated on the floor to prevent accidental movement of these objects (Fig. 3.3).

3.2.2
Alternating Magnetic Field Gradients

Part of the MR-imaging process involves alternations of the magnetic field state of the gradient magnets necessary for spatial encoding. The rate with which the change of magnetic field (B) occurs is dependent on the gradient power of the systems and is expressed as dB/dt. Gradient requirements are usually higher in high-application systems (e.g., for functional brain MRI and cardiovascular MRI), to enable sequence repetition time (TR) to be as short as possible. The United States Food and Drug Administration (FDA) has issued recommendations for dB/dt for each system to be at a level less than that required to produce peripheral nerve stimulation.

The switching of these magnetic gradients also produces high acoustic noise levels, which has been limited by the FDA to 140 dB. It is also recommended that all patients should be provided with hearing protection in the form of earplugs or headphones.

3.2.3
Bioeffects of Radiofrequency Energy

The RF energy from an imaging sequence is nonionizing electromagnetic radiation in a high-frequency range. Research has shown that the majority of the RF energy transmitted for MR imaging is dissipated as heat in the patient's tissues due to resistive losses. Such temperature changes are not felt by the patient. Nevertheless, MR imaging can potentially cause significant heating of body tissues, and the FDA recommends that the exposure to RF energy be limited. The limiting measure is the specific absorption rate (SAR) and is expressed as joules of RF energy deposited per second per kilogram of body weight (i.e., watts per kilogram). The recommended SAR limit

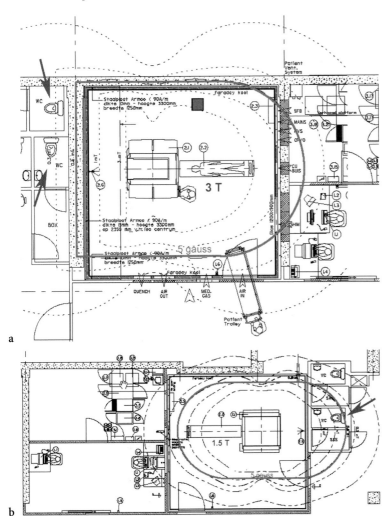

a

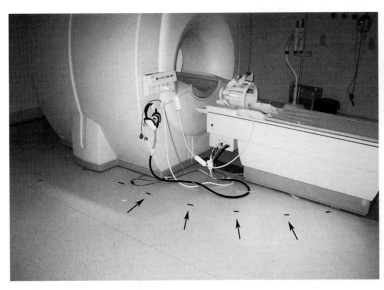

b

Fig. 3.2. a Siting diagram for a 3-T unit. The 5-gauss line is marked in *red*. Note that the public restrooms in the waiting hall (*arrows*) are separated from the magnetic field by a thick reinforced wall. **b** Similar, but less optimal siting diagram of a 1.5-T unit. The 5-gauss line extends beyond the Faraday cage into the restrooms (*arrow*). People with pacemakers are potentially in danger when using this facility

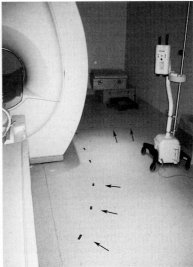

Fig. 3.3. Floor markings inside a 3-T suite mark the invisible boundary of the 10-gauss line (*arrows*). No additional monitoring unit or power injection, even MRI-compatible ones may be positioned within this line for safety purposes

depends on the anatomy being imaged. The SAR for the whole body must be less than 4 W/kg, and must be less than 3.2 W/kg averaged over the head. Any pulse sequence must not raise the temperature by more than 1°C and no greater than 38°C in the head, 39°C in the trunk, and 40°C in the extremities.

The precise mechanism of tissue heating with MRI in not completely understood. It seems to be multi-factorial in origin. Some organs are more sensitive than others to heating, and underlying medical conditions or drugs can influence the degree of heat accumulation within the human body. Normally, when heat accumulates in the body, it is dissipated by conduction, convection, evaporation, and radiation. Disease states (hypertension, diabetes) or medication (sedatives, vasodilators) can impair the normal thermoregulatory responses to a heat challenge.

The heat interaction of pure biological phenomena is negligible. However, this is not true in the case of heating in association with devices inside the MR system. Thermal injuries, up to third-degree burns, have been reported with the use of ECG leads, pulse oximeters, and monitoring devices with wires made of conductive materials. Therefore, manufacturers' guidelines should be strictly enforced, and if any doubt exists about safety of a certain device it should not be used.

If leads are used they should not be looped and should not be placed immediately on the individual's bare skin (Fig. 3.4). If available, leads with fiberoptic signal transmission and special outer shielding should be used.

3.2.4
Interaction with Medical Devices

3.2.4.1
Cardiac Pacemakers and Automatic Implantable Cardiac Defibrillators

A cardiac pacemaker is the most common electrical implant that can be found across the patient population. A commonly asked question is therefore whether or not an MR procedure can be safely performed in patients with implanted cardiac pacemakers. It is generally assumed that presence of a pacemaker is a strict contraindication for MRI.

The effects of the MR environment on pacemakers are diverse and dependent on many factors, such as the strength of the external magnetic field, the kind of sequences used, and the body area that is to be imaged.

Practical experience has taught us that though many patients with pacemakers have been inadvertently placed into MR systems in the past, hazardous or fatal outcomes have only occurred in a small number of patients. The following facts, however, summarize the many dangers of performing MRI with pacemaker patients and provide evidence that such practices should be strictly discouraged.

The metal casing of a pacemaker tends to align to the longitudinal axis of the external MR magnetic field. This gives rise to magnet-related translational attraction or torque effects. In different studies deflection angles were measured from 9° to 90° for

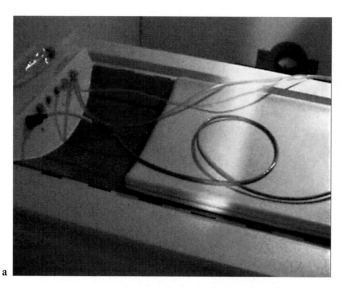
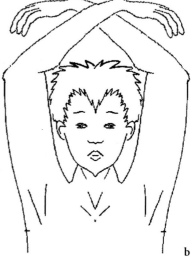

a   b

Fig. 3.4a,b. Example of conductive loops inside an MRI unit. **a** An ECG cable with a loop forms a potential hazard, since this may induce currents and cause burns when the patient's skin is in contact with this wire. **b** A patient must never cross arms or legs, since this also causes an inductive loop

long-bore and from 11° to 90° for short-bore MR systems. Such movement of the pacemaker box may be problematic for patients undergoing MRI, with possible discomfort and the potential for proximal lead fracture.

It is also known that static magnetic fields close the reed switches – tiny electrical relays – of many pacemakers. Reed switch closure has been studied for different orientations and positions relative to the main magnetic field and at different magnetic fields. If reed switches are oriented parallel to the magnetic field, they generally close at 1.0±0.2 mT and open at 0.7±0.2 mT. Different reed switch behavior has been observed at different magnetic field strengths. In low magnetic fields (<50 mT), the reed switches were found to close; while, in higher magnetic fields (>200 mT), the reed switches opened in 50% of all tested orientations. Thus, reed switch closure is not predictable with certainty in clinical situations. Despite this unpredictability of the reed switch in these experimental circumstances, tests on isolated pacemakers and in patients with AICDs using continuous monitoring of pacemaker output and temperature at the lead tip at low fields (0.5 T), have shown no pacemaker or AICD dysfunction during MR imaging, and no changes in the programmed parameters in any device tested in vivo or in vitro. Furthermore, the only consequence of reed switches closing is that the pacemaker is switched into asynchronous mode, during which a predetermined fixed pacing rate takes over. This effect can be compared with the short period of pacemaker interrogation that takes place in routine pacemaker checkups.

However, it is not the above effects alone that are responsible for the adverse outcome in patients with pacemakers during MR examinations. More concerning is induction of currents in the pacemaker lead which could cause action potentials in and subsequent contraction of the ventricle. There have indeed been reports in the literature of cardiac pacing occurring at the TR of the sequence.

Furthermore, temperature increase in the pacemaker lead is a severe and realistic problem. Studies have shown that pacemaker electrodes exposed to MR imaging can have temperature increases of up to 63°C after 90 s of scanning. The potential adverse effect of a thermal injury to the myocardium should thus be considered as the main caveat in conduction MRI examinations in these patients, especially if RF power is to be transmitted in the vicinity of the pacemaker and its leads (i.e., MR imaging of the neck, chest, and abdomen).

Despite reports in the literature that MR examinations can be performed in patients who are not pacemaker dependent and have the device switched off, it remains inadvisable to perform such examinations considering the potential hazards as stated above. If a patient is somehow accidentally exposed to the MR field, good clinical practice demands that the pacemaker function should be checked by a trained cardiologist. Relatives or other individuals with pacemakers accompanying patients should be asked to leave the MR unit.

3.2.4.2
Temporary External Pacemaker Wires

Often patients are referred early after cardiac surgery with temporary external pacemaker wires still in situ. Usually these are cut off close to the skin before discharge. This condition should not be considered as a contraindication to MRI. In our experience, the external portion of these wires should be contained in plastic, test tube-like receptacles, taped to the patient's chest. These segments of the wires (the straight wire section) can cause significant susceptibility artifacts on the anterior chest wall. This generally poses no concern for evaluation of left ventricular function for example, though the wires do interfere with image quality in the immediate region of the wire, e.g., if an evaluation of the right coronary artery is to be obtained.

3.2.4.3
Prosthetic Valves, Surgical Clips, and Osteosynthesis Materials

There are standard procedures for testing of prosthetic valves for MRI safety. The term "MRI-safe" is defined by the American Society for Testing and Materials (ASTM), Designation F 2052. *Standard test method for measurement of magnetically induced displacement force on passive implants in the magnetic resonance environment.* A device is considered to be MRI-safe when this device poses no additional risk to the patient or other individuals in a static magnetic field, but may affect the quality of the diagnostic information.

Prior to the approval of the ASTM, prosthetic valves are tested for translational attraction (average deflection angle measured in magnetic fields up to 3 T), tissue heating in the immediate vicinity of the device, and artifacts.

Most currently used prosthetic valves have been extensively tested in the past and it was found that there is very little interaction between the valves and the magnetic field, i.e., insufficient translational attraction to pose any danger, very little MRI-related heating for these implants; but artifacts characterized for these implants may be problematic if the imaging area of interest is where the implant is located. Therefore, to perform cardiac MRI in patients with artificial valves can be considered safe, but potentially uninteresting on the basis that limited diagnostic information can be gained from the perivalvular area.

Surgical clips and osteosynthesis material are not considered to be contraindications for MRI examinations, with the sole exception of cerebral aneurysm clips.

However, in the light of the constant evolution in development of medical devices, the purpose of this chapter is not to provide an exhaustive overview of compatibility of every possible bioprosthetic one may encounter. Several good reference works and pocket guides have been written on this subject and it serves recommendation to keep a copy of such a book in the MRI suite, to be consulted in case of doubt.

3.3
General Patient Preparation

3.3.1
Patient Positioning and Coil Placement

Prior to any cardiac MRI, the patient should be briefly interviewed with regard to MR contraindications. We ascertain whether the patient has a pacemaker or any other implanted device, retained pacemaker wires, or other foreign material inside the body (in particular postsurgical subarachnoid hemorrhage clips). Female patients are best advised to remove any make-up, since small metallic residues in cosmetics may cause artifacts in the images or be potentially hazardous.

In general, it is always recommended to remove jewellery and have the patient disrobe completely and wear a hospital gown (ideally without pockets!). This avoids the accidental retention of materials in trouser or shirt pockets, as patients are not always completely aware of exactly which objects pose a potential risk.

For cardiac MRI, most systems have specific cardiac or torso coils. These are often multi-element phased-array coils, required for parallel imaging. The number of elements in such dedicated coils

ranges from 4 to 8, and coils with up to 32 channels are currently under construction. These coils have anterior and posterior elements, which require accurate positioning, critical for adequate signal reception (Fig. 3.5).

The coils should always be centered over the organ of interest. It is important to note that, when imaging the heart, the coil placements should be lower than when imaging the aortic arch (e.g., in aortic coarctation). At the beginning of each examination, visual inspection of the localizer or scout images can give an indication as to whether coil placement was performed correctly (Fig. 3.6).

3.3.2
ECG Monitoring

As already stated in Chap. 1, accurate peak detection in the ECG is critically important for good quality MR scans. Most MR systems currently use advanced triggering modules based on vectorcardiography (VCG) to improve R-wave detection in the MR environment. They use a three-dimensional (3D) and orthogonal lead system. The ECG electrodes should be attached in a cross-shaped or triangular pattern, depending on the number of electrodes of the system (Fig. 3.7). Prior to application of the electrodes, the skin should be cleaned with alcoholic pads or an abrasive gel to improve surface contact. Excess gel should be carefully removed, and if necessary the chest may need to be shaved. Nonmetallic, pregelled electrodes should be used for optimal result. Note that when the electrodes are removed from their

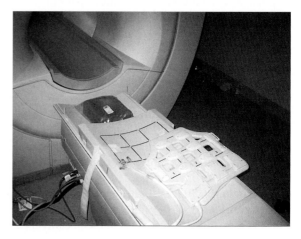

Fig. 3.5. Example of a 6-element phased-array cardiac surface coil. The markings on the coil surface facilitate adequate positioning of the coil elements with regards to the body

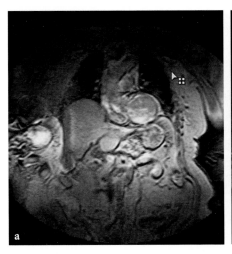 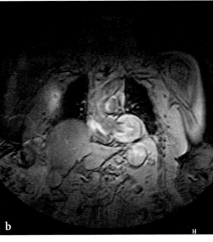

Fig. 3.6. a Coronal scout image in a patient where the coil placement is too low on the body. The erroneous placement can be clearly noted, since the area of the higher signal intensities, i.e., higher coil sensitivity, is centered under the heart. **b** After repositioning of the patient, the signal distribution in the scout image reveals better coil placement

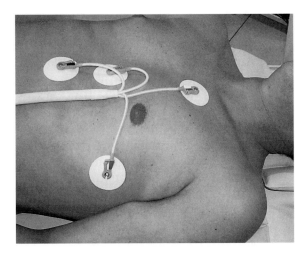

Fig. 3.7. Typical setup of vectorcardiogram (VCG) system with four skin electrodes. (Image courtesy of Philips Medical Systems, Marketing Division, Best, The Netherlands)

sealed container for a long period, the gel pad tends to dry out and lose good signal transduction.

During positioning, the quality of the ECG trace should be checked, and a constant, high-amplitude R-wave and a low T-wave identified. If the tracing is unsatisfactory, restart and reposition the electrodes.

3.3.3
Breath-Holding and Free-Breathing Scans

Prior to the placement of the cardiac or torso coil and introduction into the magnet bore, the patient should be made properly aware of what is going to happen during the MR examination.

It is essential to explain the breath-hold commands to the patient and, if necessary, to briefly rehearse these instructions. Breath-holding can be performed during inspiration or expiration. If measurements are performed during expiration, reproducibility among the different views is higher and the chance of partial volume effects due to slice misregistration is decreased; though patients generally get the impression they have less "air" and are likely to give up a breath-hold prematurely. Therefore some investigators prefer to do breath-hold studies in inspiration.

If any sequences using navigator gating are to be used, ask the patient not to move and if possible to breathe as regularly as possible, to avoid deep inspirations, and to try to avoid falling asleep. Lastly provide the patient with headphones so breath-hold commands and other communications can be efficiently conveyed. The patient is now ready for image acquisition.

3.4
Specific Patient Preparation

3.4.1
Stress Testing

As demonstrated in the following chapters, cardiac MRI offers several clinically usable approaches for the assessment of ischemic heart disease. Using echocardiography, the analysis of wall-motion abnormalities under pharmacological stress with intravenous administration of dobutamine has been established as a sensitive method. It has been shown that, using fast cine acquisition techniques, identical incremental stress protocols to those used for echo-cardiography can be applied to cardiac MRI. Other studies have focused on using physiological stress inside the MR scanner, using an MR-compatible, nonferromagnetic treadmill or bicycle, though these devices are expensive to construct, and difficult and impractical to implement.

Performing stress MRI studies requires a specific practical approach to address the potential adverse effects during a study, since physical access to the patient is more limited than in echocardiography. Using low-dose protocols, side-effects are minimal, but at higher doses side-effects can occur in 0.25% of patients, including myocardial infarction (0.07%), ventricular fibrillation (0.07%), and sustained ven-tricular tachycardia (0.1%). The MR unit should be equipped with facilities to allow a rapid extraction of the patient, such as a removable tabletop, to en-able rapid clinical assessment and treatment in case of adverse events. Resuscitation equipment and medication should be in the immediate vicinity to be administered by experienced staff in case of an emergency.

Physicians performing stress studies should be aware of the patient's medical history and strictly observe the known contraindications. These are: se-vere arterial hypertension, unstable angina pectoris, aortic stenosis, severe cardiac arrhythmias, obstruc-tive cardiomyopathy, endocarditis, and myocardi-tis. Patients are asked not to take their beta-blockers and nitrates 24 h prior to the examination.

Before a stress study is initiated, standard ECG leads are applied, as in any other cardiac MR scans. Many experienced users, however, prefer to place electrodes in such a way that permits the acquisi-tion of a standard 12-lead ECG before the MR scan; a policy that can save a considerable amount of time in case of an emergency.

It is important to be aware that ST segment changes indicating ischemia are deemed not to be reliable in the static magnetic field, so the ECG during the scans can only be used for monitoring of the cardiac frequency. Further physiology moni-toring requires the use of MR-compatible devices. Nonferromagnetic monitoring devices exist, which can be brought up to a distance of 1–2 m from the entrance of the magnet bore opening. Using such devices, blood pressure can be measured every min-ute and pulse oximetry continuously monitored (Fig. 3.8).

Furthermore, audiovisual contact with the pa-tient is maintained throughout the MR examina-

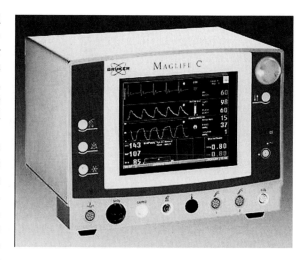

Fig. 3.8. Example of MR-compatible monitoring unit

tion, to be aware of any symptoms that may occur during the dobutamine infusion. At the same time, the acquired images are immediately assessed to de-tect wall-motion abnormalities; the most sensitive sign of a positive stress test.

Indications for termination of a stress study are: a systolic blood pressure decrease greater than 20 mmHg below baseline; a systolic blood pres-sure decrease greater than 40 mmHg from a pre-vious level; a blood pressure increase greater than 240/120 mmHg; intractable symptoms and/or new or worsening wall-motion abnormalities in at least two adjacent left ventricular segments.

3.4.2
Pediatric and Neonatal Cardiac MRI

Given the inherent benefits of tissue contrast and resolution in MRI, cardiac studies are frequently used as a complementary technique in children and infants with congenital heart disease to elucidate complex cardiac anatomy. However, the require-ment of complete immobility and the ability to follow breathing instructions is often not obtain-able in children, due to either age or developmental stage. Therefore general anesthesia or prolonged sedation is often necessary to overcome these limi-tations and to complete these procedures success-fully.

In our own centers, general anesthesia is pre-ferred due to previous experiences with failed sedation or perceived medical risk. The greatest concern during prolonged sedation is respiratory depression and hypoxemia. A study by Lamireau et al. has found an 89% incidence of oxygen desaturation in children who were sedated for endoscopic procedures. For less invasive procedures, a study performed by Malviya et al., performed in 922 children undergoing MRI or CT procedures, has found a 2.9% incidence of hypoxemia and failure rate of 7% in children who received sedation. In contrast, the procedure is successful in all of the children receiving general anesthesia, with only one incident of laryngospasm (0.7%). Although general anesthesia is a more expensive procedure than sedation, it is an essential aid in successful completion of MRI studies with a minimum of adverse events (Fig. 3.9).

3.5
MRI and Pregnancy

In 2002, the American College of Radiology Blue Ribbon Panel on MR Safety finalized its review of the MR Safe Practice Guidelines as detailed in the so-called White Paper on MR Safety. With regard to safety of MRI procedures in pregnancy, a distinction was made between health care practitioners and patients.

Pregnant health care practitioners are allowed to work in and around the MR unit throughout the entire pregnancy. This includes the positioning of patients, injecting contrast, and entering the MR scan room in response to an emergency. Pregnant MR

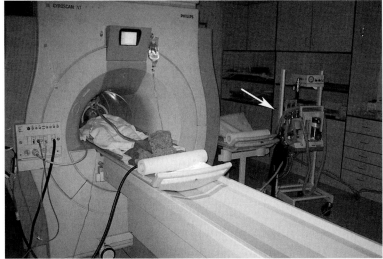

a

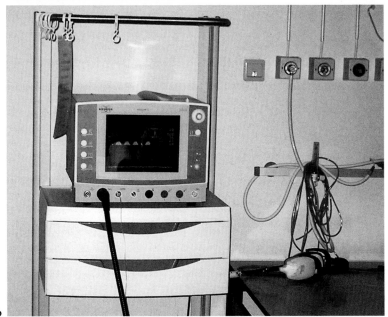

b

Fig. 3.9. a Patient installation for pediatric MR examination under general anesthesia. The child is mechanically ventilated by a nonferromagnetic gas-inhalator and covered with blankets to decrease body temperature loss. **b** Physiological parameters are constantly monitored by use of the MR-compatible unit

operators are advised not to enter the scanner room during actual data acquisition itself.

For pregnant patients, MR scans can be performed if the performing radiologist and the patient's clinician concur that the risk/benefit ratio to the patient warrants that the study be performed. This in practice means that the information provided by the MR examination cannot be acquired by another noninvasive or nonionizing investigation (e.g., ultrasound). Furthermore, it should be argued that the information derived from the MR scan has therapeutic consequences during the duration of the pregnancy. MR contrast agents should not be administered to pregnant patients, since there is insufficient data regarding the pharmacokinetics of MR contrast agents passing through the placenta.

3.6
Contraindications to MRI

Any patient with any of the following devices implanted should, on a routine basis, not be imaged by means of MRI:
- Cardiac pacemaker
- Automatic implanted cardiac defibrillator
- Aneurysm clips
- Carotid artery vascular clamp
- Neurostimulator
- Insulin or infusion pump
- Implanted drug infusion device
- Bone growth/fusion stimulator
- Cochlear, otologic, or ear implant

Furthermore, any patients presenting with the following medical conditions should also preferentially not be brought into the MRI device:
- Patients with severe claustrophobia in which medical sedation is contraindicated or unable to resolve anxiety sufficiently
- Patients with ocular foreign body (e.g., metal shavings)
- Patients with unstable angina or New York Heart Association functional class IV heart failure

Finally, the following patient groups form no contraindication for MRI but should not be administered intravenous contrast agents:
- Pregnant and lactating women
- Patients with hemoglobinopathies
- Patients with severe renal disease (creatinine clearance less than 20 ml/min)

References

Ahmed S, Shellock FG (2001) Magnetic resonance imaging safety: implications for cardiovascular patients. J Cardiovasc Magn Reson 3:171–182

Collins CM, Liu W, Wang J et al (2004) Temperature and SAR calculations for a human head within volume and surface coils at 64 and 300 MHz. J Magn Reson Imaging 19:650–656

Farling P, McBrien ME, Winder RJ (2003) Magnetic resonance compatible equipment: read the small print! Anaesthesia 58:86–87

Gimbel JR, Kanal E (2004) Can patients with implantable pacemakers safely undergo magnetic resonance imaging? J Am Coll Cardiol 43:1325–1327

Greatbatch W, Miller V, Shellock FG (2002) Magnetic resonance safety testing of a newly-developed fiber-optic cardiac pacing lead. J Magn Reson Imaging 16:97–103

Kanal E (2002) American College of Radiology white paper on MR safety. Am J Roentgenol 178:1335–1347

Kanal E (2004) Clinical utility of the American College of Radiology MR safe practice guidelines. J Magn Reson Imaging 19:2–5

Lamireau T, Dubreuil M, Daconceicao M (1998) Oxygen saturation during esophagogastroduodenoscopy in children: general anesthesia versus intravenous sedation. J Pediatr Gastroenterol Nutr 27:172–175

Luechinger R, Duru F, Zeijlemaker VA et al (2002) Pacemaker reed switch behavior in 0.5, 1.5, and 3.0 Tesla magnetic resonance imaging units: are reed switches always closed in strong magnetic fields? Pacing Clin Electrophysiol 25:1419–1423

Malviya S, Voepel-Lewis T, Eldevik OP et al (2000) Sedation and general anaesthesia in children undergoing MRI and CT: adverse events and outcomes. Br J Anaesth 84:743–748

Martin ET, Coman JA, Shellock FG et al (2004) Magnetic resonance imaging and cardiac pacemaker safety at 1.5-Tesla. J Am Coll Cardiol 43:1315–1324

Nahrendorf M, Hiller KH, Hu K, Zeijlemaker V et al (2004) Pacing in high field cardiac magnetic resonance imaging. Pacing Clin Electrophysiol 27:671–674

Partain CL, Price RR (2004) MR safety. J Magn Reson Imaging 19:1

Pohost GM. (2001) Is CMR safe? (Editor's page) J Cardiovasc Magn Reson 3:9

Shellock FG, Kanal E (1991) Policies, guidelines, and recommendations for MR imaging safety and patient management. SMRI Safety Committee. J Magn Reson Imaging 1:97–101

Shellock FG, Tkach JA, Ruggieri PM et al (2003) Cardiac pacemakers, ICDs, and loop recorder: evaluation of translational attraction using conventional („long-bore") and „short-bore" 1.5- and 3.0-Tesla MR systems. J Cardiovasc Magn Reson 5:387–397

Shellock FG (2001) Pocket guide to MR procedures and metallic objects update 2001. Lippincott Williams and Wilkins, Philadelphia

Sommer T, Vahlhaus C, Lauck G et al (2000) MR imaging and cardiac pacemakers: in-vitro evaluation and in-vivo studies in 51 patients at 0.5 T. Radiology 215:869–879

4   Cardiac Anatomy

Jan Bogaert and Andrew M. Taylor

CONTENTS

4.1
Introduction

The first widely accepted strength of magnetic resonance imaging (MRI) was its ability to non-invasively study cardiac morphology and structure. MRI provides anatomical images of the heart with high spatial and contrast resolution, in a fast and reliable fashion. These images can be acquired in every imaginable plane, without restrictions in image orientation and without the need for administration of contrast agents (Dinsmore et al. 1984; O'Donovan et al. 1984; Burbank et al. 1988). Although spin-echo (SE) imaging techniques were initially used for studying cardiac anatomy, a variety of MRI se-

J. Bogaert MD, PhD
Department of Radiology, Gasthuisberg University Hospital, Catholic University of Leuven, Herestraat 49, 3000 Leuven, Belgium
A.M. Taylor, MD, MRCP, FRCR
Cardiothoracic Unit, Institute of Child Health and Great Ormond Street Hospital for Children, London, UK

quences are now available for this task. To accurately interpret cardiac anatomy with MRI, a thorough knowledge of cardiac anatomy, with reference to both the axes of the body and the heart, and of the different cardiac MRI techniques is required, for both normal and pathological conditions. Analysis of cardiac anatomy can sometimes be very difficult. This is especially true for congenital heart disease, where a segmental approach, consisting of a careful analysis of the different components (venous structures, atria, atrioventricular valves, ventricles, ventriculo-arterial valves, and great arteries), each with its own typical characteristics, enables an accurate description of these complex hearts.

Radiologists interested in cardiac imaging are often not sufficiently familiar with cardiac anatomy and have difficulties visualizing the heart in relation to its intrinsic cardiac axes, whilst cardiologists are often not sufficiently familiar with the tomographic approach for visualization of cardiac and extracardiac structures on MR images.

In this chapter on cardiac anatomy, the specific features of the different cardiac components and their presentation on MR images will be highlighted. A detailed description of the cardiovascular anatomy on MR images in the different body axes (transverse, coronal, sagittal), and the intrinsic cardiac axis (short-axis, horizontal long-axis, vertical long-axis, left ventricular, LV, outflow tract, and right ventricular, RV, outflow tract) is available at the end of this chapter (Figs. 4.17–4.24). The strategies for cardiac image planning and slice positioning are discussed in Chap. 5.

4.2
Cardiac MRI Techniques

Assessment of cardiac anatomy with MRI is for many people still linked with the SE-MRI technique. This has a historical explanation: In the early 1980s, the SE-MRI technique was the only available sequence for studying the heart, providing "morphologic images" (HAWKES et al. 1981; HENEGHAN et al. 1982; HERFKENS et al. 1983; HIGGINS et al. 1985). Functional cardiac imaging, although possible, was very cumbersome with SE-MRI (LANZER et al. 1985; TSCHOLAKOFF and HIGGINS 1985; LONGMORE et al. 1985). It took several years before the availability of the gradient-echo (GE) technique, with short repetition times, provided a more useful method for analysis of cardiac function with MRI (FRAHM et al. 1986; HIGGINS et al. 1988).

Contrast in cardiac SE-MRI is not only generated by differences in tissue relaxation, but also by the flow phenomenon. This allows images of the heart and great vessels to be obtained without the need of contrast agent administration to visualize the blood pool. As explained in detail in Chap. 1, the excited spins within the blood pool in the image slice are replaced by non-excited spins between the excitation and read-out pulses, thus creating a "black-blood" or "dark-blood" appearance. The older SE-MRI sequences, whereby only one line of κ-space per slice, per heartbeat was acquired, have now been replaced by fast SE-MRI techniques. Newer techniques (e.g., double inversion pulse) are also available for generating better suppression of the blood signal (STEHLING et al. 1996; SIMONETTI et al. 1996; WINTERER et al. 1999). These innovations have led to an overall improvement in image quality. Image quality has become largely independent of the slice direction, slice thickness and other influencing parameters. In the analysis of the SE-MRI, one should be careful not to mistake other anatomical structures devoid of signal, such as the air-filled trachea and bronchi, for vascular structures. For a similar reason, calcium-containing structures (e.g., calcified valve leaflets) may be not detected on SE-MRI.

As mentioned above, the gradient-echo technique introduced in the late 1980s to study cardiac dynamics (e.g., function, perfusion), should be considered a very useful method for depicting cardiac anatomy. This sequence provides bright-blood images, and offers complementary information to the SE-MRI technique about cardiac morphology. With the advent of the balanced, steady-state free precession (SSFP) GE MRI sequence, combining high contrast between blood and surrounding tissues with high temporal resolution, subtle anatomical structures such as valve leaflets, tendinous chords, muscular trabeculations, and pectinate muscles can be well visualized, especially when using the cine-loop viewing mode (CARR et al. 2001). A similar sequence design is used for coronary artery imaging (Chap. 14), and contrast-enhanced three-dimensional (3D) MR angiography for great-vessel imaging (Chap. 16).

Real-time MRI is no longer a research tool, but it allows the operator to interactively navigate through the heart and rapidly determine the cardiac image planes (CASTILLO and BLUEMKE 2003). It is quite obvious that this task can only be achieved with an extensive knowledge of the 3D cardiac anatomy.

4.3
Position of the Heart in the Thorax – Gross Cardiac Anatomy

The heart has a central, ventrobasal location in the thorax and is bordered bilaterally by the lungs, anteriorly by the sternum, and inferiorly by the diaphragm (Fig. 4.1). It has an oblique position in the thoracic cavity, with the cardiac apex in the left hemithorax.

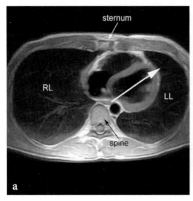 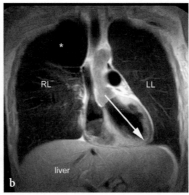 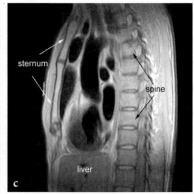

Fig. 4.1a-c. Position of the heart in the thorax. All images are obtained using a breath-hold dark-blood double inversion-recovery SE-MRI technique. **a** Transverse image; **b** coronal image; **c** sagittal image. The *arrow* on the transverse and coronal image indicates the longitudinal axis of the heart. *LL*, left lung; *RL*, right lung. *star*, bullous emphysema.

The long axis of the heart is rotated about 45° to both the sagittal and the coronal planes. In younger or slender individuals, the heart tends to be more vertical, whereas it tends to be more horizontal in obese patients. For the most part, the heart is surrounded by the pericardial sac and has no physical connections with the surrounding structures except posteriorly and superiorly where the great arteries originate and the caval and pulmonary veins drain into the atria (AMPLATZ and MOLLER 1993).

While the position of the heart in the thorax is relatively constant, the position of the different cardiac components, their intrinsic relationship, as well as their relationship with the great vessels is much more complex and prone to a large number of congenital variations, isolated or in combination with other extracardiac congenital abnormalities. Knowledge of the gross cardiac anatomy and of the specific characteristics of the different cardiac structures enables description of most complex congenital heart disease (Table 4.1)

The heart is a double, two-chambered pump, usually described in terms of "right-sided" and "left-sided" chambers. In reality, the right chambers are more anteriorly positioned within the chest, the left chambers more posteriorly, and the ventricles are more inferiorly located than the atria. This is caused by a primary important feature of the normal heart, is that its long axis is not parallel to the long axis of the body. In congenitally malformed hearts, the use of right and left might be confusing, since morphological "right" structures may occupy a left-sided position, and vice versa. The difficulty is overcome in congenitally malformed hearts by adding the description "morphological" to "right" and "left". The relationship of the right and left structures of the normal heart are further complicated by the marked twisting of the ventricular outflow tracts. The aorta, even though emerging from the left ventricle (and therefore a left component of the heart) has its valve in a right-sided position relative to the pulmonary valve (ANDERSON 2000).

4.4
Cardiac Structures

4.4.1
Atria

4.4.1.1
Morphological Right Atrium

Both atria can be divided anatomically into a venous component, a vestibule of the atrioventricular valve,

Table 4.1. Essentials of the heart

Left Atrium	Right Atrium
Receives pulmonary veins	Receives IVC / SVC – coronary sinus
Posterosuperior location	Fibromuscular webs
	Eustachian valve (IVC)
	Thebesian valve (coronary sinus)
	Crista terminalis: divides venous component from vestibule
	Prominent pectinate muscles > left atrium
Left Atrial Appendage	**Right Atrial Appendage**
Anterosuperior (over LCx)	Broad triangular
Long/narrow	Wide connection with RA
Small junction	
Left Ventricle	**Right Ventricle**
Oval or prolate ellipsoid shape	Pyramidal shape
Fine trabeculations	Coarse trabeculations[a]
Inflow and outflow in contact	No connection between inflow and outflow[a]
No infundibulum	Infundibulum[a]
Smooth septal surface	Chordal attachment of septal leaflet to septum[a]
Feeds the aorta	Feeds the pulmonary artery
	Moderator band[a]
	Tricuspid valve more apically positioned than mitral valve[a]

[a]Criteria helpful in differentiating morphological left from right ventricles

a septal component, and an appendage and are sepa-rated by the atrial septum. The right atrium forms the right heart border (Fig. 4.2). Embryologically, the right atrium is formed from the sinus venous and the primitive auricle. These two parts of the atrium are separated on the inside by a ridge, the terminal crest or crista terminalis, and on the outside by a groove, the sulcus terminalis. The sinus venosus, forming the posterior part of the right atrium, forms the venous component, which has a smooth interior because of its origin as a vessel; while the primitive auricle, having a rough trabeculated interior, will form the appendage (ANDERSON 2000). Pectinate muscles branch from the crest at right angles to run into the appendage. These muscles encircle completely the parietal margin of the vestibule of the atrioventricular valve. The venous

component receives the inferior and superior caval veins on its posterior surface, and the coronary sinus at the inferior junction with the septal component. Fibromuscular webs attach to the terminal crest in the regions of the openings of the inferior caval vein and coronary sinus. These are the so-called venous valves, the Eustachian valve in relation to the inferior caval vein, and the Thebesian valve at the coronary sinus. The coronary sinus running through the left or posterior atrioventricular groove opens into the right atrium above the postero-inferior interventric-ular groove. Sometimes, the right coronary vein, also draining into the right atrium, is visible in the ante-rior atrioventricular groove. The junction between the appendage and venous component is particular wide, and the appendage has a broad, triangular ap-pearance, positioned just ventrally to the entrance of the superior vena cava in the right atrium (Figs. 4.3 and 4.4). The vestibule is smooth walled and supports the attachments of the leaflets of the tricuspid valve. The different components, as well as the relationship to the caval veins and the coronary sinus, can be well appreciated on several imaging planes, including the transverse, coronal, and vertical long-axis or sagittal planes (MOHIADDIN et al. 1991; GALJEE et al. 1995). The terminal crest is routinely visible on dark-blood and bright-blood MRI as a mural nodular or trian-gular structure adjacent to the lateral wall that con-nects both caval veins. This muscular structure can be misinterpreted as an abnormal intra-atrial mass

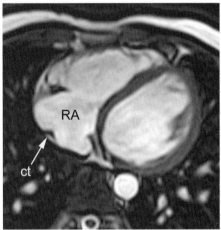

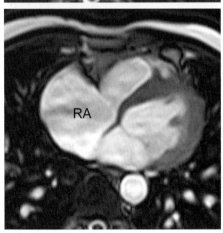

Fig. 4.2a,b. Right atrium at a end diastole and b end sys-tole. The images are obtained in the transverse axis, using a balanced steady-state free precession (SSFP) technique. The terminal crest (crista terminalis, *ct*) divides the venous component (posteromedially) from the vestibule. Note the important changes in right atrial (*RA*) volume and shape during the cardiac cycle.

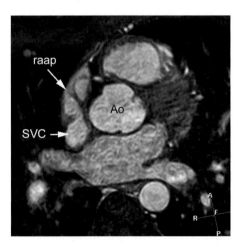

Fig. 4.3. Right atrial appendage. Transverse image using a 3D balanced-SSFP technique with submillimeter spatial resolu-tion The right atrial appendage (*raap*) is located ventrally to the superior vena cava (*SVC*) and laterally to the ascending aorta (*Ao*). The high spatial and high contrast resolution en-able depiction of the pectinate muscles that branch from the terminal crest and run at right angles to the *raap*.

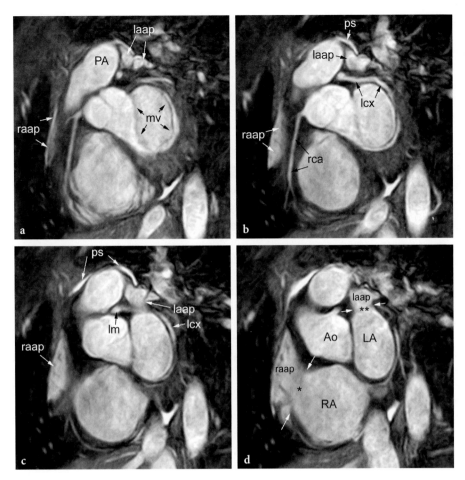

Fig. 4.4a-d. Right and left atrial appendage. Short-axis images using a 3D balanced-SSFP technique with submillimeter spatial resolution. While the right atrial appendage (*raap*) has a triangular appearance, and a broad communication (*star*) with the body of the right atrium (*RA*), the left atrial appendage (*laap*) has a narrow junction (*two stars*) and a long, tubular appearance. Note the relationship of the appendages to the coronary arteries. The *raap* is dorsally located to the right coronary artery (*rca*), while the *laap* overlies the posterior (or left) atrioventricular groove and the left circumflex coronary artery (*lcx*). *Ao*, Aorta; *LA*, left atrium; *lm*, left main stem coronary artery; *PA*, pulmonary artery; *ps*, pericardial sac.

(MENEGUS et al. 1992; MEIER and HARTNELL 1994; MIROWITZ and GUTIERREZ 1992). Bright-blood MRI techniques with submillimeter spatial resolution, such as currently used for coronary artery imaging, enable visualization of thin structures such as the pectinate muscles in the right atrial appendage. Enlargement of the right atrium will easily displace the adjacent lung, while right atrial-appendage enlargement encroaches on the upper retro-sternal air space.

4.4.1.2
Morphological Left Atrium

The morphological left atrium forms the upper posterior heart border, with its appendage extending anteromedially. It lies just beneath the carina and anterior to the esophagus. The left atrium extends cranially behind the aortic root and the proximal part of the ascending aorta. The close relationship to the esophagus makes the left atrium useful as an acoustic window during transesophageal echocardiography. Embryologically, the left atrium also

consists of sinus venosus and primitive auricle, and they form the same anatomical components as in the right atrium. The venous component, also posteriorly located and smooth-walled, receives the four pulmonary veins, one at each corner (Fig. 4.5). The vestibule supports the leaflets of the mitral valve and is also smooth-walled. The pectinate muscles, being confined in the appendage, are much less obvious than in the right atrium and never extend around the atrioventricular junction. The appendage, overlying the left atrioventricular groove and left circumflex coronary artery (LCx), has a narrow junction with the body of the left atrium and has a long, tubular-shaped appearance (ANDERSON 2000; Fig. 4.4). Imaging planes for studying the left atrium are similar to those used to study the right atrium. The relationship of the left atrium to the carina and main stem bronchi is best visualized on coronal views. The visualization of the entrance of the pulmonary veins in the left atrium (e.g., to exclude abnormal pulmonary venous return) is best done using a combination of transverse (or four-

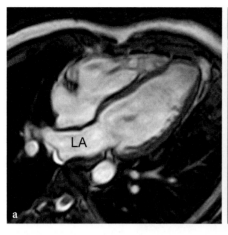 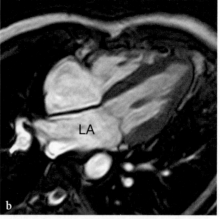

Fig. 4.5a,b. Left atrium at end diastole (**a**) and end systole (**b**). Horizontal long-axis images using a balanced SSFP technique. The entrance of the pulmonary vein from the right lower lobe in the left atrium (*LA*) can be clearly seen.

chamber) views and coronal (or short-axis) views. Enlargement of the left atrium displaces the esophagus posteriorly and widens the subcarinal angle. Massive enlargement, exceeding the space in front of the spine, results in encroachment upon the right lung such that the left atrium becomes border-forming on the right and may push the right ventricle forward. Enlargement of the left atrial appendage displaces the adjacent left lung and might be visible as an additional left border on frontal chest X-ray film.

4.4.1.3
Atrial Septum

The atrial or interatrial septum separates the left from the right atrium. In the atrial septum is an oval depression, the fossa ovalis. The floor of the fossa ovalis is the remains of the septum primum. The septal surface on its right atrial aspect is made up of the floor of the oval fossa and its postero-inferior rim. The superior rim of the fossa (the so-called septum secundum) is no more than an infolding of the atrial wall between the superior caval vein and right pulmonary veins. The septal surface is roughened on its left atrial aspect, as is the flap of the oval fossa. The flap valve, superiorly, overlaps the infolded atrial walls (the "septum secundum") so that, even if the two are not fused, there will be no shunting across the septum as long as left atrial pressure exceeds that in the right atrium. In most cases the atrial septum can be seen on SE-MRI as a thin line separating the two atria, except at the level of the foramen ovale, which is often too thin to be seen. This finding should not be misinterpreted as an atrial septal defect. Bright-blood cine MRI, providing a higher contrast between bright atrial blood and atrial walls, usually depicts this thin membrane

very well (Fig. 4.6). Sometimes fatty infiltration of the interatrial septum is observed, which can be easily differentiated from pathological masses by the characteristic signal intensity corresponding to the subcutaneous fat. It is a mostly benign, usually asymptomatic condition, with a low frequency on autopsy series. The atrial septum is best shown in horizontal and longitudinal planes through the heart (e.g., transverse or four-chamber views).

4.4.2
Ventricles

4.4.2.1
Morphological Right Ventricle

In a normal heart, the right ventricle sits above the liver and forms the inferior and anterior heart border with the exception of the apex. The morphological right ventricle can be identified externally by its

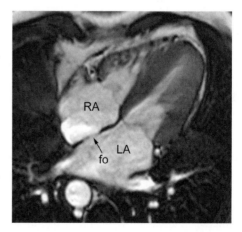

Fig. 4.6. Atrial (interatrial) septum. Horizontal long-axis image using a balanced-SSFP technique (end-systolic image).

pyramidal shape and by its coronary distribution pattern, which is distinctive and typical. The left anterior descending coronary artery (LAD) demarcates the right from the left ventricle. The right ventricle possesses an inlet component, an apical trabecular component, and an outlet component (ANDERSON 2000; Fig. 4.7). The presentation of the different components is specific for each ventricle

and essential for differentiation of the morphological right from left ventricles. The inlet component (tricuspid valve and atrioventricular septum) surrounds and supports the leaflets and subvalvular apparatus of the tricuspid valve. The leaflets can be divided into septal, anterosuperior, and inferior (or mural) locations within the atrioventricular junction. The most characteristic feature of the tricuspid valve (and thus also of the right ventricle) is the presence of tendinous chords attaching its septal leaflet to the ventricular septum. Chordal attachments to the septal surface are never seen in the morphological left ventricle. The apical trabecular portion of the right ventricle has characteristically coarse trabeculations. The infundibulum is incorporated into the right ventricle and forms the outflow tract, whereas the right ventricle proper forms the inflow tract. This completely muscular ring supports the three semilunar leaflets of the pulmonary valve. The junction between the infundibulum and the right ventricle is composed of the parietal band, the septomarginal band, and the moderator band. This moderator band, a muscular band that contains the continuation of the right bundle branch, passes from the interventricular septum to the anterior wall and is an essential characteristic of the morphological right ventricle (Fig. 4.8). The septal and moderator bands are also known as the trabeculae septomarginalis or septomarginal trabeculation. Only a small part of the infundibulum is a truly muscular septum (Fig. 4.9), while the rest of the posterior margin of the infundibulum, also called supraventricular crest (crista supraventricularis) is caused by an infolding of the roof of the ventricle (also called ventriculoinfundibular fold), and is separated from the aorta by extracardiac space. The separation of the tricuspid and pulmonary valves by the crista supraventricularis is another characteristic of the morphological right ventricle. Additional trabeculations, the septoparietal trabeculations, run around the anterior margin of the infundibulum. The internal appearance of the morphological right ventricle is specific for it, though a muscular infundibulum can be rarely from the left ventricle. The muscular trabeculations are relatively coarse, few, and straight, tending to run parallel the right ventricular (RV)

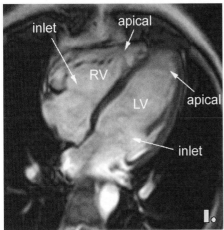

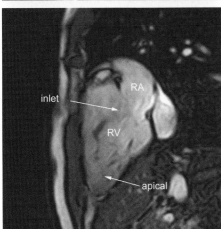

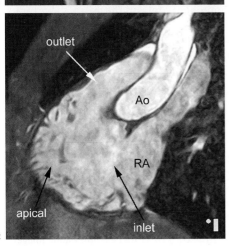

Fig. 4.7a-c. Components of the right ventricle. Horizontal long-axis image (**a**), RV vertical long-axis image (**b**), RV inflow and outflow tract image (**c**) using a balanced-SSFP technique. The inlet, apical and outlet part of the right ventricle are indicated on the different images. Ao, Aorta; LV, left ventricle; RA, right atrium; RV, right ventricle.

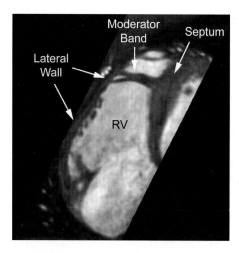

Fig. 4.8. Moderator band. Horizontal long-axis view, using the balanced-SSFP technique. This muscular structure connects the apical ventricular septum with the apical part of the *RV* free or lateral wall. *RV*, right ventricle.

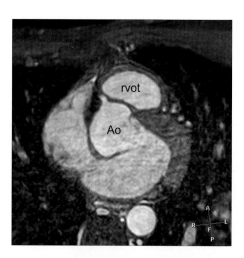

Fig. 4.9. Infundibulum. Transverse image using the balanced-SSFP technique with submillimeter spatial resolution. The right ventricular outflow tract (*rvot*) is characterized by a complete, thin muscular ring. *Ao*, Aorta.

inflow and outflow tracts. The papillary muscles of the right ventricle are relatively small (making right ventriculotomy readily possible) and numerous, and they attach both to the septal and to the free wall surfaces. Because of its numerous attachments to the RV septal surface (mostly to the posteroinferior margin of the septal band), the tricuspid valve may be described as "septophilic". The lining of the chamber becomes smooth in the infundibulum, a funnel leading to the exit from the chamber, the pulmonary trunk. The normal right ventricle is a relatively thin wall chamber with an end-diastolic wall thickness of 3–4 mm. Towards the RV apex, there is often a thinning of the free wall which is not to be mistaken for a wall thinning such as found in arrhythmogenic RV dysplasia (ARVD or ARVC; see Chap. 9). Although the RV free wall is considerably thicker than that of the right atrium, it is thinner than the wall of the left ventricle. These relative thicknesses reflect the range of pressures in the chambers. In the right atrium, the pressure is usually close to 0 mmHg; in the right ventricle, the pressure rises up to about 25 mmHg, while in the left ventricle the peak pressure is about 120 mmHg. The complex cardiac anatomy of the morphological right ventricle is best studied using a combination of different imaging planes, i.e., transverse or horizontal long-axis views in combination with short-axis views and/or RV outflow tract views. Other interesting planes to study the right ventricle are described in Chap. 5. RV enlargement reduces the retrosternal airspace. Because this space is normally limited, RV

enlargement can also displace the left ventricle leftward and posteriorly, and the apex of the heart up and back, lifting the apex of the heart off the hemidiaphragm on the frontal chest radiograph.

4.4.2.2
Morphological Left Ventricle

The morphological left ventricle in a normal heart is a thick-walled chamber that forms the apex and lower part of the left and posterior heart border. The exterior of the left ventricle is shaped like a cone. Internally, the left ventricle is demarcated by its fine trabeculations, which are numerous, fine muscular projections. Like its morphological right counterpart, the morphological left ventricle also possesses an inlet, an apical trabecular, and an outlet portion. The inlet component contains the mitral valve (or LV valve) and extends from the atrioventricular junction to the attachments of the prominent papillary muscles (Fig. 4.10). The most characteristic anatomical feature of the mitral valve is that it has no chordal attachments to the ventricular septum. There are two papillary muscles; the anterior lateral and the posterior medial (Fig. 4.11). Notably, the papillary muscles do not attach to the septum (ANDERSON 2000). Since the LV papillary muscles are large and arise only from the free wall surface, this makes left ventriculotomy difficult, except at the apex or at the high paraseptal area. In addition to the anterior descending branch of the left coronary artery (LCA), which externally marks the location of the

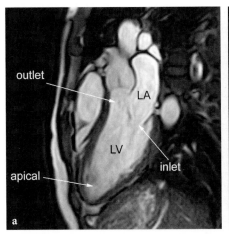

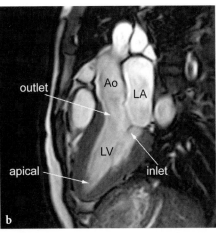

Fig. 4.10a,b. Components of the left ventricle. Left ventricular inflow–outflow tract flow view at end diastole (**a**) and end systole (**b**), using the balanced-SSFP technique. *Ao*, Aorta; *LA*, left atrium.

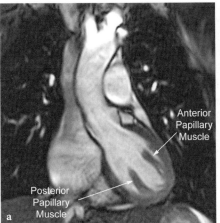

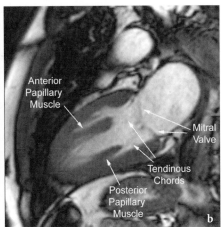

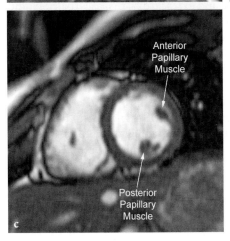

Fig. 4.11a-c. Left ventricular papillary muscles. Left ventricular outflow tract (**a**), vertical long-axis (**b**) and midventricular short-axis (**c**) view, using the balanced-SSFP technique. The papillary muscles are clearly depicted as intracavity structures attached to the posterior(medial) and anterior(lateral) LV wall. Their fibrous extensions, i.e., tendinous chords, towards the mitral valve can be seen on high-quality MR images. Note that the LV septal surface on the short-axis view is free of muscular attachments.

anterior portion of the ventricular septum, anterior and posterior obtuse marginal branches of the left coronary artery course across the LV free wall. Also known as diagonals, these branches supply the large papillary muscles and the adjacent LV free wall. The apical trabecular portion is the most characteristic feature of the morphological left ventricle, which contains the fine characteristic trabeculations. The smooth septal surface also helps in identification, since the morphological left ventricle never possesses a septomarginal trabeculation or a moderator band (Fig. 4.12). While intracavity muscular bands

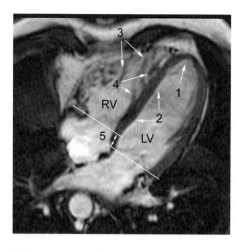

Fig. 4.12. Essential characteristics of the morphologically right and left ventricle. Horizontal long-axis view using the balanced-SSFP technique. Five essential differences can be seen on this image: *1*, fine apical trabeculations in *LV* apex; *2*, *LV* septal surface free of muscular insertions; *3*, rough apical trabeculations in *RV* apex; *4*, muscular insertions on *RV* septal surface; *5*, tricuspid valve more apically positioned than mitral valve. *LV*, left ventricle; *RV*, right ventricle.

are always present on the right as the moderator band, sometimes thin intraventricular strands can be found in the LV apex, known as false tendons. The outlet part, with the aortic valve, is in direct continuity with the inlet part, since normally there is little or no conal musculature beneath the aortic valve, which results in aortic-mitral fibrous continuity. The outlet portion of the morphological left ventricle is distinguished by its abbreviated nature. Part of two of the three leaflets of the aortic valve have muscular attachments to the outlet component. The remainder of the leaflets take origin from the fibrous tissue of the aortic root, part of this being the extensive area of fibrous continuity with the aortic leaflet of the mitral valve. This fibrous continuity is called mitral-aortic intervalvular fibrosa. It is the posterior aspect of the roof of the outlet, therefore, which is particularly short. There is no muscular segment of the ventriculoinfundibular fold in the left ventricle such as separates the arterial and the right ventricular valves. The morphological left ventricle is usually studied along the three intrinsic cardiac axes, i.e., short-axis, horizontal long-axis, and vertical long-axis view. Other interesting imaging planes are the LV outflow-tract view and the LV inflow- and outflow-tract view. These imaging planes are particularly interesting in patients with obstructive hypertrophic cardiomyopathy or to depict aortic regurgitation. Wall thicknesses are not uniform throughout the left ventricle. Most pronounced dif-

ferences are found in the longitudinal direction, with a gradual wall-thinning towards the LV apex. Compared with the lateral LV wall segments (i.e., end-diastolic wall thickness: 7–8 mm in women, 8–9 mm in men), the LV apex can be extremely thin (approximately 3 mm; Fig. 4.10). Less pronounced variations in wall thickness are seen around the LV circumference (BOGAERT and RADEMAKERS 2001). LV enlargement takes place inferiorly and to the left, displacing the left lung.

4.4.2.3
Ventricular Septum

The ventricular or interventricular septum separates the left from the right ventricle. It is mainly a thick-walled muscular layer, except in the subaortic region, where it becomes very thin ("membranous septum"). It contains muscular fibers coming from the LV as well as from the RV free wall. The position and shape of the ventricular septum are determined by the loading conditions. In the unloaded condition, the ventricular septum has a flat appearance. In normal loading conditions, the septum has a convex shape towards the right ventricle, and this shape is maintained during the cardiac cycle. Enhanced RV filling, as during onset of inspiration, may lead to a slight flattening of the ventricular septum during early diastolic filling. This phenomenon is called ventricular coupling (see Chaps. 6 and 11). In several cardiac and extracardiac diseases, pathological ventricular coupling may occur (e.g., constrictive pericarditis, cor pulmonale, atrial septal defects, severe pulmonary incompetence, pulmonary hypertension). The ventricular septum is best studied in short- and horizontal long-axis views. As with the atrial septum, a diagnosis of septal defect cannot be made on the basis of this morphological (i.e., SE-MRI) finding alone, and additional bright-blood and flow measurements should be obtained to make a definite diagnosis.

4.4.3
Valves

Two atrioventricular (AV) (or ventricular) valves connect the atria to the ventricles, a mitral and a tricuspid valve. Embryologically, the mitral valve is always connected to the morphological left ventricle, whilst the tricuspid valve is connected with the morphological right ventricle. There is a difference in positioning along the longitudinal cardiac axis between both valves. The tricuspid valve is always somewhat more apically positioned than the mitral valve, a feature that is very helpful in differentiating the ventricular morphology.

The RV (AV) valve, or tricuspid valve, has three leaflets, these being the septal, inferior, and antero-superior leaflets (Fig. 4.13). The muscular support of the tricuspid valve is made up of the anterior muscle, which is the largest and usually arises from the septomarginal trabeculation. The complex of chords supporting the anteroseptal commissure is dominated by the medial papillary muscle (of Lancisi), a relatively small muscle which arises either as a single band or as a small branch of chords from the posterior limb of the septomarginal trabeculation (ANDERSON 2000). The inferior muscle, smallest of the three, is usually single and may be represented by several small muscles.

The LV (AV) valve, or mitral valve, has aortic and mural leaflets, so named because of their re-

lationship with the leaflets of the aortic valve and the parietal atrioventricular junction, respectively (Fig. 4.13). The zone of apposition between the two leaflets has anterolateral and posteromedial ends, the so-called commissures, each supported by one of the paired LV papillary muscles which are embedded in the anterolateral and posteromedial walls of the left ventricle.

The semilunar valves of both great arteries attach across the anatomic ventriculoarterial junction and therefore lack a fibrous supporting annulus such as supports the atrioventricular valves. They have no chordal attachments. The pulmonary artery normally arises from the infundibulum of the right ventricle. The leaflets of the pulmonary valve and the leaflets of the triscuspid valve are widely separated by the infundibular musculature. The aortic valve cusps are usually described according to the origin of the coronary arteries – left, right, and non-coronary, although they may also be called anterior, and right and left poste-

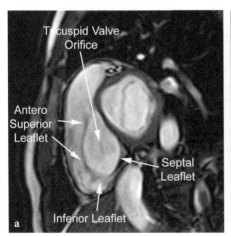
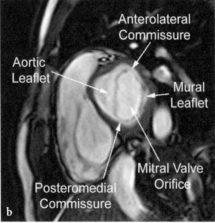

Fig. 4.13a,b. Tricuspid and mitral valve. Short-axis view through atrioventricular valves, using balanced-SSFP technique obtained during diastole. The leaflets, commissures and valve orifices can be best appreciated when the valves are opened.

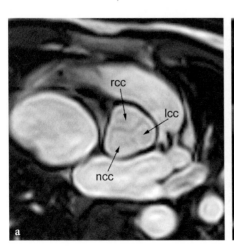
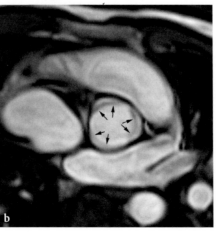

Fig. 4.14a,b. Aortic valve cusps in closed (a) and open (b) condition. The right coronary (*rcc*), left coronary (*lcc*), and noncoronary (*ncc*) cusps in closed condition are similar to a "Mercedes Benz" star. At maximal opening during systole, the cusps are nearly completely apposed to the wall of sinus of Valsalva.

rior (Fig. 4.14). Each valve cusp has a small nodule of connective tissue at its mid-point. When the great arteries are normally related, the non-coronary left coronary commissure of the aortic valve sits directly above the middle of the anterior mitral leaflet. The non-coronary right coronary commissure sits directly above the membranous septum, which in turn is located directly above the left bundle of a branch of the conduction system.

Because the valve leaflets are thin and fibrous, SE-MRI is not ideal for visualizing the cardiac valves and for studying valve pathology. Although they are often seen on SE-MRI, especially when in closed position, appreciation of small changes in thickness, structure and integrity are difficult to appreciate. Bright-blood MRI techniques demonstrate valve leaflet morphology, valve leaflet motion, abnormal valve opening, and valvular flow patterns much better (DE ROOS et al. 1995). The cardiac valves are best studied in specific imaging planes perpendicularly or longitudinally oriented through the valve of interest (see Chap. 5).

4.4.4
Coronary Arteries

Two of the sinuses of Valsalva give rise to coronary arteries. These sinuses are the ones adjacent to the pulmonary truncus.

The right coronary artery (RCA) arises from an ostium located just below the sinotubular junction, in the middle of the right (anterior) sinus of Valsalva.

(Fig. 4.15). The RCA courses into the right atrioventricular groove and provides nutrient branches to the infundibulum (infundibular or conal branch) and to the RV free wall (ANGELINI et al. 1999). The extension, and thus the myocardial perfusion territory of the RCA is highly variable. It may stop proximally in the right atrioventricular groove or may continue into the posterior interventricular groove to the apex or to the left atrioventricular groove, ending in the posterolateral LV branch. Occasionally, it might extend up to the LAD. In nearly 85–90% of cases, it is normal for the RCA to provide a posterior descending branch that follows the posterior atrioventricular groove as far as the apex of the heart but not beyond (dominant RCA), thus supplying the inferoseptal part of the LV myocardium. In only 5%, the LCx continues as posterior descending artery (dominant LCx), while, in 10% of cases, both the right coronary artery and left circumflex supply the inferior wall (balanced pattern).

The LCA originates from the middle portion of the left anterior sinus of Valsalva, just below the sinotubular junction (Fig. 4.15). The proximal vessel originating from the left ostium, called the left main stem (LM) or trunk, is only a short conductive arterial segment (±1 cm) from which the LCx and LAD arteries normally arise. The LAD courses in the anterior interventricular groove, the LCx in the left (posterior) atrioventricular groove. The LAD gives off branches to both the septum (perforator branches) and the anterolateral wall of the left ventricle (diagonal branches), and the LCx produces branches to the posterolateral wall of the left ventricle, including the

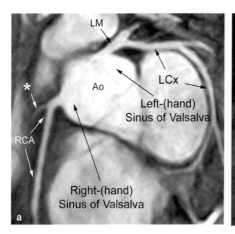

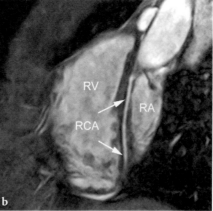

Fig. 4.15a,b. Origin and proximal course of coronary arteries. Short-axis view through the aortic root (**a**), and oblique view through anterior (or right) atrioventricular groove, using a balanced-SSFP technique with submillimeter spatial resolution. The right coronary artery (*RCA*) and left coronary artery originate from the right and left sinus of Valsalva, respectively. The major arteries as well as several branches can be readily depicted. This subject has a *LCx* dominant system. *Ao*, Aorta; *LM*, left main stem coronary artery; *RA*, right atrium; *RV*, right ventricle; star, conal branch.

posteromedial papillary muscle. The LAD terminates at the cardiac apex, or 1–2 cm before or after the apex. The perforators originate from the LAD at a grossly perpendicular angle and these branches immediately become intramural, coursing within the septum (see Chap. 14). The MRI techniques, as well as the ideal imaging planes, to study the coronary arteries are described in detail in Chaps. 5 and 14.

4.4.5
Pericardium

The pericardium envelops the heart and the origin of the great vessels and consists of an outer fibrous layer (the fibrous pericardium) and an inner serous sac (the serous pericardium). This fibrous part is attached to the sternum and diaphragm. The serous pericardium consists of an inner visceral layer (the epicardium), which is intimately connected to the heart and the epicardial fat, and an outer parietal layer, which lines the fibrous pericardium. The visceral layer is reflected from the heart and the root of the great vessels onto the inner surface of the fibrous pericardium to become continuous with the parietal layer. The pericardial cavity lies between these two layers of the serous pericardium. Two serosal tunnels can be identified: the transverse sinus, posterior to the great arteries and anterior to the atria and the superior vena cava, and the oblique sinus, posterior to the left atrium (GROELL et al. 1999). The transverse sinus is divided into the following four recesses: the superior aortic recess, inferior aortic recess, left pulmonic recess, and right pulmonic recess. Pericardial sinuses and recesses are frequently depicted on cardiac MR images (see Figs. 11.2–3). Knowledge of their locations is helpful in the differentiation of normal pericardium from pericardial effusions and mediastinal processes such as lymph nodes. Under physiologic conditions, the pericardial space contains 20–25 ml of serous fluid; however, the amount of fluid may vary considerably among individuals, particularly in children and infants. These differences may explain, at least in part, why in some patients, sinuses or recesses may or may not be seen. Moreover, clinically asymptomatic patients can have large pericardial fluid collections, especially when it accumulates over long periods, and it may be found incidentally.

On MR images, the normal pericardial sac is visible as a very thin curvilinear structure of low signal intensity surrounded by the high-intensity mediastinal and (sub)epicardial fat (SECHTEM et al. 1986a,b).

The pericardium is best visualized over the right side of the heart and cardiac apex, while it is often invisible along the LV free wall ,where it is interposed between the myocardium and the low-intensity left lung (see Fig. 11.1). In normal subjects, the pericardium has a thickness of 1.2±0.5 mm in diastole and 1.7±0.5 mm in systole (SECHTEM et al. 1986a). Similar results (i.e., 1.7 mm, range 1.5–2.0 mm) have been found by Bogaert and Duerinckx, evaluating the normal appearance of the pericardium on breath-hold MRI used to visualize coronary arteries (BOGAERT and DUERINCKX 1995). These values exceed the thickness of 0.4–1.0 mm reported for anatomical measurements of pericardial thickness. The layer of normal pericardial fluid present in the pericardial space also has a low intensity, and it likely that this thin layer of fluid contributes to the overall pericardial thickness as visualized by MRI. Because MRI is sensitive to the small amount of normal pericardial fluid and depicts its anatomical distribution, it should be valuable in detection and quantification of even small pericardial effusions (see Chap. 11). In patients with constrictive pericarditis, Sechtem et al. have found a pericardial thickness of more than 4 mm (SECHTEM et al. 1986a). Newer studies, however, have shown that constrictive pericarditis might be present in patients with a normal or near-normal pericardial thickness at surgery (TALREJA et al. 2003). Thus, in the absence of a thickened pericardium, other diagnostic criteria are needed to differentiate constrictive pericarditis patients from restrictive cardiomyopathy patients. A combination of transverse or long-axis imaging planes and short-axis views ensures the best approach for studying the entirety of the pericardial sac.

4.5
Great Vessels

The aorta has its origin from the centre point of the base of the heart and curves upwards to the aortic arch, where the brachiocephalic vessels have their origin. The junction between the aortic root containing the sinuses of Valsalva and the ascending aorta is called the sinotubular junction. The course of the aortic arch, as well as the branching pattern of the brachiocephalic vessels, can be subject to a large number of congenital variations (see Chaps. 15 and 16). The most frequent presentation is a left-sided aortic arch running over the main stem bronchus with the following branching pattern: right brachiocephalic trunk, left common carotid artery, and finally left subclavian artery (Fig. 4.16). The leaflets of the aortic valve are supported by the three sinuses of Valsalva. The pulmonary trunk orginates from the muscular pulmonary infundibulum, and bifurcates into the right and left pulmonary arteries. Two of the sinuses of the pulmonary trunk are always next to the aorta (also called facing sinuses), while the third sinus is non-facing. The ligamentum arteriosus, a fibrous remnant of the arterial duct (or "ductus arteriosus") extends from the pulmonary trunk into the descending aorta. The aortic isthmus is defined as the segment between the site of take-off of the left subclavian artery and the aortic insertion of the duct. A combination of different imaging planes is recommended to study the thoracic great vessels.

Systemic venous return to the heart is through the superior and inferior caval veins (venae cavae), which lie on the right side of the spine. The superior caval vein is formed by the confluence of the right and left innominate veins, which lie in front of the brachiocephalic artery. The inferior caval vein has only a small intrathoracic portion. After receiving the hepatic veins, it crosses the diaphragm to enter the posterior aspect of the right atrium.

There are two right and two left pulmonary veins, joining the posterior aspect of the left atrium. The right pulmonary veins enter close to the atrial septum. In patients with an atrial septal defect, the pulmonary venous blood from the right lung drains preferentially into the right atrium. The two left pulmonary veins frequently join the left atrium as a single trunk.

The great vessels are usually studied using a combination of black-blood and bright-blood techniques in different imaging planes. This combination of sequences is the best guarantee to see the vessel wall and para-aortic tissues. Often, velocity-encoded flow, cine MRI studies are performed to calculate the flow patterns in blood vessels. A good imaging plane to start with is the transverse imaging plane. Abnormalities in the course and dimensions of the great vessels are readily depicted in this imaging plane. However, to obtain accurate dimensions, an imaging plane perpendicular to the long axis of the vessel should be used. Additional imaging in other planes is often necessary to better depict the vascular abnormality (e.g., aortic coarctation) or to better visualize the consequences of valvular pathology on vascular structures (e.g., post-stenotic aortic dilatation).

The outflow tract of the right ventricle, the pulmonary trunk, and its bifurcation are well depicted

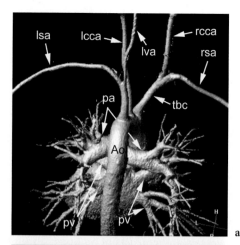
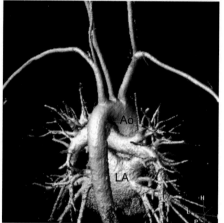
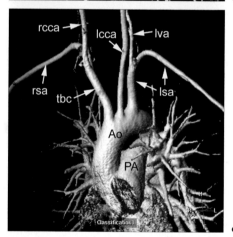

Fig. 4.16a-c. Great vessels of the thorax and neck. Contrast-enhanced MR angiography using volume rendered reconstruction, posterior-anterior view (a), posterior-anterior view with slightly oblique inclination (b), anterior-posterior view (c). The aorta (Ao), the brachiocephalic vessels (right brachiocephalic trunk (tbc), right subclavian artery (rsa), right common carotid artery (rcca), left common carotid artery (lcca), left subclavian artery (lsa) and left vertebral artery (lva)), the pulmonary artery (PA) and its major branches (pa), as well as the pulmonary veins (pv) entering the left atrium (LA), are clearly depicted.

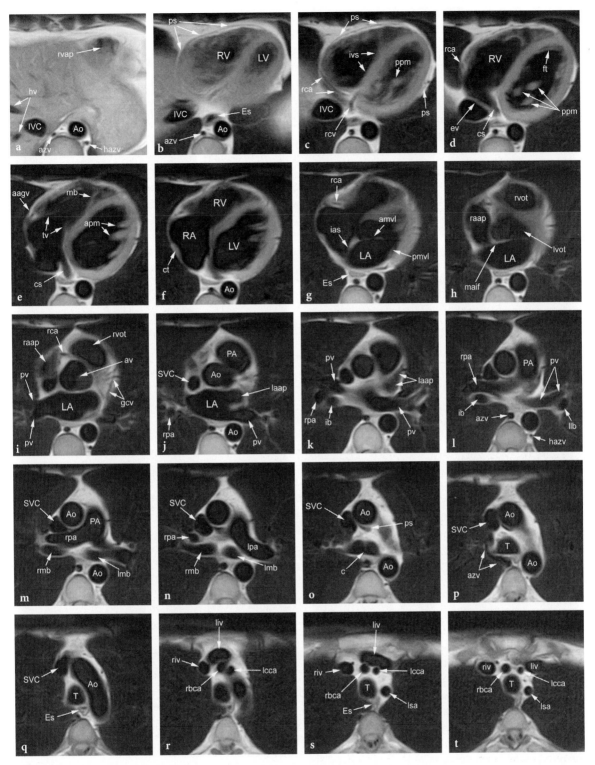

Fig. 4.17a-t. Transverse images. Abbreviations: *aavg*, anterior (or right) atrioventricular groove; *amvl*, anterior mitral valve leaflet; *Ao*, aorta; *apm*, anterior papillary muscle; *av*, aortic valve; *azv*, azygos vein; *c*, carina; *cs*, coronary sinus; *ct*, crista terminalis; *Es*, esophagus; *ev*, Eustachian valve; *ft*, false tendon; *gcv*, great cardiac vein; *hazv*, hemiazygos vein; *hv*, hepatic vein; *ias*, interatrial septum; *ib*, intermediate bronchus; *IVC*, inferior vena cava; *ivs*, interventricular septum; *LA*, left atrium; *laap*, left atrial appendage; *lcca*, left common carotid artery; *liv*, left innominate, (or brachiocephalic) vein; *llb*, left lower lobebronchus; *lmb*, left main stem bronchus; *lpa*, left pulmonary artery; *lsa*, left subclavian artery; *LV*, left ventricle; *lvot*, left ventricular outflow tract; *maif*, mitral-aortic intervalvular fibrosa; *mb*, moderator band; *PA*, pulmonary artery (or trunk); *pmvl*, posterior mitral valve leaflet; *ppm*, posterior papillary muscle; *ps*, pericardial sac; *pv*, pulmonary vein; *RA*, right atrium; *raap*, right atrial appendage; *rbca*, right brachiocephalic artery; *rca*, right coronary artery; *rcv*, right cardiac vein; *riv*, right innominate (or brachiocephalic) vein; *rmb*, right main stem bronchus; *rpa*, right pulmonary artery; *RV*, right ventricle; *rvap*, right ventricular apex; *rvot*, right ventricular outflow tract; *SVC*, superior vena cava; *T*, trachea; *tv*, tricuspid valve.

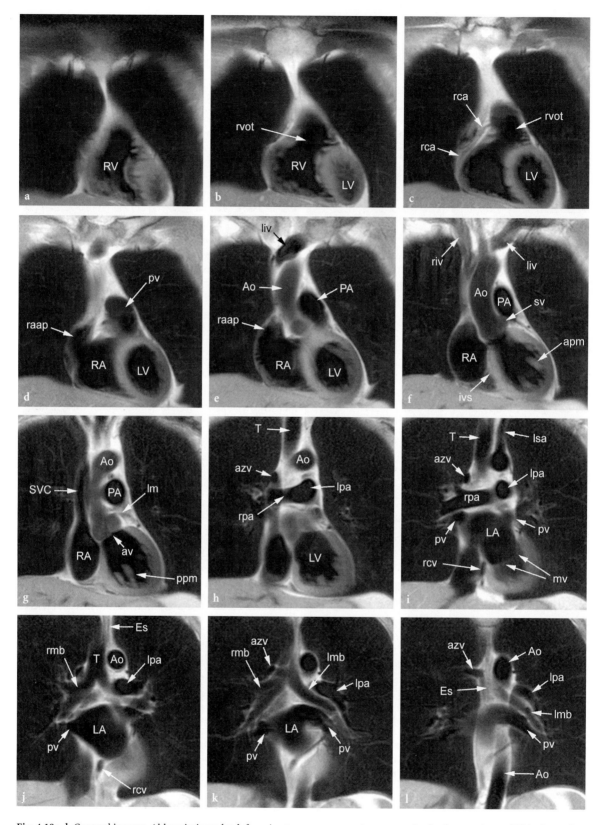

Fig. 4.18a–l. Coronal images. Abbreviations: *lm*, left main stem coronary artery; *mv*, mitral valve; *sv*, sinus of Valsalva; other abbreviations as in Fig. 4.17.

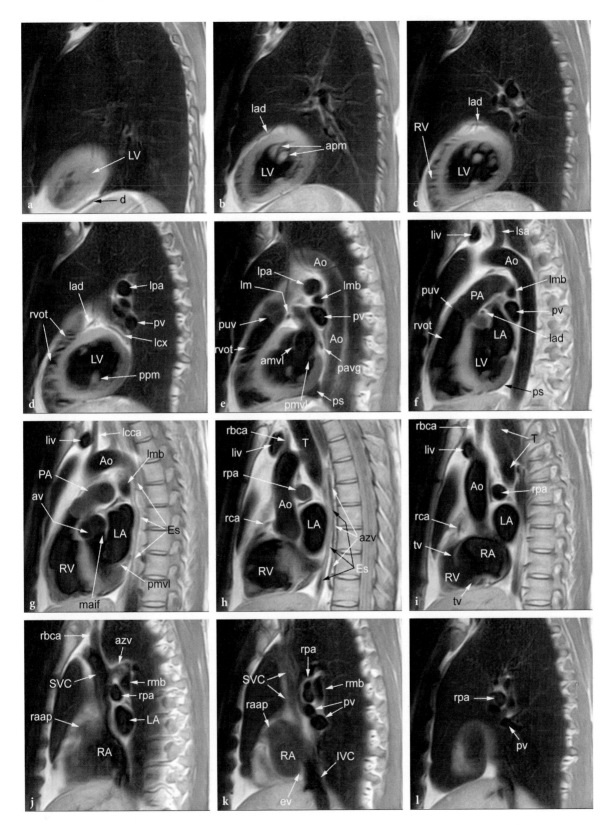

Fig. 4.19a–l. Sagittal images. Abbreviations: *lad*, left anterior descending coronary artery; *lcx*, Left circumflex artery; *pavg*, posterior (or left) atrioventricular groove; *puv*, pulmonary valve; *sv*, sinus of Valsalva; other abbreviations as in Fig. 4.17.

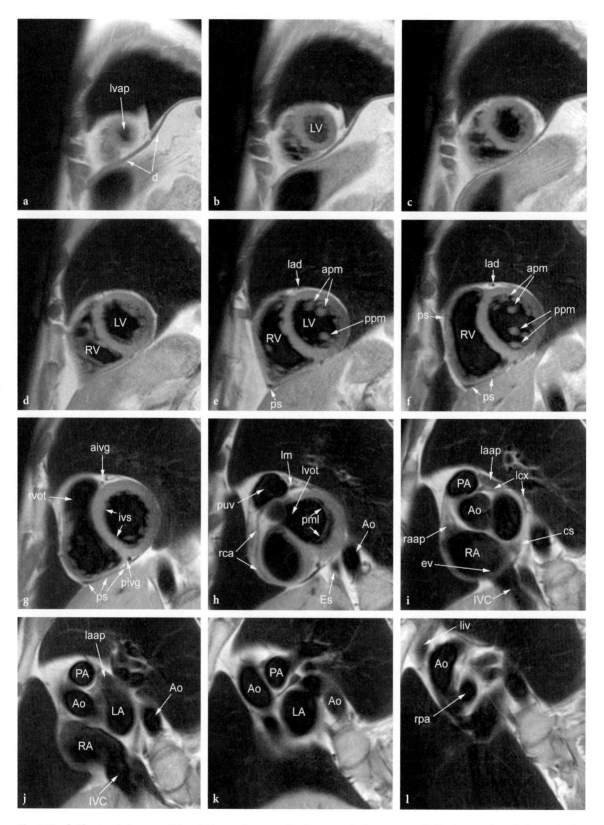

Fig. 4.20a–l. Short-axis images. Abbreviations: *aivg*; anterior interventricular groove; *d*, diaphragm; *lvap*, left ventricular apex; *pivg*, posterior interventricular groove; other abbreviations as in preceding figures.

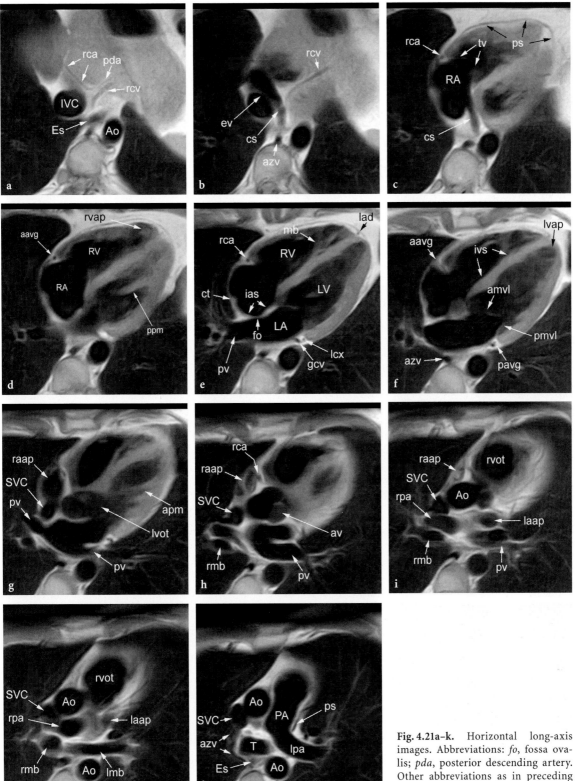

Fig. 4.21a–k. Horizontal long-axis images. Abbreviations: *fo*, fossa ovalis; *pda*, posterior descending artery. Other abbreviations as in preceding figures.

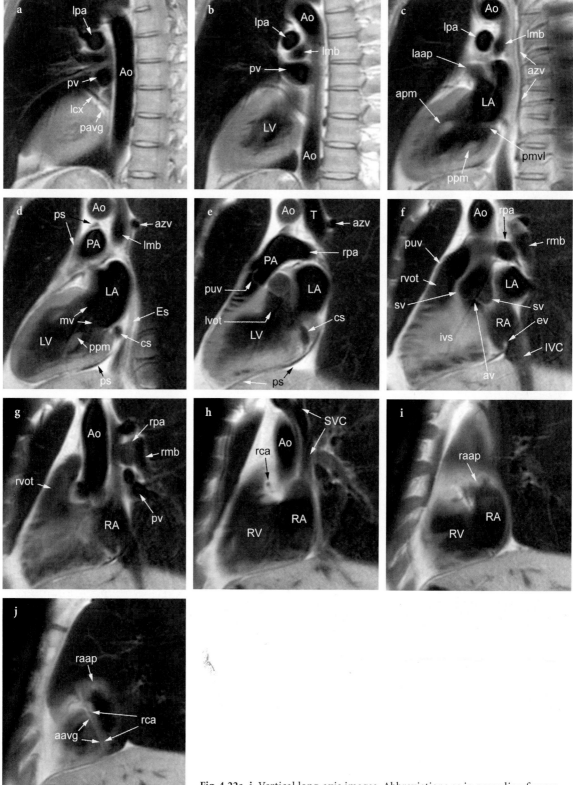

Fig. 4.22a–j. Vertical long-axis images. Abbreviations as in preceding figures.

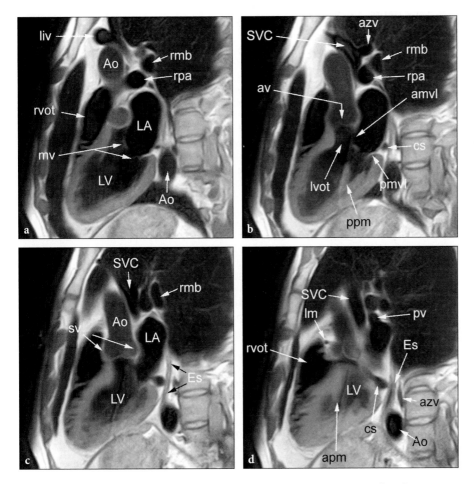

Fig. 4.23a-d. Left ventricular outflow tract images. Abbreviations as in preceding figures.

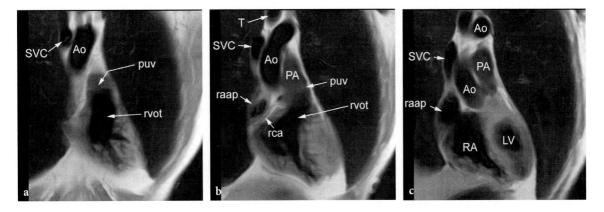

Fig. 4.24a-c. Right ventricular outflow tract images. Abbreviations as in preceding figures.

on the transverse images, while specific imaging planes in a parasagittal plane through the left and right pulmonary branches can be used for cine and flow measurements (PAZ et al. 1993; MURRAY et al. 1994; BOUCHARD et al. 1985). Although the thoracic aorta can be visualized over its entire course (FRIEDMANN et al. 1985; BYRD et al. 1985; DINSMORE et al. 1986), it is often not possible to achieve this in a single plane, because the aortic arch usually does not fall in the same plane as the ascending and descending aorta. With the advent of contrast-enhanced 3D MR angiography, depiction of thoracic vessels has been greatly facilitated (PRINCE 1996).

4.6
Key Points

- MRI is an excellent technique for evaluating cardiac anatomy, at least if the image acquisition and image interpretation are performed adequately, otherwise it is worthless
- A combination of black-blood and bright-blood techniques is advisable to study cardiac anatomy
- Moreover, a combination of imaging in different cardiac imaging planes is always helpful to better depict cardiac anatomy
- Always combine morphological evaluation with functional evaluation of the heart
- For accurate measurements of dimensions, use imaging planes perpendicular to the structure of interest, e.g., myocardial wall, ventricular cavity, vessel lumen
- Use of a systematic approach to analyze cardiac anatomy
- Each of the components of the heart has its specific characteristics, enabling the most complex congenital heart disease to be unraveled.
- The mitral valve is always connected to the morphological left ventricle, while the tricuspid valve is connected to the morphological right ventricle. The tricuspid valve is more apically positioned than the mitral valve
- The moderator band always belongs to the morphological right ventricle
- The septal surface of the LV cavity is smooth and has no insertions of muscular structures

References

Anderson RH (2000) The anatomic structure of the normal heart, and the structure of congenitally malformed hearts. A handbook prepared to support the foundation course in cardiac morphology held at the Institute of Child Health University College London on 10th and 11th February 2000, UK, pp 2–24

Angelini P, Villason S, Chan AV Jr, Diez JG (1999) Normal and anomalous coronary arteries in humans. In: Angelini P (ed) Coronary artery anomalies. A comprehensive approach. Lippincott Williams and Wilkins, Philadelphia, pp 27–79

Amplatz K, Moller JH (1993) Cardiac anatomy. In: Amplatz K, Moller JH, Radiology of congenital heart disease. Mosby Year Book, St Louis, pp 13–48

Bogaert J, Duerinckx AJ (1995) Appearance of the normal pericardium on coronary MR angiograms. J Magn Reson Imaging 5:579–587

Bogaert J, Rademakers FE (2001) Regional nonuniformity of the normal adult human left ventricle. A 3D MR myocardial tagging study. Am J Physiol Heart Circ Physiol 280:610–620

Bouchard A, Higgins CB, Byrd BF, Amparo EP, Osaki L, Axelrod R (1985) Magnetic resonance imaging in pulmonary hypertension. Am J Cardiol 56:938–942

Burbank F, Parish D, Wexler L (1988) Echocardiographic-like angled views of the heart by MR imaging. J Comput Assist Tomogr 12:181–195

Byrd FB, Schiller NB, Botvinick EH, Higgins CB (1985) Normal cardiac dimensions by magnetic resonance imaging. Am J Cardiol 55:1440–1442

Carr JC, Simonetti O, Bundy J et al (2001) Cine MR angiography of the heart with segmented true fast imaging with steady-state precession. Radiology 219:828–834

Castillo E, Bluemke DA (2003) Cardiac MR imaging. Radiol Clin North Am 41:17–28

De Roos A, Doornbos J, van der Wall EE, van Voorthuisen AE (1995) Magnetic resonance of the heart and great vessels. Nat Med 1:711–713

Dinsmore RE, Wismer GL, Levine RA, Okada RD, Brady TJ (1984) Magnetic resonance imaging of the heart: positioning and gradient angle selection for optimal imaging planes. Am J Roentgenol 143:1135–1142

Dinsmore RE, Liberthson RR, Wismer GL et al (1986) Magnetic resonance imaging of the thoracic aorta in long and short axis planes: comparison with other techniques in patients with aortic aneurysms. Am J Roentgenol 146:309–314

Frahm J, Haase A, Matthei D (1986) Rapid NMR imaging of dynamic processes using the FLASH technique. Magn Reson Med 3:321–327

Friedmann BJ, Waters J, Kwan OL, de Maria AN (1985) Comparison of magnetic resonance imaging and echocardiography in determination of cardiac dimensions in normal subjects. J Am Coll Cardiol 5:1369–1376

Galjee MA, van Rossum AC, van Eenige MJ et al (1995) Magnetic resonance imaging of the pulmonary venous flow pattern in mitral regurgitation. Independence of the investigated vein. Eur Heart J 16:1675–1685

Groell R, Schaffler GJ, Rienmueller R (1999) Pericardial sinuses and recesses: findings at electrocardiographically triggered electron-beam CT. Radiology 212:69–73

Hawkes RC, Holland GN, Moore WS, Roebuck EJ, Worthington BS (1981) Nuclear magnetic resonance (NMR) tomography of the normal heart. J Comp Assist Tomogr 5:605–612

Heneghan MA, Biancaniello TM, Heidelberger E, Peterson SB, Marsh MJ, Lauterbur PC (1982) Nuclear magnetic resonance zeugmatographic imaging of the heart: application to the study of ventricular septal defect. Radiology 143:183–186

Herfkens RJ, Higgins CB, Hricak H et al (1983) Nuclear magnetic resonance imaging of the cardiovascular system: normal and pathologic findings. Radiology 147:749–759

Higgins CB, Lanzer P, Stark D et al (1985) Assessment of cardiac anatomy using nuclear magnetic resonance imaging. J Am Coll Cardiol 5:77S–81S

Higgins CB, Holt W, Pfugfelder P, Sechtem U (1988) Functional evaluation of the heart with magnetic resonance imaging. Magn Reson Med 6:121–139

Lanzer P, Barta C, Botvinick EH, Wiesendanger HUD, Modin G, Higgins CB (1985) ECG-synchronized cardiac MR imaging: method and evaluation. Radiology 155:681–686

Longmore DB, Underwood SR, Hounsfield GN et al (1985) Dimensional accuracy of magnetic resonance in studies of the heart. Lancet I:1360–1362

Meier RA, Hartnell GG (1994) MRI of right atrial pseudo masses. Is it really a diagnostic problem? J Comput Assist Tomogr 18:398–402

Menegus MA, Greenberg MA, Spindola-Franco H et al (1992) Magnetic resonance imaging of suspected atrial tumors. Am Heart J 123:1260–1268

Mirowitz SA, Gutierrez FR (1992) Fibromuscular elements of the right atrium: pseudomass at MR imaging. Radiology 182:231–233

Mohiaddin RH, Amanuma M, Kilner PJ, Pennell DJ, Manzara C, Longmore DB (1991) MR phase-shift velocity mapping of mitral and pulmonary venous flow. J Comput Assist Tomogr 15:237–243

Murray TI, Boxt LM, Katz J, Reagan K, Barst RJ (1994) Estimation of pulmonary artery pressure in patients with primary pulmonary hypertension by quantitative analysis of magnetic resonance images. J Thorac Imaging 9:198–203

O'Donovan PB, Ross JS, Sivak ED, O'Donnell JK, Meaney TF (1984) Magnetic resonance imaging of the thorax: the advantages of coronal and sagittal planes. Am J Roentgenol 143:1183–1188

Paz R, Mohiaddin RH, Longmore DB (1993) Magnetic resonance assessment of the pulmonary arterial trunk anatomy, flow, pulsatility and distensibility. Eur Heart J 14:1524–1530

Prince (1996) Body MR angiography with gadolinium contrast agents. Magn Reson Imaging Clin North Am 4:11–24

Sechtem U, Tscholakoff D, Higgins CB (1986a) MRI of the normal pericardium. Am J Roentgenol 147:239–244

Sechtem U, Tscholakoff D, Higgins CB (1986b) MRI of the abnormal pericardium. Am J Roentgenol 147:245–252

Simonetti OP, Finn JP, White RD, Laub G, Henry DA (1996) "Black blood" T2-weighted inversion-recovery MR imaging of the heart. Radiology 199:49–57

Stehling MK, Holzknecht NG, Laub G, Bohm D, von Smekal A, Reiser M (1996) Single-shot T1- and T2-weighted magnetic resonance imaging of the heart with black blood: preliminary experience. MAGMA 4:231–240

Talreja DR, Edwards WD, Danielson GK et al (2003) Constrictive pericarditis in 26 patients with histologically normal pericardial thickness. Circulation 108:1852–1857

Tscholakoff D, Higgins CB (1985) Gated magnetic resonance imaging for assessment of cardiac function and myocardial infarction. Radiol Clin North Am 23:449–456

Winterer JT, Lehnhardt S, Schneider B et al (1999) MRI of heart morphology. Comparison of nongradient echo sequences with single-and multislice acquisition. Invest Radiol 34:516–522

5 Cardiovascular MR Imaging Planes and Segmentation

Andrew M. Taylor and Jan Bogaert

CONTENTS

5.1 Introduction

In general, structures within the body are described in relation to the "anatomical position" (subject standing upright, facing the observer). Thus, for axial cross-sectional body imaging (MR and computed tomography, CT) the convention is to describe the images as viewed from below as if facing the subject (i.e., subject's right is to the left of the image) (Fig. 5.1). This principle enables accurate description of the spatial relationship of structures within the body in terms of right/left, inferior/superior, and medial/lateral, and helps clinicians direct treatment, in particular when surgery is required.

The heart is the exception to this rule, with intracardiac anatomy described according to the axes of the heart, from the pathologist's perspective (heart

A. M. Taylor MD, MRCP, FRCR
Cardiothoracic Unit, Institute of Child Health and Great Ormond Street Hospital for Children, London WC1N 3JH, UK
J. Bogaert MD, PhD
Department of Radiology, Gasthuisberg University Hospital, Catholic University of Leuven, Herestraat 49, 3000 Leuven, Belgium

positioned on its apex, with the atria above the ventricles) – the so-called Valentine approach. Thus, though the ventricles are referred to as right and left, in the majority of subjects they occupy a more anterior and posterior position, respectively, in relation to the body axes on cross-sectional imaging.

Despite this anomaly, the heart will continue to be described in terms of reference to its own axes. In both echocardiography and nuclear scintigraphy, the heart is imaged without reference to other structures, and the use of the cardiac axes enables standard points of reference to be maintained in these imaging modalities. Cross-sectional imaging modalities should also describe the heart in terms of these frames of reference (Cerqueira et al. 2002), though more conventional cross-sectional terms of reference can still be used when describing MR and CT images.

5.2 Imaging Planes for Cardiac Structures

5.2.1 Body Axes

The transverse or axial plane (Fig. 5.1) is useful for studying morphology and the relationships of the four cardiac chambers and the pericardium. Sagittal images (see Fig. 4.19) can be used to study the connections between the ventricles and the great vessels, while frontal or coronal images are most useful for investigation of the left ventricular outflow tract (LVOT), the left atrium, and the pulmonary veins (see Fig. 4.18). The optimal planes also depend on the global positioning of the heart in the thorax, which is more vertical in young individuals and more diaphragmatic in elderly persons. It has to be stressed that, while these images are appropriate for evaluation of the overall morphology of the heart, quantitative measurements of wall thickness, cavity dimensions, and functional data cannot be obtained

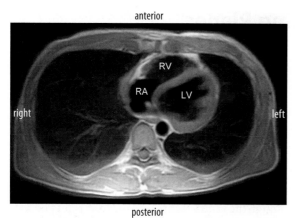

Fig. 5.1. Axial plane through the mid-thorax. Note that the right ventricle (*RV*) lies anterior and the left ventricle (*LV*) posterior. The right atrium (*RA*) is seen in this plane, but the left atrium lies superior and posterior, and is often not seen in the same axial plane as the RA (see Chap. 4)

5.2.2
Cardiac Axes

To obtain the correct inclinations for imaging in the cardiac axes, a transverse or axial scout view at the level of the left ventricle (LV) is acquired initially (BURBANK et al. 1988). On this image, a new plane is chosen running through the apex of the LV and the middle of the left atrioventricular (AV), mitral, valve. This yields the vertical long-axis (VLA) plane (Fig. 5.2b). On this image, a plane chosen to transect the LV apex and the middle of the mitral ring yields the horizontal long-axis (HLA) plane (Fig. 5.2c). The short-axis (SA) plane can now be prescribed perpendicular to both the VLA and HLA (Fig. 5.2d). From a SA plane at the level of the mitral valves, the four-chamber view can be acquired (4Ch). The plane for the 4Ch view passes from the most superior mitral valve, "anterolateral" papillary muscle to the inferior angle of the right ventricle (RV) anteriorly, usually through the mid-point of the interventricular septum (Fig. 5.2e). A true-SA plane can now be prescribed off the 4Ch view perpendicular to the interventricular septum. The inclination of short-axis slices is not always easy, since the anterior and inferior walls of the left ventricle are not exactly parallel,

accurately, since the planes are not perpendicular to the wall or the cavity, with the consequence that partial volume effects and obliqueness can introduce a large overestimation of the true dimensions. The cardiac imaging planes are more suitable for this purpose (LONGMORE et al. 1985).

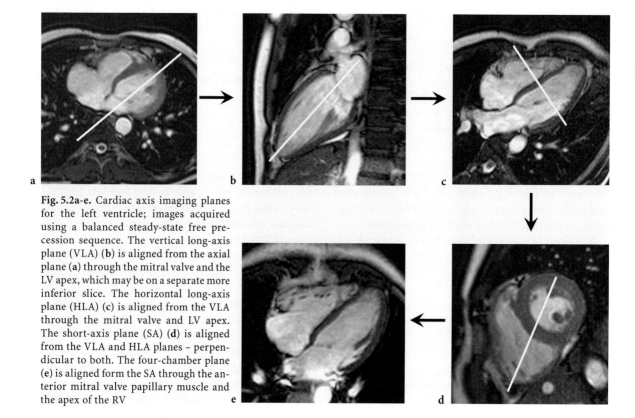

Fig. 5.2a-e. Cardiac axis imaging planes for the left ventricle; images acquired using a balanced steady-state free precession sequence. The vertical long-axis plane (VLA) (**b**) is aligned from the axial plane (**a**) through the mitral valve and the LV apex, which may be on a separate more inferior slice. The horizontal long-axis plane (HLA) (**c**) is aligned from the VLA through the mitral valve and LV apex. The short-axis plane (SA) (**d**) is aligned from the VLA and HLA planes – perpendicular to both. The four-chamber plane (**e**) is aligned form the SA through the anterior mitral valve papillary muscle and the apex of the RV

and no single plane is absolutely perpendicular to both walls. A compromise can be made, by using a short-axis plane oriented parallel to the mitral valve ring. Furthermore, when a SA stack is being prescribed for ventricular volume calculations, the imaging plane is often best positioned parallel to the AV valves, between the anterior and posterior AV grooves (Fig. 5.3).

Beside these standard cardiac imaging planes, specific planes can be chosen depending on the pathology under study. In congenital heart disease, it may be necessary to obtain multiple, nonclassical imaging planes to achieve optimal visualization.

5.2.3
Left Side of the Heart

From the short-axis plane, the VLA, HLA, and LV inflow /outflow (equivalent to the apical long-axis view acquired at echocardiography) can be acquired (Fig. 5.4). This later LV inflow /outflow image is

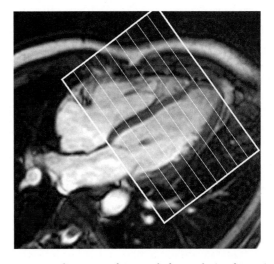

Fig. 5.3. Alignment of SA stack for analysis of ventricular volumes on the HLA. Note that the basal slice is parallel to the atrioventricular (AV) valves (between the anterior and posterior AV grooves), and almost perpendicular to the interventricular septum, though this can vary between subjects

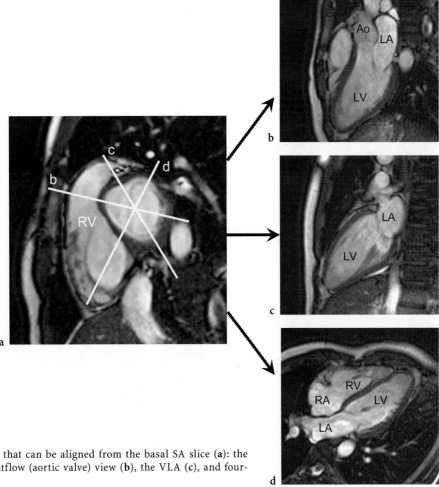

Fig. 5.4a-d. Imaging planes that can be aligned from the basal SA slice (**a**): the *LV* inflow (mitral valve)/outflow (aortic valve) view (**b**), the VLA (**c**), and four-chamber (**d**) views

acquired with a plane that passes across the center of the aortic and mitral valves on the basal SA slice, or by performing a 3-point acquisition with the first point on the LV apex, the second in the center of the mitral valve, and the third in the center of the aortic valve. This view is particularly useful for imaging septal hypertrophy and LVOT obstruction in hypertrophic cardiomyopathy. Since this view encompasses the LV inflow, concomitant mitral regurgitation in patients with LVOT obstruction can be easily depicted.

An LVOT view can be acquired by passing an imaging plane through and perpendicular to the aortic valve: oblique coronal orientation (Fig. 5.5b). This can be easily achieved by indicating on an LV inflow /outflow image a perpendicular imaging plane through the middle of the LVOT and aortic valve. Both the LVOT and LV inflow and outflow planes are well suited for evaluation of aortic valve stenosis and/or regurgitation. A plane through the aortic root ("aortic valve plane"), just above the aortic valve, perpendicular to both the LV inflow/outflow and LVOT views, can be used to assess through-plane aortic flow. This plane is used when quantifying aortic incompetence (Fig. 5.5). The morphology of the aortic valve (e.g., number of valve leaflets and fusion of leaflets), aortic valve area, and orifice can be best studied in this plane using a set of adjacent slices through the aortic valve.

The mitral valve lies in a double oblique plane. Through-plane imaging of the mitral valve to assess LV inflow curves should therefore be aligned from two views, the VLA and 4Ch (Fig. 5.6). For flow measurements, the plane should lie just beyond the mitral valve leaflets in the left ventricle.

5.2.4
Right Side of the Heart

A two-chamber view of the right side of the heart can be obtained by placing a plane through the right ventricle (RV) apex and the mid-point of the tricuspid valve on the 4Ch view (Fig. 5.7). The right ventricular outflow tract (RVOT) is visualized by aligning a plane that passes through the main pulmonary artery (PA) and the RV inferiorly from a set of axial images (Fig. 5.8c). An alternative way to obtain the RVOT view is by aligning a plane that passes through the main PA and descending aorta. This is usually a sagittal or oblique sagittal plane. A plane perpendicular to this, in an axial or oblique axial orientation, will give a second view

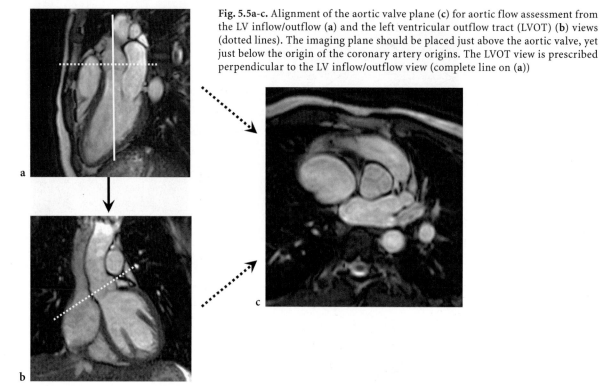

Fig. 5.5a-c. Alignment of the aortic valve plane (c) for aortic flow assessment from the LV inflow/outflow (a) and the left ventricular outflow tract (LVOT) (b) views (dotted lines). The imaging plane should be placed just above the aortic valve, yet just below the origin of the coronary artery origins. The LVOT view is prescribed perpendicular to the LV inflow/outflow view (complete line on (a))

Fig. 5.6a-c. Alignment of the mitral valve plane (c) for LV inflow assessment from the VLA (a) and the four-chamber planes (b). The imaging plane should be placed just within the LV

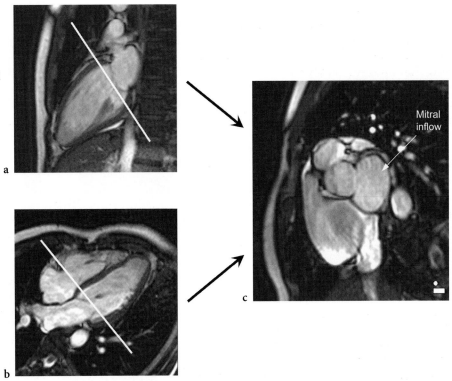

Fig. 5.7a-c. Alignment of the tricuspid valve plane (c) for RV inflow assessment from the VLA (a) and the four-chamber planes (b). The imaging plane should be placed just within the RV

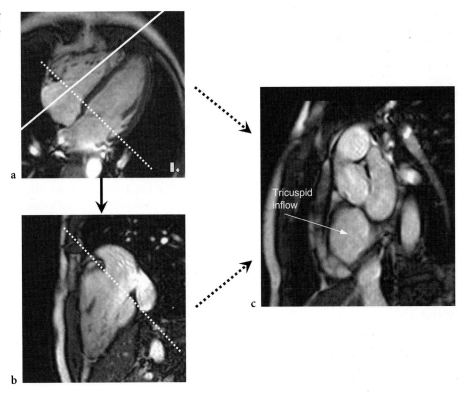

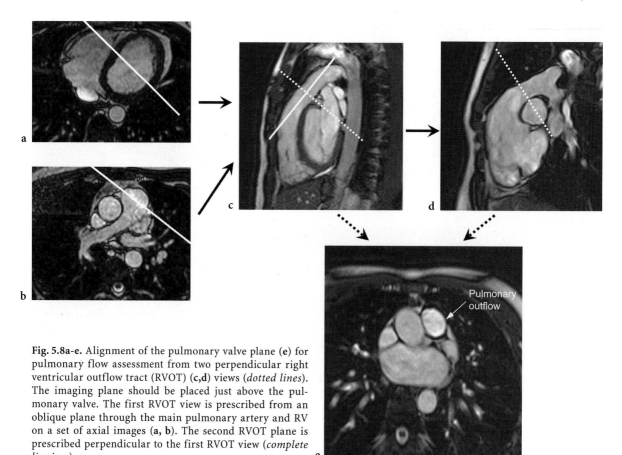

Fig. 5.8a-e. Alignment of the pulmonary valve plane (**e**) for pulmonary flow assessment from two perpendicular right ventricular outflow tract (RVOT) (**c,d**) views (*dotted lines*). The imaging plane should be placed just above the pulmonary valve. The first RVOT view is prescribed from an oblique plane through the main pulmonary artery and RV on a set of axial images (**a, b**). The second RVOT plane is prescribed perpendicular to the first RVOT view (*complete line* in **c**)

through the RVOT (Fig. 5.8d). A plane through the main PA, just above the pulmonary valve, perpendicular to both RVOT views, can be used to assess through-plane pulmonary flow. This plane is used when quantifying pulmonary incompetence (Fig. 5.8e).

An inflow/outflow plane of the RV can be acquired using a 3-point plane. The first point is placed on the tricuspid valve, the second on the RV apex, and the third on the pulmonary valve (Fig. 5.9).

As with the mitral valve, the tricuspid valve lies in a double oblique plane. Through-plane imaging of the tricuspid valve to assess RV inflow curves should therefore be aligned from two views, the RV two-chamber view and 4Ch view (Fig. 5.7c). For flow measurements, the plane should lie just beyond the tricuspid valve leaflets in the right ventricle.

5.3
Imaging Planes for Great Vessels

When performing 2D imaging through any vessel, it is essential to image in two perpendicular planes to ensure that any narrowings are real and not secondary to partial volume effects.

Furthermore, care must be taken when performing breath-hold 2D acquisitions in the axial plane, as varying degrees of breath-hold position may remove small structures from the imaging plane (Taylor et al. 1999).

5.3.1
Aorta

The aorta can be tortuous in the diseased state, and it can be difficult to align the whole aorta in a single

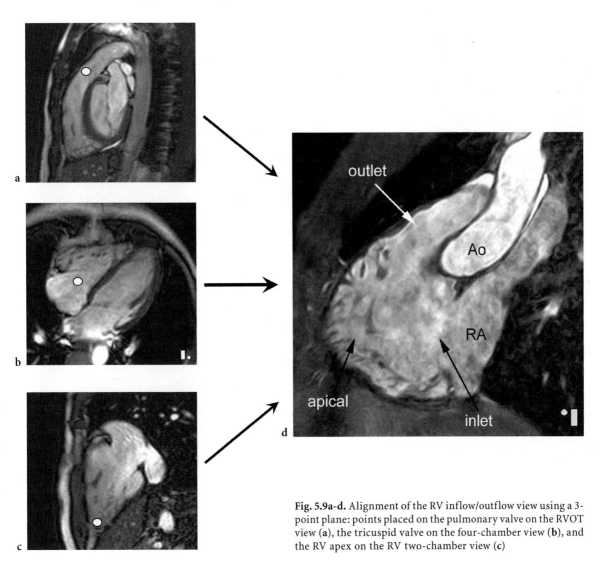

Fig. 5.9a-d. Alignment of the RV inflow/outflow view using a 3-point plane: points placed on the pulmonary valve on the RVOT view (**a**), the tricuspid valve on the four-chamber view (**b**), and the RV apex on the RV two-chamber view (**c**)

plane. However, a large section of the aortic can be aligned in an oblique sagittal plane using a 3-point plane (Fig. 5.10). This is particularly useful for in-plane imaging of aortic jets in aortic coarctation.

When performing a contrast-enhanced, 3D MR angiogram (MRA) for aortic pathology, an oblique sagittal volume is the best imaging plane for data acquisition, ensuring that the entire aorta is included in the imaging volume with the shortest acquisition time. If imaging a long section of the head and neck vessels is also required or if pathology of the sub-clavian arteries (e.g., thoracic outlet syndrome) is suspected, the imaging volume can be placed in the coronal direction, though in-plane image resolution will be reduced (increased field of view) to avoid wrapping in the left-to-right phase-encode direction.

5.3.2
Pulmonary Artery and its Branches

The main PA is usually imaged in the sagittal plane when imaging of the RVOT is performed (Fig. 5.7b). Imaging in an axial plane, perpendicular to the RVOT view, enables imaging of the PA bifurcation (Fig. 5.11a).

The right pulmonary artery (RPA) is best imaged in a coronal plane (Fig. 5.11b) and the left pulmonary artery in a sagittal plane (Fig. 5.11c), both of which can be aligned from the axial images. Branch pulmonary artery flow planes can be prescribed off two perpendicular images for both arteries (axial and coronal for the RPA, axial and sagittal for the LPA), to ensure perpendicular velocity vectors for accurate flow mapping.

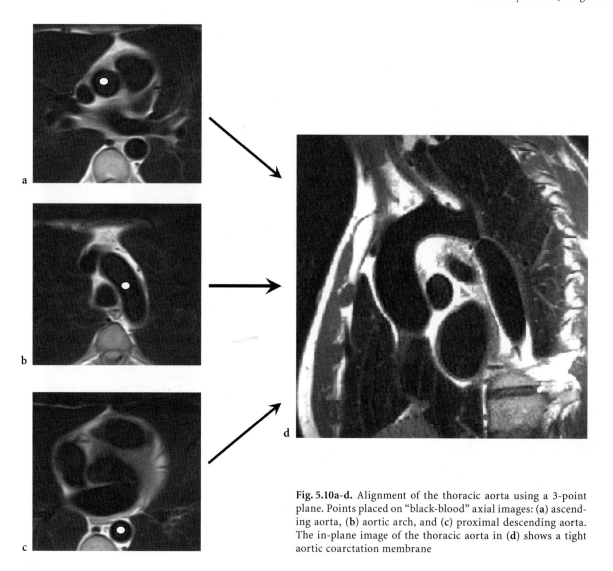

Fig. 5.10a-d. Alignment of the thoracic aorta using a 3-point plane. Points placed on "black-blood" axial images: (**a**) ascending aorta, (**b**) aortic arch, and (**c**) proximal descending aorta. The in-plane image of the thoracic aorta in (**d**) shows a tight aortic coarctation membrane

When performing an MRA of the pulmonary vasculature, a coronal volume is the best imaging plane for data acquisition. Care must be taken to ensure that the right-to-left field of view is sufficiently large to avoid wrapping in the phase-encode direction.

5.4
Imaging Planes for Coronary Arteries

MR coronary angiography can be performed by aligning a narrow 3D volume along the length of each artery.

The right coronary artery (RCA) plane is aligned using a 3-point-plane scan, applied on axial images. The points are placed on the RCA origin, the mid-

point of the RCA in the anterior AV groove, and distally in the inferior portion of the RCA as it passes toward the crux (Fig. 5.12). These 3 points define the geometry of the center plane of the imaged 3D volume, subsequently applied for the submillimeter coronary MR angiography sequence (STUBER et al. 1999). This 3D volume covers not only the anterior AV groove, but also the posterior AV groove containing the left circumflex artery.

To image the left coronary tree, two scans are performed. The first plane is referred to as the "tangential view" and images the proximal course of the left main stem (LM), the bifurcation into the left anterior descending (LAD) and left circumflex coronary artery (LCx) arteries, and their subsequent proximal course. The plane is aligned using a 3-point-plane scan, using points placed on the LM

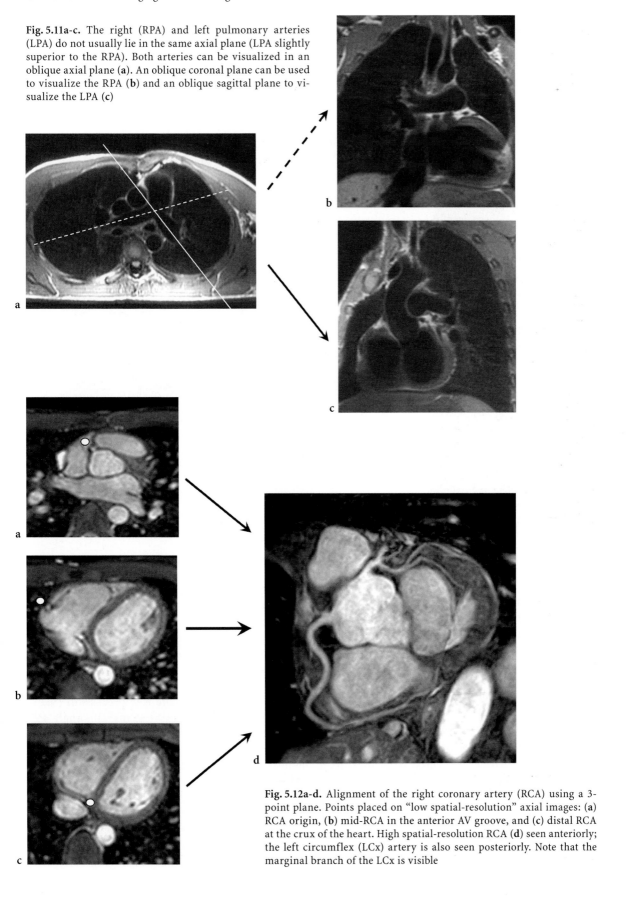

Fig. 5.11a-c. The right (RPA) and left pulmonary arteries (LPA) do not usually lie in the same axial plane (LPA slightly superior to the RPA). Both arteries can be visualized in an oblique axial plane (**a**). An oblique coronal plane can be used to visualize the RPA (**b**) and an oblique sagittal plane to visualize the LPA (**c**)

Fig. 5.12a-d. Alignment of the right coronary artery (RCA) using a 3-point plane. Points placed on "low spatial-resolution" axial images: (**a**) RCA origin, (**b**) mid-RCA in the anterior AV groove, and (**c**) distal RCA at the crux of the heart. High spatial-resolution RCA (**d**) seen anteriorly; the left circumflex (LCx) artery is also seen posteriorly. Note that the marginal branch of the LCx is visible

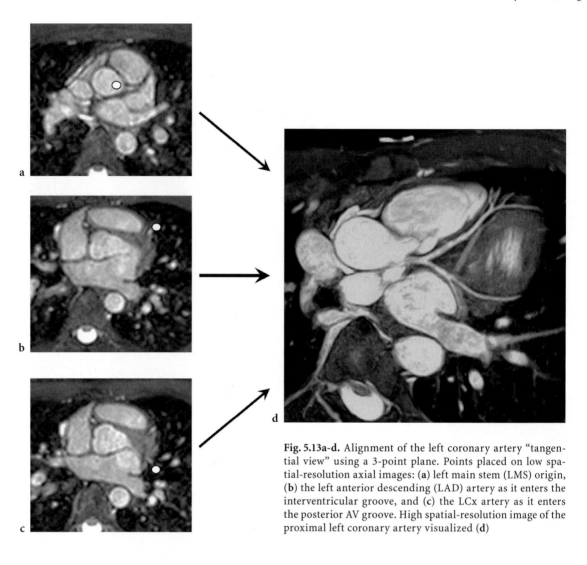

Fig. 5.13a-d. Alignment of the left coronary artery "tangential view" using a 3-point plane. Points placed on low spatial-resolution axial images: (**a**) left main stem (LMS) origin, (**b**) the left anterior descending (LAD) artery as it enters the interventricular groove, and (**c**) the LCx artery as it enters the posterior AV groove. High spatial-resolution image of the proximal left coronary artery visualized (**d**)

origin, the mid-point of the LAD, and the mid-point of the LCx (Fig. 15.13). The landmarks on the LAD and LCx should be positioned carefully to assure the longest coverage of the left coronary tree, including the diagonal branching vessels. The second plane is referred to as the "perpendicular view" and passes through the LM and entire length of the LAD. Three-point planning is again used, with the points placed on the LM origin, the mid-LAD, and the distal LAD (Fig. 15.14). On the perpendicular view, the small, septal branches of the LAD are often visualized. In this way, the LM, LCx, and LAD (but not the RCA) are scanned in two perpendicular directions. As a result, longer segments of the left coronary artery tree and more of its branching vessels are visualized. Also, the visualization and description of stenotic lesions benefits from this approach, as lesions are scanned in-plane (better resolution) in at least one direction.

5.5
Interactive Imaging for Definition of Imaging Planes

Interactive/real-time sequences are increasingly used in cardiovascular MRI (BARKHAUSEN et al. 2002; LEE et al. 2002; HORI et al. 2003; MUTHURANGU et al. 2004). The sequence used is a "white-blood" steady-state free precession (SSFP) sequence (TR=2.9 ms, TE=1.45 ms; flip angle 45°) and has a temporal resolution of 10–14 frames/s and a lower spatial resolution than conventional SSFP cine images (matrix 128×128, FOV 250–350 mm) (Fig. 5.15). Imaging is performed without cardiac or respiratory gating.

Interactive cardiovascular MR allows flexible application of imaging planes in any direction, including 3-point prescription, in real time, and in many ways it is more akin to imaging with echo-

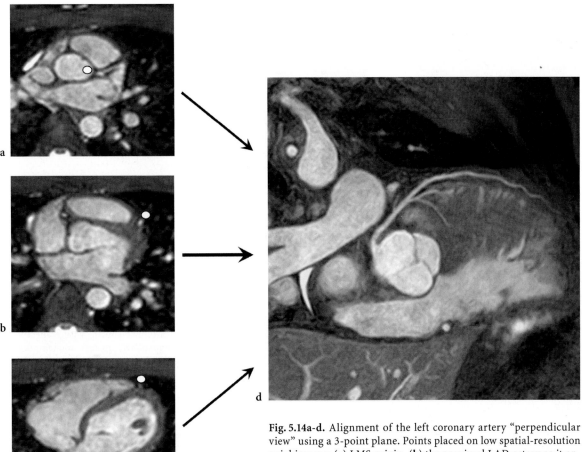

Fig. 5.14a-d. Alignment of the left coronary artery "perpendicular view" using a 3-point plane. Points placed on low spatial-resolution axial images: (**a**) LMS origin, (**b**) the proximal LAD artery as it enters the interventricular groove, and (**c**) the distal LAD artery in the interventricular groove toward the LV apex. High spatial-resolution image of the LMS and LAD visualized (**d**). Note septal branches of the LAD can be seen

cardiography than conventional cross-sectional imaging. Imaging planes can be stored and used to acquire high spatial and temporal resolution images during subsequent scanning. For uncooperative patients, interactive imaging can be of sufficient resolution to define cardiac structure for accurate diagnosis.

5.6
Segmentation of the Left Ventricle

For imaging the left ventricle, there is a need for standardization of imaging modalities to assure that accurate intra- and cross-modality comparisons can be made for patient management and research (nuclear cardiology, cardiac ultrasound, cardiovascular MR, cardiovascular CT, and cardiac catheter-

ization). Such methods are also important to enable comparison between the various cardiovascular MR techniques. Thus, wall motion abnormalities in one particular segment can be matched with perfusion and/or late-enhancement patterns in the same region of the heart.

A 17-segment frame of reference is used (CERQUEIRA et al. 2002). The heart is divided into three SA planes along the long axis of the LV: basal, mid-cavity, and apical (Fig. 5.16). These SA planes are then divided radially into 6 segments for the basal and mid-cavity SA slices, and 4 segments for the apical slice (Fig. 5.17); the 17th segment is the apex itself and is visualized on the long-axis images (VLA, HLA). The radial segments commence at the anterior junction of the LV and RV on the SA image and are then numbered in an anti-clockwise fashion in equal-sized segments around the LV. Thus, the anterior basal segment is segment 1, and the inferior

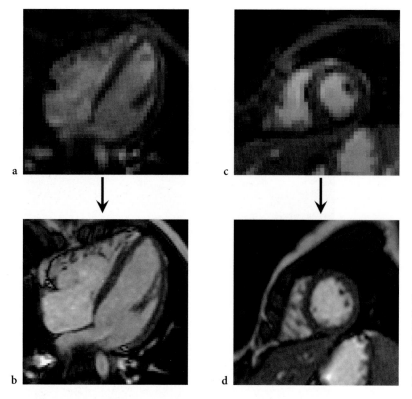

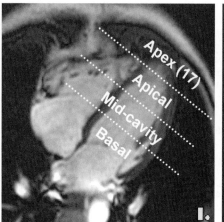

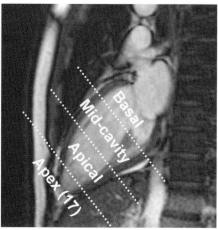

Fig. 5.15a-d. Low spatial- and temporal-resolution real-time, interactive images in the four-chamber (**a**) and SA planes (**c**) are shown, with respective, subsequent high spatial- and temporal-resolution balanced steady-state free precession images (**b, d**)

Fig. 5.16. Division of the LV into basal, mid-cavity, and apical SA segments for subsequent segment numbering (see Fig. 5.17) on four-chamber and VLA views. Segment 17, the apex, is seen on these long-axis views

lateral segment is segment 16 (Fig. 5.17). It should be noted that, with a slice thickness of 6–10 mm, the number of SA slices obtained with MRI exceeds the standardized division of the long-axis of the LV in three sections. Thus, in practice, the papillary muscles are used as anatomical landmarks to distinguish the mid-cavity SA slices from the apical and basal slices.

The entire 17 segments can be represented in a single image using a bull's-eye plot (Fig. 15.18) (Post et al. 1999). Furthermore, the segments can be related to the most common distribution of coronary artery anatomy in an attempt to correlate regional wall motion, perfusion, and/or late-enhancement abnormalities to specific coronary artery territories (see Fig. 8.9) (Schiller et al. 1989; Post et al. 1999).

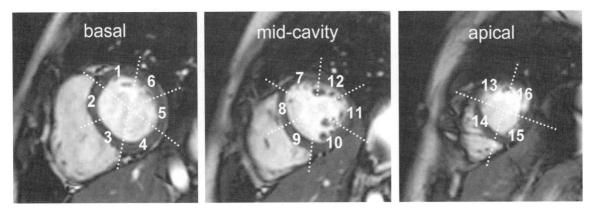

Fig. 5.17. Subsequent division of SA slices into 6 basal, 6 mid-cavity, and 4 apical segments, with segment 17 being the apex seen on the long-axis views (see Fig. 5.16). *Basal: 1,* anterior; *2,* anteroseptal; *3,* inferoseptal; *4,* inferior; *5,* inferolateral; *6,* anterolateral. *Mid-cavity: 7,* anterior, *8,* anteroseptal; *9,* inferoseptal; *10,* inferior; *11,* inferolateral; *12,* anterolateral. *Apical: 13,* anterior; *14,* septal; *15,* inferior; *16,* lateral

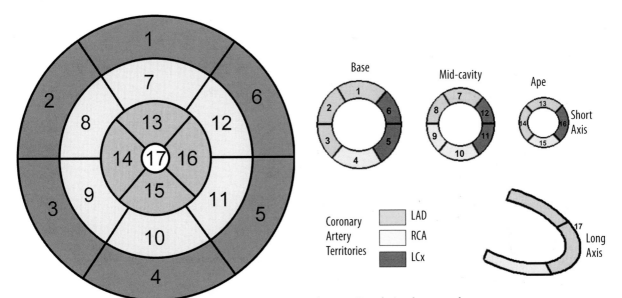

Fig. 5.18. Bull's-eye plot representation of all segments of the left ventricle. The segments numbers refer to the same segments as described in Fig. 5.17

Fig. 5.19. Correlation between the most common coronary artery distribution pattern and the seven segments of the left ventricle. Note there is tremendous variability in coronary blood supply to myocardial segments, in particular the apex (segment 17), which depens on right or left dominance.

5.7
Conclusion

An understanding of imaging planes in relation to both the axes of the body and the axes of the heart is necessary when imaging the heart with cardiovascular MR. This enables accurate description of cardiovascular anatomy and reliable standardization between the various cardiovascular imaging modalities.

References

Barkhausen J, Goyen M, Ruhm SG, et al (2002) Assessment of ventricular function with single breath-hold real-time steady-state free precession cine MR imaging. AJR Am J Roentgenol 178:731–735

Burbank F, Parish D, Wexler L (1988) Echocardiographic-like angled views of the heart by MR imaging. J Comput Assisted Tomogr 12:181–195

Cerqueira MD, Weissman NJ, Dilsizian V et al (2002) Standardized myocardial segmentation and nomenclature for tomographic imaging of the heart. Circulation 105:539–542

Hori Y, Yamada N, Higashi M, Hirai N, Nakatani S (2003) Rapid evaluation of right and left ventricular function and mass using real-time true-FISP cine MR imaging without breath-hold: comparison with segmented true-FISP cine MR imaging with breath-hold. J Cardiovasc Magn Reson 5:439–450

Lee VS, Resnick D, Bundy JM, et al (2002) Cardiac function: MR evaluation in one breath hold with real-time true fast imaging with steady state precession. Radiology 222:835–842

Longmore DB, Underwood SR, Hounsfield GN et al (1985) Dimensional accuracy of magnetic resonance in studies of the heart. Lancet I:1360–1362

Meier RA, Hartnell GG (1994) MRI of right atrial pseudo masses. Is it really a diagnostic problem? J Comput Assist Tomogr 18:398–402

Muthurangu V, Taylor AM, Andriantsimiavona R et al (2004) A novel method of quantifying pulmonary vascular resistance utilizing simultaneous invasive pressure monitoring and phase contrast MR flow. Circulation (in press)

Post S, Berman D, Garcia E et al (1999) Imaging guidelines for nuclear cardiology procedures: part 2. J Nucl Cardiol 6:49–84

Schiller N, Shah P, Crawford M et al (1989) A recommendation for quantification of the left ventricle by two-dimensional echocardiography. J Am Soc Echocardiogr 5:358–367

Stuber M, Botnar RM, Danias PG et al (1999) Double-oblique free-breathing high resolution three-dimensional coronary magnetic resonance angiography. J Am Coll Cardiol 34:524–531

Taylor AM, Keegan J, Jhooti P, et al (1999) Differences between normal subjects and patients with coronary artery disease for three different MR coronary angiography respiratory suppression techniques. J Magn Reson Imaging 9:786–793

6 Cardiac Function

Jan Bogaert

J. Bogaert MD, PhD
Department of Radiology, Gasthuisberg University Hospital, Catholic University of Leuven, Herestraat 49, 3000 Leuven, Belgium

6.1 Introduction

Since many cardiac diseases have an impact on the performance of the cardiac pump activity, assessment of cardiac performance (*cardiac function*) in an accurate and reproducible way is crucial to determine the disease severity and to evaluate the efficacy of treatment. This task, however, appears to be far more complicated than initially expected. For decades, investigators have explored different pathways and strategies to quantify global and regional cardiac performance, using a variety of techniques, ranging from the injection of dye for determining cardiac output to assessment of myocardial deformation by implantation of metallic beads. With the availability of noninvasive cardiac imaging modalities such as echocardiography and cardiac scintigraphy, assessment of cardiac function became part of the routine clinical examination. This urged for clinically useful functional parameters and the need to determine normal values and their physiological ranges.

The potential of magnetic resonance imaging (MRI) to study physiological phenomena such as cardiac pump activity was already evident in the mid-1980s (Matthaei et al. 1985). Thanks to major progress in MR hard- and software, MRI has emerged in less than two decades to be a preferred imaging modality to evaluate cardiac function. The cardiological community is becoming rapidly convinced of the opportunities offered by MRI. The combination of an excellent spatial, contrast, and temporal resolution, providing high-quality morphological images of the heart throughout the cardiac cycle, enables truly volumetric quantification and regional functional analysis. Velocity-encoded MRI techniques ("velocity mapping") allow assessment of flow profiles through cardiac valves and analysis of myocardial motion patterns. MR myocardial tagging techniques offer unique information about myocardial wall deformation and the mechanisms of myocardial contraction, while the new real-time sequences will further expand the clinical value of MRI. Although the principal aim of this textbook is to provide the reader with guidelines about how to use cardiac MRI in daily clinical routine, we feel that the role of MRI cannot be well understood without a brief discussion of the complexity of myocardial contraction and relaxation processes (Fig. 6.1).

6.2
Systolic Function

6.2.1
Mechanisms of Ventricular Contraction and Ejection

The heart can be considered as a highly sophisticated muscle, conceived to be the central circulatory pump. Anatomically, the main component of the ventricles is a thick-walled myocardium that surrounds the ventricular cavities. Electrical stimulation of individual myofibers leads to an increase in fiber tension and fiber shortening. At myocardial level, this fiber shortening is translated in a myocardial deformation or "strain" and a myocardial motion. At ventricular level, the myocardial deformation and motion is translated into a rise of ventricular pressure, and subsequent volume reduction of the ventricular cavities with *ejection* of blood into the great vessels (Fig. 6.2). This part of the cardiac cycle is defined as the contraction and ejection phase. Contraction starts after electrical stimulation and encompasses mitral valve closure, isovolumic contraction, and early ejection as long as left ventricular (LV) pressure is higher than aortic pressure.

Most fascinating in this cascade of events, is the efficiency of the ventricular pump function. With a myofiber shortening of approximately 10–15%, about 70% of the ventricular content is ejected.

To elucidate this apparent discrepancy, a brief description of the complex fiber anatomy and of the transmural fiber interaction is necessary. The individual myofibers are grouped in fiber bundles. Anatomically, the direction of these fiber bundles throughout the myocardial wall is highly variable. While the midwall fibers in the LV wall have a circumferential course, the fiber orientation progressively becomes oblique toward the endo- and epicardium, but are directed in an opposite direction (Streeter et al. 1969; Greenbaum et al. 1981). As a consequence, the epi- and endocardial oblique fibers are almost perpendicularly oriented toward each other. Truly longitudinally oriented fibers are, except in the papillary muscles and the endocardial trabeculations, sparse in the LV wall. As a direct consequence of this complex fiber orientation, contraction of the myofibers results in a complex myocardial and ventricular deformation. Contraction of the midwall fibers is responsible for a circumferential shortening with a centripetal wall motion, while longitudinal ventricular shortening is largely the result of the contraction of the oblique epi- and endocardial fibers. Myocardial wall thickening, though partly the result of centripetal wall motion by the circumferential shortening, is mainly due to an interaction between the oblique epi- and endocardial fibers. This transmural interaction, called "myocardial tethering," is based on a predominance of the torque of the epicardial fibers on the torque of the endocardial fibers. Shortening of the epicardial fiber bundles forces the endocardial fiber bundles to passively reorder, with shortening along the epicardial fiber direction, nearly perpendicular to the endocardial fiber direction. The magnitude of this "cross-fiber" endocardial shortening largely exceeds the endocardial fiber shortening. Based on the principle of conservation of mass, shortening of a volume in two directions necessitates lengthening in the remaining direction, i.e., wall thickening in the radial direction. Myocardial tethering can

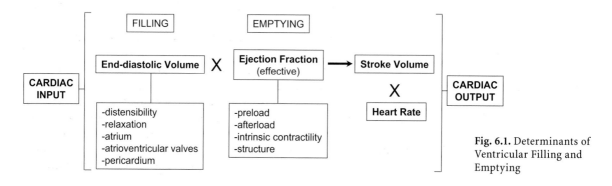

Fig. 6.1. Determinants of Ventricular Filling and Emptying

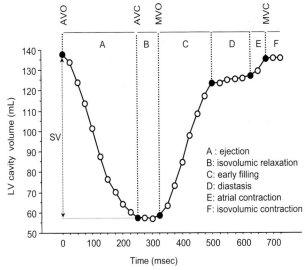

Fig. 6.2. Volume–time curve of the left ventricle during the cardiac cycle in a 27-year-old normal volunteer. Cine MRI, using the balanced steady-state free precession (b-SSFP) technique, in cardiac short-axis using contiguous 8-mm-thick slices, and 2-mm slice gap. Temporal resolution 24 ms. The different phases of the cardiac cycle (A–F) can be easily recognized on the volume–time curve. The onset of ejection (A) (characterized by decrease in left ventricular (LV) volume coincides with the aortic valve opening (AVO). At aortic valve closure (AVC), the minimal LV volume is obtained. The difference in volume between AVO and AVC represents the stroke volume (SV). The time period between AVC and MVO is the isovolumic relaxation (B). At the moment of mitral valve opening (MVO), ventricular filling start. This is characterized by an early, fast-filling phase (C), a period with nearly no filling, called "diastasis" (D), and a final phase of filling caused by the atrial contraction (E). The last part, i.e., isovolumic contraction, starts with mitral valve closure (MVC) and ends with AVO

A : ejection
B : isovolumic relaxation
C : early filling
D : diastasis
E : atrial contraction
F : isovolumic contraction

thus be considered a highly effective mechanism to improve the efficiency of the individual myocardial layers. Although deformation is the largest in the inner part of the myocardium, this deformation is directed by the outer myocardial wall. For instance, it has been shown that destruction of the epicardial fibers leads to an abolishment of endocardial cross-fiber shortening and wall thickening. In a normal human heart, the midwall circumferential shortening in the left ventricle is 30%, with higher values in the endocardial layers (approximately 44%), and lower in the epicardial layers (approximately 21%) (Palmon et al. 1994). Longitudinal shortening of the left ventricle is about 17% and radial wall thickening about 40–50% (Rogers et al. 1991; Bogaert and Rademakers 2001) (Figs. 6.3 and 6.4). This complex myocardial wall deformation and inward motion results in a volume reduction of LV cavity of approximately 70% at end-systole. It is important to emphasize that in pathological conditions, such as myocardial ischemia, the impact may not be the same on the different mechanisms of myocardial deformations. Since the subendocardium is particularly sensitive to myocardial ischemia, the long-axis function, largely reflecting the subendocardial function, may be a useful parameter to early detect ischemia (Brecker 2000).

Another intriguing phenomenon of the left ventricle is the torsion or twisting. The left ventricle exhibitis a counterclockwise rotation (when viewed from the apex), which is a component of normal systolic function (Buchalter et al. 1990, 1994). This wringing or rotational motion increases the longer the distance from the base (up to ±28° of rotation),

but the spread is fairly homogeneous from base to apex. Although the precise mechanism is unknown, it is probaly related to an imbalance between fibers with a left-hand and fibers with a right-hand obliquity, with dominance of epifibers over endofibers. Torsion leads to an increased efficiency of transmural myocardial function by equalizing fiber stress and function, and can therefore be considered as a necessary component of wall thickening and ejection (Arts et al. 1991). Moreover, it has been shown that torsion has a major role in normal myocardial relaxation. Contrary to what would be expected, return to the end-diastolic situation or untwisting does not occur during ventricular filling but starts much earlier, during isovolumic relaxation, and sometimes in the latter part of ejection. This leads to a clear dissociation between ventricular untwisting and filling (Rademakers et al. 1992; Dong et al. 2001). This dissociation is believed to be a potent mechanism in the suction of blood during early diastole. Although torsion was depicted and initially quantified using invasive methods, e.g., implanted beads and transducers, nowadays it can be noninvasively quantified with the use of MR myocardial tagging techniques.

Assessment of the performance of the entire ventricle not only consists of the evaluation of the contribution of the differents parts of the ventricle, but also involves analysis of the synchronization of events between different segments. It is well known that inhomogeneities in both magnitude and timing of deformation are present in the normal ventricle. In several disease states, such as myocardial ischemia or infarction, both synchronization of events and re-

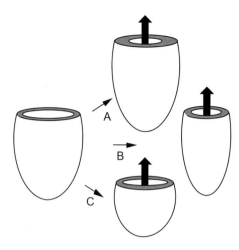

Fig. 6.3. Mechanisms of (left) ventricular ejection. On the *left* is shown the ventricle at end-diastole, and on the *right* the ventricle at end ejection: *A–C* represent three different hypothetical mechanisms of ventricular ejection: *A*, pure wall thickening; *B*, circumferential shortening; *C*, longitudinal ventricular shortening. Normal ventricular ejection relies on a combination of these three mechanisms

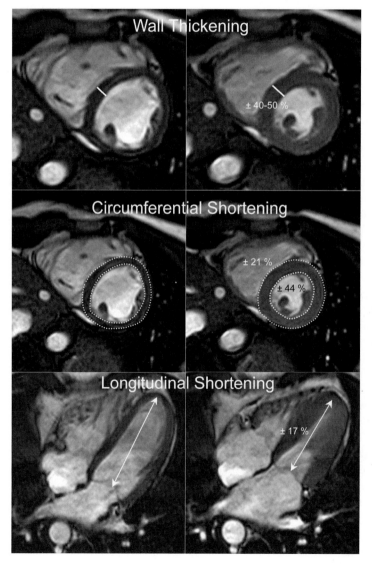

Fig. 6.4. Mechanisms of (left) ventricular ejection, studied with cine MRI. Cine MRI, using the b-SSFP technique, in the cardiac short-axis (*upper and middle row*), and horizontal long-axis (*bottom*), at end-diastole (*left*) and end-systole (*right*). The *upper row* represents the mechanism of wall thickening (mean value, approximately 40–50%), the *middle row* shows the mechanism of circumferential shortening, which is larger at the endocardium (mean value approximately 44%) than at the epicardium (mean value approximately 21%). The *lower row* shows the mechanism of longitudinal ventricular shortening (mean value approximately 17%).

gional nonuniformity may be disrupted (BOGAERT and RADEMAKERS 2001). Use of a single timepoint for end-systole is not sufficient to elucidate this temporal inhomogeneity, nor to assess the maximal extent of deformation. Although there is one single timepoint where the ventricle reaches its smallest volume and ejection ends, maximal deformation for every segment of the ventricle does not necessarily occur at that specific timepoint. For instance, post-systolic contraction is a well-know phenomenon in ischemically diseased myocardium (Fig. 6.5). Use of multiple timepoints during the cardiac cycle from the second half of systole to the end of isovolumic relaxation enables elucidation and quantification of this inhomogeneity.

6.2.2
Ventricular Volumes, Function and Mass

6.2.2.1
Parameters of
Global Ventricular Function and Ventricular Mass

Assessment of global ventricular function generally includes measuring the adequacy of the ventricles to eject blood into the great vessels. Since the ventricles exhibit a repetitive process of ejection and filling, the filling process should be considered part of the global ventricular performance. For the sake of simplicity, the diastolic ventricular function is discussed separately (see Sect. 6.3). Although ideally the changes in ventricular volumes and the velocity of these changes during systole should be assessed

to obtain a complete description of the global ventricular performance, in clinical routine only the ventricular volumes at maximal filling, i.e., at end-diastole, and maximal emptying, i.e., at end-systole, are usually quantified. From these two volumetric parameters, i.e., end-diastolic volume and end-systolic volume, all other global functional parameters can be deduced. Subtracting the end-systolic volume from the end-diastolic volume yields the stroke volume (Table 6.1). The stroke volume divided by the end-diastolic volume gives the ejection fraction. The stroke volume multiplied by the heart rate gives the cardiac output. Moreover, from these values, normalized values can be calculated. It is evident that the reliability of the deduced global ventricular parameters is only as good as the accuracy by which the end-diastolic and end-systolic volumes are determined. Another important parameter of global ventricular performance, and an independent predictor of morbidity and mortality from coronary

Table 6.1. Global functional parameters

EDV – ESV = SV (ml)
SV/EDV = EF (%)
SV x HR = CO (ml/min)
EDV$_{INDEX}$ = EDV/BSA (l/m^2)
ESV$_{INDEX}$ = ESV/BSA (ml/m^2)
CO/BSA = CI (l/min/m^2)

BSA, body surface area; CI, cardiac index; CO, cardiac output; EDV, end-diastolic volume; EF, ejection fraction; ESV, end-systolic volume; HR, heart rate; SV, stroke volume

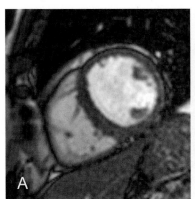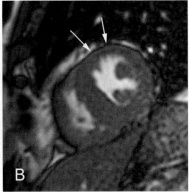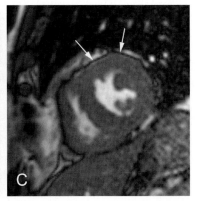

Fig. 6.5a–c. Postsystolic contraction during dobutamine-atropine stress MRI study in a patient with significant stenosis in the proximal left anterior descending coronary artery (LAD) coronary artery. Cine MRI, using the b-SSFP technique, in the midventricular cardiac short-axis at end-diastole (**a**), end-systole (**b**), and isovolumic relaxation (**c**). During systole (**b**), the ischemic myocardium in the anterior wall is akinetic (*arrows*). However, during isovolumic relaxation (**c**), while the nonischemic regions start to relax, myocardial thickening can be clearly seen in the ischemic anterior LV wall (*arrows*).

heart disease, is the ventricular or myocardial mass (LEVY et al. 1990).

6.2.2.2
Geometric Assumptions versus Volumetric Ventricular Quantification

Two different approaches are currently available to obtain the ventricular volumes, global function, and myocardial mass, i.e., geometric assumptions and volumetric ventricular quantification. Geometric assumptions compare the ventricular cavity with a geometrical model. Using a (limited) number of standardized measurements of the ventricular cavity, the corresponding volumes are calculated. For the left ventricle, either short-axis views, e.g., hemisphere cylinder model, modified Simpson's technique, or Teichholz model; either long-axis views, e.g., biplane ellipsoid and single-plane ellipsoid model; or a combination of long- and short-axis views is used for calculations of ventricular volumes (DULCE et al. 1993; THIELE et al. 2002) (Fig. 6.6). Geometric assumptions are used in planar imaging techniques, such as contrast ventriculography and radionuclide scintigraphy, as well as in echocardiography (M-Mode and 2D). They have the advantage of rapidly obtaining ventricular volumes and LV mass, but they are only reliable as long the geometrical model corresponds to the true ventricular cavity or myocardial wall, which might not be the case in focally diseased ventricles (Fig. 6.7). Moreover, their role is limited in assessing small but significant changes in global ventricular function. With the advent of new tomographic cardiac imaging techniques, e.g., 3D-echocardiography, computed tomography (CT), and MRI, true volumetric quantification became feasible. Volumetric quantification is based on the Simpson's rule. The volume of a complex structure such as a ventricle can be quantified by dividing this structure into several smaller, less complex subvolumes (Fig. 6.6). Volume quantification of all subvolumes yields the total volume of the complex structure. In practice, this is obtained by using a stack of parallel slices encompassing the entire ventricle. By delineation of the endocardial contours, multiplication of the area by the thickness of the imaging plane and the interslice distance, and addition of these (sub)volume slices yields the total ventricular volume. Volumetric quantifcation has the advantage of quantifying more reliably the ventricular volumes and being more easily reproducible than the geometric assumptions techniques, but is, on the other hand, usually more time-con-

suming both for image acquisition and postprocessing. Recently, Thiele and colleagues have proposed a new combined triplane geometric model, using a combination of short-axis, and vertical and horizontal long-axis to estimate LV volumes (THIELE et al. 2002) (Fig. 6.6). In comparison with the volumetric data set, this geometric model in combination with the b-SSFP GE technique yields the best accuracy and reproducibility, even in patients with regional dysfunction. Notwithstanding the superiority of true volumetric approaches, in clinical practice the use of geometric assumptions may be useful, for instance if something goes wrong in the volumetric data acquisition or as a fast check for the validity of results obtained by the volumetric approach. For example, the use of a simple geometric formula $(L1 \times L2 \times L3 \times \Pi)/6$, where L1 represents the long-axis diameter of the LV (obtained on vertical or horizontal long-axis images), and L2 and L3 represent the maximal short-axis diameters in two perpendicular views, can be recommended for these purposes.

For calculation of ventricular mass, using the volumetric approach, the same stack of images (preferably in the short-axis direction) is used on which the epicardial and endocardial contours are delineated with inclusion of the papillary muscles (AURIGEMMA et al. 1992; LIMA et al. 1993; FORBAT et al. 1994; GERMAIN et al. 1992). Taking into account slice thickness and interslice distance, LV mass can be obtained by multiplication of the volume with the specific density of myocardium, 1.05 g/cm^3. To obtain the most reliable estimates of ventricular volumes and masses, several issues, discussed in the following paragraphs, should be taken into consideration.

6.2.2.3
MRI Sequence Design

Although the spin-echo (SE) MRI technique can be used for quantification of global ventricular function and ventricular mass (PATTYNAMA et al. 1992), this technique is time-consuming, and the single-phase, multislice approach is less convenient, since the different slices through the ventricle are obtained at different phases of the cardiac cycle (CAPUTO et al. 1990). Even if, with the newer turbo SE and half-Fourier single-shot turbo SE (HASTE), image acquisition is much faster and images can be obtained at a specific timepoints during the cardiac cycle, the SE technique is primarily used in cardiac imaging for morphological analysis. In

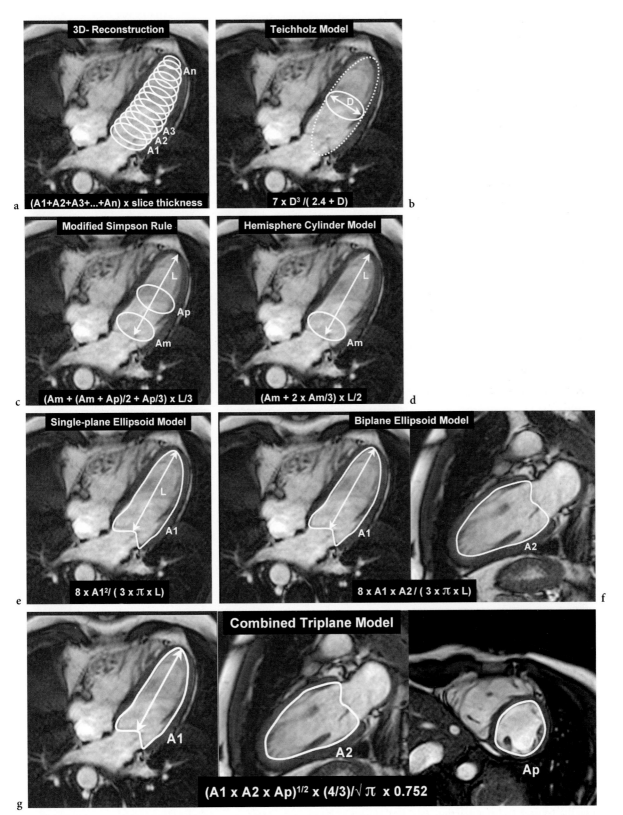

Fig. 6.6a–g. Geometric assumptions versus volumetric ventricular quantification. (**a**) 3D volumetric quantification; (**b**) Teichholz method; (**c**) modified Simpson's method; (**d**) hemisphere cylinder method; (**e**) single-plane ellipsoid model; (**f**) biplane ellipsoid model; (**g**) combined triplane model. The formula for each of the different techniques is shown at the bottom of each figure. Abbreviations: *A*, area; *Am*, area at mitral level; *Ap*, area at papillary level; *D*, diameter; *L*; length

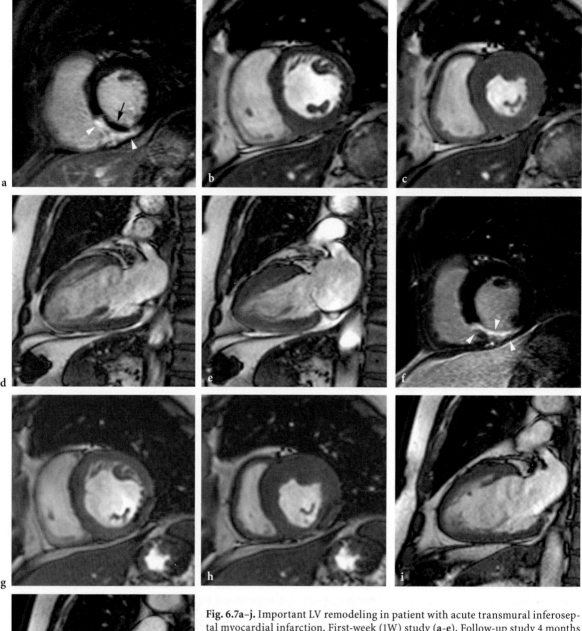

Fig. 6.7a–j. Important LV remodeling in patient with acute transmural inferoseptal myocardial infarction. First-week (1W) study (**a-e**), Follow-up study 4 months (4M) after the acute event (**f-j**). Contrast-enhanced inversion-recovery MRI with late imaging in cardiac short-axis (**a, f**). Cine MRI, using b-SSFP technique, in cardiac short-axis at end-diastole (**b, g**) and end-systole (**c, h**); and in vertical long-axis at end-diastole (**d, i**) and end-systole (**e, j**). During the acute event, contrast-enhanced MRI (**a**) shows transmural enhancement inferoseptally in the mid-basal part of the left ventricle (*white arrowheads*). Presence of an important no-reflow zone with more than 50% transmural extension (*black arrow*). The infarct area is edematously thickened and shows severe hypokinesia on cine MR images (**b-e**). At 4 months, the fibrotic, old infarction is well defined on contrast-enhanced MR images (*arrowheads*) (**f**). Due to scar formation, the transmural infarct area has become thin and is functionally akinetic (**g-j**). Assessment of global LV function using the 3D volumetric approach shows moderately decreased function the 1st week (ejection fraction, EF, 54%). However, due to an important remodeling of the ventricle, at 4 months after the acute event, end-diastolic and mainly end-systolic volumes are increased, while stroke volume and ejection fraction show an important decrease (EF 40.5%). Although most of the geometric assumption techniques show a decrease in global function (EF), they obviously underestimate the severity of the LV remodeling.

▷ ▷

contrast, the spoiled gradient-echo (GE) MRI technique, i.e., fast low flip-angle single-shot (FLASH) or fast field-echo (FFE) sequence, overcomes many of the limitations of the SE technique (SECHTEM et al. 1987; UTZ et al. 1987; BUSER et al. 1989). The use of shorter repetition times, e.g., 30–40 ms, with small flip angles enables one to obtain images at multiple, consecutive timepoints during the cardiac cycle within a certain image slice. Loading the images into a cine or movie loop provides information about the cardiac dynamics, e.g., myocardial motion and deformation, ventricular contraction and filling, valve leaflet motion. Blood–myocardium contrast in the spoiled GE-technique is based on inflow enhancement, i.e., repetitive excitation progressively suppresses the stationary tissues in the image slice, while the blood pool is continuously refreshed by inflow of fully relaxed spins into the image slice. As a result, the ventricular blood pool is shown as bright, the surrounding myocardium as gray. The best blood–myocardium contrast is obtained in short-axis images (largest through-plane flow), while long-axis planes may suffer from in-plane saturation especially toward the LV apex. Although the introduction of the spoiled GE-technique in cardiac imaging allowed the noninvasive study of cardiac dynamics, its clinical use to study cardiac patients was limited, because this sequence was too time-consuming (i.e., acquisition time of several minutes per image slice).

The real breakthrough of MRI in the clinical evaluation of ventricular function coincided with the introduction of the fast, segmented spoiled-GE sequences in the early 1990s (ATKINSON and EDELMAN 1991; BLOOMGARDEN et al. 1997). By acquiring multiple lines of κ-space per heartbeat (i.e., "segmented approach"), use of very short repetition times and low flip angles, imaging time could be reduced to the length of a breath-hold, at the expense, however, of a longer acquisition window. Breath-hold segmented κ-space cine MRI is not only an effective means to speed up image acquisition but also to reduce substantially the respiratory motion artifacts (SCHULEN et al. 1996). As a result, 8–12 breath-holds are sufficient to encompass the left ventricle in the short-axis direction (using a slice thickness of 8 mm and a slice gap of 2 mm), making this technique appealing for clinical use. Using the breath-hold segmented cine MRI technique, the best compromise between breath-hold duration and acquisition window has to be determined (see Sect. 6.2.2.7). For years, this segmented κ-space cine MRI sequence has been recommended to study the global and regional ventricular function in rest and stress conditions, and to visualize valvular regurgitation and stenosis (SAKUMA et al. 1993; BOGAERT et al. 1995).

Low contrast between myocardium and blood-filled ventricular cavities with the spoiled-GE cine MRI technique, however, severely impedes the ability to use automated edge-detection algorithms (ROMIGER et al. 1999). Accordingly, time-consuming and tedious manual tracing of epi-and endocardial contours is the only alternative. Although several authors have advocated the use of intravascular contrast agents to increase the blood–myocardium contrast (STILLMANN et al. 1997; ALLEY et al. 1999), the recent introduction of the b-SSFP GE sequence in cardiac imaging (BARKHAUSEN et al. 2001; CARR et al. 2001; THIELE et al. 2001) is very probably the ideal solution to solve this intrinsic limitation of the spoiled-GE technique. Several papers have convincingly shown the superiority of the b-SSPF cine MRI compared with the spoiled-GE cine MRI technique; and nowadays this sequence has become the standard sequence with which to study cardiac function (PLEIN et al. 2001; THIELE et al. 2001; MOON et al. 2002; LEE et al. 2002; FIENO et al. 2002; ALFAKIH et al. 2003; HORI et al. 2003; SPUENTRUP et al. 2003). Tissue signal in the b-SSFP sequence is based on T2/T1 relaxation behavior and is largely inflow-independent. As a result, a high contrast is created between blood-filled ventricular cavities (high signal) and myocardium (low signal), allowing a significantly better detection of the endocardial border than the spoiled-GE technique (BARKHAUSEN et al. 2001). Whereas the endocardial border is usually smoothed by a slow flow phenomenon using the spoiled-GE technique, yielding the risk of overestimation of the true myocardial wall thickness, the individual trabeculations can be clearly differentiated from the surrounding blood on the b-SSFP technique. Moreover, on long-axis images particu-

Fig. 6.7a–j. (Continued)

	EDV (ml)		ESV (ml)		SV (ml)		EF (%)	
	1W	4M	1W	4M	1W	4M	1W	4M
3D volumetric	158	171	73	102	85	69	54.0	40.5
Modified Simpson	182	195	87	105	95	100	52.2	51.2
Hemisphere	196	209	99	112	97	97	49.4	46.4
Teichholz	167	173	83	93	84	80	50.2	46.2
Single-plane	202	195	73	83	129	112	63.9	57.4
Biplane	206	200	78	88	128	112	62.1	56.0
Combined triplane	205	208	81	97	124	111	60.5	53.3

larly, in-plane saturation of the ventricular blood-pool signal intensity with the spoiled-GE sequence is absent with the b-SSFP technique. The consequence of the improved endocardial border visualization and absence of saturation effects on ventricular volume and mass calculations is a significant increase in ventricular volumes, and otherwise a decrease in myocardial mass compared with the spoiled-GE technique (Moon et al. 2002; Alfakih et al. 2003) (Table 6.2). As a consequence, automated image-segmentation techniques should also benefit from the increased discrimination of the blood–myocardium interface with the b-SSFP technique, thereby reducing the manual correction of the delineated contours.

Table 6.2. Influence of MRI sequence on LV volume and mass calculations in controls and patients. Adapted from Moon et al. (2002)

	Spoiled-GE	b-SSFP	Difference		p-value
CONTROLS (n=10)					
EDV (ml)	133 ± 37	151 ± 37	18	(13%)	<0.001
ESV (ml)	46 ± 14	55 ± 18	9	(17%)	0.001
EF (%)	66 ± 3	64 ± 4	−2	(−3%)	0.19
LV MASS (g)	145 ± 46	120 ± 37	−25	(−19%)	<0.001
PATIENTS (n=10)					
EDV (ml)	202 ± 78	208 ± 69	6	(4%)	0.25
ESV (ml)	116 ± 65	123 ± 65	8	(6%)	0.001
EF (%)	44 ± 14	43 ± 17	−2	(−4%)	0.27
LV mass (g)	202 ± 46	181 ± 51	−21	(−11%)	<0.001

Spoiled-GE: spoiled gradient-echo, b-SSFP: balanced steady-state free-precession

6.2.2.4
Correction for Through-Plane Motion

Through-plane motion represents a major challenge to achieve accurate volume measurements of the ventricular cavities during the cardiac cycle. The currently used 2D tomographic MRI techniques with fixed imaging planes are limited to studying organs with complex 3D motion patterns such as the cardiac ventricles. As a result of through-plane motion, the position of the heart toward a fixed imaging plane will continuously change during the cardiac cycle, and different parts of the heart will be visualized on consecutive images in this imaging plane. Through-plane motion is most obvious on cardiac short-axis images in the base of the heart, at the interface of the atria and ventricles. This is the result of pronounced longitudinal shortening of the ventricles (approximately 15% in normal ventricles), whereby the base of the heart moves toward the cardiac apex (ROGERS et al. 1991). As a consequence of this long-axis shortening, a short-axis slice positioned through the base of the left ventricle at end-diastole will be located in the left atrium during systole (Fig. 6.8). Without correction for through-plane motion, end-systolic volumes are significantly overestimated, and stroke volumes underestimated (MARCUS et al. 1999a). An added difficulty is the delineation of the left ventricle toward the left atrium, since it is not always possible to accurately identify the mitral valve. Often the mitral valve ring plane is used, which slightly overestimates LV volumes.

Although correction for through-plane motion may be directly achieved with slice-tracking, this promising feature is not yet clinically available (KOZERKE et al. 1999, 2001). So, correction techniques need to be applied during image postprocessing, or alternative approaches need to be used where

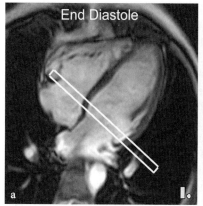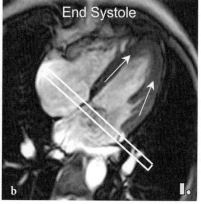

Fig. 6.8a,b. Effect of through-plane motion. Horizontal long-axis cine MRI, using the b-SSFP technique, at end-diastole (a) and end-systole (b). As a consequence of longitudinal shortening (arrows) of the ventricle during systole, a short-axis slice through the basal part of the left ventricle at end-diastole will be positioned in the left atrium at end-systole

the effects of through-plane motion are not present or at least less pronounced. The slice-omission technique omits the slices that are atrially located at end-systole. Based on LV morphology, short-axis slices with a complete muscular ring are considered as "ventricular," while incomplete muscular rings with less than 75% myocardium or thin-walled rings are regarded as "atrial." This slice-ommission approach, although easy to apply, is not entirely correct, since the mitral valve anatomy is not taken into account. A second approach is to measure the longitudinal LV shortening on a (vertical or horizontal) long-axis view and use this information to correct the short-axis images at end-systole. For example, when measuring a longitudinal shortening of 10 mm, the most basal slice (using a slice thickness of 8 mm and gap of 2 mm) at end-diastole will be atrially located at end-systole and needs to be omitted to obtain a reliable estimate. Therefore, it is important to position the most basal slice at end-diastole perfectly through the most basal part of the left ventricle. Another, but more difficult approach, necessitating experience, is using a priori knowledge about cardiac morphology during delineation of the images, e.g., exclusion of the mitral valve area but inclusion of the LV outflow tract region into the ventricular cavity. Other potentially interesting approaches include the use of a different cardiac image plane or a combination of different image planes, e.g., radial approach (see Sect. 6.2.2.5). Since correction for through-plane motion has a major impact on the calculated ventricular volumes, a consistent approach is definitely necessary for repeated studies.

6.2.2.5
Cardiac Image Plane

The choice of imaging plane is another important issue in assessing ventricular function. Although most studies in literature recommend the short-axis imaging plane, it may be worth comparing the advantages and limitations of the different options in imaging planes. The short-axis imaging plane has several advantages: most of the left ventricle, except the most basal and apical portion, can be very easily studied. The papillary muscles as well as the smaller msucular trabeculations are well definable, and the short-axis plane allows analysis of regional function in 16 of the 17 standardized wall segments (except the LV apex or segment 17; see Chap. 5) (CERQUEIRA et al. 2002). The major limitation of the short-axis plane is the difficulty in assessing the mitral valve, and the interface between left

ventricle and left atrium. Taking into account the important through-plane motion occurring in the LV base, any inaccuracy in defining the atrioventricular interface will have a significant impact on the global left ventricular volume. For instance, using a slice thickness of 1 cm, the most basal LV slice has a volume of 17 ± 9 ml and 9 ± 4 ml at end-diastole and end-systole, respectively (normal volunteers; unpublished data). If the LV has an end-diastolic volume of 130 ml and an end-systolic volume of 45 ml, inclusion or exclusion of the basal slice leads to change in volume of 13% and 20%, respectively. Toward the LV apex, the curving of the lateral walls leads to partial volume effects which may influence the reliability of wall mass calculations, as well as the assessment of myocardial wall thickness and systolic wall thickening (see Sect. 6.2.3).

Scanning in the transverse or horizontal long-axis plane has the major advantage that the mitral valve and the interface between left ventricle and left atrium, as well as the LV apex, are clearly visible. These advantages are also valid for the right ventricle. Even if some through-plane motion occurs at the anterior and inferior wall, and at the region of the aortic valve, the impact is far less pronounced than the basal ventricular motion in the short-axis plane. Volumes and volume changes in the image slice just below the aortic valve, i.e., LV outflow tract, are much smaller than in the basal LV slice on short-axis views, i.e., 6 ± 1 ml at end-diastole, 5 ± 1 ml at end-systole (unpublished data). Thus, inaccuracies to correct for the volume changes in this slice will have only a minimal impact on LV volume calculations. The largest shortcomings of scanning in these imaging planes are the risk of under- or overestimation of ventricular volumes by inconsistency in breath-hold position during the repetitive breath-holds, a problem that may be overcome by using a single breath-hold regime; and the risk of partial volume effects, occurring at the anterior and inferior LV wall, and in the neighborhood of the papillary muscles.

A combination of imaging planes may overcome at least some of the inaccuracies related to the use of a single imaging plane approach. A combination of long-axis and short-axis images, for instance, whereby short-axis information is used for the main, central part of the left ventricle, and the long-axis information for assessment of the apical and basal part of the left ventricle, may be a good alternative. Fusion of the short- and long-axis information, however, is still quite problematic. Another interesting approach, described by Bloomer and colleagues, is a radial approach with long-axis views, whereby the image plane is oriented radially around the long-axis center line of the left ventricle (BLOOMER et al. 2001; CLAY et al. 2004). This approach, especially in combination with the b-SSFP cine MRI technique, has several advantages. The aortic valve, mitral valve and LV apex are clearly visible; effects of through-plane motion as well as partial volume effects are minimal; and interobserver variability is low (variability <2.3%).

6.2.2.6
Endo- and Epicardial Borders, Endocardial Trabeculations, and Papillary Muscles

Precise delineation of the endo- and epicardial ventricular borders is crucial for accurate quantification of ventricular mass and volumes. As discussed in Sect. 6.2.2.3, visualization of the endocardial borders is closely related to the type of cine MRI sequence. Visualization of the external myocardial border is often impeded at regions where the difference in signal intensity between myocardium and adjacent tissue, such as lung parenchyma and subdiaphragmatic tissues, is minimal. As a rule of thumb, endo- and epicardial border visualization can be enhanced using the ventricular dynamics, i.e., by means of using the cine viewing mode.

Anatomical structures such as the papillary muscles and endocardial muscular trabeculations have a significant impact on ventricular volume and mass calculations (Table 6.3). Therefore, it should be decided whether or not to include these structures either in the myocardium or in the ventricular cavity, and consistency is necessary in follow-up studies (Fig. 6.9). Though there are no absolute recommendations, it may be advisable to include the papillary muscles in the myocardium in patients with hypertensive diseases, hypertrophic cardiomyopathy, or myocardial storage diseases, because of concomitant hypertrophy of the papillary muscles. This ap-

Table 6.3. Inclusion or exclusion of papillary muscles and trabeculae into the LV cavity and the influence on global functional parameters and left ventricular mass

	Papillary muscles and trabeculae included	Papillary muscles excluded	Trabeculae excluded
EDV (ml)	130.8 ± 33.4	120.8 ± 31.7	101.1 ± 27.8*
ESV (ml)	51.2 ± 15.5	42.4 ± 14.3	32.6 ± 11.1*
EF (%)	60.9 ± 3.7	65.2 ± 4.4	68.2 ± 4.8*
Mass (g)	110.6 ± 23.1	118.7 ± 23.0	129.7 ± 25.1*

*(p<0.001)
IBRAHIM et al. 1999

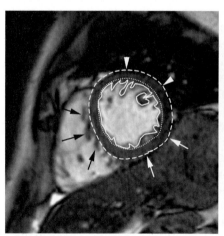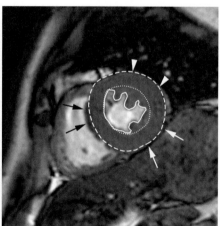

a   b

Fig. 6.9a,b. Impact of endocardial trabeculations and papillary muscles on calculations of LV volumes, mass, and function. Midventricular short-axis cine MRI, using the b-SSFP technique, at end-diastole (a) and end-systole (b). The *continuous line* shows the endocardial border, including the papillary muscles and trabeculations into the myocardium. The *fine dashed line* shows the endocardial border, excluding the above structures from the myocardium. The *coarse dashed line* shows the epicardial LV border. Note that the interface with the adjacent lung (*white arrowheads*) and infradiaphragmatic structures (*white arrows*) impedes the visualization of the epicardial contours. Compaction of the endocardial trabeculations in the right ventricle to the ventricular septum at end-systole (*black arrows*) may lead to an overestimation of the true septal wall thickness and thus of the LV mass.

	EDV (ml)	ESV (ml)	SV (ml)	EF (%)	Mass (g)
Papillary muscles/trabeculations included in myocardium	134	39	95	71	138
Papillary muscles/trabeculations included in LV cavity	161	59	102	63	114

proach yields the best quantification of the exact myocardial mass. On the other hand, assessment of regional myocardial morphology and function usually benefits from the exclusion of the trabeculations and especially of the papillary muscles. Since these structures "pollute" the regional functional data, exclusion is the best guarantee to provide homogeneous data throughout the ventricle (see Sect. 6.2.3). Automated contouring programs often struggle with the recognition and delineation of the papillary muscles. This is mainly related to the complex anatomy, and problems often arise when the papillary muscles are not in contact with the myocardial wall.

6.2.2.7
Temporal and Spatial Resolution

Functional cardiac imaging with MRI is constrained by several parameters. One important parameter is definitely total acquisition time. With breath-hold techniques, acquisition times are limited by patient comfort and capability, and should be less than 16–20 s for most patients. With implementation of segmented κ-space methods, multiple κ-lines per heartbeat per image are acquired, reducing the total imaging time to the length of a breath-hold period. Total acquisition time can be traded for temporal resolution. For example, increasing the number of κ-lines per heartbeat from 7 to 9, using 128 phase-encoding steps and a TR of 9 ms, reduces the breath-hold length from 18 to 14 heartbeats, but involuntarily the temporal resolution increases from 63 to 81 ms. Thus, shortening of the breath-hold duration allows faster imaging and increases patient comfort but yields the risk of increased blurring due to cardiac motion. With acquisition windows that are too long (e.g., 80–100 ms), only a few images per cardiac cycle can be obtained, reducing not only the quality of the dynamic views, but also volume calculations, especially at end-systole, might be less accurate because of rapid changes in volume occurring at the temporal boundary of the images (SETSER et al. 2000). Since end-systole only lasts for as little as 40–50 ms, incorrect determination of end-systole will lead to a slight overestimation of end-systolic volumes, and underestimation of stroke volumes and ejection fractions (BARKHAUSEN et al. 2002; MILLER et al. 2002). One way to overcome this problem is echo- or view-sharing (Foo et al. 1995). Using echo-sharing the effective temporal resolution can be improved, i.e., doubled, without changing the true temporal resolution or acquisition time (number of

κ-lines × TR). The principle of echo-sharing is based on reconstructing new images with a timing exactly in between two original images. The reconstructed intermediate image is obtained by using the second half of the κ-lines from the previous original image and the first half of the κ-lines from the next original image. Another way to achieve a better temporal resolution is the use of echo-planar readout schemes (LAMB et al. 1996; BORNSTEDT et al. 2001). Temporal (or spatial) resolution can also be improved by combining the fast b-SSFP sequences with parallel imaging (i.e., simultaneous acquisition of spatial harmonics or sensitivity encoding) (SODICKSON and MANNING 1997; GRISWOLD et al. 1999; WEIGER et al. 2000). The speed of these techniques results from reducing the number of phase-encoding gradient steps by extracting spatial information contained in a radiofrequency (RF) coil array (see Chap. 1). Because of the excellent contrast-to-noise ratios, b-SSFP sequences are well suited to these approaches (BARKHAUSEN et al. 2002).

Spatial resolution, both in-plane and through-plane, has a significant impact on ventricular volume and mass calculations (MILLER et al. 2002). Normally, an in-plane pixel size of 1–2 mm can be achieved in a reasonable breath-hold period while maintaining high temporal resolution. A significant change in LV end-diastolic volume, as much as 11%, occurs when pixel size is increased to 3 mm (MILLER et al. 2002). However, no significant change in LV mass is found with increasing pixel size. Slice thickness and slice spacing are important not only to determine the total measurement time but have an impact on determining regional and global function parameters. Use of thinner slices is benefical to reduce partial volume effects occurring at the blood–myocardium interface, especially toward the LV apex, and thus to obtain sharper depiction of the myocardial borders. The disadvantage is that more slices (and thus more breath-holds) are required to encompass the ventricle, increasing the total acquisition time and postprocessing time. Although thinner slices yield the risk of decreased signal-to-noise ratio with lower acccuracy rates, the effect is counteracted by the high intrinsic contrast-to-noise ratios with the b-SSFP cine MRI technique. In practice, 6- to 10-mm-thick slices in adults and 5- to 8-mm-thick slices in children with the b-SSFP technique can be recommended. Use of noncontiguous slices to encompass the ventricle is beneficial to reduce total imaging and postprocessing time; although, in a comparative study, DEBATIN and colleagues (1992a) have shown that use of contiguous slices is more accurate than increased slice spacing to calculate ventricular volumes, COTTIN et al. (1999) have found in a more recent study that an intersection gap as large as 10 mm has no signficant influence of the accuracy of volume measurements.

6.2.2.8
Real-time MRI

The availability of MR scanners with stronger gradients and faster gradient-switching capabilities, improved field shimming, new sequences such as b-SSFP MRI, new technologies such as parallel imaging, and different κ-space fill-in strategies such as partial κ-space filling or spiral κ-space filling have offered the possibility of studying cardiac dynamics in real-time without the necessity of ECG triggering (SETSER et al. 2000; KAJI et al. 2001; BARKHAUSEN et al. 2002; LEE et al. 2002; SPUENTRUP et al. 2003). Since imaging is extremely fast, examination time can be reduced, and patient discomfort and cost be minimized. No data averaging of several heartbeats is needed. This makes it possible to scan patients with absolute arrhythmia or frequent premature ventricular complexes, or to assess the influence of hemodynamic maneuvers (NAGEL et al. 2000). In combination with interactive planning tools, real-time planning and adaptation of imaging planes is feasible. For ventricular volume calculations, it is possible to image with real-time MRI the complete ventricle within one breath-hold which might further improve the diagnostic accuracy of MR stress testing. In patients unable to hold their breath, such as small children or incooperative patients, even non-breath-hold real-time MRI can be applied for ventricular volume calculations. Hori and colleagues have found a close correlation between non-breath-hold real-time b-SSFP and the breath-hold multislice, segmented b-SSFP technique (HORI et al. 2003). The dramatic reduction of data-acquisition time in real-time MRI, however, requires compromises in spatial and/or temporal resolution. As outlined above, the best compromise needs to be determined in order to obtain the most reliable estimates. Currently, the temporal resolution as short as 60 ms per image in combination with an in-plane spatial resolution of 2–3 mm is feasible.

6.2.2.9
Right Ventricular Volumes, Function, and Mass

Accurate quantification of right ventricular (RV) volumes, function, and mass is important in congenital and acquired cardiac diseases involving the right ventricle, such as tetralogy of Fallot, transposition of the great arteries, single ventricle, arrhythmogenic RV dysplasia, and pulmonary hypertension (e.g., chronic obstructive pulmonary disease and chronic pulmonary thromboemboli) (KATZ et al. 1993; TARDIVON et al. 1994; CASALINO et al. 1996; MARCUS et al. 1998; KROFT et al. 2000; HOEPER et al. 2001). The necessity of using volumetric quantification techniques such as MRI to quantify RV volumes and function is even more important than for the left ventricle, because of its complex geometry (MARKIEWICZ et al. 1987a). The value of echocardiography and other imaging techniques that use geometric assumptions to estimate RV function and ejection fraction is limited. Most of the problems and challenges to obtain accurate measurements, discussed in the previous paragraphs, are also valid for the right ventricle. However, some features specific for the right ventricle need to be highlighted. A first issue is the imaging plane that is best suited for RV volumetric and mass analysis. Due to its complexicity, probably no single imaging plane is well suited to study the right ventricle. The short-axis imaging plane, commonly used to study the left ventricle, is not ideal to study the right ventricle. On short-axis images, the interface between right ventricle and right atrium is nearly invisible, and strategies used for the left ventricle are not useful for the right ventricle. JAUHIAINEN and colleagues (2002) recommend the use of a transverse or a RV inflow view (imaging plane perpendicular to the axis drawn from the RV apex through the middle of the tricuspid annulus) to quantify RV ventricular volumes and mass. In the absence of RV hypertrophy, the RV wall is very thin, i.e., 2–4 mm, and therefore difficult to quantify. In contrast to the three-layered LV wall (i.e., oblique endo- and epicardial layer, circumferential midwall), the RV wall has a two-layered appearance: oblique epicardial fibers, and longitudinally oriented endocardial fibers, whereby the endocardial fibers follow the direction of the inflow and outflow tract. For RV wall mass calculations, the ventricular septum is usually excluded. For the normal values for RV volumes, function, and mass, see Table 6.7.

6.2.2.10
Assessment of Ventricular Stroke Volumes with Phase-Shift MRI

An alternative technique to quantify ventricular function is the assessment of the forward flow volumes (or stroke volumes) in the ascending aorta or pulmonary artery with velocity-encoded cine or phase MR imaging ("velocity mapping"; Kondo et al. 1991) (Fig. 6.10). Kondo et al. found a close correlation between the measurements of aortic and pulmonary stroke volumes and the stroke volumes determined by volumetric ventricular quantification using short-axis cine MR images. Theoretically, also the inflow volumes in the tricuspid valve and mitral valve should be useful to determine stroke volume. Velocity-encoded cine MRI is fast and simple to perform, and can be used as a control for the volumetrically determined stroke volumes. It should be mentioned that the velocity-encoded cine MR images provide no information about the (absolute) ventricular volumes or ejection fraction. Use of velocity-encoded stroke volumes in the ascending aorta and pulmonary artery is the best way to noninvasively quantify a cardiac shunt (Arheden et al. 1999; Beerbaum et al. 2001; Powell et al. 2003). The ratio of the pulmonary artery stroke volume to the ascending aorta stroke volume is an indication of the severity of the shunt, and usually a cut-off value of 1.5 is taken to consider surgical intervention. In patients with single or multiple valvular regurgitation, a combination of volumetrically determined ventricular volumes and velocity-encoded flow volumes over the different valves allows to perfectly quantify the severity of valvular insufficiency (see Chap. 13, Valvular Heart Disease).

6.2.2.11
Variability of Measurements

How large a disparity between measurements of two sequential examinations with MRI should there be before we can decide that there is a real change? If, in a follow-up study, in the same patient 118 g and 132 g are obtained for measurements of the LV myocardial mass, would this be a real increase in weight, or could this difference be explained by observer variability? Changes over time can be the result of technical issues reflecting reproducibility, the result of biological day-to-day variation, and the result of disease evolution or effects of treatment. The overall variability should be assessed to define the confidence limits for individual measurements, before real changes within a subject over time can be detected (Semelka et al. 1990a, 1990b; Yamaoka et al. 1993; Pattynama et al. 1993, 1995; Bogaert et al. 1995). This can be done with a variance component analysis providing a measure of total variability of repeated MRI measurements, taking into account the relative contributions of interstudy, interobserver, and intraobserver error (or variability). It allows to calculate the confidence intervals for measurements. Besides the estimation of the total variance, determination of the "within-subject standard deviation" indicates the limits around a single measurement that must be regarded as possible values for the true measurement. The "95% range for change" indicates how much measurements from serial examinations should at least differ to infer a real change. In Table 6.4 are shown the mean values, the percentage contribution of the intraobserver, interobserver, and interstudy variability to the overall variability, the total variance, within-subject standard deviation, and 95% range for change, using the spoiled-GE cine MRI technique in the short-axis to assess LV volume, function, and mass. For instance,

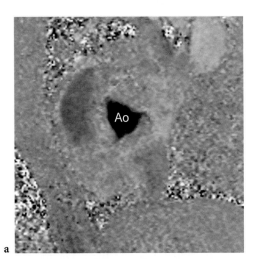

a

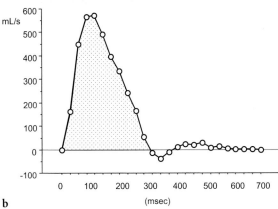

b

Fig. 6.10a,b. Assessment of LV stroke volume by measurement of the forward flow in the ascending aorta. Velocity-encoded cine MRI through the aortic valve (*Ao*) (**a**). Corresponding flow versus time curve of the aortic flow (**b**). The *dashed area* under the curve of the systolic forward flow represents the stroke volume. In the absence of valve regurgitation or interventricular shunt, quantification of the ventricular filling by means of LV inflow through the mitral valve should yield similar values (not shown)

for LV mass calculations, a 16% change is necessary to be sure that this is related to a real change in LV mass. So the change in LV mass in the above-mentioned patient (14 g or 11%) does not reflect a real increase. The same authors performed also a variance component analysis for RV measurements (Pattynama et al. 1995) (Table 6.4). Whereas for the left ventricle the interstudy variability has the largest contribution to the overall variability, for the right ventricle the intraobserver and interobserver errrors are particular large, indicating that observer subjectivity is the limiting factor in the interpretation of the MR images of the right ventricle.

Table 6.4. Variability of ventricular measurements obtained with cine MRI. Data obtained from Pattynama et al. (1993, 1995)

Parameter	Mean	Sources of variability IA	IO	IS	Total variance (%)	Within subject SD (%)	95% Range for change (%)
Left ventricle							
EDV	161 ml	20	0	80	125	7	20
ESV	57 ml	25	4	72	38	11	31
SV	104 ml	16	1	83	91	9	26
CO	6.5 l	8	1	91	0.69	13	36
EF	64 %	16	8	76	13	4	10
Mass	127 g	30	8	62	53	6	16
Right ventricle							
EDV	161 ml	66	0	34		13	37
ESV	82 ml	93	7	0		8	22
EF	49 %	76	2	22		6	16
Mass	37 g	88	0	12		6	16

IA, intraobserver variability; IO, interobserver variability; IS, interstudy variability; CO, cardiac output; EDV, end-diastolic volume; EF, ejection fraction; ESV, end-systolic

The reproducibility of an imaging technique determines the sample size required to demonstrate a clinical change, which is a major cost in pharmaceutical trials (Bottini et al. 1995; Bellenger et al. 2000b). Compared with echocardiography using geometric models to quantify LV volumes and mass, breath-hold cine MRI with volumetric ventricular quantification has a much higher reproducibility values, thus requiring smaller samples sizes to detect changes in volumes, mass, and function than echocardiography (Table 6.5). In a recent study, the Brompton group evaluated the interstudy reproducibility of MRI to assess RV volumes, function, and mass (Grothues et al. 2004). They found reproducibility values similar but generally lower than those for the left ventricle, indicating that sample sizes for RV studies need to be larger than those for LV studies.

Table 6.5. Sample size required to detect the same change in LV mass and function by echocardiography and MRI with a power of 90% and $p<0.05$. Adapted from Bellenger et al. (2000b)

Clinical change	Echocardiography SD	N	MRI SD	N	Reduction in sample size(%)
EDV, 10 ml	23.8	121	7.4	12	90
ESV, 10 ml	15.8	53	6.5	10	81
EF, 3% (abs)	6.6	102	2.5	15	85
mass, 10 g	36.4	273	6.4	9	97

EDV, end-diastolic volume; EF, ejection fraction; ESV, end-systolic volume; LV, left ventricle

6.2.2.12
Comparison with other Cardiac Imaging Techniques

Since the early publications on quantification of cardiac function with MRI, study results have been compared with those obtained with other established techniques, such as contrast ventriculography, echocardiography, radionuclide imaging, or indicator dilution or thermodilution techniques (Longmore et al. 1985; Stratemeier et al. 1986; Kaul et al. 1986; Mogelvang et al. 1986; Dilworth et al. 1987; Markiewicz et al. 1987b; van Rossum et al. 1988a,b; Culham and Vince 1988; Debatin et al. 1992b; Gopal et al. 1993; Herregods et al. 1994; Bavelaar-Croon et al. 2000; Chuang et al. 2000; Bellenger et al. 2000a, 2002; Chuang et al. 2000; Rajappan et al. 2002; Sierra Galan et al. 2003; Ichikawa et al. 2003). None of these techniques, however, has the gold standard to quantify ventricular volumes and function, and thus question the value of these kind of comparisons. Probably more important is the issue of how the results obtained by the different techniques relate and if the results are interchangeable. In patients with heart failure and with cardiac transplants, Bellenger and colleagues have found that measurements of ejection fraction by echocardiography, contrast ventriculography, radionuclide ventriculography, and MRI are not interchangeable (Bellenger et al. 2000a, 2002). Echocardiography systematically overestimates the LV ejection fraction and shows poor agreement with other techniques. Contrast ventriculography overestimates LV function, and its routine use does not add to information gained from noninvasive studies. Rajappan and colleagues have found a reasonable correlation between MRI and gated PET (Rajappan et al. 2002). The same results have been found between MRI and gated SPECT (Bavelaar-Croon et al. 2000). In patients with dilated cardiomyopathy, volumetric MRI and volumetric echocardiographic measures of LV volumes and function agree well and give similar results when used to stratify patients with dilated cardiomyopathy. Agreement is poor between biplane and volumetric methods, and worse between biplane methods, which assigns 40% of patients to different categories according to LV ejection fraction (CHUANG et al. 2000).

6.2.3
Regional Ventricular Function

Assessment of the contribution of the different parts of the ventricular wall to the global ventricular performance is important in many cardiac diseases. Clinically used parameters to express regional ventricular function are myocardial wall thickness, systolic wall thickening, and circumferential and longitudinal wall motion or shortening. Myocardial thickness can be measured on long- and short-axis images. When images are acquired at end-diastole and end-systole, the absolute or percentual wall thickening can be calculated. Preserved wall thickness is a good indicator of the presence of viable myocardium in the setting of a chronic infarction (BAER et al. 1994), while thickening provides a powerful measure of regional LV performance, which is independent of any external reference point and can be used for assessment during pharmacological stress. Although, for daily clinical use, often a

visual analysis is used to regionally score the systolic wall thickening (i.e., normal, diminished, absent, wall thinning, or eventually increased wall thickening), a quantitative approach is definitely preferable. Although simple measurements of wall thickness can be performed, a better quantitiative approach is the use of the epicardial and endocardial contours to define wall thickness, either by using perpendicular lines between the two contours or by using segmental areas divided by the length of the segment, yielding mean thickness values. These techniques use only 2D information (available in the short-axis image) for the wall thickness measurements and are therefore somewhat limited in their accuracy. First, the wall is somewhat tilted toward the LV apex and is no longer perpendicular to the parallel short-axis images (Fig. 6.11). Some degree of partial volume effect and overestimation therefore comes into play, and only a 3D reconstruction can completely compensate for this deviation and deliver an exact wall thickness (AURIGEMMA et al. 1992; LIMA et al. 1993; FORBAT et al. 1994). Second, to yield accurate measurements of wall thickening, a correction for through-plane motion should be applied (PATTYNAMA et al. 1992). The influence of papillary muscles and trabeculations on wall thickness and thickening measurements also need some consideration. To obtain the most homogeneous results in wall thickness and thickening around the LV circumference, it is preferable to exclude the papillary muscles from the LV wall. With the advent of

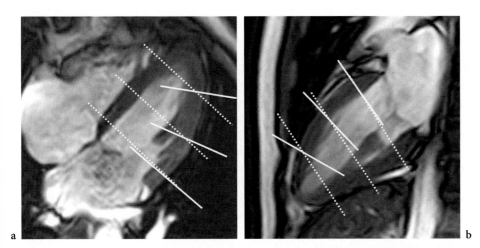

a   b

Fig. 6.11a,b. Overestimation of true myocardial wall thickness using nonperpendicular imaging through LV myocardial wall. Horizontal long-axis (**a**) and vertical long-axis (**b**) cine MRI at end-systole. Though a short-axis stack of images (*dashed lines*) cuts the LV wall almost perpendicularly in the basal part of the LV, this is no longer valid for more apical slices. Due to the curved appearance toward the LV apex of, for instance, the lateral wall on horizontal long-axis images (**a**) or the anterior wall on vertical long-axis views (**b**), the myocardium is cut obliquely (*dashed lines*) rather than perpendicularly (*full lines*), yielding overestimation of the true wall thickness

the b-SSFP cine MRI technique, visualization of the thin endocardial trabeculations has substantially improved. However, compaction of these endocardial trabeculations at end-systole yields the risk of overestimation of the true myocardial wall thickness and systolic wall thickening (Fig. 6.9).

A comprehensive evaluation of regional function should also include assessment of circumferential and longitudinal shortening. On a short-axis plane, the inward motion of the endocardium can be evaluated which corresponds with the endocardial circumferential shortening. As mentioned above, this is the result of both wall thickening and epicardial inward motion. According to the principle of conservation of mass, extensive wall thickening, as seen in a short-axis plane of the LV wall (approximately 50%), can only occur when myocardial mass moves into the imaging plane, i.e., when substantial long-axis shortening is present. Visual analysis using semi-quantitative scoring for regional wall motion assessment is often used clinically. Different grades for wall motion are used: normokinesis (i.e., normal wall motion), hypokinesis (i.e., decreased wall motion), akinesis (i.e., absent wall motion), and dyskinesis (i.e., wall motion in the opposite direction), and hyperkinesis (i.e., increased wall motion) (Fig. 6.12). Hypokinesis can be subdivided according to severity (e.g., slight, moderate, severe). Although wall motion is often visually assessed, contouring of endo- and epicardial borders may be helpful to quantitate motion (e.g., amount of centripetal motion of endocardial border during systole). Accurate segmental quantitification of circumferential and long-axis shortening necessitates the use of myocardial markers (such as MR tags); anatomical landmarks (RV insertions, papillary muscles) can also be used but only to a limited extent. Myocardial tags enable tracking of 2D or 3D motion and differentiation between motion related to true myocardial deformation and gross cardiac motion.

Another issue in the regional contribution to ejection is the relative importance of wall thickening versus epicardial inward motion. Ejection of blood from the cavity is the result of a coordinated inward motion of the endocardium. This can be accomplished by wall thickening while the epicardium remains stationary or, as in most normal conditions, moves slightly inwards; the latter, however, depends on the reference point that is used. Everyone is familiar with eccentric interventricular septal thickening after cardiac surgery where adequate septal thickening is obvious but the motion of the endocardium toward the LV cavity is diminished, absent, or

even reversed. Sometimes, as in the postinfarct situation, wall thickening can be very reduced but partially compensated by increased subepicardial deformation and inward motion, resulting in a greater contribution of that segment to global ejection than could be expected from wall thickening alone. Even in the normal heart, the relative contribution of wall thickening and epicardial inward motion to regional ejection differs from region to region, another example of ventricular inhomogeneity (BOGAERT and RADEMAKERS 2001).

6.2.4
Myocardial Wall Deformation, Myocardial Tagging, and Strain Analysis

During the cardiac cycle, the heart deforms in a very complex pattern. Besides its intrinsic deformation, the cardiac deformation is also influenced by the attached and neighboring structures and it displays a whole body motion, including rotation and translation. To quantify only the *intrinsic deformation*, myocardial markers are essential. Implanted beads, strain gauges, and coils have been used for this purpose in animal models and posttransplant patients (HANSEN et al. 1988; WALDMAN et al. 1985, 1988), but their application to study human hearts is limited for obvious reasons. Although MRI, as outlined above, enables noninvasive assessment of regional wall motion, it does not correct for gross cardiac motion. Accurate myocardial deformation analysis became possible with the introduction of MRI myocardial tagging by Elias Zerhouni in 1988 (ZERHOUNI et al. 1988) and Leon Axel in 1989 (AXEL and DOUGHERTY 1989a, 1989b). Since then many more modalities of tagging have been used, e.g., (C)-SPAMM [(complementary) spatial modulation of magnetization] tagging, line tagging, radial tagging, and ring tagging (FISCHER et al. 1993; RYF et al. 2002). All tagging techniques have the same purpose, i.e., to have 2D or 3D regional information about the shape and dimensions of the heart cavities and its walls at different timepoints throughout the cardiac cycle, enabling the calculation of strains (normal and shear), regional function, and shape.

6.2.4.1
Principles of Myocardial Tagging

Myocardial tagging relies on the spatial-selective destruction of the magnetization of the myocardium by means of excitation pulses prior to the

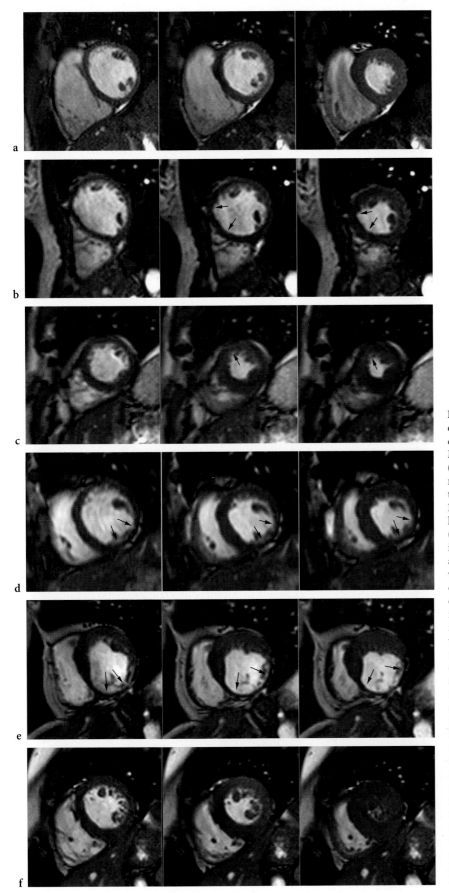

Fig. 6.12a-f. Visual assessment of wall motion patterns, using cardiac short-axis b-SSFP cine MRI. For each motion pattern (**a-f**), an end-diastolic (*left*), mid-systolic (*middle*), end-systolic (*right*) image is shown. (**a**) Normokinesia; (**b**) minor hypokinesia in ventricular septum (*arrows*); (**c**) severe hypokinesia in anterior LV wall (*arrows*); (**d**) akinesia of the inferolateral LV wall in an old transmural myocardial infarction (*arrows*); (**e**) dyskinesia of the inferior wall in a patient with an old transmural myocardial infarction with aneurysm formation (*arrows*); (**f**) hyperkinesia of the entire LV wall in a patient with a severe congenital aortic stenosis. For each motion pattern, analyze carefully the motion of the endocardial and epicardial border, and the concomitant changes in wall thickness in the normal and abnormal regions. Dynamic assessment using the cine viewing mode is very helpful in this analysis. Note the outward motion of the aneurysm in the patient with the dyskinetic wall motion pattern (**e**), and the subtotal occlusion of the LV cavity in the patient with the hyperkinetic wall motion pattern (**f**)

imaging process. The creation of tags, as described by ZERHOUNI and colleagues in 1988, consists of the application of RF pulses in one or more planes perpendicular to the imaging plane, prior to the application of the RF pulses required for imaging (Fig. 6.13) (ZERHOUNI et al. 1988). In this way, the signal of the tissue in the tag planes is destroyed immediately prior to the imaging procedures (the tissue in the tag planes is said to be "saturated"). During the subsequent MRI procedure, no signal is obtained from these protons, and they appear as hypointense or black areas. Since the crossing of two perpendicular planes is a line, tag lines can be imprinted on the myocardium. When imprinted at end-diastole, the tags subsequently deform with the myocardium on which they were inscribed. By measuring tag displacement and deformation, actual myocardial deformation can be analyzed (YOUNG and AXEL 1992; YOUNG et al. 1993). Tags are therefore truly noninvasive myocardial markers. Tag lines are a temporary phenomenon. Immediately after the tag preparation pulse, the fully saturated protons will gradually return to their normal energy level. This means that the difference between the tagged and the nontagged myocardium will progressively disappear in subsequent acquisitions later in the cardiac cycle. The rate of the loss of tag visibility is determined by the relaxation parameters of the myocardium (T1) and is a function of the imaging parameters used (BOSMANS et al. 1996). With the newer tagging sequences such as C-SPAMM, myocardial tag persistance throughout the entire cardiac cycle is achievable, thus enabling the study of not only the systolic but also the diastolic myocardial deformation (FISCHER et al. 1993). Accuracy of the myocardial deformation can be improved, especially about the midwall deformation, using a finer

grid and thinner grid or tag lines (BOLSTER et al. 1990; PIPE et al. 1991; ROGERS et al. 1991; McVEIGH and ATALAR 1992; HENDRICH et al. 1994; MOORE et al. 1994; O'DELL et al. 1995; PERMAN et al. 1995; BOSMANS et al. 1996). The principle of presaturating pulses can be combined with different types of ECG-triggered MRI sequence type, i.e., SE, breath-hold spoiled-GE sequences and the newer b-SSFP GE sequences. It is important that the first image is acquired as close as possible to the mitral valve closure (i.e., true end-diastole) to ensure assessment of the myocardial deformation during the isovolumic contraction phase, during which the ventricle builds pressure to open the aortic valve. Although the LV cavity volume does not change during the isovolumic contraction phase (see Fig. 6.2), a significant amount of myocardial deformation occurs.

Different types of myocardial tagging techniques are currently available. Whereas initially two types of tagging techniques were proposed, several variations have been added over the years. The SPAMM technique, introduced by Leon Axel in 1989 (AXEL and DOUGHERTY 1989a, 1989b), is probably the most frequently used tagging technique (Fig. 6.14). It uses two perpendicular sets of parallel stripes which form a rectangular grid on the image that can be tracked through the cardiac cycle. The grid can be defined and inscribed in a very short time, but its exact location on the heart is not as easily controlled. The myocardial deformation is basically 2D, although 3D approaches have been proposed (KUIJER et al. 2002). The other tagging technique, as originally described by E. Zerhouni in 1988, uses specific presaturation planes to define the tags and can be obtained in different geometric patterns (ZERHOUNI et al. 1988). A good approach to study the left ventricle consists of a radial orientation of the tag lines in the

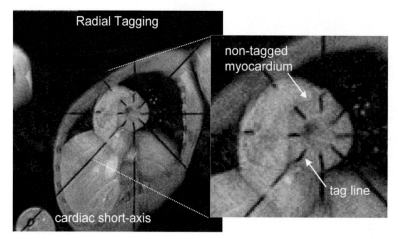

Radial Tagging

non-tagged myocardium

tag line

cardiac short-axis

Fig. 6.13. Creation of tag lines of the myocardium, using radial tagging technique. Short-axis view (*left*) and enlarged view (*right*) using spoiled gradient-echo (GE) technique. Tag prepulses, in four tag planes perpendicular on the short-axis plane crossing in the center of the left ventricle, create eight tag lines on the myocardium. These tag lines are in contrast with the nontagged myocardium and allow analysis of the myocardial deformation during the cardiac cycle

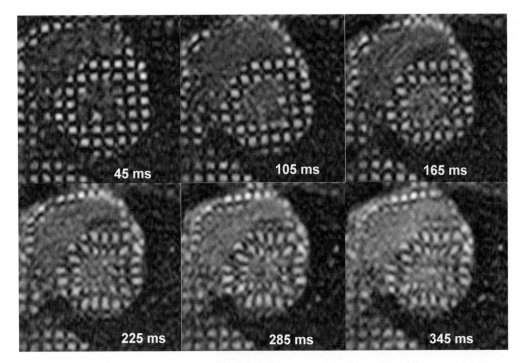

Fig. 6.14. Spatial modulation of magnetization (SPAMM)-tagging creates a grid on the myocardium. Example of short-axis SPAMM tagging. Six timepoints are shown during cardiac systole (45–345 ms). The original grid at end-diastole is rapidly deformed by the myocardial deformation. Note that, in the subendocardial layers, deformation is significantly larger than in the subepicardial layers

short-axis plane crossing each other in the center of LV cavity, while, in the long-axis plane, parallel-oriented tags are used (see Fig. 6.15). Combinations of the two types of technique exist, e.g., use of striped radial tags where the radial tag planes are subject tot the SPAMM technique to give a line composed of separate dots rather than a solid line; in this way information on radial inhomogeneity of deformation can be obtained which is otherwise impossible with radial tagging (BOLSTER et al. 1990; MCVEIGH and ZERHOUNI 1991). As outlined above, tag survival is crucial to study the myocardial deformation throughout the cardiac cycle. This was achieved with the introduction of the C-SPAMM techniques. Recently it became possible to generate a 3D tagging grid, using a C-SPAMM technique in three spatial directions (RYF et al. 2002). Ring-tagging, introduced by the Zürich group, is a variant of classic radial tagging (SPIEGEL et al. 2003), enabling more accurate assessement of the midwall circumferential fiber shortening, especially in hypertrophied heart, where the endocardial ejection indices lead to an overestimation of the contractility. Although most studies have focused on tagging of the left ventricle, tagging can perfectly be applied on the right ventricle as well (NAITO et al. 1995); for instance to study

myocardial deformation in patients with congenital heart diseases. The complex RV geometry and the presence of a thin RV wall (at least in normal circumstances) makes tagging technically more difficult. For completeness, it should be added that MRI tagging techniques are not exclusively used to study the myocardium, but can also be applied to evaluate pericardial adhesions, differentiate slow flow from thrombus, or to differentiate solid structures (e.g., differentiate muscular tissue from tumor) (HATABU et al. 1994; KOJIMA et al. 1999).

Radial tagging has the advantage of easier merging of short- and long-axis images in a truly 3D data set (Fig. 6.15). The distribution of markers or tagging points is more homogeneously distributed spread over the myocardium, and the endo- and epicardial borders are easier delineated. However, radial tagging is not part of standard, commercially available software; no or minimal information is obtained about the midwall dynamics, and no postprocessing packages are commercially available. SPAMM sequences are usually part of the extended cardiac MRI software packages, some commercially available postprocessing packages are available, and they provide information about the midwall dynamics. However, especially on the first image immediately

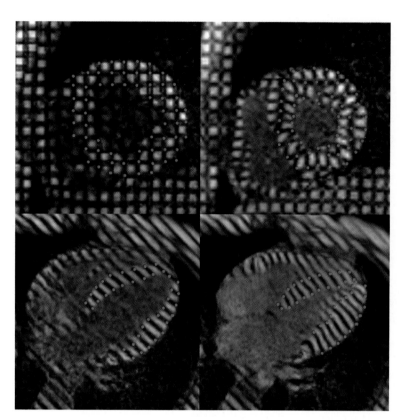

Fig. 6.15. 2D Tagging analysis. Tagging in cardiac short-axis (*upper row*) and horizontal long-axis (*lower row*), end-diastolic (*right*) and end-systolic time frame (*left*). Tracking of the grid intersections (indicated in *red*) on the short-axis views, and the intersections of the tags with the endo- and epicardial border (indicated in *red*) on the long-axis views, allows to analyze the local myocardial deformation

after the tag implementation, the delineation of the endo- and epicardial contours is often obscured. A variable amount of grid-crossing is available at different sites of the myocardium which is unevenly spread throughout the myocardial wall. Finite element analysis may solve this problem. And, although 3D SPAMM techniques exist, only 2D SPAMM techniques are commercially available.

6.2.4.2
Strain Analysis

The goal of MRI myocardial tagging, whatever technique used, is the 2D or preferably 3D analysis and quantification of myocardial deformation, expressed by normal, shear, and principal strains (WALDMAN et al. 1985, 1988) (Figs. 6.15–17). With radial tagging, using a combination of tagging in five short-axis levels and four long-axis levels, where the tag planes in the short-axis imaging plane are used as imaging planes for the long-axis views (and vice versa), the left ventricle can be divided into 32 small, cuboidal volume elements (see Fig. 6.17). Typical dimensions of such a myocardial cuboid are 17 mm (circumferentially) × 10 mm (radially) × 14 mm (longitudinally). The crossing points of the tag lines with the endo-or epicardial borders form the corner or node

points of the cuboids. The 3D spatial displacement of these node points during the cardiac cycle can be accurately determined after merging the information from long- and short-axis images (thus allowing a four-dimensional analysis of myocardial deformation) (GOSHTASBY and TURNER 1996).

Although, an external coordinate system, i.e., the coordinate system of the magnet (*XYZ*) can be chosen for strain analysis, description of the 3D deformation using a local cardiac coordinate system contributes much more to the understanding of cardiac mechanics (Fig. 6.17). In this local cardiac coordinate system (RCL), two of axes are oriented tangential to the LV wall, i.e., circumferential (C) and longitudinal (L), and the third axis is perpendicular to the LV wall, i.e., radial (R). R, C, and L are perpendicular to each other. This RCL coordinate system is thus specific for each epi- and endocardial node point. Due to the taper of the apex, the radial axis points slightly down and the longitudinal axis slightly outward in this region. To increase our understanding of how the basic action of the fibers relates to the regional and global deformation of the wall during contraction and relaxation, the RCL coordinate system can be transformed into a local fiber coordinate system (RFX), using standard fiber angle orientations obtained from autopsy studies

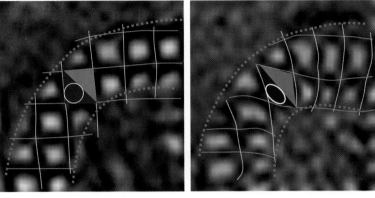

Fig. 6.16a,b. 2D principal strain analysis ("Moore's principle"). Short-axis SPAMM tagging at end-diastole (**a**) and end-systole (**b**). The circle that fits in the equiangular triangle at end-diastole, is transformed by the underlying myocardial deformation into an oval at end-systole. This oval is defined by two axes. The short-axis correspond with the first principal strain. This is a shortening strain and corresponds to the circumferential shortening. The long-axis of the oval represents the third principal strain. This strain is a positive strain and corresponds to the radial strain (systolic wall thickening). The principle axes reflect the direction of the principal strains. The axis of shortening and lengthening correspond closely to the direction of circumferential shortening and wall thickening, respectively. The *green dashed lines* represent the endo- and epicardial borders

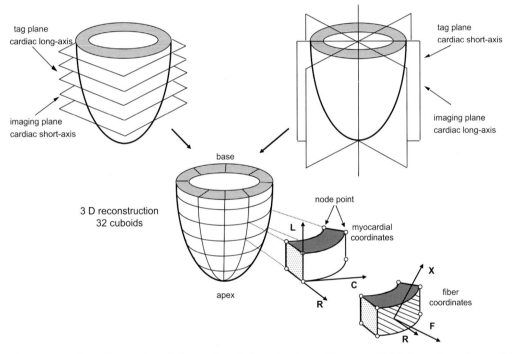

Fig. 6.17. Merging of long-axis and short-axis radial tagging into a 3D myocardial deformation scheme. Using a combination of long- and short-axis tagging, the LV myocardium can be divided into small blocks of myocardial tissue (cuboids) defined by the node points in 3D space. Their coordinates can be expressed in a local cardiac [(radial (R),circumferential (C), longitudinal (L)] or in a fiber (radial-fiber (R), cross-fiber (X)) coordinate system. This approach allows calculation of 3D strains during the cardiac cycle. *F*, fiber direction

(low intersubject variation). The F or fiber direction indicates the fiber direction along the endocardial or epicardial surface. The X or cross-fiber direction, defines the direction along the endo-or epicardial surface perpendicular to the fiber direction, while R (radial) remains the same as in the RCL system. This RFX coordinate system allows us to quantify

the most basic component of myocardial deformation, i.e., fiber shortening. Strain analysis enables the decomposition of the complex 3D myocardial deformation into three normal and three shear strains (MOORE et al. 1992; PIPE et al. 1991; YOUNG and AXEL 1992; YOUNG et al. 1993, 1994; BOGAERT 1997) (Fig. 6.18). Normal strains quantify the dis-

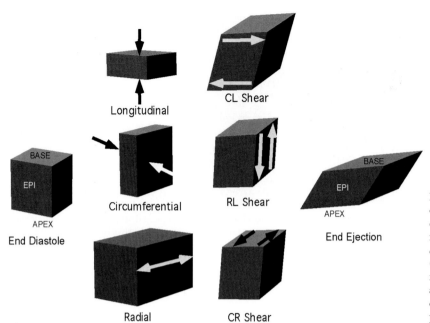

Fig. 6.18. Decomposition of the complex deformation of the myocardial cuboid during systole into three normal strains (*middle left*), and three shear strains (*middle right*). Nondeformed myocardial cuboid at end-diastole (*left*) and same cuboid at end-systole (*right*). *EPI*, echoplanar imaging

placements or changes in length along a coordinate system. Three normal strains are therefore defined for each coordinate system, three in the local cardiac coordinate system (RR, CC, LL) and three in the local fiber coordinate system (RR, FF, XX), in which the radial strain RR remains the same. Myocardial strains can be positive or negative, for example positive radial strains represent wall thickening, while negative strains represent segment shortening, e.g., circumferential shortening or fiber shortening. Shear strains quantify the displacements of two adjacent node points along another coordinate system. They are defined in the plane between two axes of the coordinate system and describe the deformation of a square to a parallelogram. For the RCL coordinate system, the shear strains are RC, LR, CL (Fig. 6.18). The circumferential-longitudinal shear strain describes the LV twisting and can be used to quantify the ventricular torsion (BUCHALTER et al. 1990; LORENZ et al. 2000).

Myocardial deformation can also be described independently from a Cartesian coordinate system using three principal strains and three principal angles or axes of deformation (WALDMAN et al. 1985; AZHARI et al. 1993; CROISILLE et al. 1999) (Fig. 6.16). The principal strains are ranked at end-systole from smallest, i.e., most negative, to largest, i.e., most positive. The first principal strain is a shortening strain. The second principal strain is often a negligible but sometimes a substantial shortening, especially near the endocardium. The third principal strain is usually positive or thickening, cor-

responding to the radial strain. The principle axes reflect the direction of the three principal strains. While, at the subepicardium, the principal axes of shortening corresponds to the direction of active shortening of the obliquely oriented myofibers, at the subendocardium this axis is nearly perpendicular to the endocardial fiber shortening, suggesting substantial interactions between neighboring fibers in the LV wall, leading to the phenomenon of cross-fiber shortening (WALDMAN et al. 1985, 1988; RADEMAKERS et al. 1994).

6.2.4.3
Regional Ejection Fraction

The local deformation of the myocardial wall has as ultimate goal the ejection of blood by the ventricle. MRI myocardial tagging can be used to assess this regional performance or "regional ejection fraction," by quantifying the contribution of each myocardial cuboid to global ejection of blood by the left ventricle (BOGAERT et al. 1999, 2000; BOGAERT and RADEMAKERS 2001; RADEMAKERS et al. 2003) (Fig. 6.19). With the radial tagging technique, the short-axis tags are radially oriented with the crossing of the tag lines in the center of the LV cavity. Therefore, each cuboid defines an intracavitary triangular volume where the endocardial surface is the base of the triangle and the center of the LV is the apex. The inward motion and deformation (circumferentially and longitudinally) of the endocardium determines the changes in intracavitary trian-

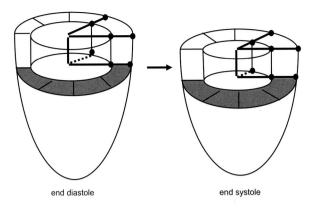

end diastole   end systole

Fig. 6.19. Regional ejection fraction. Two adjacent radial tag lines on two adjacent levels describe an intracavitary triangle with the apex in the center of the left ventricle and the base on the endocardial surface. In this way, one cuboid describes a triangular volume which permits calculation and quantification of the regional ejection fraction for this cuboid

gular volume. Subtraction of the end-systolic from the end-diastolic triangular volume divided by the end-diastolic volume defines the regional ejection fraction. Similarly, the regional ejection fraction at the epicardium can be computed, but the changes in cuboid volume are added to the changes in intracavitary volume. Endocardial regional ejection fraction thus can be viewed as a composite measure of the local contribution to ejection. Since it is a percentage, it does not describe the absolute amount of ejected blood, but rather the relative change at each cuboid. Nearer the apex, for example, the triangular volumes are somewhat smaller and a larger ejection fraction could still represent a smaller absolute volume change than at the base.

6.2.4.4
Myocardial Tagging and Ventricular Morphology

MRI myocardial tagging techniques, especially radial tagging and to a lesser extent SPAMM tagging, enable the obtaining of accurate information on local ventricular morphology, i.e., myocardial wall thickness, as well as radii of curvature. This enables us to directly relate regional morphology to regional deformation and local function (see Sect. 6.4). True myocardial wall thickness is obtained in a 3D fashion, by adjusting the tag length for wall curvature in the longitudinal direction (LIMA et al. 1993) (see also Table 6.11). Circumferential and longitudinal radius of curvature are calculated in each cuboid using the cord and arc lengths fitting a model. A small

radius of curvature denotes a curved surface, while a large radius of curvature is representative of a flat surface. The radii of curvature can be computed for the epicardial and endocardial border in both the longitudinal and the circumferential direction. Very similar longitudinal and circumferential radii of curvature represent a structure close to a sphere, whereas very different radii are typical for an ellipsoid. In a cylinder one of the radii of curvature is infinite. Changes in these radii of curvature during the cardiac cycle denote regional shape changes of the ventricle and can be used together with wall thickness to calculate wall stresses (BEYAR et al. 1993).

6.2.5
Myocardial Wall Velocity Mapping

Myocardial wall deformation is not only characterized by the amount of deformation but also by the speed or velocity of deformation ("strain rate"). With the advent of tissue Doppler imaging, enabling the quantification of myocardial velocities, it became evident that assessment of myocardial velocity patterns is important in many cardiac diseases. Phase imaging, although initially proposed as an alternative to myocardial tagging for quantification of myocardial deformation and motion (WEDEEN 1992; WEDEEN et al. 1995), should be fitted to quantify myocardial velocity patterns. Normally, the amount of received signal ("magnitude") is used to reconstruct MR images. Using the "phase" information, the velocity can be measured (Fig. 6.20). This technique is routinely used for flow quantification in blood vessels and through the cardiac valves (FIRMIN et al. 1989; HIGGINS et al. 1992; KILNER et al. 1991), but can also be applied to quantify 2D or 3D myocardial motion and velocity (CONSTABLE et al. 1994). With its specific properties, phase imaging may overcome some limitations of myocardial tagging, such as better persistance throughout the cardiac cycle and quantification of myocardial deformation in the entire wall, rather than in the areas destroyed by the tagging pulses. Although the temporal resolution of phase imaging is currently far below the frame rate achievable with tissue Doppler imaging, phase imaging is spatially not restricted, e.g., to the posterior LV wall, but can quantify 2D or 3D the velocity patterns throughout the LV wall. To date, myocardial velocity mapping is a research rather than a clinical tool, but it has the potential to become more widely integrated into clinical imaging protocols in the near future.

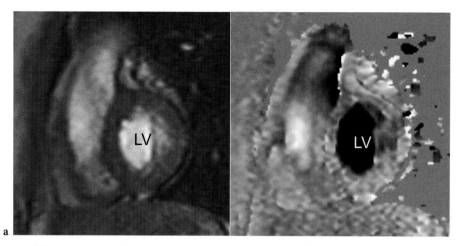

a

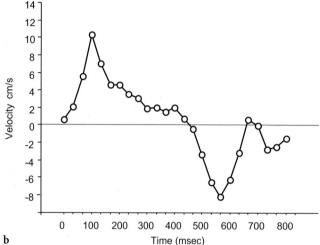

b

Fig. 6.20a,b. Assessment of myocardial velocities using velocity mapping technique in a 27-year-old healthy woman. Short-axis, magnitude (*left*) and phase (*right*) image. Myocardial velocities quantified in the inferior LV wall represents the through-plane, i.e., longitudinal, velocities (**b**). During systole, shortening of the left ventricle is shown by the positive velocities. Ventricular lengthening during diastole is biphasic, with a large velocity caused by early, fast filling, and a smaller velocity peak during atrial contraction

6.3
Diastolic Function

Heart failure, caused by a predominant abnormality in diastolic function (i.e., *diastolic heart failure*) is considered to be responsible for at least one-third of all patients with congestive heart failure (PAELINCK et al. 2002). However, the diagnosis of diastolic dysfunction and diastolic heart failure is still challenging because of controversy surrounding the definition of diastolic dysfunction and the criteria for diastolic heart failure. "Diastolic dysfunction" refers to a condition in which abnormalities in mechanical function are present during diastole. Abnormalities in diastolic function can occur in the presence or absence of a clinical syndrome of heart failure and with normal or abnormal systolic function. "Diastolic dysfunction" describes an abnormal mechanical property, "diastolic heart failure" describes a clinical syndrome (ZILE and BRUTSAERT 2002).

6.3.1
Mechanisms of Ventricular Relaxation and Filling

Diastole represents the filling phase of the ventricles. Mechanically, based on valvular events, diastole is the period between mitral valve opening and mitral valve closure. Filling, however, is the end-product of the underlying mechanisms of myocardial relaxation, atrial contraction, and the compliance of the ventricle and the atrium. Thus, physiologically and conceptually, diastole encompasses the time period during which the myocardium loses its ability to generate force and shorten, and returns to an unstressed length and force. Ventricular relaxation begins when myofiber tension starts to decline during late ejection, proceeds rapidly as pressure falls during isovolumic relaxation, and continues through the period of early filling. Active myocardial relaxation encompasses the processes of calcium removal from the contractile elements mainly into the sarcoplasmic reticulum, the presence of restoring forces inside or outside the myocytes, and the interaction with load. With the onset of myocardial relaxation, the ventricular pressure drops and continues to drop until a pressure is reached below the pressure of the atrium even after filling has started, due to the active relaxation process and the presence of restoring forces. It is thought that, during contraction and early ejection, part of the energy is stored in the cytoskeleton of the myocytes or in the collagen matrix, as potential energy to be used subsequently during relaxation as restoring forces, lowering ventricular pressure and drawing blood from the atrium. Blood enters the ventricle through the atrioventricular valve at the moment the ventricular pressure drops under the atrial pressure. Depending also on the compliance and distensibility of the ventricle, the local gradients across the atrioventricular valve will switch, and blood flow will be decelerated and only continue through diastasis, dependent on momentum. With atrial contraction, a new gradient and acceleration is created, further filling the ventricle, depending on atrial and ventricular compliance and force of atrial contraction. Active relaxation is thus only responsible for the first part of fast filling in the normal ventricle, but its influence can be prolonged in the case of abnormal, prolonged relaxation, i.e., in ischemia. Compliance, on the contrary, is important throughout filling but, due to the shape of the passive pressure–volume ratio of the ventricle, it plays its most important role at the end of fast filling and during atrial contraction.

6.3.2
Assessment of Diastolic Function and Dysfunction

For several reasons, assessment of diastolic (dys)-function is definitely more challenging and complicated than evaluation of systolic (dys)function. Since different physiological mechanisms contribute to ventricular filling, the study of diastolic (dys)function is hampered by the absence of an easily obtained global parameter such as ejection fraction used to express global systolic function. The ventricular relaxation process is difficult to assess by noninvasive means, because imaging methods cannot directly measure cavity pressure changes. Echocardiographic, Doppler, and radionuclide pa-

rameters of diastolic function are derived from rates of inflow of blood or outward movement of the myocardium. However, the process of relaxation occurs mostly during the diastolic isovolumic period of the cardiac cycle, before blood flow or wall motion begins. Indexes measured later in the cycle examine only the final stages of relaxation. Furthermore, these parameters are subject to "pseudonormalization," because the variation in atrial pressure profoundly affects filling dynamics and thus confounds attempts to indirectly estimate the relaxation rate (DONG et al. 2001; HEES et al. 2004). In normal subjects, aging has a significant impact on RV and LV filling patterns (IWASE et al. 1993). Although Doppler echocardiography is currently the noninvasive imaging technique used to assess diastolic function (MANDINOV et al. 2000), MRI is emerging as a valuable alternative, having the unique potential of 3D function analysis with great accuracy and reproducibility (BELLENGER et al. 2000a; PAELINCK et al. 2002).

6.3.2.1
Ventricular Mass and Volumes

Since ventricular mass is one the major determinants of diastolic function and filling, MRI can be considered the preferred imaging modality to accurately and precisely quantify the myocardial mass. In contrast to M-mode and 2D echocardiography, which make assumptions about shape and geometry of the ventricle that often lead to large errors, MRI does not make any assumption but images and measures the entire volume and mass, providing highly accurate values with very good intra- and interobserver variability (see Sect. 6.2.2.12). The new b-SSFP cine MRI technique in combination with parallel imaging allows dynamic cardiac imaging with temporal resolutions as short as 10 ms. This should enable accurate tracking of changes in RV and LV volumes throughout the cardiac cycle, and measurement of the ventricular filling curves and their derivative with peak rates and time to peak rate (FUJITA et al. 1993; SOLDO et al. 1994; KUDELKA et al. 1997) (Fig. 6.2). Moreover, MRI can potentially provide interesting information with regard to the timing and rate of wall thinning. This interesting (but underused) parameter is very helpful to differentiate normal from pseudonormal inflow patterns, but necessitates a tedious, and often time-consuming delineation of the epi- and endocardial borders. Finally, MRI allows quantification of atrial volumes, providing information on atrial filling and emptying curves in normal, diseased, and transplanted hearts (JARVINEN et al. 1994a, 1994b; MOHIADDIN and HASEGAWA 1995; LAUERMA et al. 1996).

6.3.2.2
Ventricular Inflow Patterns

During the last two decades, Doppler-echocardiography has emerged as an important clinical tool, providing reliable and useful data on diastolic performance. A combination of the transmitral and pulmonary venous flow, intraventricular filling patterns and measuring the duration of isovolumic relaxation is routinely used. Similar measurements can be made on the right side at the tricuspid valve and in the subhepatic veins and the inferior vena cava. Using velocity-encoded or phase-contrast cine MRI techniques, MRI can accurately measure the flow in the mitral and tricuspid valve, and pulmonary and caval veins (MOHIADDIN et al. 1990, 1991; MOSTBECK et al. 1993; GALJEE et al. 1995; KROFT and DE ROOS 1999). The advantage of MRI over Doppler-echocardiography is that MRI quantifies the volume flow over the entire region, i.e., valve area or vessel, in contrast to Doppler assessing the flow and flow velocity in a relatively small area. Since the flow is not homogeneous over such a region, different positioning of the Doppler sample volume can yield different values, with possible impact on the interpretation (FYRENIUS et al. 1999). With the advent of real-time MRI techniques, also available for velocity-encoded cine MRI, it has become feasible to quantify in real-time the ventricular inflow, as well as the flow patterns in the great vessels (VAN DEN HOUT et al. 2003). This should allow evaluation of the impact of respiratory motion on ventricular filling, e.g., an essential feature to differentiate patients with restrictive cardiomyopathy from those with constrictive pericarditis (GIORGI et al. 2003).

The transmitral (or transtricuspid) velocity pattern is easy to acquire and can rapidly categorize patients with normal or abnormal diastolic function by E/A ratio (early to late filling velocity). In healthly, young individuals, most diastolic filling occurs in early diastole, so that the E/A ratio is greater than 1 (Fig. 6.21). When relaxation is impaired (e.g., myocardial hypertrophy, ischemia), early diastolic filling decreases progressively, and a vigorous compensatory atrial contraction ("atrial kick") occurs. This results in a reversed E/A ratio (E/A ratio less than 1: "delayed relaxation" pattern), increased deceleration time, and increased isovolumic relaxation time (Fig. 6.22). However, with increasing age, the myocardial relaxation is prolonged, and the myocardial and chamber stiffness increases, resulting also in a decrease of the E/A ratio. If the ventricular compliance is reduced (e.g., restrictive cardiomyopathy), the filling pressures increase, leading to a compensatory augmentation of the atrial pressure with an increase in early filling despite a concomitant impaired relaxation, so that filling looks relatively similar to a normal pattern ("pseudo-normalization" pattern: E/A >1). This pattern, however, represents abnormalities of both relaxation and compliance and is distinguished from normal filling by a shortened early deceleration time. In patients with severe decrease in ventricular complicance, atrial pressure

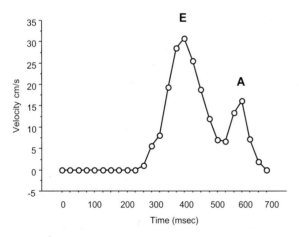

Fig. 6.21. Mitral inflow pattern in a 24-year-old normal subject. The fast, early-filling velocity (*E*) is almost twice as large as the flow velocity during atrial contraction (*A*)

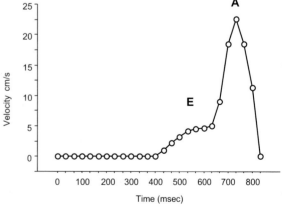

Fig. 6.22. Severe myocardial relaxation disturbance leading to a reversal of the E/A ratio. The early-filling velocities are strongly decreased (*E*), whereas the late-filling velocities are increased (*A*).

is markedly elevated and compensates with vigorous early diastolic filling for impaired relaxation. This "restrictive" filling pattern (E/A >>1) is consistent with an abnormal rise in ventricular pressure and an abrupt deceleration of flow with little additional during mid-diastole and atrial contraction (MANDINOV et al. 2000).

Analysis of the venous flow patterns in the pulmonary veins or caval veins also provides valuable information about the LV or RV diastolic function, respectively. The S-wave, occurring during ventricular systole, depends on the atrial relaxation and longitudinal ventricular shortening with subsequent motion of the atrioventricular valve annulus. The D-wave occurring during ventricular diastole reflects ventricular filling, and the A-wave, which has an opposite direction to the other waves, occurs during atrial contraction and reflects ventricular compliance. Whereas, in younger subjects, the D-wave velocity is larger than the S-wave velocity, with aging

the D-wave velocity decreases as a result of the prolonged and impaired myocardial relaxation, while the A-wave increases in magnitude (Fig. 6.23). With the progressive decrease in ventricular compliance, the returning venous flow shows a diminution of the systolic forward flow with an enhanced early diastolic flow and a reversal of the atrial flow. The latter is the result of the contraction against an increased afterload due to an elevated diastolic filling pressure or an increased ventricular stiffness. Accordingly blood is preferentially ejected in the pulmonary or caval veins, resulting in a venous A-wave that is high in magnitude and long in duration.

6.3.2.3
Ventricular Coupling

Although the left and right ventricles are physically separate in man, the two ventricles are anatomically and functionally bound together in many ways. They share a common ventricular septum and ventricular, myocardial bundles and are enclosed and bound together by the common pericardium. In addition, the left ventricle indirectly connects with the right ventricle via the pulmonary circulation (so-called series interaction). There is a close functional interaction between the right and left ventricles, not only in diastole but also in systole. This ventricular interaction is reflected by the position and configuration of the ventricular septum, which is determined by the pressure difference between the left and right ventricle, i.e., the transseptal pressure gradient. In normal loading conditions, the septum has a concave shape toward the left ventricle due to a positive left-to-right transseptal pressure gradient, and this shape is maintained during the cardiac cycle (WEYMAN et al. 1976; BRINKER et al. 1980; GUZMAN et al. 1981; LIMA et al. 1986). The phenomenon whereby the function of one ventricle is altered by changes in the filling of the other is called "ventricular coupling" or "interventricular dependence". Pathological ventricular coupling occurs when there is an acute or chronic imbalance between the left and right ventricular loading conditions, e.g., constrictive pericarditis, mitral stenosis, cor pulmonale (WEYMAN et al. 1977; JESSUP et al. 1987; GIORGI et al. 2003). In these circumstances, this imbalance will lead to an abnormal motion and configuration of the ventricular septum. Ventricular coupling is moreover significantly influenced by respiration (HATLE et al. 1989; KLEIN et al. 1993; HURRELL et al. 1996). During inspiration, the intrathoracic pressure decreases, leading to a diminished pulmonary venous return and a

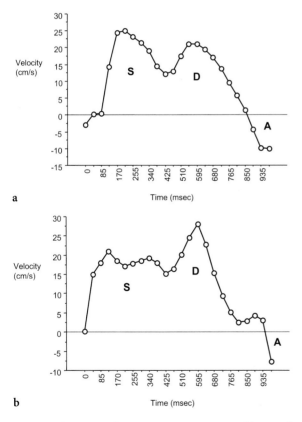

Fig. 6.23a,b. Venous flow patterns in a 39-year-old normal subject through the inferior vena cava (a) and pulmonary vein (b). In the inferior vena cava, the systolic (S) forward-flow velocity is slightly larger than the diastolic (D) flow. A represents the reversed flow caused by the atrial contraction. In the pulmonary vein (a), diastolic forward-flow velocities slightly exceed systolic forward velocities

decreased left ventricular filling, and an increased systemic venous return and right ventricular filling, while the opposite phenomenon is found during expiration. Assessment of the impact of respiration on ventricular coupling is, for example, crucial to differentiate patients with constrictive pericarditis from those with restrictive cardiomyopathy.

At present, Doppler-echocardiography is the image modality of choice to assess the influence of respiration on ventricular inflow and septal motion (HATLE et al. 1989). With the advent of MRI systems with stronger gradient systems, faster gradient switching capabilities, and new cine MRI sequences in combination with parallel imaging, data acquisition has shortened considerably, enabling real-time dynamic evaluation of ventricular septal motion and configuration throughout the cardiac cycle. This has opened new opportunities for cardiac MRI to become competitive with echocardiography. In a preliminary study, Francone and colleagues were able to assess the impact of respiration on ventricular filling in normals as well as in patients with restrictive inflow pattern and in patients with chronic cor pulmonale (FRANCONE et al., unpublished data). In patients with constrictive pericarditis, a ventricular septal flattening or inversion was found on real-time MR images during early ventricular filling (see Chap. 11). The intensity of the abnormalities was most pronounced during the first heartbeat after onset of inspiration, rapidly decreased during the next heartbeats, and completely disappeared during expiration. This pattern was absent in patients with restrictive cardiomyopathy.

6.3.2.4
Ventricular Relaxation

Cardiac catherization with simultaneous pressure and volume measurements is the gold standard for asssesing ventricular relaxation and ventricular compliance. The myocardial or ventricular relaxation can be quantified by calculation of the time constant (tau, τ) of myocardial relaxation. High-fidelity, manometer-tipped catheters measure the intraventricular pressure changes. The pressure from time of aortic valve closure to mitral valve opening is fitted to a monoexponential equation. Tau is 30–40 ms in normal humans, and relaxation is considered to be "complete" after three time constants (90–120 ms). Assessment of ventricular relaxation by noninvasive means, e.g., Doppler-echocardiography and radionuclide methods, is difficult because imaging methods cannot directly measure cavity

pressure. The measured indexes of rates such as inflow of blood or outward movement of the myocardium reflect only the final stages of relaxation. MRI myocardial tagging, however, allows accurate and noninvasive measurement of the global and regional deformation and shape of the heart and its cavities throughout the cardiac cycle, enabling the calculation of strains (normal and shear). One shear-strain parameter that has a particular importance for diastolic function is the circumferential-longitudinal shear or torsion, expressing wringing motion of the left ventricle (RADEMAKERS et al. 1992; DONG et al. 1999). Counterclockwise torsion develops during ejection, but the clockwise recoil of torsion or untwisting is a deformation that occurs largely during isovolumic relaxation, before mitral valve opening. This recoil is associated with the release of restoring forces that have been accumulated during systole and is thought to contribute to diastolic suction (ROBINSON et al. 1986). The extent of torsion is correlated with cavity pressure, and its recoil rate is closely related to the rate of pressure fall and the relaxation time constant (τ) (DONG et al. 2001). Recently HEES et al. (2004), studying changes in recoil rate with aging using myocardial tagging, remarkably have found that the decrease in early filling velocities with aging was rather related to changes in left atrial pressure than to changes in myocardial relaxation behavior. Untwisting may be abnormal in timing and extent in several pathologies, including heart failure from various causes, myocardial infarction, hypertrophy due to hypertension, or aortic disease (MATTER et al. 1996; STUBER et al. 1999).

6.3.2.5
Atrial Volumes and Function

Most MRI studies as so far have mainly focused on determining the optimal criteria for quantification of ventricular function. However, atrial volumes and changes during the cardiac cycle can be measured in a similar way as for the ventricles, providing important information about ventricular filling (JARVINEN et al. 1994a,b; LAUERMA et al. 1996; MOHIADDIN and HASEGAWA 1995). Probably the transaxial or horizontal long-axis imaging planes can be recommended for atrial volume quantification, since these planes visualize well the atrioventricular valve(s), the atrial septum, and the lateral and dorsal atrial walls. In analogy to echocardiography, also anteroposterior and lateral diameters might be an easy method of estimating atrial volumes.

6.4
Stress–Strain Relation

6.4.1
Wall Stress

Wall stress, or the force generated by the intraventricular cavity pressure on the surrounding myocardial wall, is a major determinant of the systolic myocardial deformation and ventricular ejection. Moreover, myocardial oxygen consumption is closely related to wall stress. Since wall stress cannot be measured, it has to be assumed (ARTS et al. 1991). Several assumptions for wall stress have been proposed, the one more complex than the other, but most of them are based on the measurable parameters, i.e., wall thickness, radii of curvature, and systolic blood pressure; while other parameters such as influence of fiber direction or anisotropy are usually ignored (WONG and RAUTAHARJU 1968; STREETER et al. 1970; JANZ 1982). For a similar cavity pressure, wall stress decreases if the wall becomes more curved or if the wall thickness increases. This explains why the LV apex, which is highly curved, can sustain high systolic pressures without bulging or rupturing. Because of the lower wall stress in the LV apex, the systolic strains and thus the contribution to the ventricular ejection are proportionally larger in the apex than in other segments of the left ventricle (BOGAERT and RADEMAKERS 2001). The transmural spread of wall stress is inhomogeneous, with the highest wall stresses in the subendocardium, making this area especially vulnerable to ischemia. Wall stress gradually decreases toward the subepicardium.

With the advent of MRI, and especially MRI myocardial tagging techniques, accurate information can be obtained on regional morphology, i.e., wall thickness and circumferential and longitudinal radii of curvature. MRI diffusion techniques have been shown to noninvasively depict myocardial fiber directions, and even to quantitate myocardial fiber shortening (HSU et al. 1998; SCOLLAN et al. 1998; TSENG et al. 2000). This should allow more accurate estimates of regional wall stresses and determination of the regional stress–strain relationship (RADEMAKERS et al. 2003). Using a simple formula for wall-stress estimations, based on wall thickness (corrected for angulation), circumferential and longitudinal radii of curvature, and systolic blood pressure rather than the true measured intraventricular pressure, RADEMAKERS and colleagues (2003) recently have found a close, inverse relation between the regional systolic wall stress and the corresponding amount of deformation. Since systolic wall stress is also a major determinant of myocardial relaxation, quantification may be helpful in unraveling the regional pattern in myocardial relaxation. The same principles are also valid for assessment of RV wall stress, which is even more difficult to estimate, mainly because of its complex shape (NAITO et al. 1995; YIM et al. 1998). And as mentioned above, better knowledge of wall stress would also help to better understand the mechanism of ventricular coupling and the impact on ventricular filling.

6.4.2
Intrinsic Myocardial Contractility

All clinically used parameters to express ventricular function, such as stroke volume, ejection fraction, fractional shortening or rate of ejection, and velocity of circumferential or fiber shortening (Vcf), are determined not only by the intrinsic myocardial contractility but also by load-dependent parameters, i.e., the ventricular pre- and afterload (STREETER et al. 1970; MIRSKY et al. 1988; LEGGET 1999). Knowledge of the intrinsic myocardial contractility, however, is essential in many disease states. Most techniques used to assess myocardial contractility are elaborative and require a variation of the afterload to assess the ventricular response, e.g., fractional shortening, shortening velocities. The inverse linear relation between both is a means to quantify the myocardial contractility (MIRSKY et al. 1988). This is accomplished by leg lifting, pharmacological interventions, or static exercise (handgrip). This approach is used to assess the real level of myocardial contractility and can be used, for example, in patients with reduced ejection fraction to distinguish between reduced myocardial shortening due to excessive afterload (aortic stenosis) and that due to depressed myocardial contractility (BOROW et al. 1992; LEGGET 1999). Rather than varying the end-systolic LV wall stress to determine the myocardial contractility, Rademakers and colleagues used the regional inhomogeneity of LV wall stress to determine the LV stress–strain relation and thus the myocardial contractility at a single global LV load level (RADEMAKERS et al. 2003). They found a close inverse linear relationship between regional wall stress (or load) and regional wall strain (or performance), expressed by the regional ejection fraction (Fig. 6.24). Regions with a higher end-systolic load show lower strains and regional ejection fractions and vice versa (FUJITA et al. 1993).

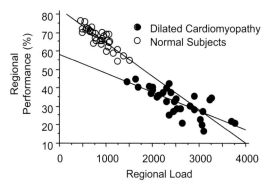

Fig. 6.24. Inverse relation between regional load and regional performance in a group of normal subjects ($n=87$) and patients with idiopathic dilated cardiomyopathy ($n=12$). The regional load (or wall stress) is obtained using the radii of curvature in the long- and short-axis direction, wall thickness and intraventricular pressure. The regional performance represents the regional ejection fraction (see Fig. 6.19). The R^2 of the correlation in normal subjects is 0.76 and in patients with dilated cardiomyopathy 0.58. (Partially adapted from BOGAERT 1997 and RADEMAKERS et al. 2003)

The tight link between regional stress and strain is indicative for a highly uniform myocardial contractility throughout the left ventricle. Although the afterload is similar for the entire LV, the regional loading conditions vary significantly depending on the regional morphology, i.e., wall thickness, and circumferential and longitudinal radii of curvatures. While the contractility is uniform, the corresponding ventricular response at regional level is highly inhomogeneous (BOGAERT and RADEMAKERS 2001).

6.5
MRI Stress Imaging

In patients with coronary artery disease, myocardial function at rest is often within normal limits. However, during periods of increased oxygen consumption, e.g., during physical exercise, the oxygen supply through a stenotic coronary artery might be insufficient to cover the increased needs, leading to regional or more global myocardial ischemia (see Chaps. 7 and 8). A series of events, i.e., the ischemic cascade, occurs after the onset of disturbances in myocardial blood flow, starting with diastolic and systolic functional abnormalities, followed by changes on the ECG and later symptoms of angina. With the new imaging

modalities, earlier manifestations of ischemia can be used as markers of significant coronary artery disease. Although clinically still underused, MRI has probably the biggest potential as a stress imaging technique. For this purpose, stress perfusion, stress cine MRI, stress myocardial tagging, and even stress aortic flow measurements have been applied (PENNELL et al. 1990, 1992, 1995; BAER et al. 1992, 1993, 1994; CIGARROA et al. 1993; VAN RUGGE et al. 1993a,b, 1994; HARTNELL et al. 1994, CROISILLE et al. 1999).

6.6
Postprocessing and Delineation Techniques

Fast and accurate analysis of image data is a prerequisite for each imaging modality to be implemented into clinical routine. The success of other imaging techniques, such as radionuclide imaging, is exactly the availability of postprocessing techniques with fast, automated extraction of ventricular volumes, function, and mass. Although MRI has all the intrinsic qualities to be considered as a reference technique for assessment of global and regional cardiac function, mainly the lack of easily usable postprocessing and delineation techniques still hampers a thorough clinical use (YOUNG et al. 2000). One of the major strengths of MRI, i.e., the superb depiction of cardiac morphology, is unfortunately the largest challenge for most automated delineation techniques. Another impediment is the discrimination between atria and ventricles because of difficulties in defining the atrioventricular valve position. Different methods have been reported for automatic segmentation of the endocardial border, including region growing, edge detection, adaptive thresholding, and fuzzy logic (SINGLETON and POHOST 1997; FURBER et al. 1998; BALDY et al. 1994; LALANDE et al. 1999; SANTARALLI et al. 2003). Results have been ambiguous. VAN DER GEEST et al. (1997) have concluded that LV functional parameters can be obtained with a high degree of accuracy with semiautomatic contour detection; ROMIGER et al. (1999) have reported that semiautomatic evaluation is erroneous and manual correction of these contours takes more time than manual contour tracing alone. Use of the same software on the b-SSFP technique has provided, in contrast, accurate cardiodynamic measurements (BARKHAUSEN

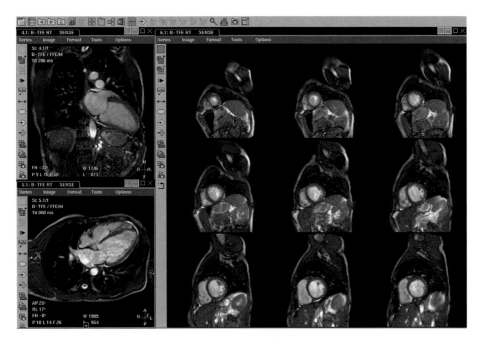

Fig. 6.25. Viewing of a functional cardiac MRI study on an off-line workstation (Easy-Vision, Philips Medical Systems, Best, The Netherlands). Routinely, the left ventricle is studied using a combination of a vertical (*upper left*) and horizontal (*lower left*) long-axis view, and a set of contiguous short-axis image encompassing the entire left ventricle (*right*)

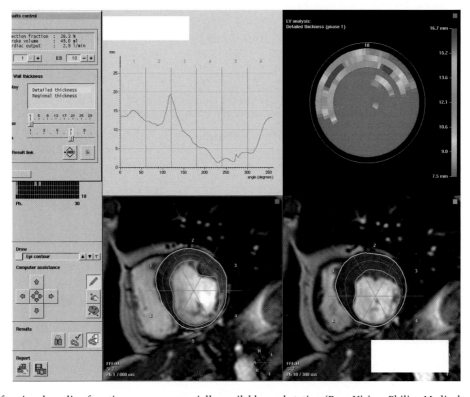

Fig. 6.26. Assessment of regional cardiac function on a commercially available workstation (Easy-Vision, Philips Medical Systems, Best, The Netherlands) in a patient with a large, inferior aneurysm following a transmural myocardial infarction. After contouring epi- and endocardial contours, several parameters such as wall thickness, absolute and relative systolic wall thickening, and endocardial wall motion can be assessed. The results can be shown numerically, graphically (*upper left*) or as a bull's eye view (*upper right*), allowing a better appreciation of the spread of data throughout the left ventricle

et al. 2001). Currently, most vendors of MRI have dedicated postprocessing packages available (Figs. 6.25, 6.26). Also, other companies have specialized in commercial software for analysis of cardiac MRI studies, including analysis of myocardial tagging studies. Because of the growing interest in cardiac MRI, postprocessing tools will certainly improve in the near future. One way to accomplish this task is by using a priori knowledge of the ventricular anatomy and function patterns (preferably of both ventricles) in normal subjects and a series of different cardiac disease states. This approach would probably be very useful in improving the reliability of (semi)-automated delineation techniques.

6.7
Normal Values for Cardiac Function

Before the cardiac performance in a patient can be defined as abnormal, the normal values for ventricular volumes, function, and mass, as well as their physiological ranges, need to be known. Normal values are influenced not only by body constitution, age, sex, or level of training or fit-

ness, but also by technical issues such as MRI sequence design, use of imaging plane, image analysis, etc. (MARCUS et al. 1999b). In several tables in this chapter, a compilation of data from the currently available literature is provided. To improve the convenience of these tables for routine clinical use, normalized data (i.e., indexed to body surface area), confidence limits, separate data for women and men, or different age groups, as well as the type of MRI sequence and imaging plane are given (Tables 6.6 and 6.7). Normal MRI values in children are shown in Table 6.8. Values for endurance athletes are shown in Table 6.9. Normal values for LV wall thickness and chamber dimensions are shown in Table 6.10. In Table 6.11 is shown the regional variation in myocardial wall thickness and myocardial strains in a normal population group (BOGAERT 1997). Since most studies are single-center studies, based on a relatively small number of normal subjects (MOON et al. 2002; ALFAKIH et al. 2003), there is definitely need for a large, multicenter study using a standardized approach for data acquisition and analysis. However, taking into account the huge progress in the field of cardiac MRI in the last years, it will be difficult to determine the ideal timing and the best protocol of such a study.

Table 6.6. LV volumes, function and mass values in normal adult population, obtained with MRI

Study (year)	n	Sex – Age Mean/Range	View	Sequence	EDV ml(ml/m²)	ESV ml(ml/m²)	SV ml(ml/m²)	EF %	Mass g(g/m²)	CO (l/min)
LORENZ et al. (1999)	47	M 28 (8-57)	SA	SPOILED-GE	136 (69)	45	92 (47)	67	178 (91)	5.8 (3.0)
		(95% confidence limits)			*77-195*	*19-72*	*51-133*	*56-78*	*118-238*	*2.8-8.2*
	28	F 28 (8-57)			96 (61)	32	65 (41)	67	125 (79)	4.3 (2.8)
		(95% confidence limits)			*52-141*	*13-51*	*33-97*	*56-78*	*75-175*	*2.6-6.0*
SANDSTEDE et al. (2000)	36	TOTAL	SA	SPOILED-GE	108 (58)	35 (19)		68	132 (71)	5.2 (2.8)
	9	M 32 (22-44)			133 (66)	47 (23)		65	158 (79)	5.7 (2.8)
	9	F 27 (22-44)			103 (60)	33 (19)		69	109 (64)	4.8 (2.8)
	9	M 59 (45-74)			103 (52)	34 (17)		68	152 (77)	5.1 (2.6)
	9	F 57 (45-74)			91 (53)	26 (15)		72	111 (66)	5.1 (3.0)
SALTON et al. (2002)	63	M 57 (38-72)	SA	SPOILED-GE	115 (58)	36 (18)	79 (40)	69	155 (78)	
		(95% upper limit)			*169 (80)*	*65 (31)*	*104 (49)*	*59**	*201 (95)*	
	79	F 58 (36-78)	SA	SPOILED-GE	84 (50)	25 (15)	69 (35)	70	103 (61)	
		(95% upper limit)			*117 (65)*	*41 (24)*	*76 (41)*	*60**	*134 (75)*	
ALFAKIH et al. (2003)	30	M	SA	b-SSFP	168 (82)	61	108	64	133 (65)	
	30	F			135 (78)	49	86	64	90 (52)	
CLAY et al. (2004)	20	M 32 (18-59)	Radial	b-SSFP	181 (91)	71		61	162 (68)	
		(95% confidence limits)			*121-242*	*62-120*		*49-73*	*95-177 (50-86)*	
	20	F 37 (21-54)	Radial	b-SSFP	145 (81)	52		64	96 (54)	
		(95% confidence limits)			*103-187*	*28-77*		*54-73*	*65-127 (36-72)*	

b-SSFP, steady-state free precession; CO, cardiac output; EDV, end-diastolic volume; ESV, end-systolic volume; EF, ejection fraction; SA, short-axis; Spoiled-GE, spoiled gradient-echo; SV, stroke volume. Values between brackets are normalized to body surface area; *the 5th percentile (lower) limits for EF

Table 6.7. RV volumes, function and mass values in normal adult population, obtained with MRI

Study (year)	n	Sex – Age Mean/Range	View	Sequence	EDV ml(ml/m²)	ESV ml(ml/m²)	SV ml(ml/m²)	EF %	Mass g(g/m²)	CO (l/min)
LORENZ et al. (1999)	47	M 28 (8-57)	SA	Spoiled-GE	157 (80)	63	95 (48)	60	50 (26)	
		(95% confidence limits)			*88-22*	*23-10*	*52-138*	*47-74*	*30-70*	
	28	F 28 (8-57)			106 (67)	40	66 (42)	63	40 (25)	
		(95% confidence limits)			*58-154*	*12-68*	*35-98*	*47-80*	*24-55*	
SANDSTEDE (2000)	36	Total	SA	Spoiled-GE	115 (62)	43 (23)		64	45 (24)	5.2 (2.8)
	9	M 32 (22-44)			143 (71)	57 (29)		60	50 (25)	5.7 (2.8)
	9	F 27 (22-44)			109 (63)	38 (22)		65	39 (23)	4.8 (2.8)
	9	M 59 (45-74)			119 (59)	50 (24)		60	54 (27)	5.1 (2.6)
	9	F 57 (45-74)			91 (53)	26 (15)		72	39 (23)	5.1 (3.0)
HOEPER et al. (2001)	6		SA	Spoiled-GE	120	47	73	61	44	
JAUHIAINEN et al. (2002)	12		TA	Spoiled-GE	120 (67)	57 (32)	63 (35)	53	38 (26)	
ALFAKIH et al. (2003)	30	M	SA	b-SSFP	176	79	98	55		
	30	F			131 (75)	52	78	60		

b-SSFP, steady-state free precession; EDV, end-diastolic volume; ESV, end-systolic volume; EF, ejection fraction; Spoiled-GE, spoiled gradient-echo; SV, stroke volume; TA, transaxial. Values between brackets are normalized to body surface area

Table 6.8. LV and RV Volumes, Function and Mass Values in Normal Children, obtained with MRI

Study (year)	n°	Sex – Age	View	Sequence	EDV ml(ml/m²)	ESV ml(ml/m²)	SV ml(ml/m²)	EF %	CO (CI) l/min(l/min/m²)
Left Ventricle									
HELBING 1995	22	5-16	TA	Spoiled-GE	89 (69)	26 (20)	62 (47)	70	
LORENZ 2000	8	7-20	SA	Spoiled-GE	(67)		(44)		(3.2)
Right Ventricle									
HELBING 1995	22	5-16	TA	Spoiled-GE	92 (70)	27 (21)	63 (48)	70	
LORENZ 2000	8	7-20	SA	Spoiled-GE	(70)		(43)		

Abbreviations: EDV, end-diastolic volume; EF, ejection fraction; ESV, end-systolic volume; SV, stroke volume; CI, cardiac index. Values between brackets are normalized to body surface area.

Table 6.9. Differences in LV and RV Volumes, Function and Mass between Endurance Athletes and Untrained Control Subjects

	EDV ml(ml/m²)	ESV ml(ml/m²)	SV ml	EF %	Mass g(g/m²)	CO l/min(l/min/m²)
Endurance Athetes (n: 21 / mean age: 27 ± 4 years)						
Left Ventricle	167 (89)	68 (36)	99	59	200 (107)	5.2 (2.8)
Right Ventricle	160 (86)	58 (31)	102	63	77 (41)	
Untrained Control Subjects (n: 21 / mean age: 26 ± 3 years)						
Left Ventricle	125 (67)	51 (27)	74	59	148 (79)	4.9 (2.6)
Right Ventricle	128 (68)	49 (26)	79	62	56 (30)	

Adapted from SCHARHAG et al., 2002.
A breath-hold ECG-triggered spin-echo technique was used for wall mass calculations. A breath-hold segmented spoiled-GE technique was used for functional evalution of right and left ventricle. All sequences were obtained in the cardiac short-axis. Between brackets are shown the values normalized to BSA.

Table 6.10. Normal Values of LV wall thickness and chamber dimensions.

Study – Year	n°	Sequence	PWT mm(mm/m²)	IVS mm(mm/m²)	EDD mm(mm/m²)	2-ChL mm(mm/m²)	4-ChL mm(mm/m²)
SALTON – 2002	63 M	Spoiled-GE	9.9 (5.0)	10.1 (5.1)	50.2 (25.3)	82.3 (41.3)	81.9 (41.5)
		(95% upper limit)	*11.2 (6.0)*	*11.7 (6.2)*	*58.5 (29.7)*	*93.8 (46.8)*	*93.0 (47.7)*
	79 F	Spoiled-GE	8.7 (5.2)	8.9 (5.3)	45.6 (27.1)	73.2 (43.5)	71.7 (42.7)
		(95% upper limit)	*9.8 (6.3)*	*10.1 (6.4)*	*51.1 (31.8)*	*83.7 (48.4)*	*81.5 (47.8)*

Between brackets is shown the values normalized to body surface area. All results are shown at end diastole.
Abbreviations: 2-ChL, two-chamber length; 4-ChL, four-chamber length; EDD, end-diastolic diameter; IVS: thickness interventricular septum; PWT: posterior wall thickness.

Table 6.11. Regional variation in LV wall thickness and myocardial strains in a normal population, using 3D MRI myocardial tagging

	Basal	Mid	Apical
End-diastolic Wall Thickness (mm)			
- Septum	9.1	9.3	8.0
- Inferior	9.3	9.3	8.1
- Lateral	9.6	9.6	8.2
- Anterior	9.6	9.2	7.6
Radial Thickening (%)			
- Septum	32	38	40
- Inferior	36	37	38
- Lateral	36	35	44
- Anterior	35	45	53
Circumferential Shortening (%)			
- Septum	28	34	39
- Inferior	36	40	43
- Lateral	36	42	46
- Anterior	28	38	42
Longitudinal Shortening (%)			
- Septum	14	17	18
- Inferior	21	18	20
- Lateral	21	19	21
- Anterior	18	15	17
Circumferential-Longutidinal Shear Strain (%)			
- Septum	10	11	12
- Inferior	14	6	6
- Lateral	12	6	5
- Anterior	11	11	11

The study group consists of 87 normal subjects (31 females), ranging 21 – 75 years (Data from BOGAERT 1997). Data are obtained using radial tagging technique, dividing the LV myocardium in 32 cuboids. These data are meaned to 12 regions, ie 4 segments (septum, inferior, lateral, anterior) per level (basal, mid, apical). The longitudinal and circumferential shortening strain represent the endocardial strain. The circumferential-longitudinal shear strain quantifies LV torsion.

6.8
Key Points

- Assessment of cardiac function involves evaluation of both systolic and diastolic function. MRI can be considered together with echocardiography as the primary imaging modality to assess cardiac function.
- The efficiency of the single myofiber shortening during systole is strongly enhanced by the complex fiber anatomy, leading to transmural fiber interaction. As a result, the LV undergoes a circumferential and longitudinal ventricular shortening, and extensive wall thickening during systole, allowing us to obtain an ejection fraction of ±70% with a fiber shortening of only ±10%.

- Cine MRI, using the new b-SSFP technique, is probably the best technique to quantify ventricular volumes, function, and mass.
- Be aware of different parameters, such as through-plane motion, anatomical structures, temporal and spatial resolution, that have a major impact on the results. Use therefore a consistent approach when performing functional cardiac MRI studies.
- 3D-volumetric ventricular quantification is superior to geometric assumptions, but is more time-consuming for data acquisition and analysis.
- Use a combination of short-axis and long-axis (horizontal and vertical) views to study the regional LV function. Because of its complex shape, the RV can be best studied using a combination of short-axis and longitudinal (axial or horizontal long-axis) views.
- Myocardial tagging is an ideal technique to analyze myocardial deformation and thus to unravel the mechanisms of myocardial contraction in normal and pathological conditions.
- MRI has an arsenal of techniques to assess cardiac function. Flow patterns through the atrioventricular valves, and systemic and pulmonary veins can be easily assessed by means of velocity mapping techniques. Moreover, myocardial tagging is probably the only technique allowing noninvasive assessment of the myocardial relaxation process.
- There is need for more sophisticated automated analysis programs for functional cardiac evaluation.

Acknowledgements: the author would like to thank F.E. Rademakers for the collaboration in the field of myocardial tagging and his expertise in myocardial strain analysis.

References

Alfakih K, Plein S, Thiele H et al (2003) Normal human left and right ventricular dimensions for MRI as assessed by turbo gradient echo and steady-state free precession imaging sequences. J Magn Reson Imaging 17:323–329
Alley MT, Napel S, Amano Y et al (1999) Fast 3D cardiac cine MR imaging. J Magn Reson Imaging 9:751–755
Arheden H, Holmqvist C, Thilen U et al (1999) Left-to-right shunts: comparison of measurement obtained with MR velocity mapping and with radionuclide angiography. Radiology 211:453–458
Arts T, Bovendeerd PHM, Prinzen FW, Reneman RS (1991) Relation between left ventricular cavity pressure and

volume and systolic fiber stress and strain in the wall. Biophys J 59:93–102

Atkinson DJ, Edelman RR (1991) Cineangiography of the heart in a single breath hold with a segmented turboflash sequence. Radiology 178:357–360

Aurigemma G, Davidoff A, Silver K, Boehmer J (1992) Left ventricular mass quantitation using single-phase cardiac magnetic resonance imaging. Am J Cardiol 70:259–262

Axel L, Dougherty L (1989a) Heart wall motion: improved method for spatial modulation of magnetization for MR imaging. Radiology 172:349–350

Axel L, Dougherty L (1989b) MR imaging of motion with spatial modulation of magnetization. Radiology 171:841–845

Azhari H, Weiss JL, Rogers WJ, et al (1993) Noninvasive quantification of principal strains in normal canine hearts using tagged MRI images in 3-D. Am J Physiol Heart Circ Physiol 264:33–41

Baer FM, Smolarz R, Jungehulsing M et al (1992) Feasibility of high-dose dipyridamole MRI for detection of coronary artery disease and comparison with coronary angiography. Am J Cardiol 69:51–56

Baer FM, Theissen P, Smolarz K et al (1993) Dobutamine versus dipyridamole-magnetic resonance imaging: safety and sensitivity for the diagnosis of coronary artery stenoses. Z Kardiol 82:494–503

Baer FM, Theissen P, Schneider CA, et al (1994) Magnetic resonance imaging techniques for the assessment of residual myocardial viability. Herz 19:51–64

Baldy C, Duke P, Crossville P, et al (1994) Automated myocardial edge detection from breath-hold cine MR images: evaluation of left ventricular volumes and mass. Magn Reson Imaging 12:589–598

Barkhausen J, Ruehm SG, Goyen M, et al (2001) MR evaluation of ventricular function: true fast imaging with steady-state precession versus fast low-angle shot cine MR imaging: feasibility study. Radiology 219:264–269

Barkhausen J, Goyen M, Rühm SG et al (2002) Assessment of ventricular function with single breath-hold real-time steady-state free precession cine MR imaging. Am J Roentgenol AJR 178:731–735

Bavelaar-Croon CDL, Kayser HWM, Wall EE van der et al (2000) Left ventricular function: correlation of quantitative gated SPECT and MR imaging over a wide range of values. Radiology 217:572–575

Beerbaum P, Köperich H, Barth P, et al (2001) Noninvasive quantification of left-to-right shunts in pediatric patients. Phase-contrast cine magnetic resonance imaging compared with invasive oxymetry. Circulation 103:2476–2482

Bellinger NG, Burgess MI, Ray SG et al (2000a) Comparison of left ventricular ejection fraction and volumes in heart failure by echocardiography, radionuclide ventriculography and cardiovascular magnetic resonance. Are they interchangeable? Eur Heart J 21:1387–1396

Bellinger NG, Davies LV, Francis JM, et al (2000b) Reduction of sample size for studies of remodeling of heart failure by the use of cardiovascular magnetic resonance. J Cardiovasc Magn Reson 2:271–278

Bellenger NG, Francis JM, Davies CL, Coats AJ, Pennell DJ (2000c) Establishment and performance of a magnetic resonance cardiac function clinic. J Cardiovasc Magn Reson 2:271–278

Bellenger NG, Marcus NJ, Rajappan K, et al (2002) Comparison of techniques for the measurement of left ventricular function following cardiac transplantation. J Cardiovasc Magn Reson 4:255–263

Beyar R, Weiss JL, Shapiro EP, et al (1993) Small apex-to-base heterogeneity in radius-to-thickness ratio by three-dimensional magnetic resonance imaging. Am J Physiol Heart Circ Physiol 264:133–140

Bloomer TN, Plein S, Radjenovic A et al (2001) Cine MRI using steady state free precession in the radial long axis orientation is a fast and accurate method for obtaining volumetric data of the left ventricle. J Magn Reson Imaging 14:685–692

Bloomgarden DC, Fayad ZA, Ferrari VA, Chin B, Sutton MGA (1997) Global cardiac function using fast breath-hold MRI: validation of new acquisition and analysis techniques. Magn Reson Med 37:683–692

Bogaert J (1997) Three-dimensional strain analysis of the human left ventricle. PhD dissertation, Catholic University, Leuven, Belgium

Bogaert J, Rademakers FE (2001) Regional nonuniformity of the normal adult human left ventricle. A 3D MR myocardial tagging study. Am J Physiol Heart Circ Physiol 280:610–620

Bogaert J, Bosmans H, Rademakers F et al (1995) Left ventricular quantification with breath-hold MR imaging: comparison with echocardiography. Magma 3:5–12

Bogaert J, Maes A, Van de Werf F et al (1999) Functional recovery of subepicardial myocardial tissue in transmural myocardial infarction after successful reperfusion. Circulation 99:36–43

Bogaert J, Bosmans H, Maes A, et al (2000) Remote myocardial dysfunction following acute anterior myocardial infarction. Impact of LV shape on regional function. J Am Coll Cardiol 35:1525–1534

Bolster BJ, McVeigh ER, Zerhouni EA (1990) Myocardial tagging in polar coordinates with use of striped tags. Radiology 177:769–772

Bornstedt A, Nagel E, Schalla S, et al (2001) Multi-slice dynamic imaging: complete functional cardiac MR examination within 15 seconds. J Magn Reson Imaging 14:300–305

Borow KM, Neumann A, Marcus RH, Sareli P, Lang RM (1992) Effects of simultaneous alterations in preload and afterload on measurements of left ventricular contractility in patients with dilated cardiomyopathy: comparisons of ejection phase, isovolumetric and end-systolic force-velocity indexes. J Am Coll Cardiol 20:787–795

Bosmans H, Bogaert J, Rademakers FE et al (1996) Left ventricular radial tagging acquisition using gradient-recalled-echo techniques: sequence optimization. Magma 4:123–133

Bottini PB, Carr AA, Prisant M, et al (1995) Magnetic resonance imaging compared to echocardiography to assess left ventricular mass in the hypertensive patient. Am J Hypertens 8:221–228

Brecker SJD (2000) The importance of long axis ventricular function. Heart 84:577–579

Brinker JA, Weiss JL, Lappe DL et al (1980) Leftward septal displacement during right ventricular loading in man. Circulation 61:626–633

Buchalter MB, Weiss JL, Rogers WJ (1990) Noninvasive quantification of left ventricular rotational deformation in normal humans using magnetic resonance imaging myocardial tagging. Circulation 81:1236–1244

Buchalter MB, Rademakers FE, Weiss JL, et al (1994) Rotational deformation of the canine left ventricle measured by magnetic resonance tagging: effects of catecholamines, ischemia,, and pacing. Cardiovasc Res 28:629–635

Buser PT, Auffermann W, Holt WW et al (1989) Noninvasive evaluation of global left ventricular function with use of cine nuclear magnetic resonance. J Am Coll Cardiol 13:1294–1300

Caputo GR, Suzuki JI, Kondo C et al (1990) Determination of left ventricular volume and mass with use of biphasic spin-echo MR imaging: comparison with cine MR. Radiology 177:773–777

Carr JC, Simonetti O, Bundy J et al (2001) Cine MR angiography of the heart with segmented true fast imaging with steady-state precession. Radiology 219:828–834

Casalino E, Laissy JP, Soyer P, Bouvet E, Vachon F (1996) Assessment of right ventricle function and pulmonary artery circulation by cine MRI in patients with AIDS. Chest 110:1243–1247

Cerqueira MD, Weissman NJ, Dilsizian V et al (2002) Standardized myocardial segmentation and nomenclature for tomographic imaging of the heart. J Cardiovasc Magn Reson 4:203–210

Chuang ML, Hibberd MG, Salton CJ (2000) Importance of imaging method over imaging modality in noninvasive determination of left ventricular volumes and ejection fraction. J Am Coll Cardiol 35:477–484

Cigarroa CG, Filippi C de, Brickner ME, et al (1993) Dobutamine stress echocardiography identifies hibernating myocardium and predicts recovery of left ventricular function after coronary revascularization. Circulation 88:430–436

Clay SR, Alfakih K, Radjenovic A et al (2004) Normal human left ventricular dimensions using steady state free precession MRI in the radial long-axis orientation (abstract). J Cardiov Magn Reson 6:231

Constable RT, Rath KM, Sinusas AJ, Gore JC (1994) Development and evaluation of tracking algorithms for cardiac wall motion analysis using phase velocity MR imaging. Magn Reson Med 32:33–42

Cottin Y, Touzery C, Guy F et al (1999) MR imaging of the heart in patients after myocardial infarction: effect of increasing intersection gap on measurements of left ventricular volume, ejection fraction and wall thickness. Radiology 213:513–520

Croisille P, Moore CC, Judd RM et al (1999) Differentiation of viable and nonviable myocardium by the use of three-dimensional tagged MRI in 2-day-old reperfused canine infarcts. Circulation 99:284–291

Culham J, Vince DJ (1988) Cardiac output by MR imaging: an experimental study comparing right ventricle and left ventricle with thermodilution. J Can Assoc Radiol 39:247–249

Debatin JF, Nadel SN, Sostman HD, et al (1992a) Magnetic resonance imaging-cardiac ejection fraction measurements: phantom study comparing four different methods. Invest Radiol 27:198–204

Debatin JF, Nadel SN, Paolini JF et al (1992b) Cardiac ejection fraction: phantom study comparing cine MR imaging, radionuclide blood pool imaging and ventriculography. J Magn Reson Imaging 2:135–142

Dilworth LR, Aisen AM, Mancini J, Lande I, Buda AJ (1987) Determination of left ventricular volumes and ejection fraction by nuclear magnetic resonance imaging. Am Heart J 113:24–32

Dong SJ, Hees PS, Huang WM, et al (1999) Independent effects of preload, afterload, and contractility on left ventricular torsion. Am J Physiol Heart Circ Physiol 277:1053–1060

Dong SJ, Hees PS, Siu CO, Weiss JL, Shapiro EP (2001) MRI assessment of LV relaxation by untwisting rate: a new isovolumic phase measure of τ. J Cardiovasc Magn Reson 281:2002–2009

Dulce MC, Mostbeck GH, Friese KK, Caputo GR, Higgins CB (1993) Quantification of the left ventricular volumes and function with cine MR imaging: comparison of geometric models with three-dimensional data. Radiology 188:371–376

Fieno DS, Jaffe WC, Simonetti OP, Judd RM, Finn JP (2002) TrueFISP: assessment of accuracy for measurement of left ventricular mass in an animal model. J Magn Reson Imaging 15:526–531

Firmin DN, Klipstein RH, Hounsfield GL, Paley MP, Longmore DB (1989) Echo-planar high-resolution flow velocity mapping. Magn Reson Med 12:316–327

Fischer SE, McKinnon GC, Maier SE, Boesiger P (1993) Improved myocardial tagging contrast. Magn Reson Med 30:191–200

Foo TK, Bernstein MA, Aisen AM, et al (1995) Improved ejection fraction and flow velocity estimates with use of view sharing and uniform repetition time excitation with fast cardiac techniques. Radiology 195:471–478

Forbat SM, Karwatowski SP, Gatehouse PD, et al (1994) Technical note: rapid measurement of left ventricular mass by spin echo magnetic resonance imaging. Br J Radiol 67:86–90

Furber A, Balzer P, Cavaro-Menard C et al (1998) Experimental validation of an automated edge-detection method for a simultaneous determination of the endocardial and epicardial borders in short-axis cardiac MR images: application in normal volunteers. J Magn Reson Imaging 8:1006–1014

Fujita N, Duerinckx AJ, Higgins CB (1993) Variation in left ventricular regional wall stress with cine magnetic resonance imaging: normal subjects versus dilated cardiomyopathy. Am Heart J 125:1337–1345

Fyrenius A, Wigstrom L, Bolger AF et al (1999) Pitfalls in Doppler evaluation of diastolic function: insights from 3-dimensional magnetic resonance imaging. J Am Soc Echocardiogr 12:817–826

Galjee MA, Rossum AC van, Eenige MJ van, et al (1995) Magnetic resonance imaging of the pulmonary venous flow pattern in mitral regurgitation. Independence of the investigated vein. Eur Heart J 16:1675–1685

Germain P, Roul G, Kastler B, et al (1992) Inter-study variability in left ventricular mass measurement. Comparison between M-mode echography and MRI. Eur Heart J 13:1011–1019

Giorgi B, Matton N, Dymarkowski S, Rademakers FE, Bogaert J (2003) Assessment of ventricular septal motion in patients clinically suspected of constrictive pericarditis, using magnetic resonance imaging. Radiology 228:417–424

Gopal AS, Keller AM, Rigling R, King DL Jr, King DK (1993) Left ventricular volume and endocardial surface area by three-dimensional echocardiography: comparison with two-dimensional echocardiography and nuclear magnetic resonance imaging in normal subjects. J Am Coll Cardiol 22:258–270

Goshtasby AA, Turner DA (1996) Fusion of short-axis and long-axis cardiac MR images. Comput Med Imaging Graph 20:77–87

Greenbaum RA, Ho SY, Gibson DG, Becker AE, Anderson RH (1981) Left ventricular fibre architecture in man. Br Heart J 45:248–263

Griswold MA, Jakob PM, Chen Q et al (1999) Resolution enhancement in single-shot imaging using simultaneous acquisition of spatial harmonics (SMASH). Magn Reson Med 41:1236–1245

Grothues F, Moon JC, Bellenger NG, et al (2004) Interstudy reproducibility of right ventricular volumes, function, and mass with cardiovascular magnetic resonance. Am Heart J 147:218–223

Guzman PA, Maughan WL, Yin FC et al (1981) Transseptal pressure gradient with leftward septal displacement during the Mueller manoeuvre in man. Br Heart J 46:657–662

Hansen DE, Daughters G, Alderman EL, Ingels NJ, Miller DC (1988) Torsional deformation of the left ventricular midwall in human hearts with intramyocardial markers: regional heterogeneity and sensitivity to the inotropic effects of abrupt rate changes. Circ Res 62:941–952

Hartnell G, Cerel A, Kamalesh M et al (1994) Detection of myocardial ischemia, value of combined myocardial perfusion and cineangiographic MR imaging. Am J Roentgenol 163:1061–1067

Hatabu H, Gefter WB, Axel L (1994) MR imaging with spatial modulation of magnetization in the evaluation of chronic central pulmonary thromboemboli. Radiology 190:791–796

Hatle LK, Appleton CP, Popp RL (1989) Differentiation of constrictive pericarditis and restrictive cardiomyopathy by Doppler echocardiography. Circulation 79:357–370

Hees PS, Fleg JL, Dong SJ, Shapiro EP (2004) MRI and echocardiographic assessment of the diastolic dysfunctin of normal aging: altered LV pressure decline or load? Am J Physiol Heart Circ Physiol 286:782–788

Hendrich K, Xu Y, Kim S, Ugurbil K (1994) Surface coil cardiac tagging and (31)P spectroscopic localization with B-1-insensitive adiabatic pulses. Magn Reson Med 31:541–545

Herregods M, Paep G de, Bijnens B et al (1994) Determination of left ventricular volume by two-dimensional echocardiography: comparison with magnetic resonance imaging. Eur Heart J 15:1070–1073

Higgins CB, Caputo G, Wendland MF, Saeed M (1992) Measurement of blood flow and perfusion in the cardiovascular system. Invest Radiol 2:66–71

Hoeper MM, Tongers J, Leppert A, et al (2001) Evaluation of right ventricular performance with a right ventricular ejection fraction thermodilution catheter and MRI in patients with pulmonary hypertension. Chest 102:502–507

Hori Y, Yamada N, Higashi M, Hirai N, Nakatani S (2003) Rapid evaluation of right and left ventricular function and mass using real-time true-FISP cine MR imaging without breath-hold: comparison with segmented true-FISP cine MR imaging with breath-hold. J Cardiovasc Magn Reson 5:439–450

Hsu EW, Muzikant AL, Matulevicius SA, Penland RC, Henriquez CS (1998) Magnetic resonance myocardial fiber-orientation mapping with direct histologic correlation. Am J Physiol Heart Circ Physiol 274:1627–1634

Hurrell DG, Nishimura RA, Higano ST et al (1996) Value of dynamic respiratory changes in left and right ventricular pressures for the diagnosis of constrictive pericarditis. Circulation 93:2007–2013

Ibrahim T, Weniger C, Schwaiger M et al (1999) Effect of papillary muscles and trabeculae on left ventricular parameters in cine-magnetic resonance images (MRI) (abstract). J Cardiovasc Magn Reson 1:319

Ichikawa Y, Sakuma H, Kitagawa K et al (2003) Evaluation of left ventricular volumes and ejection fraction using fast steady-state cine MR imaging: comparison with left ventricular angiography. J Cardiovasc Magn Reson 5:333–342

Iwase M, Nagata K, Izawa H (1993) Age-related changes in left and right ventricular filling velocity profiles and their relationship in normal subjects. Am Heart J 126:419–426

Janz RF (1982) Estimation of local myocardial stress. Am J Physiol Heart Circ Physiol 242:875–881

Jarvinen VM, Kupari MM, Hekali PE, Poutanen VP (1994a) Assessment of left atrial volumes and phasic function using cine magnetic resonance imaging in normal subjects. Am J Cardiol 73:1135–1137

Jarvinen VM, Kupari MM, Hekali PE, Poutanen VP (1994b) Right atrial MR imaging studies of cadaveric atrial casts and comparisons with right and left atrial volumes and function in healthy subjects. Radiology 191:137–142

Jauhiainen T, Järvinen VM, Hekali PE (2002) Evaluation of methods for MR imaging of human right ventricular heart volumes and mass. Acta Radiol 43:587–592

Jessup M, Sutton MS, Weber KT, Janicki JS (1987) The effect of chronic pulmonary hypertension on left ventricular size, function, and interventricular septal motion. Am Heart J 113:1114–1122

Kaji S, Yang PC, Kerr AB et al (2001) Rapid evaluation of left ventricular volume and mass without breath-holding using real-time interactive cardiac magnetic resonance imaging system. J Am Coll Cardiol 38:527–533

Katz J, Whang J, Boxt LM et al (1993) Estimation of right ventricular mass in normal subjects and in patients with primary pulmonary hypertension by nuclear magnetic resonance imaging. J Am Coll Cardiol 21:1475–1481

Kaul S, Wismer GL, Brady TJ (1986) Measurement of normal left heart dimensions using optimally oriented MR images. Am J Roentgenol 146:75–79

Kilner PJ, Firmin DN, Rees RSO et al (1991) Valve and great vessel stenosis: assessment with MR jet velocity mapping. Radiology 178:229–235

Klein AL, Cohen GI, Pietrolungo JF et al (1993) Differentiation of constrictive pericarditis from restrictive cardiomyopathy by Doppler transesophageal echocardiographic measurements of respiratory variations in pulmonary venous flow. J Am Coll Cardiol 22:1935–1943

Kojima S, Yamada N, Goto Y (1999) Diagnosis of constrictive pericarditis by tagged cine magnetic resonance imaging. N Engl J Med 341:373–374

Kondo C, Caputo GR, Semelka R, et al (1991) Right and left ventricular stroke volume measurements with velocity-encoded cine MR imaging: In vitro and in vivo validation. Am J Roentgenol 157:9–16

Kozerke S, Scheidegger MB, Pedersen EM, Boesiger P (1999) Heart motion adapted cine phase-contrast flow measurements through the aortic valve. Magn Reson Med 42:970–978

Kozerke S, Schwitter J, Pedersen EM, Boesiger P (2001) Aortic and mitral regurgitation: quantification using moving slice velocity mapping. J Magn Reson Imaging 14:106–112

Kroft LJ, Roos A de (1999) Biventricular diastolic cardiac function assessed by MR flow imaging using a single angulation. Acta Radiol 40:563–568

Kroft LJM, Simons P, Laar JM van, Roos A de (2000) Patients with pulmonary fibrosis: cardiac function assessed with MR imaging. Radiology 216:464–471

Kudelka AM, Turner DA, Liebson PR, et al (1997) Comparison of cine magnetic resonance imaging and Doppler echocardiography for evaluation of left ventricular diastolic function. Am J Cardiol 80:384–386

Kuijer JPA, Marcus JT, Götte MJW, Rossum AC van, Heethaar RM (2002) Three-dimensional myocardial strains at end-systole and during diastole in the left ventricle of normal humans. J Cardiovasc Magn Reson 4:341–351

Lalande A, Legrand L, Walker PM et al (1999) Automatic detection of left ventricular contours from cine magnetic resonance imaging using fuzzy logic. Invest Radiol 34:211–217

Lamb HJ, Doornbos J, Velde EA van der, et al (1996) Echo planar MRI of the heart on a standard system: validation of measurements of left ventricular function and mass. J Comput Assist Tomogr 20:942–949

Lauerma K, Harjula A, Jarvinen V, Kupari M, Keto P (1996) Assessment of right and left atrial function in patients with transplanted hearts with the use of magnetic resonance imaging. J Heart Lung Transplant 15:360–367

Lee VS, Resnick D, Bundy JM, et al (2002) Cardiac function: MR evaluation in one breath hold with real-time true fast imaging with steady-state precession. Radiology 222:835–842

Legget ME (1999) Usefulness of parameters of left ventricular wall stress and systolic function in the evaluation of patients with aortic stenosis. Echocardiography 16:701–710

Levy D, Garrison RJ, Savage DD, Kannel WB, Castelli WP (1990) Prognostic implications of echocardiographically determined left ventricular mass in the Framingham Heart Study. N Engl J Med 322:1561–1566

Lima JA, Guzman PA, Yin FC et al (1986) Septal geometry in the unloaded living human heart. Circulation 74:463–468

Lima JAC, Jeremy R, Guier W et al (1993) Accurate systolic wall thickening by nuclear magnetic resonance imaging with tissue ragging: correlation with sonomicrometers in normal and ischemic myocardium. J Am Coll Cardiol 21:1741–1751

Longmore DB, Underwood SR, Hounsfield GN (1985) Dimensional accuracy of magnetic resonance in studies of the heart. Lancet 15:1360–1362

Lorenz CH (2000) The range of normal values of cardiovascular structures in infants, children and adolescents measured by magnetic resonance imaging. Pediatr Cardiol 21:37–46

Lorenz CH, Walker ES, Morgan VL, Klein SS, Graham TP Jr (1999) Normal human right and left ventricular mass, systolic function, and gender differences by cine magnetic resonance imaging. J Cardiovasc Magn Reson 1:7–21

Lorenz CH, Pastorek JS, Bundy JM (2000) Delineation of normal human left ventricular twist throughout systole by tagged cine magnetic resonance imaging. J Cardiovasc Magn Reson 2:97–108

Mandinov L, Eberli FR, Seiler C, Hess OM (2000) Diastolic heart failure. Cardiovasc Res 45:813–825

Marcus JT, Vonk Noordegraaf A, Vries PM de et al (1998) MRI evaluation of right ventricular pressure overload in chronic pulmonary disease. J Magn Reson Imaging 8:999–1005

Marcus JT, Götte MJW, DeWaal LK et al (1999a) The influence of through-plane motion on left ventricular volumes measured by magnetic resonance imaging: implications for image acquisition and analysis. J Cardiovasc Magn Reson 1:1–6

Marcus JT, DeWaal LK, Götte MJ,et al (1999b) MRI-derived left ventricular function parameters and mass in healthy young adults: relation with gender and body size. Int J Card Imaging 15:411–419

Markiewicz W, Sechtem U, Higgins CB (1987a) Evaluation of the right ventricle by magnetic resonance imaging. Am Heart J 113:8–15

Markiewicz W, Sechtem U, Kirby R, et al (1987b) Measurement of ventricular volumes in the dog by nuclear magnetic resonance imaging. J Am Coll Cardiol 10:170–177

Matter C, Nagel E, Stuber M, Boesiger P, Hess OM (1996) Assessment of Systolic and diastolic LV function by MR myocardial tagging. Basic Res Cardiol [Suppl 2] 91:23–28

Matthaei D, Frahm J, Haase A, Hanicke W (1985) Regional physiological functions depicted by sequences of rapid magnetic resonance images. Lancet 19:893

McVeigh ER, Atalar E (1992) Cardiac tagging with breath-hold cine MRI. Magn Reson Med 28:318–327

McVeigh ER, Zerhouni EA (1991) Noninvasive measurement of transmural gradients in myocardial strain with MR imaging. Radiology 180:677–683

Miller S, Simonetti OP, Carr J, Kramer U, Finn JP (2002) MR imaging of the heart with cine true fast imaging with steady-state precession: influence of spatial and temporal resolutions on left ventricular functional parameters. Radiology 223:263–269

Mirsky I, Corin WJ, Murakami T, et al (1988) Correction for preload in assessment of myocardial contractility in aortic and mitral valve disease. Application of the concept of systolic myocardial stiffness. Circulation 78:68–80

Mogelvang J, Thomsen C, Mehlsen J, et al (1986) Evaluation of left ventricular volumes measured by magnetic resonance imaging. Eur Heart J 7:1016–1021

Mohiaddin RH, Hasegawa M (1995) Measurement of atrial volumes by magnetic resonance imaging in healthy volunteers and in patients with myocardial infarction. Eur Heart J 16:106–111

Mohiaddin RH, Wann SL, Underwood R, Firmin DN, Rees S, Longmore DB (1990) Vena caval flow: assessment with cine MR velocity mapping. Radiology 177:537–541

Mohiaddin RH, Amanuma M, Kilner PJ, et al (1991) MR phase-shift velocity mapping of mitral and pulmonary venous flow. J Comput Assist Tomogr 15:237–243

Moon JCC, Lorenz CH, Francis JM, Smith GC, Pennell DJ

(2002) Breath-hold FLASH and FISP cardiovascular MR imaging: left ventricular volume differences and reproducibility. Radiology 223:789–797

Moore CC, O'Dell WG, McVeigh ER, Zerhouni EA (1992) Calculation of three-dimensional left ventricular strains from biplanar tagged MR images. J Magn Reson Imaging 2:165–175

Moore CC, Reeder SB, McVeigh ER (1994) Tagged MR imaging in a deforming phantom: photographic validation. Radiology 190:765–769

Mostbeck GH, Hartiala JJ, Foster E, et al (1993) Right ventricular diastolic filling: evaluation with velocity-encoded cine MRI. J Comput Assist Tomogr 17:245–252

Nagel E, Schneider U, Schalla S et al (2000) Magnetic resonance real-time imaging for the evaluation of left ventricular function. J Cardiovasc Magn Reson 2:7–14

Naito H, Arisawa J, Harada K, et al (1995) Assessment of right ventricular regional contraction and comparison with the left ventricle in normal humans: a cine magnetic resonance study with presaturation myocardial tagging. Br Heart J 74:186–191

O'Dell WG, Moore CC, Hunter WC, Zerhouni EA, McVeigh ER (1995) Three-dimensional myocardial deformations: calculation with displacement field fitting to tagged MR images. Radiology 195:829–835

Paelinck BP, Lamb HJ, Bax JJ, Van der Wall EE, Roos A de (2002) Assessment of diastolic function by cardiovascular magnetic resonance. Am Heart J 144:198–205

Palmon LC, Reichek N, Yeon SB et al (1994) Intramural myocardial shortening in hypertensive left ventricular hypertrophy with normal pump function. Circulation 89:122–131

Pattynama PM, Doornbos J, Hermans J, Wall EE van der, Roos A de (1992) Magnetic resonance evaluation of regional left ventricular function. Effect of through-plane motion. Invest Radiol 27:681–685

Pattynama PM, Lamb HJ, Velde EA van der, Wall EE van der, Roos A de (1993) Left ventricular measurements with cine and spin-echo MR imaging: a study of reproducibility with variance component analysis. Radiology 187:261–268

Pattynama PM, Lamb HJ, Velde EA van der, Geest RJ van der, Wall EE van der, Roos A de (1995) Reproducibility of MRI-derived measurements of right ventricular volumes and myocardial mass. Magn Reson Imaging 13:53–63

Pennell DJ, Underwood SR, Ell PJ, Swanton RH, Walker JM, Longmore DB (1990) Dipyridamole magnetic resonance imaging: a comparison with thallium-201 emission tomography. Br Heart J 64:362–369

Pennell DJ, Underwood SR, Manzara CC et al (1992) Magnetic resonance imaging during dobutamine stress in coronary artery disease. Am J Cardiol 70:34–40

Pennell DJ, Firmin DN, Burger P et al (1995) Assessment of magnetic resonance velocity mapping of global ventricular function during dobutamine infusion in coronary artery disease. Br Heart J 74:163–170

Perman WH, Creswell LL, Wyers SG, Moulton MJ, Pasque MK (1995) Magnetic resonance imaging during dobutamine stress in coronary artery disease. Am J Cardiol 70:34–40

Pipe JG, Boes JL, Chenevert TL (1991) Method for measuring three-dimensional motion with tagged MR imaging. Radiology 181:591–595

Plein S, Bloomer TN, Ridgway JP, et al (2001) Steady-state free precession magnetic resonance imaging of the heart: comparison with segmented κ-space gradient-echo imaging. J Magn Reson Imaging 14:230–236

Powell AJ, Tsai-Goodman B, Prakash A, Greil GF, Geva T (2003) Comparison between phase-velocity cine magnetic resonance imaging and invasive oxymetry for quantification of atrial shunts. Am J Cardiol 91:1523–1525

Rademakers FE, Buchalter MB, Rogers WJ et al (1992) Dissociation between left ventricular untwisting and filling: accentuation by catecholamines. Circulation 85:1572–1581

Rademakers FE, Rogers WJ, Guier WH et al (1994) Relation of regional cross-fiber shortening to wall thickening in the intact heart. Three-dimensional strain analysis by NMR tagging. Circulation 89:1174–1182

Rademakers FE, Marchal G, Mortelmans L, Werf F van de, Bogaert J (2003) Evolution of regional performance after an acute anterior myocardial infarction in humans using magnetic resonance tagging. J Physiol (Lond) 546:777–787

Rajappan K, Livieratos L, Camici PG, Pennell DJ (2002) Measurement of ventricular volumes and function: a comparison of gated PET and cardiovascular magnetic resonance. J Nucl Med 43:806–810

Robinson TF, Factor SM, Sonnenblick EH (1986) The heart as a suction pump. Sci Am 254:84–91

Rogers WJ, Shapiro EP, Weiss JL et al (1991) Quantification of and correction for left ventricular systolic long-axis shortening by magnetic resonance tissue tagging and slice isolation. Circulation 84:721–731

Romiger MB, Bachmann GF, Geuer M et al (1999) Accuracy of right and left ventricular heart volume and left ventricular muscle mass determination with cine MRI in breath holding technique. Rofo Fortschr Geb Rontgenstr Neuen Bildgeb Verfahr 170: 54–60

Ryf S, Spiegel MA, Gerber M, Boesiger P (2002) Myocardial tagging with 3D-CSPAMM. J Magn Reson Imaging 16:320–325

Sakuma H, Fujita N, Foo TK et al (1993) Evaluation of left ventricular volume and mass with breath-hold cine MR imaging. Radiology 188:377–380

Salton CJ, Chuang ML, O'Donnell CJ et al (2002) Gender differences and normal left ventricular anatomy in an adult population free of hypertension. J Am Coll Cardiol 39:1055–1060

Sandstede J, Lipke C, Beer M, et al (1999) Age- and gender-specific differences in left and right ventricular cardiac function and mass determined by cine magnetic resonance imaging. Eur Radiol 10:438–442

Santaralli MF, Positano V, Michelassi C, Lombardi M, Landini L (2003) Automated cardiac MR image segmentation: theory and measurement segmentation. Med Eng Phys 25:149–159

Scharhag J, Schneider G, Urhausen A, et al (2002) Athlete's heart. Right and left ventricular mass and function in male endurance athletes and untrained individuals determined by magnetic resonance imaging. J Am Coll Cardiol 40:1856–1863

Schulen V, Schick F, Loichat J et al (1996) Evaluation of κ-space segmented cine sequences for fast functional cardiac imaging. Invest Radiol 31:512–522

Scollan DF, Holmes A, Winslow R, Forder J (1998) Histological validation of myocardial microstructure obtained from diffusion tensor magnetic resonance imaging. Am J Physiol Heart Circ Physiol 275:2308–2318

Sechtem U, Pflugfelder PW, Gould RG et al (1987) Measurement of right and left ventricular volumes in healthy individuals with cine MR imaging. Radiology 163:697–702

Semelka RC, Tomei E, Wagner S et al (1990a) Interstudy reproducibility of dimensional and functional measurements between cine magnetic resonance studies in the morphologically abnormal left ventricle. Am Heart J 119:1367–1373

Semelka RC, Tomei E, Wagner S et al (1990b) Normal left ventricular dimensions and function: interstudy reproducibility of measurements with cine MR imaging. Radiology 174:763–768

Setser RM, Fischer SE, Lorenz CH (2000) Quantification of left ventricular function with magnetic resonance images acquired in real-time. J Magn Reson Imaging 12:430–438

Sierra-Galan LM, Ingkanisorn WP, Rhoads KL, Agyeman KO, Arai AE (2003) Qualitative assessment of regional left ventricular can predict MRI or radionuclide ejection fraction: an objective alternative to eyeball estimates. J Cardiovasc Magn Reson 5:451–463

Singelton HR, Pohost GM (1997) Automatic cardiac MR image segmentation using edge detection by tissue classification in pixel neighborhoods. Magn Reson Med 37:418–424

Sodickson DK, Manning WJ (1997) Simultaneous acquisition of spatial harmonics (SMASH): fast imaging with radiofrequency coil arrays. Magn Reson Med 38:591–603

Soldo SJ, Norris SL, Gober JR, et al (1994) MRI-derived ventricular volume curves for the assessment of left ventricular function. Magn Reson Imaging 12:711–717

Spiegel MA, Luechinger R, Schwitter J, Boesiger P (2003) Ring tag: ring-shaped tagging for myocardial centerline assessment. Invest Radiol 38:669–678

Spuentrup E, Schroeder J, Mahnken AH et al (2003) Quantitative assessment of left ventricular function with interactive real-time spiral and radial MR imaging. Radiology 227:870–876

Stillmann AE, Wilke N, Jerosch-Herold M (1997) Use of an intravascular T1 contrast agent to improve MR cine myocardial-blood pool definition in man. J Magn Reson Imaging 7:765–767

Stratemeier EJ, Thompson R, Brady TJ (1986) Ejection fraction determination by MR imaging: comparison with left ventricular angiography. Radiology 158:775–777

Streeter DD, Spotnitz HM, Patel DP, Ross J, Sonnenblick EH (1969) Fiber orientation in the canine left ventricle during diastole and systole. Circ Res 24:339–347

Streeter DD, Vaishnav RN, Patel DJ, et al (1970) Stress distribution in the canine left ventricle during diastole and systole. Biophys J 10:343–363

Stuber M, Scheidegger MB, Fischer SE et al (1999) Alterations in the local myocardial motion pattern in patients suffering from pressure overload due to aortic stenosis. Circulation 27:361–368

Tardivon AA, Mousseaux E, Brenot F et al (1994) Quantification of hemodynamics in primary pulmonary hypertension with magnetic resonance imaging. Am J Respir Crit Care Med 150:1075–1080

Thiele H, Nagel E, Paetsch I et al (2001) Functional cardiac MR imaging with steady-state free precession (SSFP) significantly improves endocardial border delineation without contrast agents. J Magn Reson Imaging 14:362–367

Thiele H, Paetsch I, Schnackenburg B et al (2002) Improved accuracy of quantitative assessment of left ventricular volume and ejection fraction by geometric models with steady-state free precession. J Cardiovasc Magn Reson 4:327–339

Tseng W-Y I, Reese TG, Weisskoff RM, Brady TJ, Wedeen VJ (2000) Myocardial fiber shortening in humans: initial results of MR imaging. Radiology 216:128–139

Utz JA, Herfkens RJ, Heinsimer JA et al (1987) Cine MR determination of left ventricular ejection fraction. AJR Am J Roentgenol 148:839–843

Van den Hout RJ, Lamb HJ, Aardweg JG van den et al (2003) Real-time MR imaging of aortic flow: influence of breathing on left ventricular stroke volume in chronic obstructive pulmonary disease. Radiology 229:513–519

Van der Geest RJ, Buller VG, Jansen E et al (1997) Comparison between manual and semiautomated analysis of left ventricular volume parameters from short-axis MR images. J Comput Assist Tomogr 21:756–765

Van Rossum AC, Visser FC, Sprenger M, et al (1988a) Evaluation of magnetic resonance imaging for determination of left ventricular ejection fraction and comparison with angiography. Am J Cardiol 15:628–633

Van Rossum AC, Visser FC, Eenige MJ van, Valk J, Roos JP (1988b) Magnetic resonance imaging of the heart for determination of ejection fraction. Int J Cardiol 18:53–63

Van Rugge FP, Holman ER, Wall EE van der, et al (1993a) Quantitation of global and regional left ventricular function by cine magnetic resonance imaging during dobutamine stress in normal human subjects. Eur Heart J 14:456–463

Van Rugge FP, van der Wall EE, de Roos A, Bruschke AVG (1993b) Dobutamine stress magnetic resonance imaging for detection of coronary artery disease. J Am Coll Cardiol 22:431–439

Van Rugge FP, Wall EE van der, Spanjersberg SJ et al (1994) Magnetic resonance imaging during dobutamine stress for detection and localization of coronary artery disease: quantitative wall motion analysis using a modification of the centerline method. Circulation 90:127–138

Waldman LK, Fung YC, Covell JW (1985) Transmural myocardial deformation in the canine left ventricle. Normal in vivo three-dimensional finite strains. Circ Res 57:152–163

Waldman LK, Nosan D, Villarreal F, Covell JW (1988) Relation between transmural deformation and local myofiber direction in canine left ventricle. Circ Res 63:550–562

Wedeen VJ (1992) Magnetic resonance imaging of myocardial kinematics. Technique to detect, localize, and quantify the strain rates of the active human myocardium. Magn Reson Med 27:52–67

Wedeen VJ, Weisskoff RM, Reese TG et al (1995) Motionless movies of myocardial strain-rates using stimulated echoes (erratum in Magn Reson Med 1995, 33:743). Magn Reson Med 33:401–408

Weiger M, Pruessmann KP, Boesiger P (2000) Cardiac real-time imaging using SENSE: sensitivity encoding scheme. Magn Reson Med 43:177–184

Weyman AE, Wann S, Feigenbaum H, Dillon JC (1976) Mechanism of abnormal septal motion in patients with right ventricular volume overload: a cross-sectional echocardiographic study. Circulation 54:179–186

Weyman AE, Heger JJ, Kronik TG, et al (1977) Mechanism of paradoxical early diastolic septal motion in patients with mitral stenosis: a cross-sectional echocardiographic study. Am J Cardiol 40:691–699

Wong AYK, Rautaharju PM (1968) Stress distribution within the left ventricular wall approximated as a thick ellipsoidal shell. Am Heart J 75:649–662

Yamaoka O, Yabe T, Okada M et al (1993) Evaluation of left ventricular mass: comparison of ultrafast computed tomography, magnetic resonance imaging, and contrast left ventriculography. Am Heart J 126:1372–1379

Yim PJ, Ha B, Ferreiro JI et al (1998) Diastolic shape of the right ventricle of the heart. Anat Rec 250:316–324

Young AA, Axel L (1992) Three-dimensional motion and deformation of the heart wall: estimation with spatial modulation of magnetization – a model-based approach. Radiology 185:241–247

Young AA, Axel L, Dougherty L, Bogen DK, Parenteau CS (1993) Validation of tagging with MR imaging to estimate material deformation. Radiology 188:101–108

Young AA, Kramer CM, Ferrari VA, Axel L, Reichek N (1994) Three-dimensional left ventricular deformation in hypertrophic cardiomyopathy. Circulation 90:854–867

Young AA, Cowan BR, Thrupp SF, Hedley WJ, Dell'Italia LJ (2000) Left ventricular mass and volume: fast point calculation with guide-point modeling on MR images. Radiology 216:597–602

Zerhouni EA, Parish DM, Rogers WJ, Yang A, Shapiro EP (1988) Human heart: tagging with MR imaging - a new method for noninvasive assessment of myocardial motion. Radiology 169:59–63

Zile MR, Brutsaert DL (2002) New concepts in diastolic dysfunction and diastolic heart failure. 1. Diagnosis, prognosis and measurements of diastolic function. Circulation 105:1387–1393

7 Myocardial Perfusion

Nidal Al-Saadi and Jan Bogaert

CONTENTS

7.1
Introduction

Assessment of the regional myocardial perfusion is of crucial importance in the evaluation and therapeutic decision-making in patients with known or suspected ischemic heart disease. Although conventional catheter-based angiography is the reference to study morphologically the epicardial coronary arteries, this technique provides limited information on the functional impact of a stenosis on the myocardial perfusion distally to the lesion (HARRISON et al. 1984; GOULD and KELLEY 1982). Such information would be most valuable in reducing the number of unnecessary invasive angiographic procedures. Moreover, because coronary artery disease (CAD) is the most important, potentially preventable cause of congestive heart failure, early recognition and adequate intervention would lead to a better patient outcome and to a decrease in the cost of care for cardiovascular disease. With the advent of faster magnetic resonance imaging (MRI) techniques in the early 1990s, assessment of myocardial perfusion by means of MRI has become feasible (ATKINSON et al. 1990; MANNING et al. 1991). Evaluation of myocardial perfusion with MRI is intrinsically appealing because of its noninvasive nature and other strengths such as high spatial, contrast, and temporal resolution. Moreover, first-pass myocardial MR perfusion studies (during rest and stress) are clinically appealing because they may be integrated into a more comprehensive MR approach to study ischemic heart disease patients, including functional imaging, myocardial viability imaging, and eventually coronary MR angiography (PLEIN et al. 2003). Unfortunately, myocardial MR perfusion is facing serious challenges, which explains why perfusion imaging is less well integrated into routine clinical evaluation of ischemic heart disease patients than other applications such as functional imaging or myocardial viability assessment. The main purpose of this chapter is to highlight the complexity of the myocardial perfusion issue and to focus on the practical solutions that have been developed to cope with these problems.

N. AL-SAADI, MD
Institute for Cardiac Magnetic Resonance Tomography, Berlin, Nuernberger Str. 67, 10787 Berlin, Germany
J. BOGAERT, MD, PhD
Department of Radiology, Gasthuisberg University Hospital, Catholic University of Leuven, Herestraat 49, 3000 Leuven, Belgium

7.2
Pathophysiology of Myocardial Perfusion

A unique feature of the myocardium is its oxidative metabolism with a limited and short-lived capacity for anaerobic metabolism. Therefore, any consideration of myocardial perfusion needs to stress the pivotal relationship between myocardial oxygen requirements and coronary blood flow. In normal conditions, there is a balance between oxygen demand and oxygen supply. Oxygen demand is primarily influenced by wall stress, heart rate, and contractility, while oxygen supply is determined by the coronary blood flow and the oxygen extraction. The oxygen extraction in the myocardial microcirculation is high under basal conditions (i.e., with an oxygen saturation of coronary sinus blood of only 20–30%). Therefore, it is mandatory that changes in myocardial oxygen demand result from similar changes in coronary flow.

The increase in coronary blood flow primarily relies on vasodilation. A normal coronary circulation may increase its flow in resting conditions by a factor of 4–6. Quantitative perfusion measurements performed by positron-emission tomography (PET) studies show a baseline myocardial blood flow of 0.7–1.25 ml $min^{-1} g^{-1}$, while the flow in the hyperemic myocardium is 3.7–6.7 ml $min^{-1} g^{-1}$. The capacity to increase the coronary flow or the *coronary flow reserve* is defined by the ratio of flow during maximum vasodilation to flow under resting conditions and is normally in a range of 3.5–5 (Araujo et al. 1991; Uren et al. 1994; Bergmann et al. 1989; Czernin et al. 1993; Sambuceti et al. 1993). There are also transmural differences in oxygen demand. The oxygen demand is greater in the subendocardium than in the subepicardium, with a greater flow and oxygen extraction in the inner myocardial layers. Therefore, and because of the fact that oxygenated blood supply begins in the subepicardium and ends in the subendocardium, the subendocardial layers are much more vulnerable to ischemia, and myocardial necrosis starts in the inner layers with a variable transmural spread depending on the severity of ischemia (Reimer and Jennings 1979).

Conditions with an imbalance between oxygen demand and oxygen supply are primarily the result of coronary atheromatosis with one or several stenoses on the coronary arteries. This imbalance causes myocardial ischemia, and, if prolonged, myocardial necrosis. Perturbations in the myocardial microcirculation with angiographically normal coronary arteries (i.e., syndrome X), may also lead to myocardial ischemia but are less frequent. The flow profile across a stenosis has a close relation with the degree of stenosis. A lumen-narrowing of a coronary artery below 70% has only a minimal influence on the flow resistance; while, with a narrowing greater than 70%, the resistance increases sharply, leading

to a significant pressure drop across the stenosis (Uren et al. 1994; Gould et al. 1990). The effects of a coronary artery stenosis on myocardial perfusion are closely related to the flow hemodynamics in the coronary arteries. In resting conditions, the myocardial perfusion is not altered until the coronary artery has an 85–90% stenosis. This is the result of progressive arteriolar vasodilation distal to the stenosis, which compensates for the effects of coronary stenoses under basal conditions and allows coronary flow to be maintained (Uren et al. 1994). However, with increasing coronary stenosis, vasodilatory capacity gets partially or completely exhausted and flow cannot be increased adequately during stress conditions. The coronary reserve is reduced or diminished and cannot be induced by vasodilatory stimulus. Under these circumstances, the myocardium distal to less severe coronary stenosis (i.e., between 50% and 85%) may become ischemic and the coronary artery stenosis is considered as hemodynamically significant although rest perfusion is preserved (Gould 1978, 1990). Thus, stress testing is generally considered as a prerequisite for assessment of the functional significance of coronary artery stenoses.

7.3
Modalities to Assess Myocardial Perfusion

Numerous techniques have been developed for measuring coronary flow and myocardial perfusion in experimental and clinical settings; these include electromagnetic flowmeters, coronary sinus indicator dilution techniques, velocity probes, inert gas washout analysis, labeled particles administered into the coronary arteries or the left ventricle (radioactive microspheres), and radionuclides trapped in the myocardium. In the clinical setting, only radionuclide imaging is routinely used to assess myocardial perfusion. More recently, new clinically useful techniques such as contrast echocardiography and myocardial MR perfusion imaging have become available.

7.3.1
Nuclear Medicine

Nuclear medicine is currently a cornerstone in the assessment of myocardial perfusion in CAD patients. Most cardiologists are well aware of the possibilities of this technique. Nuclear medicine techniques are well validated and their role in risk stratification for major adverse cardiac events is well established. Most often the single photon-emission computed tomography (SPECT) technique is used to diagnose and evaluate the severity of CAD (SHAW and ISKANDRIAN 2004), while PET is more accurate but also more expensive and less available (BACHARACH et al. 2004).

7.3.1.1
Single Photon-Emission Computed Tomography

Following intravenous administration of radionuclides [such as thallium201(^{201}Tl), technetium 99m (^{99m}Tc) sestamibi (MIBI), and ^{99m}Tc teboroxime], the relative myocardial distribution of these radionuclides is measured. Different protocols are used for ^{201}Tl and ^{99m}Tc-MIBI because, in contrast to ^{201}Tl, ^{99m}Tc-MIBI exhibits little or no redistribution within the first 1–2 h after administration. ^{201}Tl is injected during stress, while redistribution of the tracer is measured at rest after a delay (e.g., 4 h). ^{99m}Tc-MIBI SPECT is performed by means of an injection of tracer during stress and a second injection at rest (or vice versa). In regions with an abnormal myocardial perfusion, this will result in a lower number of counts (i.e., a defect) compared with normally perfused regions. The myocardial perfusion, however, remains unchanged unless the coronary artery has a stenosis of more than 85%. To detect less severe stenoses (between 50% and 85%), stress protocols (e.g., exercise, dipyridamole, dobutamine) are used. In these conditions, the stenosis will limit an increase in perfusion and decrease counts in the abnormal region. Thus, the defect on stress that is absent at rest (reversible defect) identifies an ischemic region that is usually supplied by a coronary artery with a 50–85% reduction in lumen diameter (i.e., redistribution on ^{201}Tl SPECT). Fixed defects (i.e., no redistribution at rest) are interpreted as myocardial scar or necrosis. The severity of the defect (i.e., reduction in counts) is related to the severity of the stenosis, while the area of the defect is related to the mass of myocardium dependent on the stenotic artery (PATTERSON et al. 1994).

Although SPECT is widely used in clinical practice, certain pitfalls should be mentioned. It has been demonstrated that, in patients with severe coronary artery stenosis, a lesion may appear as a fixed defect even though there is still viable, hibernating myocardium. This suggests that ^{201}Tl scintigraphy can fail to distinguish viable from nonviable myocardium.

Furthermore, the correlation between ^{201}Tl defect severity score and the descriptors of coronary stenosis have been shown to improve when patients with collateral vessels are excluded. (HADJIMILTIADES et al. 1989). This suggests that ^{201}Tl scintigraphy may not be sensitive enough for the detection of low-range collateral flow in ischemic myocardium, although the potential of ^{201}Tl for detection of extensive collateral flow cannot be dismissed (NIENABER et al. 1987). In a recent study by Wagner et al., comparing SPECT with contrast-enhanced, inversion-recovery MR with late imaging, subendocardial infarcts were systematically missed with SPECT because of the lack of spatial resolution, while MRI matched very well with histological findings (WAGNER et al. 2003).

Interpretation of ^{210}Tl scintigraphy scans requires substantial expertise and experience (HENKIN et al. 1994). False-positive studies are common, as thallium depends very much on body habitus. It is not uncommon for the female breast shadow to be interpreted as a septal defect. Incorrect selection of the long axis of the left ventricle during reconstruction may result in areas of decreased activity which do not correspond to anatomical lesions (HENKIN et al. 1994). False-negative results from ^{201}Tl scintigraphy may occur when a lesion appears to cause significant luminal narrowing but is not hemodynamically significant. In patients with multivessel disease, hypoperfusion of the entire myocardium may mask regional abnormalities resulting from a fall in blood flow below a critical threshold to maintain viability. Since there has to be at least a 30–40% blood flow reduction to be detectable with ^{210}Tl scintigraphy, mild perfusion changes cannot be discerned. By contrast, Kivelitz et al. were able to demonstrate in patients that changes of 20% in blood flow during rest can be detected with MR perfusion imaging, and this may explain the smaller rate of false-positive results compared with ^{201}Tl scintigraphy (KIVELITZ et al. 1997a,b). Moreover, substantial interobserver variability has been reported due to a lack of uniformly accepted standards for quantification of myocardial perfusion with ^{201}Tl scintigraphy. The reproducibility of quantitative planar ^{201}Tl scintigraphy is inversely related to the size of perfusion abnormalities (SIGAL et al. 1991), a finding shared with other imaging modalities and pointing to the importance of good spatial resolution.

7.3.1.2
Positron-Emission Tomography

PET is very useful for assessing myocardial perfusion and metabolism (Schweiger 1994; Gould 1990). Assessment of myocardial perfusion with PET can be performed with nitrogen-13 ammonia, oxygen-15 H_2O, rubidium-82, or carbon-11 acetate. PET has several advantages over SPECT, such as a higher spatial resolution (Bacharach et al. 2003). Moreover, the absolute myocardial blood flow (MBF) can be measured (in milliliters per minute per gram), while SPECT can only measure the relative blood flow. This is advantageous in patients with balanced ischemia caused by left main- or three-vessel CAD in which the maximal MBF is reduced in all regions of the left ventricle, or in patients in whom the myocardial ischemia is not caused by large-vessel CAD, such as syndrome X. It is furthermore considered the method of choice for determining the extent of viable myocardium. The drawbacks of PET are that the patient is exposed to radiation, PET is costly, the spatial resolution of cardiac PET images is substantially less than that presently achievable with myocardial MR perfusion, and it is not likely that PET scanners will be widely available in the near future. Recently, it has been reported that misregistration of attenuation and emission images, due to diaphragmatic displacement, body mass index, and heart size, is common in cardiac PET imaging and causes artifactual, false-positive myocardial perfusion defects (Loghin et al. 2004). The value of PET in the evaluation of myocardial ischemia has been reported in several studies (Schweiger 1994; Araujo et al. 1991; Go et al. 1990; Demer et al. 1989; Muzik et al. 1998).

7.3.2
Myocardial Contrast Echocardiography

Another means to obtain qualitative or quantitative information on myocardial perfusion is myocardial contrast echocardiography (MCE). Intravenous or intracoronary injection of microbubbles provides good estimates of coronary blood flow and can be used to detect CAD (Meza et al. 1996; Wei et al. 1998). Advantages of MCE are the real-time mode, the absence of injection of radioactive tracers, and the good spatial resolution. Its role in the clinical setting, however, needs to be further established. In patients with known or suspected CAD, the information obtained by MCE on the location of perfu-

sion abnormalities and their physiological relevance (reversible or irreversible) is comparable with that provided by SPECT (Kaul et al. 1997). Determination of endocardial-to-epicardial blood flow ratios during myocardial ischemia, however, is problematic with MCE (Vatner 1980). Different semiquantitative parameters have been proposed for the assessment of perfusion with MCE (Unger et al. 1994; Wei 2002), not all of which are good measures of blood flow changes. With MCE the quality of regional intensity time courses is compromised by shadowing artifacts, which impose the need to use low dosages of echo contrast agent. Both triggered, high mechanical-index (second harmonic) imaging and real-time, low mechanical-index approaches have led to improvements in this respect (Porter et al. 2001; Masugata et al. 2001), but it has not been demonstrated that capturing an adequate arterial input function for modeling is feasible.

7.3.3
Magnetic Resonance

Compared with the radionuclide techniques, myocardial MR perfusion imaging has several advantages, including higher spatial resolution, no radiation exposure, and no attenuation problem related to overlying breast shadow, elevated diaphragm, or obesity (Saeed et al. 1995; Al-Saadi et al. 2000a; Schwitter et al. 2001). Most myocardial MR perfusion imaging approaches are currently mainly based on the changes in myocardial signal intensity (SI) during the first pass of an intravenously injected contrast agent (*first-pass imaging*) (Fig. 7.1).

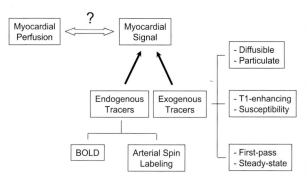

Fig. 7.1. Different strategies for myocardial MR perfusion imaging. Myocardial MR perfusion is based on changes in myocardial signal intensity caused by use of endogenous or exogenous tracers. These changes are assumed to reflect myocardial perfusion. *BOLD*, blood oxygenation level-dependent

For this purpose fast MR sequences are imperative (fast gradient-echo, GE, techniques, echo-planar imaging, EPI, parallel imaging) to acquire images of myocardium every, or at least every second, heart beat (Table 7.1). These MR pulse sequences can be either T1- (inversion-recovery, saturation-recovery, or partial saturation-recovery pulse) or T2-sensitive (driven equilibrium). Contrast media for these studies are T1-enhancing contrast agents and magnetic-susceptibility agents (T2* contrast agents), respectively. Perfusion studies for detection of regional ischemia are accomplished using low doses of MR contrast media and multislice measurements along different axes of the heart (WENDLAND et al. 1993a,b). Depending on the technique used, the ischemic area is identified as a zone either low signal in T1-weighted sequences or of high signal in T2-weighted sequences (ATKINSON et al. 1990; BJERNER et al. 2001; WENDLAND et al. 1993a,b; YU et al. 1992) (Fig. 7.2).

While quantification of absolute myocardial blood flow is extensively validated by means of PET (SCHWEIGER 1994; KLOCKE 1983; KLONER et al. 1992;

Table 7.1. Requirements for myocardial first-pass perfusion MRI

- Temporal resolution (i.e., one image per heart beat)
- Acquisition window as short as possible
  (i.e., less than 100 ms)
- Constant magnetization per image or per slice
- Spatial resolution (transmural discrimination)
- Coverage of the left ventricle
- Relationship between signal intensity and contrast dose
  (i.e., input function) that is quantifiable (linear)
- Contrast- and signal-to-noise ratios that are sufficiently
  high to allow discrimination between normal and
  ischemic regions of the myocardium
- Correction for respiration (total measurement time 45–60 s)

KRAITCHMAN et al. 1996), this is true to a much lesser degree for MRI. However, the superior spatial and temporal resolution of first-pass MRI and the use of stable and well-tolerated MR contrast agents provide compelling reasons for the study of transmural variations in blood flow and the detection of perfusion abnormalities confined to the subendocardium (KROLL et al. 1996; LAUB and SIMONETTI 1996; AL-SAADI et al. 2000a; LEE et al. 2004).

7.4
Techniques for
Myocardial MR Perfusion Imaging

7.4.1
Principles and Assumptions for Quantification

Although hypoperfused myocardium may be easily identified by visual analysis and yield sufficient diagnostic accuracy in experienced readers, this simple approach is not always sufficient and subtle differences may escape the eye as might be needed for follow-up examination or to evaluate therapeutic effects on myocardial perfusion. Furthermore, quantitative evaluation will be more objective than subjective assessment by eye. More quantitative information can be obtained from SI-versus-time (SI–time) curves generated from data obtained during early passage of contrast agent. In normally perfused myocardium, the curve starts from a baseline SI level and increases to maximum during the passage of contrast agent through the myocardium. The downslope of the curve is interpolated by a new upslope corresponding to recirculation of the contrast agent (Fig. 7.3).

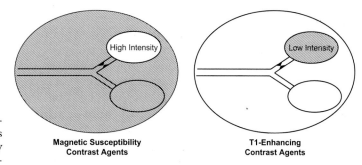

Fig. 7.2. T1-enhancing versus magnetic-susceptibility contrast agents. This figure shows the differences in myocardial signal intensity after administration of magnetic-susceptibility contrast agents (*left*) and T1-enhancing contrast agents (*right*). Following bolus injection of magnetic-susceptibility MR contrast agents, such as dysprosium or iron oxide particles, the normally perfused myocardium will show a drop in signal intensity; this is not the case for the hypoperfused myocardium, which therefore appears as a bright area with high signal. In contrast, T1-enhancing contrast agents (e.g., gadolinium) show an enhancement of the normal myocardium that is absent in hypoperfused myocardial regions; the latter thus appear as an area with low signal

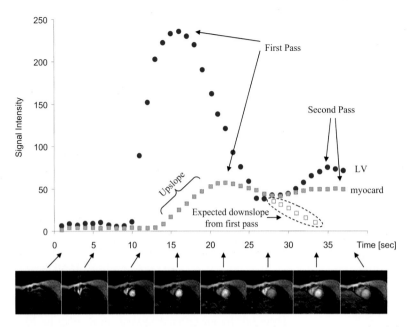

Fig. 7.3. MR myocardial perfusion study in a normal volunteer. First pass of gadolinium-diethylene triamine penta-acetic acid (Gd-DTPA; 0.1 mmol/kg body weight) through the heart using a gradient-echo–EPI sequence *(left to right, a selection of short-axis images)*. The signal of the myocardium is nulled by a saturation pulse. First, the right ventricular cavity is strongly enhanced, followed by the left ventricular cavity and the myocardium. The signal intensity-versus-time curve shows the changes in signal intensity due to the first pass in the left ventricular *(LV)* cavity, and the myocardium. Approximately 20 s later, a smaller second peak is visible, representing the second pass. The enhancement in the myocardium is much less pronounced and characterized by the absence of a sharp decline in signal intensity and of a second peak. The latter phenomena are caused by rapid extravasation of Gd-DTPA into the interstitium, which is responsible for a slow washout

In general, quantification of myocardial perfusion is done in two steps. First, a concentration-versus-time curve has to be obtained from the SI–time curve. The second step of quantification is to extract parameters of myocardial perfusion from the concentration–time curve.

Quantification of myocardial perfusion using first-pass MR perfusion imaging faces a lot of challenges that have to be overcome. A straightforward quantification needs some general requirements: (a) a nondiffusable tracer, (b) a complete washout of the tracer from the myocardium, (c) a single-spike (point-shaped) input function, and (d) a linear correlation between the tracer and the SI. These requirements are not fulfilled with gadolinium (Gd)-DTPA: (1) the contrast agent diffuses rapidly from the intravascular into the interstitial space and remains there until complete clearance. The diffusion is flow-dependent. While in normally perfused myocardium the extraction fraction varies from 40 to 60%, it can decrease to only 20% with increasing flow (TONG et al. 1993b); (2) the injection of the contrast agent in a peripheral vein leads to dilution of contrast agent with a slow and spread input curve (KEIJER et al. 1995); (3) a linear correlation

between the tracer and the SI is not maintained in all contrast agent concentrations (BURSTEIN et al. 1991; MANNING et al. 1992; SCHWITTER and Debatin 1995; FRITZ-HANSEN et al. 1996). Thus, to attempt myocardial perfusion quantification from dynamic tomographic MR images the kinetics of the tracer in the tissue must be known and described with an appropriate model of distribution. Furthermore, the blood-pool input function must be correctly defined. It has to be kept in mind that with MR the effects of Gd-DTPA on proton relaxivity rather than the concentration of gadolinium-DTPA in the myocardium is detected. This makes the acquired signal dependent on water exchange rates between the different compartments (JUDD et al. 1995a; DONAHUE et al. 1997; LANDIS et al. 2000; LARSSON et al. 2001) and leads to signal intensities which are not necessarily proportional to the concentration of the agent (MAUSS et al. 1985; BURSTEIN et al. 1991; WENDLAND et al. 1994; DONAHUE et al. 1994; JUDD et al. 1995a). Thus, MR perfusion techniques do not measure the absolute quantity of contrast medium either in the myocardium or in the blood. Wedeking and coworkers have noted that at low contrast-agent concentration, the concentration of the contrast agent can be calculated from the SI (WEDEKING et al. 1992). Increasing the dose leads to a saturation of signal enhancement and extravasation of the contrast agents which obscures the clearance phase of the first pass (WENDLAND et al. 1994). In practice, at concentrations between 0.2 and 1.2 mmol/l, the SI displays a linear progression compared with the Gd-DTPA concentrations. Above this limit, the signal increase becomes nonlinear as full relaxation is approached due to ever-decreasing T1 and due to signal loss induced by the T2* effect. Above 5.0 mmol/l, increasing Gd-DTPA concentrations result in a drop in SI as the signal losses induced by the T2* effect become dominant (BURSTEIN et al. 1991; CANET et al. 1995; MANNING et al. 1992; SCHWITTER and Debatin 1995; WENDLAND et al. 1994; KEIJER et al. 1995, TONG et al. 1993)

At the present time, myocardial MR perfusion research makes several, in part hypothetical, simplified assumptions that are incorporated into models for quantification of myocardial perfusion: (a) myocardial water is freely diffusible between the different compartments (intravascular, interstitial, and intracellular); (b) extravascular gadolinium agents enhance myocardial signal monoexponentially (i.e., the regional SI time courses change linearly with the amount of contrast agent injected); (c) MR contrast media behave as a blood component of physiological interest in its flow patterns; (d) MR contrast agents do not perturb the physiological parameters being measured; (e) the measured parameters are constant in the MR images used for calculation (SAEED et al. 1995). Two models have been used for quantification of myocardial perfusion by MR for intra- and extravascular contrast agents: the central volume model and the modified Kety model. Both models are highlighted in detail in Sect. 7.6.2.

Quantification has been attempted by several groups and also validated in animals and small numbers of patients (BURSTEIN et al. 1991; TONG et al. 1993; DIESBOURG et al. 1992; FRITZ-HANSEN et al. 1998 JEROSCH-HEROLD and Wilke 1997; HARRIS et al. 1997; LARSSON et al. 1994, 1996; TOFTS 1997; VALLEE et al. 1997; WILKE et al. 1994; JEROSH-HEROLD et al. 2002). Nevertheless, quantification of MR myocardial perfusion is still based on many assumptions and simplified models, giving rather an estimate that correlates to myocardial blood flow than a true quantitative measure of myocardial blood flow.

To circumvent the problems associated with quantitative analysis of myocardial perfusion, semiquantitative parameters have been used such as the upslope (AL-SAADI et al. 2000a), mean transit time (KEIJER et al. 1995), maximal SI (SCHAEFER et al. 1992), and time to 50% maximal SI (TAYLOR et al. 2004). Semiquantitative parameters should mainly be derived from the early wash-in phase of the contrast agent, because Gd-DTPA is an extracellular agent that leaks out of the vascular bed rapidly (approximately 30-50% during the first pass) (TONG et al. 1993). Thus, the early part of the SI-time curve is mainly influenced by perfusion and to a lesser extent by diffusion; whereas the later parts are increasingly influenced by diffusion (AL-SAADI et al. 2000a, 2001). Compared with other semiquantitative parameters of the first-pass SI–time curve, a linear fit of the upslope has been shown to be the most reliable parameter for evaluating myocardial perfusion (AL-SAADI et al. 2001) and seems to be a very sensitive semiquantitative parameter for alterations of myocardial perfusion (KROLL et al. 1996 ; JUDD et al. 1999; JEROSH-HEROLD et al. 2003). The upslope is easy to determine, is highly reproducible, with low inter- and intraobserver variability (AL-SAADI et al. 2000a), and has been evaluated and validated by several groups (AL-SAADI 2000a,b, 2001, 2002; IBRAHIM et al. 2002; SCHWITTER et al. 2001, 2004; NAGEL et al. 2004a; THIELE et al. 2003). Since such a fit does not depend on the downslope of the SI–time curve, it can be determined from a peripheral injection of Gd-DTPA. Whereas the upslope or the maximal SI may be sufficient for the detection of severe coronary artery stenosis with a rest perfusion study, the differences between normal and ischemic segments are small and a great overlap is found (AL-SAADI et al. 2000a; LAUERMA et al. 1997). Therefore myocardial perfusion reserve (MPR) calculated as an index from semiquantitative parameters has been proposed by several groups (AL-SAADI et al. 2000a; IBRAHIM et al. 2002). MPR index is calculated as the relative difference of perfusion before and after vasodilatation with dipyridamole or adenosine (AL-SAADI et al. 2000a; MATHEIJSSEN et al. 1996; LAUERMA et al. 1997; CULLEN et al. 1999; WILKE et al. 1997) (Fig. 7.4). Others have used semiquantitative parameters, which were derived only from a stress perfusion study without the need of a rest study (SCHWITTER et al. 2001). All semiquantitative parameters and the calculated MPR indices show an underestimation of perfusion estimates that seems to be less when evaluating the upslope (IBRAHIM et al. 2002, JEROSH-HEROLD et al. 2003). The degree of underestimation is dependent on the dose of contrast agent and the type of sequence used.

For all kinds of perfusion analysis, an accurate delineation of the input function is required.

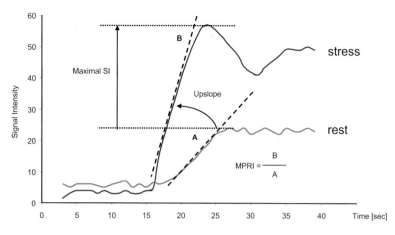

Fig. 7.4. Alterations of the signal intensity time curves after stress testing. The figure shows Gd-DTPA first-pass curves of the same myocardial segment at rest and after vasodilation with adenosine. After vasodilation maximal signal intensity increases and the upslope becomes steeper. A myocardial perfusion reserve index (*MPRI*) can be calculated from these alterations by dividing the parameter at stress through the same parameter at rest

Evaluated parameters and estimates of myocardial perfusion need a correction for the input function to adjust for different hemodynamic conditions and different kinetics of bolus applications. This allows for inter- and intraindividual comparisons and the calculation of MPR, which is derived from a rest and stress study with different hemodynamic conditions. However, at commonly used doses, contrast-agent concentrations in the blood pool are very high. The signal loses linearity to contrast-agent concentration and T2* effects may become dominant (Fig. 7.5). This makes an adequate evaluation of the blood-pool SI curve very inexact. The input function is the main obstacle needs to be overcome in quantitative and semiquantitative evaluation of MR myocardial perfusion.

7.4.2
Myocardial MR Perfusion Sequence Design

Any myocardial MR perfusion sequence designed to monitor the first pass of a contrast medium must meet several requirements (Table 7.1). It must: (a) simultaneously collect data of the entire heart, (b) provide sufficient temporal coverage to characterize wash-in and washout kinetics of the contrast agent bolus with a multi-slice acquisition every or at least every other heartbeat, (c) render sufficient spatial resolution for accurate localization and detection of small perfusion deficits, (d) cover the heart from base to apex (spatial coverage requires at least six short-axis views), (e) be sensitive to the signal changes brought about by the bolus with a signal and contrast-to-noise ratios that are sufficient to allow discrimination between normal and ischemic myocardium, and (f) provide a relation-

ship between SI and contrast concentration that is quantifiable and is preferably linear. A compact bolus of MR contrast media is necessary for perfusion studies to obtain pure first-pass transit of contrast through the myocardium. Currently, assessment of myocardial perfusion can be obtained by means of fast techniques such as spoiled gradient-echo (GE), echoplanar imaging (EPI) techniques, and balanced steady-state free precession (b-SSFP).

Fast spoiled gradient-echo (spoiled-GE) technique sequences are widely used. They usually have small flip angles with very short repetition times and a preparatory prepulse. Magnetization prepa-

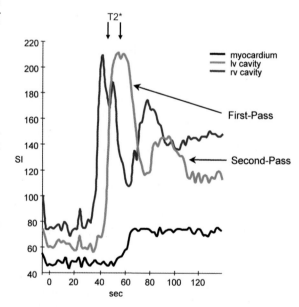

Fig. 7.5. First-pass signal intensity–time curves of the RV cavity, LV cavity, and the myocardium. Note the notch at peak signal intensity in the RV- and LV-cavity curves (*arrows*), depicting the T2* effect that results from the higher concentrations of contrast agent achieved

ration with an inversion (180°) pulse needs an inversion time of approximately 400 ms to initially zero SI of the myocardium. Thus the myocardium is initially dark, which enlarges the range of signal intensities of the myocardium before and after applying contrast agents. Due to short TR/TE and addition of preparatory pulses (inversion-recovery, saturation-recovery, or partial saturation-recovery pulses), they usually provide T1-weighted images. This fast acquisition mode allows the imaging of dynamic phenomena such as the first pass of contrast through the heart. The longer the total acquisition time in comparison with the length of the heart beat, the more the images will be blurred by cardiac motion.

EPI is most frequently used for T2-weighted perfusion studies. EPI acquires all the data for an image after a single excitation pulse, which reduces the acquisition times to between 50 and 100 ms for each image (MANSFIELD 1977). EPI has the potential to image the heart with sufficient temporal resolution and is therefore perfectly suited to study fast and dynamic phenomena such as the myocardial perfusion following bolus injection of contrast media. The spatial resolution can be improved, and the spatial distortion reduced, by using a multishot data acquisition (WETTER et al. 1995). SCHWITTER and colleagues (1997) have reported the use of this multishot EPI to assess myocardial perfusion in normal volunteers. The complete heart could be covered, with five to seven contiguous axial slices, every two heartbeats. Similarly to fast GE sequences, the spatial and temporal resolution with EPI are sufficient to evaluate perfusion of the subendocardial, midepicardial, and subepicardial layer of the heart distinctly (EDELMAN and LI 1994). While T2*-weighted GE EPI suffers from bolus-induced susceptibility problems, contrast dynamics can be best studied with T1-weighted spin-echo EPI using an pulse preparation (mostly saturation pulse) to induce T1 weighting in the subsequent signals and dephasing gradients to null the contribution from the cavity (EDELMAN and LI 1994). An obvious drawback of EPI is the need for extensive hardware modifications that only recently have become commercially available.

Further optimization of image quality and acquisition time can be obtained by means of using fast spoiled-GE techniques in combination with EPI readout. For instance using a repetition time of 8 ms and an EPI factor of 11, the acquisition time per image can be reduced to less than 100 ms. Imaging time can also be shortened using new techniques such as parallel imaging (HEIDEMANN et al. 2003). Another approach for reduction in acquisition time is using acquisition strategy where only a part of the κ-space is filled during every heartbeat, such as segmented κ-space acquisitions or "keyhole" imaging (WALSH et al. 1995, REEDER et al. 1999). The latter technique samples only a limited segment of the center of the κ-space corresponding to the low spatial frequencies during the first pass of contrast medium, thus significantly reducing the acquisition time. Because of the very fast T1-weighted sequences needed for the evaluation of myocardial perfusion, images show rather low signal-to-noise and contrast-to-noise ratios. This is not finally due to the very short repetition times which come at the cost of widening bandwidth and reducing signal-to-noise ratio. Additionally in conventional spoiled-GE pulse sequences, all transverse magnetization is destroyed before the next phase-encoding step.

Several groups have recently explored the use of the b-SSFP technique for myocardial perfusion imaging (SCHREIBER et al. 2002; HUNOLD et al. 2004; LEE et al. 2004). Although the contrast of these sequences depends on the T2/T1 properties of the tissue, the use of inversion or saturation prepulse combined with the ultrafast data readout results in predominantly T1-weighted images. They report higher signal-to-noise and contrast-to-noise ratios, and improved image quality compared with the spoiled-GE technique. However, it has been shown that this sequence is more susceptible to artifacts at the border of myocardium and contrast-enhanced blood of the ventricles than spoiled-GE sequences (FENCHEL et al. 2004). This might influence the evaluation of subendocardial perfusion defects significantly. Thus, the clinical value in assessing CAD patients needs to be assessed.

To null the signal of the myocardium and to obtain an improved T1 weighting, different strategies are available. Best known is the use of an *inversion-recovery* (180°) preparation pulse with a subsequent delay (e.g., 300-400 ms) to null the signal of myocardium. In patients with a constant heart rate, the extent of T1 relaxation between images is constant. However, in patients with arrhythmias, the change in R-R interval allows a different amount of T1 relaxation to occur between images. As a consequence, the SI and contrast detected as a function of time are modulated by sources other than the passage of the contrast agent. Moreover, use of long delay or inversion times interferes with the acquisition of multiple slices per heartbeat, and thus with the coverage of the heart. TSEKOS et al. (1995) have introduced the AICE (i.e., arrhythmia-insensitive contrast enhancement) technique to produce T1 weighting that is independent of the magnitude of longitudinal magnetization at the moment of the ECG trigger pulse. The magnetization preparation is started with a non-section-selective 90° RF pulse (*saturation recovery*) that nulls the longitudinal magnetization followed by a gradient crusher pulse that dephases the transverse magnetization. Although saturation-recovery prepulses provide less strong T1-weighting than inversion-recovery prepulses, they are less vulnerable to artifacts through triggering difficulties in arrhythmias. Moreover, they are advantageous in multi-slice scanning because of the shorter time between prepulse and data acquisition (routinely 200 ms). An intrinsic problem with the use of a single inversion or saturation pulse for a multi-slice approach is that the time between preparation pulse and data acquisition will be different for each slice. As a consequence, T1 relaxation and signal-to-noise and contrast-to-noise ratios will be different for each slice. A possible solution is presented by a notch pulse saturation technique, where a slice-selective 90° preparation pulse is applied for each slice (DING et al. 1998, SLAVIN et al. 2001). In this way, the "dead" inversion time is used for imaging in adjacent slice positions, allowing for higher flip angles and longer inversion times, leading to improved coverage and signal-to-noise ratios. The notched saturation pulse allows long magnetization recovery times without sacrificing section coverage, and yields excellent contrast between normal and ischemic myocardium. JUDD et al. (1995b) have replaced the inversion pulse in the inversion recovery turbo-fast low flip-angle single-shot technique (FLASH) sequence by a train of preparatory RF pulses. These nonselective preparatory RF pulses drive the magnetization to a steady state prior to the image acquisition. To obtain T2-weighting, the same type of acquisitions can be used with other preparation pulses, such as 90°–180°–90° triplets (ANDERSON and BROWN 1993).

7.4.3
Coverage of the Entire Ventricle

One of the main limitations of myocardial MR perfusion imaging in comparison with radionuclide imaging has been the restricted coverage of the myocardium. Although 3D MRI sequences have been developed, such as for imaging of the coronary arteries, myocardial MR perfusion sequences are basically two-dimensional (2D). Taking into account the rapid extravasation of extracellular contrast agents

and the necessity for MRI to scan during the first pass of the bolus, a single 2D approach will only cover a small part of the ventricle. It can be shown that single-slice acquisition can sufficiently detect myocardial ischemia in very selected patients with proximal high-grade coronary stenoses (AL-SAADI et al. 2000a). However, single-slice acquisition is not feasible for clinical routine. To cover a much larger part of the myocardium, different strategies have been developed. Either multi-slice imaging or multiple injections can be used, but clearly the former is more elegant and time efficient, particularly during stress imaging (TAYLOR and PENNELL 1996). MATHEIJSSEN et al. (1996) have shown that a double-slice approach enhances the detection of coronary artery lesions in five of ten patients. WALSH et al. (1995) have used a modification of keyhole imaging by sampling a limited segment of the center of the κ-space for a series of slices, such that after each two heartbeats the center of κ-space can be completed for all the slices, while WILKE et al. (1997) have used an ultrafast saturation-recovery GE acquisition. In this way up to five slices through the heart can be simultaneously obtained in a patient with a heart rate of 65 beats/minute (or less). With the advent of ultrafast EPI techniques, the entire ventricle can be studied following a single injection of contrast medium. SCHWITTER and colleagues (1997) were able to obtain seven slices through the left ventricle. From a clinical point of view, a minimum of three short-axis slices covering the basal, mid, and apical part of the left ventricle is recommended. Further increasing the number of slices is not a priori advantageous (NAGEL et al. 2003) and depends on the type of sequence and preparatory pulses chosen for acquisition. Regardless of the type of preparation used, the magnetization recovery time plays a major role in determining contrast, signal-to-noise ratio, and the maximum number of slices that can be acquired. A short recovery time permits the acquisition of more sections per cardiac cycle but sacrifices signal-to-noise ratio and contrast owing to minimal relaxation. A long TI provides higher signal-to-noise ratio and better contrast, but the delay inserted between preparation and acquisition reduces the maximum number of slices that can be acquired. The notched saturation pulse allows long magnetization recovery times without sacrificing section coverage (SLAVIN et al. 2001). An approach to increase the number of slices can be achieved by decreasing the sample frequency. Thus, the number of slices can be doubled by acquisition of two sets of slices, each acquired alternately every other heartbeat (AL-SAADI et al. 2003a). Moreover, increasing the numbers of slices necessitates obtaining images not only during diastole (preferable) but also during systole, which may impede analysis of the perfusion images. Another drawback in comparison with SPECT is that the cardiac short-axis, which is most frequently used to assess myocardium perfusion, does not provide information on the perfusion of the LV apex. Ideally one has to use a combination of both cardiac short-axis and long-axis views, which is difficult in practice. At the intersection of both planes, the signal in the tissue will recover less completely in between successive acquisitions.

7.4.4
Compensation for Respiratory Motion

Suppression of the gross cardiac motion due to respiration is strongly recommended during first-pass perfusion imaging. Because it is impossible for most patients to hold their breath for 45 s to 1 min, alternative strategies have to used. A first approach, yielding good clinical results, is to ask the patients to hold the breath just before the start of and during the first seconds after the injection of contrast agent in a cubital vein. Just before the arrival of contrast in the heart, the patient is asked to stop breathing as long as possible. If the patient is no longer able to stop breathing, he is allowed to breath shallowly till the end of the measurement. Shallow breathing during the entire examination, is a more patient-friendly approach but impedes visual as well as quantitative analysis. Elastic matching techniques are helpful to correct for respiratory-induced cardiac motion.

7.4.5
Contrast Media for MR Myocardial Perfusion

Most techniques for assessing myocardial perfusion with MRI rely on the administration of exogenous contrast media (e.g., paramagnetic gadolinium chelates, manganese gluconate, iron oxide particles, deuterium, or magnetic-susceptibility agents such as dysprosium, Dy) (SCHAEFER et al. 1989; ATKINSON et al. 1990; MITCHELL and OSBAKEN 1991; CANET et al. 1993; KANTOR et al. 1994). Alternative techniques include the use of endogenous tracers such as deoxyhemoglobin (i.e., BOLD technique) or spin tagging of arterial water (ATALAY et al. 1993; WILLIAMS et al. 1993; WACKER et al. 2003) (Fig. 7.1). Exogenous contrast media are usually classified according to their

distribution pattern (i.e., extracellular and intravascular contrast media) (Table 7.2) or to their effects on the longitudinal or transverse relaxation [T1-enhancing contrast agents and magnetic-susceptibility agents (T2* contrast agents), respectively].

Table 7.2. Extracellular versus intravascular contrast agents

	Extracellular	Intravascular
Examples		
T1-enhancing	Gd-DTPA Gd-DOTA Gd-BOPTA	Dextran-(Gd-DTPA) Albumin-(Gd-DTPA) Polylysine-(Gd-DTPA) USPIO
Magnetic-susceptibility (T2*)	Dy-DTPA	Albumin-(Dy-DTPA) MION SPIO USPIO
Molecular weight (daltons)	<1,000	>50,000
Distribution	Intravascular Interstitial	Intravascular
Distribution volume	30–40%	5–10%
Intravascular half-life	20 min	180 min (MION)
Excretion	Renal	Renal/MPS[a]
Application(s)		
T1-enhancing CM	Most widely and clinically used MR contrast agent	- Blood volume - Tissue perfusion - Capillary integrity - MR angiography
T2* CM	Detection of ischemia and early infarction and differentiation between occlusive and reperfused myocardial Infarction	- See T1-enhancing CM
MR perfusion imaging	First-pass imaging	First-pass imaging Steady-state imaging

CM, Contrast media; DTPA, diethylene-triamine pentaacetic acid; Dy, dysprosium; Gd, gadolinium; MION, monocrystalline iron oxides; MPS, mononuclear phagocytic system; SPIO, superparamagnetic iron oxides; USPIO, ultrasmall superparamagnetic iron oxides
[a]Iron oxide molecules are accumulated into the MPS system

7.4.5.1
Extracellular Contrast Media

Extracellular contrast agents or low molecular weight contrast agents (e.g., Gd-DTPA, Gd-BOPTA, and Gd-DOTA) are small molecules (<1000 Da) that rapidly diffuse through the capillary walls into the interstitium (WEINMANN et al. 1983). Their kinetic modeling is complex and has to take into account various flow- and tissue-dependent variables such as extraction fraction and partition coefficient (BURSTEIN et al. 1991; DIESBOURG et al. 1992; WENDLAND et al. 1994). Because of the rapid redistribution of extracellular contrast agents, rapid imaging techniques are required to image the inflow of the contrast agent following a bolus injection (i.e., first-pass study) (SCHAEFER et al. 1992). Bolus injection of extracellular contrast media results in typical first-pass effects, i.e., a sudden signal increase in the right ventricular blood pool, followed by a similar SI increase in the left ventricular blood pool, and subsequently a slower SI increase in the left ventricular myocardium. This increase is followed by a delayed decrease in SI, which may be attributed to the extravasation of Gd-DTPA through the capillary bed (WENDLAND et al. 1994). On the first pass through the capillary bed, up to 50% of circulating Gd-DTPA diffuses from the intravascular compartment into the extravascular compartments (TONG et al. 1993, BRASCH 1992). The optimum contrast dose for Gd-DTPA is 0.03–0.1 mmol/kg body weight (depending on the sequence used) with an injection time of 3–8 s (SCHAEFER et al. 1992; MATHEIJSSEN et al. 1996; SCHWITTER et al. 1997; AL-SAADI et al. 2000a). At higher doses the maximal relative increase in SI begins to saturate, thus hindering quantitative evaluation (SCHWITTER et al. 1997). Furthermore, saturation also affects the downslope of the SI–time curve and obscures the washout phase of the contrast medium, and may result in a plateau-shaped curve. The choice of the dose is mainly dependent on the sequence used and the method of evaluation. Quantitative approaches need smaller doses to avoid saturation or even signal drop due to T2*, whereas visual assessment needs high contrast between normally and hypoperfused myocardium to depict perfusion defects by eye, thus higher doses are necessary. A recent study could demonstrate inferiority of visual analyses compared with semiquantitation when a small dose of contrast agent was given (NAGEL et al. 2003). At the present time, clinical assessment of myocardial perfusion is largely restricted to the use of these extravascular contrast media because the use of most intravascular contrast agents is still not allowed in humans.

7.4.5.2
Intravascular Contrast Media

Intravascular contrast agents (also called bloodpool agents, macromolecular MR contrast media, or nondiffusible agents) are typically gadolinium molecules bound to large molecules such as albumin, polylysine, and dextrans (>50,000 Da). The relatively large size of these molecules confines them to the intravascular space for a significant period. A second type of intravascular contrast media are molecules that are removed from the vascular space by the mononuclear phagocytic system, such as superparamagnetic iron oxide particles (CANET et al. 1993; REVEL et al. 1996; JOHANSSON et al. 1998; PANTING et al. 1999; REIMER et al. 2004). These contrast media allow an easier kinetic modeling and have significant advantages over extracellular MR contrast media. They can be used for accurate assessment of tissue perfusion, measurement of relative blood volume, and the detection of abnormal capillary leakage (ROSEN et al. 1990; WEISKOFF et al. 1993; TONG et al. 1993; WENDLAND et al. 1994; ARTEAGA et al. 1994). Unfortunately, most of these intravascular contrast agents are currently not available for clinical use. A distinct advantage of intravascular contrast agents over extracellular contrast agents in the assessment of myocardial perfusion is that first-pass imaging is not strictly required, because these contrast agents remain much longer in the vascular compartment (i.e., steady-state myocardial perfusion instead of first-pass myocardial perfusion) (DEWEY et al. 2004). An intrinsic limitation is the smaller distribution volume, leading to lower signal-to-noise ratios compared with the extracellular contrast agents. Figure 7.6 illustrates the difference in distribution between intra- and extracellular contrast media.

7.4.5.3
T1-Enhancing and
Magnetic Susceptibility MR Contrast Media

MR contrast media act by influencing the relaxation times of the neighboring resonating protons. Several magnetic materials, such as manganese, gadolinium, dysprosium, and iron, are used. Their effect can be either a shortening of the longitudinal relaxation (i.e., T1 enhancing), a shortening of the transversal

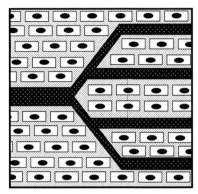
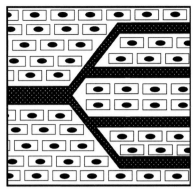

Extravascular   Intravascular

Fig 7.6. Distribution of intravascular and extracellular contrast media in the myocardium. Note that the distribution volume for extracellular contrast media in the vascular bed and the interstitial space is much larger than that of the intravascular contrast media, with a distribution volume of approximately of only 10%. This results in much lower signal-to-noise ratios in the myocardium for intravascular contrast

relaxation (i.e., magnetic susceptibility), or a combination of both. For example, gadolinium chelates at low doses are strong relaxivity (T1)-enhancing agents, causing a myocardial signal enhancement on T1-sensitive sequences, whereas at higher doses susceptibility effects become dominant and can be detected as signal loss on either T2*- or T2-sensitive sequences (SAEED et al. 1995). Thus on MR myocardial perfusion imaging, hypoperfused myocardial regions will be visible as dark areas with low SI using T1-enhancing contrast agents and as bright areas with high SI using magnetic-susceptibility MR contrast agents (YU et al. 1993) (Fig. 7.2). While gadolinium is most frequently used as a T1-enhancing contrast agent, dysprosium is a typical magnetic-susceptibility contrast agent (WENDLAND et al. 1993b). Ultrasmall superparamagnetic iron oxide particles (USPIO) can be used for both T1-weighted and T2*-weighted MR myocardial perfusion studies (PANTING et al. 1999; BJERNER et al. 2001; REIMER et al. 2004).

7.5
Stress Imaging

Except for high-grade coronary artery stenosis, perfusion abnormalities occur only under stress conditions (UREN et al. 1994; DICARLI et al. 1995; GOULD 1978; GALLAGHER et al. 1982). In the presence of a hemodynamically significant stenosis, the area in jeopardy may not be evident during the first pass in the basal state. When the flow is challenged by infusion of a vasodilator, the area in jeopardy becomes visible during the first pass of gadolinium chelates (AL-SAADI et al. 2000a; SCHWITTER et al. 2001; SAEED et al. 1994) (Fig. 7.7). Thus, stress imaging is essential to accurately assess hypoperfused myocardium. Stress can usually be induced by physical exercise or standardized stress protocols with pharmacological agents such as dipyridamole, adenosine infusion, or dobutamine/atropine. Exercise causes motion artifacts in MR images that are not obtained in real time, and is, therefore, currently not well suited for

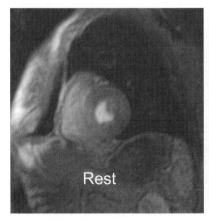
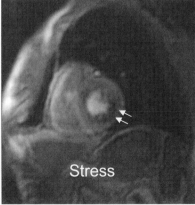

Rest   Stress

Fig. 7.7. Stress myocardial MR perfusion imaging using adenosine. Hemodynamically significant stenosis (50–85% lumen narrowing) may be undetected during resting conditions (*left*). During stress conditions (*right*), such as after the administration of adenosine, the myocardium supplied by the stenotic coronary artery becomes hypoperfused and will be visible as an area with low signal intensity using T1-enhancing contrast agents (lateral segment, *arrows*)

MR stress testing. However, pharmacological agents have been shown to be safe, well tolerated, and to reproducibly induce myocardial ischemia. In clinical practice, dipyridamole and adenosine are the most commonly used pharmacological vasodilators, both which have been applied and studied extensively for myocardial perfusion evaluation by SPECT and PET (Cerqueira et al. 1994). Dipyridamole indirectly causes coronary vasodilatation without increasing the workload of the heart by increasing the interstitial levels of adenosine, which activates the α_2 receptors (PENNELL 1994). The infusion regimen commonly used is 0.56 mg/kg intravenously, spread over 4 min. The increase in coronary flow after dipyridamole reaches its zenith approximately 2 min after the end of the 4-min infusion, and it is at this time that a myocardial contrast agent should be given. It is well known that, with maximal vasodilation, coronary blood flow in healthy subjects increases four- to fivefold over the baseline value of approximately 0.8–1.2 ml min^{-1} g^{-1}, and there is an average blood volume increase of ~50% in the myocardium (WILSON et al. 1990). The hemodynamic response is prolonged and the half-life of reduction in coronary flow is of the order of 30 min. Side-effects (e.g., chest pain, headache, dizziness, and nausea) and ischemia are reversible with aminophylline. An alternative to dipyridamole is adenosine. In contrast to dipyridamole, adenosine causes vasodilation by direct activation of the α_2 receptors. Adenosine is infused at 0.140 μg kg^{-1}min^{-1} for 4 min (0.84 mg/kg total dose). After 2–3 min, the adenosine reaction peaks and the heart rate increases. Coronary flow velocity returns to basal levels within 1–2 min. Adenosine has a very good safety profile; whereas minor side effects, such as flush, warmth, or headaches are common (81%), severe side-effects are very rare. In 9,256 patients evaluated, there were no deaths, one myocardial infarction, and seven episodes of severe bronchospasm and one episode of pulmonary edema. AV-block occurs in <1% and is mainly a lower-degree AV-block. AV block resolves spontaneously after termination of adenosine infusion (CERQUEIRA et al. 1994). Adenosine and dipyridamole seems to be equally effective in producing myocardial ischemia. However, the short half-life (<10 s) and more reliable action of adenosine compared with dipyridamole makes this drug very suitable for stress testing. Even though the risk is small, emergency precautions such as trained evacuation procedures and trained personal for resuscitation should be followed. Both pharmacological stressors are approved by the US Food and Drug Administration (FDA) for inducing

coronary hyperemia (SIEBERT et al. 1998). In case of contraindication for adenosine or dipyridamole, a dobutamine stress can be preformed for the evaluation of myocardial perfusion; however, this test is less sensitive than vasodilators (AL-SAADI 2002). Care has to be taken that patients have refrained from beverages or food containing caffeine before a dipyridamole or adenosine test. Beta-blocker should be discontinued at the day of examination with a dobutamine stress test.

7.6
Myocardial Perfusion Analysis

7.6.1
Visual Analysis

Visual assessment of first-pass myocardial perfusion imaging is the most frequently used approach to qualitatively assess the myocardial perfusion status. Although semiquantitative or preferably quantitative perfusion analysis is the goal and will enable competition in a more precise way with nuclear medicine, visual analysis performed by an experienced reader may provide very useful information. Moreover, the (semi)quantitative approaches are still very time-consuming and tedious. Without automated tracking software that corrects the cardiac position for respiratory-induced shifts, manual correction of several hundreds of images per perfusion study may be necessary, which is not feasible in a clinical setting. A true myocardial perfusion defect caused by CAD has the following characteristics: It becomes visible as a nonenhancing part of the myocardium during the first pass of contrast medium through the myocardium (i.e., after appearance of contrast agent in the LV cavity), it is pronounced in the subendocardium, it resolves from the edge to the center of the perfusion defect (from subpericardium to subendocardium), it obeys anatomical borders and respects the course of blood supply by coronary arteries (Figs. 7.8, 7.9). Depending on the severity of the coronary artery stenosis and eventually the presence of collateral vessels, the duration of the defect ranges from brief (i.e., a few heartbeats) to prolonged (i.e., persistent until the second pass). Abnormalities are most pronounced in the subendocardium, and the transmural spread is variable. The size of a perfusion defect is determined by the position of the stenosis in the coronary artery. Depending on the coronary artery involved, the perfusion defect has typical fea-

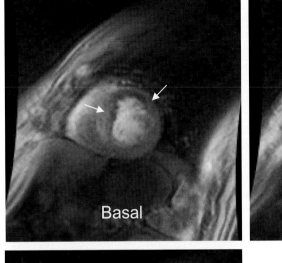

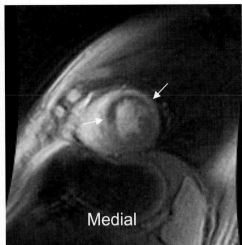

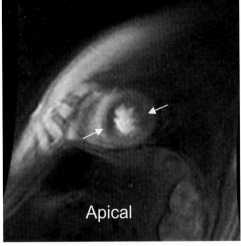

Fig. 7.8. Qualitative assessment of myocardial first-pass perfusion. Example of a large anterior perfusion defect. The perfusion defect is visible in all three (basal, medial, and apical) short-axis slices, reflecting the large perfusion territory of this coronary artery (*arrows* point to the border of the perfusion defect). The perfusion defects show a clear subendocardial pronunciation and demonstrate highest degree of transmurality in the center of the perfusion defect two typical characteristics of perfusion defects reflecting myocardial ischemia

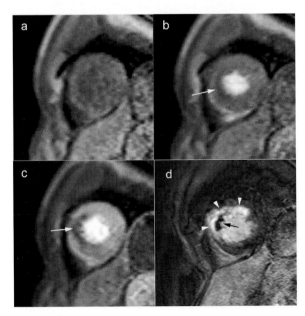

Fig. 7.9a-d. First pass of a Gd-DTPA bolus in a patient with an anteroseptal myocardial infarction. **a** Baseline image before the arrival of the contrast agent. Due to the prepulse, which nulls the signal in the myocardium, very little contrast is usually present in these images. A clear differentiation between myocardium and LV cavity is difficult. **b** Wash-in of the contrast agent in the myocardium showing an subendocardial perfusion defect in the anteroseptal segment. **c** The perfusion defect persists even after the wash-in period, a sign for severe hypoperfusion. **d** Late images using an inversion-recovery gradient-echo sequence for delayed enhancement imaging showing the necrotic area with a nonenhanced core, reflecting microvascular obstruction. Note the match between the size of the perfusion defect during first pass and the necrosis as determined by delayed enhancement

tures. A perfusion defect caused by a lesion in the left anterior descending (LAD) coronary artery is often stripe-like and involves typically one or more of the LV anteroseptal, anterior, or anterolateral segments. Right coronary artery (RCA) lesions cause typically inferobasal perfusion defects that are crescent-shaped, while left circumflex (LCx) lesions involve the lateral LV wall and may have a speckled appearance. Since perfusion defects always respect vascular territories, involvement of two or more coronary arteries will be visible as separate perfusion defects. If a contiguous subendocardial defect is visible that is not respecting the perfusion territories, first rule out susceptibility artifacts, and then consider microvascular disease, which usually appears as a contiguous, faint subendocardial perfusion defect. When performing stress–rest perfusion studies, perfusion defects caused by hemodynamically significant stenoses are usually only visible on stress perfusion imaging, or are at least more pronounced during stress compared with rest imaging. Perfusion defects at stress and rest can be encountered in patients with a recent myocardial infarction in whom the infarct-related artery is occluded or who have a no-reflow zone (i.e., microvascular obstruction area in the infarct territory) (Taylor et al. 2004). In patients with a prior history of myocardial infarction, it is advisable to start with the stress study, since delayed enhancement in the infarcted area may obscure concomitant presence of residual stenosis during the stress perfusion study if stress images are acquired after rest. In patients with a chronic myocardial infarction and scar formation, often perfusion-like defects are found in the scar region, even if they have open coronary arteries. This is related to a lower capillary density in fibrotic tissue compared with normal myocardium. Usually the size of the perfusion-like defect on first-pass perfusion matches well with the late-enhancement area. If, however, a larger perfusion defect is encountered, this may reflect a residual, potentially treatable coronary artery stenosis.

When performing stress–rest perfusion studies, it is advisable to analyze the stress and rest studies simultaneously in a standardized way. Next, perfusion abnormalities can be best described using a segmental approach (e.g., 16- or 17-segment model) (see Chaps. 5 and 8).

A first requisite is to perform a good-quality myocardial perfusion study. However, even in trained hands, artifacts are often present. Knowledge of these artifacts and assessment of their impact on myocardial perfusion may be very helpful not to misinterpret artifacts as true perfusion defects. Therefore,

it is recommended to start the image analysis by carefully evaluating the images for artifacts, such as susceptibility artifacts, motion artifacts, gibbs ringing, stripe artifacts, infolding artifacts, blurring, respiratory motion, and mistriggering. If artifacts are too severe, myocardial perfusion will become unevaluable. Susceptibility artifacts often occur during perfusion studies and are caused by differences in relaxivity between tissues. Moreover, these artifacts are usually enhanced during hyperemia (stress perfusion), which may yield the impression of true perfusion defects. They typically occur at the edges between blood pool and myocardium, and are visible as soon as the contrast arrives in the ventricular cavity (i.e., before the start of the myocardial enhancement) (Fig. 7.10). Because they represent no true perfusion defects, they often appear darker than the nonenhanced myocardium. They typically rapidly decrease in severity and disappear during the washout of contrast in the ventricular cavity, but may reoccur during the second pass, albeit with a lower intensity. Susceptibility artifacts are usually most pronounced in the basal part of the left ventricle, in the septum and around the papillary muscles. It is important to consider that susceptibility artifacts may be superimposed on a true perfusion

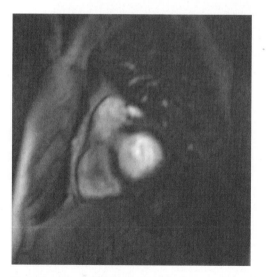

Fig. 7.10. An early image of a first-pass perfusion study (beginning of myocardial wash-in of a Gd-DTPA bolus, 0.1 mmol/kg body weight) in a basal slice. The high contrast-agent concentrations in the LV cavity result in susceptibility artifacts at the border to the myocardium. Susceptibility artifacts may be mistaken for subendocardial perfusion defects. In contrast to perfusion defects, susceptibility begins to appear before the contrast agent even arrives in the myocardium. Note the circumferential distribution of the susceptibility artifact, which does not match the supply of a coronary artery (basal short-axis slice)

defect. Other artifacts such as stripe or infolding artifacts are usually easier to differentiate from true perfusion defects, but they may hamper the interpretation of the perfusion studies. Inappropriate triggering leads to images acquired at different time points during the cardiac cycle, which often makes interpretation impossible. Respiration artifacts are often annoying, especially for (semi)quantitative analysis, and, as discussed above, it is advisable to suspend breathing at least for the relatively short period that covers the wash-in of contrast agents (AL-SAADI et al. 2000a, JEROSCH-HEROLD et al. 2004).

7.6.2
Semiquantitative and Quantitative Analysis

A first, semiquantitative approach to assess myocardial perfusion is to tract the changes in SI over time in the myocardium during the first pass of contrast through the heart. Usually this is done by contouring the endo- and epicardial borders, excluding the papillary muscles from analysis. The LV wall can be divided in several segments, and each segment can be assessed as a single unit, or can be divided in different layers (e.g., endocardial and epicardial layer) (Fig. 7.11). The analysis of these SI–time curves can be performed in different ways. The signal intensities before injection of the agent at the time T_{null} are averaged and used as offset. The following parameters can easily be calculated (Fig. 7.12): (a) the rate of increase in SI after the bolus injection of contrast agent (upslope), using a linear fit; (b) the maximum SI increase; (c) the time from T_{null} to the maximum SI increase; (d) the time from appearance of contrast agent in the LV cavity to appearance in the myocardium (contrast appearance time); (e) time to 50% of maximal SI; (f) the SI decrease after the

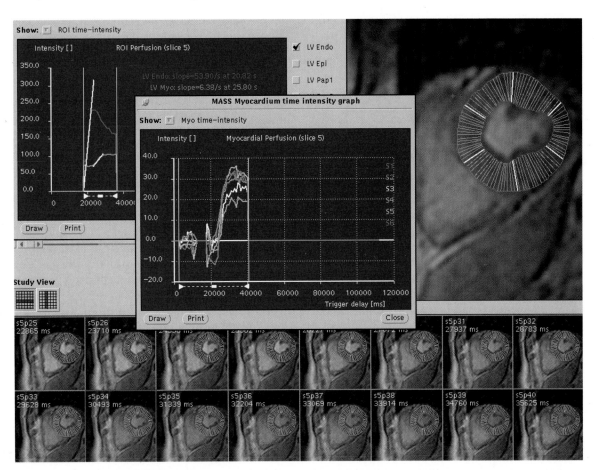

Fig. 7.11. For generating signal intensity–time curves, first the endo- and epicardial contours of the myocardium have to be drawn and corrected in each image for shift and motion (lower and right upper images). In each slice the myocardium is divided into 6 segments (right upper image). The signal intensity–time curves of each segment can be displayed (center image). Out of the signal intensity curves, different semiquantitative parameters can be derived, such as the upslope (left upper image). Courtesy of Eike Nagel and Nidal Al-Saadi, Berlin, Germany

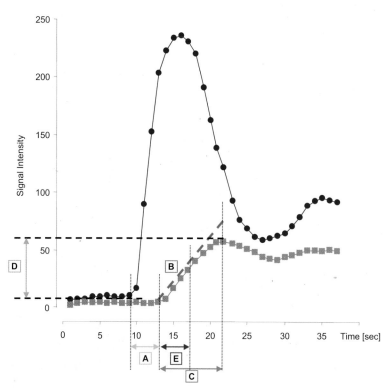

Fig. 7.12. Analysis of the signal intensity–time curve. After a series of precontrast images to acquire baseline signal intensity, the signal intensity increases in the LV cavity and, with a delay called "contrast appearance time" (*A*), in the myocardium. The rate of increase in signal intensity is measured by the upslope (*B*). After 5–10 s (time to peak; *C*) the signal intensity peaks (maximal signal intensity; *D*). Another semiquantitative parameter is the time to 50% of maximal signal intensity (time to 50%; *E*)

peak SI (downslope) ; or (g) the mean transit time using an exponential fit (AL-SAADI et al. 2000a,b, 2001; SCHWITTER et al. 2001; IBRAHIM et al. 2002; PEARLMANN et al. 2000; MATHEIJSSEN et al. 1996; MANNINNG et al. 1991; KEIJER at al. 1995). Some approaches require the application of more complex fitting procedures, such as the gamma variate fit. Such fit procedures are, however, sensitive to noise, sampling rate, and maximal signal achieved, and may result in an additional source of error when extracting semiquantitative parameters out of the fitted curve (BENNER et al. 1997).

As the upslope and maximum signal enhancement after contrast-agent administration are accepted parameters describing myocardial perfusion (MANNING et al. 1991; AL-SAADI et al. 2000a; SCHWITTER et al. 2001, NAGEL et al. 2003), the sampling rate (i.e., the number of time points on the upslope or from the onset of signal enhancement to maximum SI increase) is of paramount importance. The time of inflow of contrast medium is typically in the range of 7–12 s. If the sampling rate is too low, this will result in a large variation in measured upslope or maximum signal enhancement (AL-SAADI et al. 2003b). Further, the range from which to calculate the upslope should be in a range presenting fast wash-in of the contrast agent and should be calculated from a linear fit of four consecutive

data points acquired every heart beat. Thus, if the upslope is calculated from a range with too many data points, the upslope will be underestimated, because the SI–time curve flattens before maximal SI is reached. Applying the fit to only a few data points (i.e., two or three data points), the upslope calculation will be unreliable, because the noise will affect the measurement significantly (AL-SAADI et al. 2003c). Because the contrast medium rapidly diffuses out of the blood pool into the extravascular space, the processes of myocardial perfusion and diffusion occur almost simultaneously. It is generally believed that the upslope best reflects the wash-in or true perfusion phase of contrast in the myocardium. The interpretation of MR perfusion studies with a large number of images can be simplified by the development of automated programs for motion correction of the heart, automated pixel-based analysis programs, and the creation of parametric myocardial perfusion maps (BIDAUT and VALLÉE 2001; PENZKOFER et al. 1999, GERMAIN et al. 2001; PANTING et al. 2001) (Fig. 7.13).

During hyperemia there is a shortening of the rise time to peak SI, higher peak SI, and a clear descending limb after the peak signal, reflecting the higher perfusion rate due to the induced vasodilation and hyperemia (Fig. 7.4). In addition to the coronary flow reserve, the MPR can also be deter-

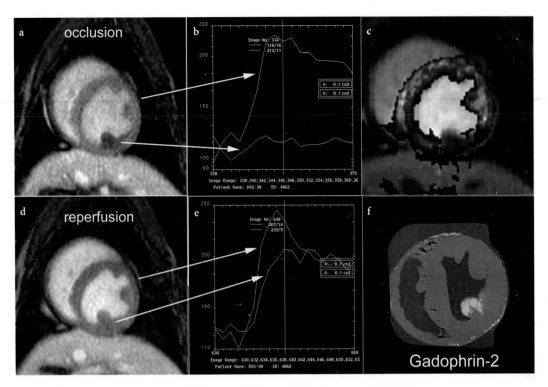

Fig. 7.13a-f. First-pass perfusion images of an experimental occlusion (**a**) and after reperfusion (**d**) with the corresponding signal intensity–time curves of an ischemic segment compared with a normally perfused segment in the same slice (**b** and **e**). Note the very flat appearance of the signal intensity curve in the ischemic segment during occlusion (**b**) and the improvement after reperfusion (**e**) when compared with normal signal intensity curves. Even improved after reperfusion, the upslope and the maximal signal intensity remain lower than the normally perfused control segment (**e**). The parametric display (**c**) shows a spared area of color, reflecting the hypoperfused segment that matches the necrosis as shown by delayed enhancement imaging (**f**)

mined as an index, being defined as the ratio of regional myocardial blood flow under hyperemic conditions to that under resting conditions (see Sect. 7.7). This ratio, however, may deviate from the coronary flow reserve, depending on the level of collateral blood flow (GOULD et al. 1990). The differences in regional perfusion can be quantified by defining a relative myocardial perfusion index as the ratio of the myocardial perfusion in the territory of the stenosed coronary artery to the myocardial perfusion in a remote normal zone (GOULD et al. 1990). Such an approach is not preferred, because patients with even severe multi-territorial ischemia may have a normal ratio and thus their ischemia would go undetected.

Analysis of SI–time curves is a semiquantitative approach to assess myocardial perfusion, since only relative and no absolute data are obtained on myocardial perfusion. More fundamental parameters can also be extracted from perfusion measurements (LE BIHAN 1995). Many attempts have been made for

more quantitative analyses of the SI–time curves. As mentioned above, quantification of myocardial perfusion is based on two different models: the *central volume principle* and the *modified Kety model*.

The central volume principle (ZIERLER et al. 1962) has been derived from the indicator-dilution theory as described by W. F. Hamilton and colleagues, in 1932, with the assumption that the indicator does not move into the tissue, a condition that is fulfilled by intravascular contrast agents. The Stewart-Hamilton equation relates the flow (F) through an organ with the total amount of injected tracer (M) and the tracer concentration as measured in the draining veins $c_d(t)$:

$$F = \frac{M}{\int_0^\infty C_d(t)\mathrm{d}t} \tag{7.1}$$

A number of assumptions are, however, necessary:

1. The tracer is not extracted from the blood pool
2. The flow should not be affected by the tracer
3. The tracer must be thoroughly mixed with the blood
4. It must be corrected for recirculation of the tracer

Additional information is obtained from the mean transit time (MTT), which represents the time the contrast agent needs to pass the myocardium, which is calculated as follows (MEIER and ZIERLER 1954):

$$MTT = \frac{\int_0^\infty t.c_d(t)d}{\int_0^\infty c_d(t)d} \qquad (7.2)$$

Here it is presumed that the tracer is injected as a bolus, but corrections can be made for a longer injection. Equation 7.3 further relates this MTT with the volume V occupied by the tracer in the myocardium (myocardial blood volume) and the flow (BOCK et al. 1995):

$$MTT = \frac{V}{F} \qquad (7.3)$$

Thus, the theory states that the MTT (which is the normalized first moment of the output concentration curve) is the ratio of the tissue blood volume to its blood flow. Assuming tissue blood volume remains constant, MTT will be directly correlated to myocardial blood flow and, thus, presents a semi-quantitative parameter that correlates better to myocardial perfusion than the previously discussed parameters.

$$MTT \sim \frac{1}{F} \qquad (7.4)$$

If myocardial blood volume could be calculated in absolute numbers, quantification of myocardial blood flow would be possible. However, only a relative value of myocardial blood volume can be derived from the first-pass curve by determining the area under the curve which is proportional to myocardial blood volume for blood-pool agents (LE BIHAN and TURNER 1992).

However, it has to be borne in mind that the central volume principle applies to the output concentration curve. MR measures venous outflow at the coronary sinus with insufficient resolution to analyze local venous flow from the myocardial wall. Therefore the residue detection method is used (LASSEN and PERL 1979). In that method contrast concentration in the myocardium derived from in the SI–time curves is converted to an output function. However, this condition needs an instantaneous contrast-agent injection. The decrease in contrast-agent concentration should be equal to the amount of contrast agent leaving the system. Therefore, the input function should be shorter than the transfer function through the myocardium. Such an instantaneous injection of contrast agent cannot be achieved noninvasively (KEIJER et al. 1995). For that reason calculation of the MTT cannot be easily determined without making several assumptions. Therefore, the use of MTT for the evaluation of myocardial perfusion by MR as proposed by some groups (WILKE et al. 1993) has been criticized (WEISKOFF et al. 1993). Models for calculation are required, such as the multiple pathway, axillary distributed model of blood tissue exchange that integrates the effects of the myocardial vascular architecture and the flow distribution (KROLL et al. 1996). JEROSH-HEROLD has described the converted tissue SI curve to be represented as convolution of the tissue impulse response with the arterial input. The initial amplitude of the tissue impulse response equals the tissue blood flow. However, deconvolution is very sensitive to noise and constraints need to be applied to stabilize the mathematical process of deconvolution. The susceptibility to noise can be reduced by constraining the deconvolution with a parameterized model for probability distribution of tracer residence times in a region of interest. The Fremi function has been applied as an empirical model for the impulse response (Fremi constrained deconvolution) (JEROSCH-HEROLD et al. 1998). Subsequently the same group has introduced a model-independent approach (JEROSCH-HEROLD et al. 2002). Both approaches could show sufficient correlation to microsphere measurements.

The second approach to quantify myocardial perfusion is derived from the Kety model (KETY 1951), which applies, in contrast to the central volume principle, only for extravascular contrast agents. Extravascular agents distribute in two compartments: the intravascular and the extracellular space. A two-model compartment with necessary derivations of equations applied for MR have used the term "modified Kety model" or "single capillary model" (DIESBOURG et al. 1992; LARSSON et al. 1994, 1996). This model assumes that the capillary bed can be seen as a tube with uniform distribution and permeability of contrast agent. The lateral diffusion of the contrast agent is not considered in this model (KETY 1951). The axial diffusion is proportional to the difference of concentration across capillary membrane and to a coefficient E that describes nonequilibrium effects, the extraction efficiency. The equation describes the relation between myocardial blood flow (MBF) and local myocardial contrast-agent concentration (CM), the myocardial extraction efficiency of the contrast agent (E), the arterial blood concentration of the contrast agent (C_a), and the partition coefficient between the vascular and the extracellular volume of distribution of the contrast agent (λ), which is equivalent to the interstitial space volume fraction (LARSSON et al. 1994; DIESBOURG et al. 1992).

$$CM = MBF.E._\mu C_a.e^{-[MBF.E/\lambda]}$$

The concentration can be expressed as deconvolution of the arterial input function with the residual impulse function:

$$MBF.E.e^{-[MBF.E/\lambda]}$$

The residual function depends on three parameters: myocardial blood flow, extraction efficiency, and the partition coefficient. Whereas E is defined as (according to Kety):

$$E = 1 - \exp(-PS/MBF)$$

Where PS is the permeability surface area product that describes the diffusion of the contrast agent through the capillary membrane. Because E and MBF present a product with two variables that depend on each other in a way to vary generally in opposite direction, it is very difficult to extract MBF from the equation. In general the product $E.MBF$ is measured. This product is called the unidirectional transfer constant (K_i).

$$K_i = F.E$$

For low flow, E will be high. The transport across the capillaries is more flow limited than diffusion limited and the product $E.F$ is more sensitive to flow. Severe ischemia is one exception in which E and F change in the same direction. For high-flow conditions, the transport of the contrast agent will be more diffusion limited than flow limited (VALLEE et al. 1997). However, the product $E.F$ increases with high flow but tends to plateau for very high flows. In conclusion, the determined parameters describe

not only myocardial perfusion, but also mainly the first-order transfer constant from the blood to the myocardium and the distribution volume of contrast agent in the myocardium.

Quite often, an assessment of quantitative parameters over a particular organ shows regional heterogeneities that provide clinically useful information. For a thorough quantitative evaluation of perfusion from currently available MR images, the following corrections have to be considered:

1. Tracer concentrations have to be calculated from signal intensities in MR images. The relation between concentration of Gd and SI is usually not known. In practice, a calibration is necessary for all sequences with their applied parameters (TR/TE/flip angle/time delays, etc.)
2. Most contrast agents used in clinical practice diffuse rapidly from the intravascular to the extravascular space. This effect can be incorporated in more difficult models that prescribe an organ as consisting of different compartments that mutually interact
3. Correction for recirculation is usually performed using a gamma-variate fit of the arterial input function
4. The effects of a finite contrast-agent injection can be corrected using deconvolution based on the same arterial input function

7.7
Applications of Myocardial Perfusion MRI

Since the early 1990s, numerous myocardial perfusion MRI studies have been performed in isolated hearts, animals, normal volunteers, CAD patients, and patients with a history of myocardial infarction (see Table 7.3). The spoiled GE technique is currently the best-validated one; other groups have explored the use of EPI techniques (both gradient-recalled EPI and inversion-recovery EPI) (SCHWITTER et al. 1997; PANTING et al. 2001), while recently the value of b-SSFP techniques for myocardial perfusion imaging has been evaluated by several groups (KLOCKE et al. 2001; SCHREIBER et al. 2002; LEE et al. 2004). The commercially available extracellular Gd chelates (e.g., Gd-DTPA, Gd-DOTA, Gd-BOPTA) have been used as contrast agents in most studies in both animals and humans. The optimal dose for myocardial perfusion imaging is 0.03–0.1 mmol/kg body weight and differs for different sequences.

Table 7.3. Review of MR myocardial perfusion studies in animals and humans

Author/year	Study group	MR sequence	Contrast agent	Dose (mmol/kg)	Stress	No. of Slices	Cardiac axis	Sensitivity (%)	Specificity (%)	Gold standard	Comments
Atkinson et al. (1990)	Rats/volunteers	GE	EC (Gd)	0.05-0.1	No	1	Ax	–	–	–	
Burstein et al. (1991)	Isolated hearts	GE	EC (Gd)	Var.	No	1	Ax	–	–	–	
Manning et al. (1991)	Patients	GE	EC (Gd)	0.04	No	1	SA	–	–	CA	
van Rugge et al. (1991)	Volunteers	GE	EC (Gd)	0.05	No	1	SA	–	–	–	
Schaefer et al. (1992)	Patients	GE	EC (Gd)	0.04	DIP	1	SA	–	–	201Tl	
Canet et al. (1993)	Dogs	GE	IV (Fe)	0.02	No	1	SA	–	–	–	
Klein et al. (1993)	Humans	GE	EC (Gd)	0.05	DIP	1	SA	77/81	75/100	99mTc/angio	
Wendland et al. (1993b)	Rats	EPI	EC (Dys)	Var.	No	1	Ax	–	–	–	
Wendland et al. (1993a)	Rats	EPI	EC (Gd)	Var.	No	1	Ax	–	–	–	
Wilke et al. (1993)	Dogs	GE	EC (Gd)	0.05	DIP	1	SA	–	–	Microspheres	
Arteaga et al. (1994)	Rabbits	GE	IV (Gd)	0.01	No	1	SA	–	–	–	
Edelman and Li (1994)	Humans	EPI	EC (Gd)	<0.2	No	1	Ax/SA	–	–	–	
Eichenberger et al. (1994)	Patients	GE	EC (Gd)	0.05	DIP	3	SA	64	76	201Tl/angio	
Hartnell et al. (1994)	Patients	GE	EC (Gd)	0.04	DIP	2	SA	92	100	201Tl/angio	Cine MRI
Kantor et al. (1994)	Dogs	EPI	EC (Gd)	0.1	DIP	1	Ax	–	–	–	
			EC (Dys)	0.1	DIP	1	Ax	–	–	–	
Wendland et al. (1994)	Rats	EPI	IV (Gd)	Var.	No	1	Ax	–	–	–	
			EC (Gd)	Var.	No	1	Ax	–	–	–	
Canet et al. (1995)	Patients	GE	EC (Gd)	Var.	No	1	SA	–	–	–	
Lima et al. (1995)	Patients	GE	EC (Gd)	0.1	No	4	SA	–	–	201Tl	
Walsh et al. (1995)	Patients	GE	EC (Gd)	0.05-0.1	DIP	3-4	SA	–	–	201Tl/99mTc	
Kraitchman et al. (1996)	Dogs	GE	IV (Gd)	0.005	DOB	1	SA	–	–	Microspheres	MR tagging
Matheijssen et al. (1996)	Patients	GE	EC(Gd)	0.05	DIP	2	SA	–	–	99mTc/angio	
Revel et al. (1996)	Dogs	GE	IV(Fe)	Var	No	1	SA	–	–	–	
Schwitter et al. (1997)	Volunteers	EPI	EC(Gd)	Var.	No	5-7	Ax	–	–	–	
Wilke et al. (1997)	Pigs/Humans	GE	EC(Gd)	0.04/0.025	AD	3-5	SA	–	–	Echo	
Cherryman et al. (1998)	Patients	GE	EC(Gd)	0.05	No	3	SA	–	–	ECG/Echo /99mTc	
Chung (1998)	Cats	GE	IV (Gd)	0.01	ATP	1	?	–	–	–	
Johansson et al. (1998)	Volunteers	GE	IV (Fe)	Var.	No	1	SA	–	–	–	
Panting et al. (1999)	Humans	GE/EPI	IV(Fe)	Var.	DIP	1	SA	–	–	–	

Author/year	Study group	MR sequence	Contrast agent	Dose (mmol/kg)	Stress	No. of Slices	Cardiac axis	Sensitivity (%)	Specificity (%)	Gold standard	Comments
Penzkofer et al. (1999)	Patients	GE	EC(Gd)	0.05	No	3	SA	77	97	99mTc	Cine MRI
Cullen et al. (1999)	Patients	GE	EC(Gd)	0.05	AD	3	SA	-	-	angio	
Wintersperger et al. (2000)	Patients	GE	EC(Gd)	0.05	No	3	SA	-	-	99mTc	
Al-Saadi et al. (2000a)	Patients	GE	EC(Gd)		DIP		SA	90	83	angio	
Al-Saadi et al. (2000b)	Patients	GE	EC(Gd)	o.o25	DIP	1	SA	89	82	angio	
Keijer et al. (2000)	Patients	GE	EC(Gd)	0.03	DIP	1	SA	-	-	201Tl	
Panting et al. (2001)	Patients	EPI	EC(Gd)	0.05	AD	1	SA	79	83	201Tl	
Bjerner et al. (2001)	Patients	T2w-TSE	IV(Fe)	3 mg/kg	-	1	SA/LA	-	-	-	
Klocke et al. (2001)	Dogs	b-SSFP	EC(Gd)	0.025	AD	1	SA/LA	-	-	Microspheres	
Germain et al. (2001)	Patients	GE	EC(Gd)	0.04	DIP	3	SA	-	-	Tetrofosmine SPECT	
Schwitter et al. (2001)	Patients/Volunteers	Gd-EPI	EC(Gd)	0.1	DIP	4	SA	91/87	94/85	PET/angio	
Al-Saadi et al. (2002)	Patients	GE	EC(Gd)	0.025	DOBU	1	SA	81	73	angio	
Ibrahim et al. (2002)	Patients	GE	EC(Gd)	0.05	AD	3	SA	69	89	PET/angio	
Kraitchman et al. (2002)	Pigs	GE-EPI	IV(Gd)	0.1	DIP	4-6	SA	-	-	99mTc	
Gerber et al. (2002)	Pigs	EPI	IV(Gd)	0.05	DIP	5-6	SA	-	-	Microspheres/99mTc	
			EC(Gd)	0.1	DIP	5-6	SA	-	-	Microspheres/99mTc	
Sensky et al. (2002)	Patients	GE	EC(Gd)		AD	3	SA	77	97	angio	
Panting et al. (2002)	Patients	GE	EC(Gd)	0.05	AD	2	SA	-	-	-	
Nagel et al. (2003)	Patients	GE-EPI	EC(Gd)	0.025	AD	5	SA	88	90	angio	
Ishida et al. (2003)	Patients	GE-EPI	EC(Gd)	0.1	DIP	3-6	SA	90	85	99mTc /angio	
Jerosh-Herold et al. (2003)	Pigs	GE	IV		AD	1	SA	-	-	-	
Kwong et al. (2003)	Patients	GE-EPI	EC(Gd)	0,1	No	3-6	SA	84	85	angio	
Reimer et al. (2004)	Volunteers	GE	IV(Fe)	Var.	No	1?	SA	-	-	-	
Lee et al. (2004)	Dogs	b-SSFP	EC(Gd)	0.05	AD	1	SA	-	-	Microspheres/99mTc/201Tl	
Dewey et al. (2004)	Pigs	b-SSFP	IV(Gd)	0.013	No	1	SA	-	-	-	
Taylor et al. (2004)	Patients	GE-EPI	EC(Gd)	0.1	No	3	SA	-	-	-	

AD, adenosine; ATP, adenosine triphosphate; Ax, axial; angio, coronary angiography; b-SSFP, balanced steady-state free-precession; CE-IR MRI, contrast-enhanced inversion-recovery MRI with late imaging; DIP, dipyridamole; DOB, dobutamine; Dys, dysprosium; EC, extracellular; Echo, echocardiography; EPI, echoplanar; IV, intravascular contrast agent; GE, gradient echo; Fe, ferritic particle (iron oxide); LA, long axis; SA, short axis; Var, variable dose of contrast agent

Furthermore, generally the dose has to be adjusted whether a visual analysis (higher dose required) or a quantitative approach is desired for evaluation, which generally requires smaller doses of contrast agent to avoid strong T2* effects. The correlation between the dose of contrast agent and the effects on the myocardial SI changes have been studied by several groups (BURSTEIN et al. 1991; WENDLAND et al. 1993a, b, 1994; CANET et al. 1995; SLAVIN et al. 2001).

The role of intravascular or blood-pool contrast agents to assess myocardial perfusion has been investigated by several groups in animals and humans (CANET et al. 1993; REVEL et al. 1996; KRAITCHMAN et al. 1996, 2002; JOHANSSON et al. 1998; PANTING et al. 1999; BJERNER et al. 2001; GERBER et al. 2002; REIMER et al. 2004; DEWEY et al. 2004). Blood-pool agents have several intrinsic advantages for myocardial perfusion imaging. Since they remain in the vascular space for a considerable time, first-pass imaging is not hampered by the rapid diffusion of the contrast agent to the interstitial space, and thus the changes in SI better reflect the true myocardial perfusion. Another advantage of the prolonged intravascular half-life is that first pass is not strictly required to assess myocardial perfusion (CHUNG et al. 1998; DEWEY et al. 2004; GERBER et al. 2002;). However, since the blood-pool agents remain confined to the vascular space, counting for only 10% of the tissue volume, signal-to-noise ratios will be lower than with the diffusible (extracellular) contrast media (see Fig. 7.6). This is the major drawback of intravascular contrast agents. Increasing the dose of intravascular contrast agents may increase signal-to-noise ratio in the myocardium, but results in strong susceptibility and T2* artifacts in the LV cavity. Ultrasmall paramagnetic iron oxide (USPIO) particles produce signal changes in T1- and T2*-weighted images and, because of their long intravascular half-life, are well suited for myocardial perfusion studies as well as for contrast-enhanced 3D MR angiography (JOHANSSON et al. 1998: PANTING et al. 1999; BJERNER et al. 2001; REIMER et al. 2004). The role of magnetic-susceptibility MR contrast agents (such as dysprosium) in the assessment of myocardial perfusion has also been evaluated (WENDLAND et al. 1993b; KANTOR et al. 1994).

The value of qualitative, visual analysis in the detection of coronary artery stenosis has been shown to achieve good diagnostic accuracy as compared to coronary angiography or SPECT (AL-SAADI et al. 2003d; ISHIDA et al. 2003; SENSKI et al. 2002; NAGEL et al. 2003). However, most studies have focused on more objective evaluation of myocardial perfusion using a semiquantitative or quantitative approach. Several groups have measured the myocardial perfusion in baseline conditions and during maximal hemodynamic stress, enabling calculation of MPR, using dipyridamole or adenosine as pharmacological stress agent (CULLEN et al. 1999; AL-SAADI et al. 2000a,b; NAGEL et al. 2003). Cullen et al. (1999) have calculated the perfusion reserve index based on a more quantitative approach by measuring the unidirectional transfer constant (K_i) and found in normal subjects an MPR index of 4.21±1.16 versus 2.02±0.7 in patients with angiographically proven CAD ($p<0.02$). The MPR index was inversely related to the severity of the coronary artery stenosis. Remarkably, MPR index was also lower in non-flow-limiting stenosis (<40% diameter) than in volunteers. In another study a MPR index could be determined from the upslope in normal myocardial segments of 2.33±0.41 versus 1.08±0.23 in ischemic segments ($p<0.001$). A cutoff value of 1.5 (mean minus 2 SD of normal segments) enabled discrimination of normal from ischemic segments with good sensitivity and specificity (90% and 83%, respectively) (AL-SAADI et al. 2000a). The usefulness of this approach has been confirmed and applied in several studies (AL-SAADI et al. 2000b, 2001; THIELE et al. 2003, IBRAHIM et al. 2002). NAGEL et al. have applied this technique to a large patient population ($n=84$). Using a somewhat lower threshold (MPR index of 1.1) in a multislice approach and a peripheral contrast agent injection, this approach yields a sensitivity of 88% and a specificity of 90%. Schwitter et al. have assessed the SI upslope only at stress (vasodilation with adenosine) as a measure of myocardial perfusion (SCHWITTER et al. 2001). The subendocardial upslope revealed a sensitivity and specificity of 91% and 94%, respectively, for the detection of CAD as defined by PET (flow reserve minus 2 SD of controls), and a sensitivity of 87% and 85%, respectively, in comparison with quantitative coronary angiography (diameter stenosis ≥50%). Other studies have reported improved accuracy when combining myocardial perfusion with cine MRI to detect associated wall-motion abnormalities.(HARTNELL et al. 1994; PENZKOFER et al. 1999), or with myocardial tagging enabling assessment of concomitant changes in regional myocardial function and principal strains (KRAITCHMAN et al. 1996).

Several studies have stressed the advantages of myocardial MR perfusion imaging compared with radionuclide imaging for obtaining information on the heterogeneous transmural enhancement (sub-epi-, mid-, and subendocardium), which may reflect the variability in myocardial perfusion across the wall (EDELMAN and LI 1994; LEE et al. 2004; KEIJER et al. 2000). In a recent study by Lee et al., first-pass MRI identified better than ^{201}Tl and ^{99m}Tc SPECT imaging regional reductions in full-thickness myocardial blood flow during global coronary vasodilation over the full range of vasodilation (using microspheres as gold standard). Moreover, transmural flow gradients can be identified, and their magnitude increases progressively as flow limitations become more severe and endocardial flow is increasingly compromised (LEE et al. 2004).

The value of MR perfusion measurements has been also shown valuable for clinical and scientific evaluation such as studying the effects of balloon angioplasty as compared to stenting in patients with significant coronary artery stenosis (AL-SAADI et al. 2000b), to evaluate myocardial perfusion in patients treated with angiogenesis (LAHAM et al. 2002), patient with transmyocardial laser reveascularization (GALINANES et al. 2004), and patients after transplantation (MUEHLING et al. 2003). In patients with a recent reperfused acute myocardial infarction, MRI myocardial perfusion imaging is helpful to assess the patency of the infarct-related artery and to assess the presence of microvascular obstruction ("no-reflow" area) in the infarct territory (LIMA et al. 1995; TAYLOR et al. 2004) as well as to evaluate reversible functional perfusion abnormalities (microvascular stunning) (AL-SAADI et al. 2003e) (see Chap. 8).

7.8
Key Points

- The advent of rapid MRI techniques has made it possible to study in real-time physiological events such as myocardial perfusion.
- Myocardial MR perfusion imaging is or can be part of a more comprehensive approach to study ischemic heart disease (IHD) patients.
- The ideal MR perfusion sequence is an ultrafast sequence that entirely covers the heart during the first pass of contrast, yielding high contrast between normal and hypoperfused myocardium.
- The ideal contrast agent for myocardial perfusion assessment is not yet available. Extracellular contrast agents are hampered by their rapid diffusion into the interstitial space. Intravascular contrast agents are intrinsically appealing but

yield lower signal-to-noise ratios because of the smaller distribution volume and are yet not commercially available.

- Although semiquantitative and quantitative perfusion analysis is possible, visual assessment remains clinically the most often used analysis tool.
- Use a systematic approach for visual perfusion analysis. Start by ruling out and grading the influence of artifacts on the perfusion study. Perfusion defects caused by CAD have typical appearances.
- Semiquantitative and quantitative evaluation needs further improvement of postprocessing tools to allow for an automated self-detection of myocardial contours.
- Assessment of the MPR is a promising tool to detect and assess the severity of CAD.

References

Al-Saadi N, Nagel E, Gross M, et al. (2000a) Noninvasive detection of myocardial ischemia from perfusion reserve based on cardiovascular magnetic resonance. Circulation 101(12):1379–1383

Al-Saadi N, Nagel E, Gross M, et al. (2000b) Improvement of myocardial perfusion reserve early after coronary intervention: assessment with cardiac magnetic resonance imaging. J Am Coll Cardiol 36(5):1557–1564

Al-Saadi N, Gross M, Bornstedt A, et al. (2001) Comparison of various parameters for determining an index of myocardial perfusion reserve in detecting coronary stenosis with cardiovascular magnetic resonance tomography. Z Kardiol 90(11):824–834

Al-Saadi N, Gross M, Paetsch I, et al. E (2002) Dobutamine induced myocardial perfusion reserve index with cardiovascular MR in patients with coronary artery disease. J Cardiovasc Magn Reson 4(4):471–480

Al-Saadi N, Abdelaty H, Friedrich M (2003a) Magnetic resonance first pass myocardial perfusion: Influence of spatial and temporal coverage on qualitative evaluation (abstract). J Cardiovasc Magn Reson 5:106

Al-Saadi N, Abdelaty H, Messroghli D, Friedrich M (2003b) Influence of interslice gap and sample frequency on semiquantitative evaluation of first pass myocardial perfusion with magnetic resonance. J Cardiovasc Magn Reson 5:72–73

Al-Saadi N, Abdelaty H, Messroghli D, Friedrich M (2003c) Factors influencing semiquantitative evaluation of magnetic resonance first pass myocardial perfusion (abstract). J Cardiovasc Magn Reson 5:222

Al-Saadi N, Wassmuth R, Friedrich M (2003d) Qualitative evaluation of myocardial perfusion for the detection of coronary artery disease. Circulation 108:IV–402

Al-Saadi N, Dechend R, Taylor A, Abdel-Aty H, Freidrich M (2003e) Glycoprotein Iib/IIIa antagonist reduces the extent of irreversible microvascular injury in patients with reperfused acute myocardial infarction. Circulation 108:IV-580

Anderson CM, Brown JJ (1993) Cardiovascular magnetic resonance imaging: evaluation of myocardial perfusion. Coron Artery Dis 4:354-360

Araujo LI, Lammertsma AA, Rhodes CG, et al. (1991) Noninvasive quantification of regional myocardial blood flow in coronary artery disease with oxygen 15 labeled carbon dioxide inhalation and positron emission tomography. Circulation 83:875-885

Arteaga C, Canet E, Ovize M, Janier M, Revel D (1994) Myocardial perfusion assessed by subsecond magnetic resonance imaging with a paramagnetic macromolecular contrast agent. Invest Radiol 29:54-57

Atalay MK, Forder JR, Chacko VP, Kawamoto S, Zerhouni EA (1993) Oxygenation in the rabbit myocardium: assessment with susceptibility-dependent MR imaging. Radiology 189:759-764

Atkinson DJ, Burstein D, Edelman RR (1990) First-pass cardiac perfusion: evaluation with ultrafast MR imaging. Radiology 174:757-762

Bacharach SL, Bax JJ, Case J, et al. (2004) PET myocardial glucose metabolism and perfusion imaging: part 1 – guidelines for patient preparation and data acquisition. J Nucl Cardiol 10:543-554

Benner T, Heiland S, Erb G, Forsting M, Sartor K (1997) Accuracy of gamma-variate fits to concentration-time curves from dynamic susceptibility-contrast enhanced MRI: influence of time resolution, maximal signal drop and signal-to-noise. Magn Reson Imaging 15(3):307-317

Bergmann SR, Herrero P, Markham J, Weinheimer CJ, Walsh MN (1989) Noninvasive quantitation of myocardial blood flow in human subjects with oxygen 15 labeled water and positron emission tomography. J Am Coll Cardiol 14:639-652

Bidaut LM, Vallée JP (2001) Automated registration of dynamic MR images for the quantification of myocardial perfusion. J Magn Reson Imaging 13:648-655

Bjerner T, Johansson L, Ericsson A, et al. (2001) First-pass myocardial perfusion MR imaging with outer-volume suppression and the intravascular contrast agent NC100150 injection: preliminary results in eight patients. Radiology 221:822-826

Bock JC, Henrikson O, Gotze AH, et al. (1995) Magnetic resonance perfusion imaging with gadolinium-DTPA. A quantitative approach for the kinetic analysis of first-pass residue curves. Invest Radiol 30(12):693-699

Brasch RC (1992) New directions in the development of MR imaging contrast media. Radiology 183:1-11

Burstein D, Taratuta E, Manning WJ (1991) Factors in myocardial "perfusion" imaging with ultrafast MRI and Gd-DTPA administration. Magn Reson Med 20:299-305

Canet E, Revel D, Forrat R, et al. (1993) Superparamagnetic iron oxide particles and positive enhancement for myocardial perfusion studies assessed by subsecond T-1-weighted MRI. Magn Reson Imaging 11:1139-1145

Canet E, Doulk P, Janier M, et al. (1995) Influence of bolus volume and dose of gadolinium chelate for first-pass myocardial perfusion MR imaging studies. J Magn Reson Imaging 5:411-415

Cerqueira MD, Verani MS, Schwaiger M, Heo J, Iskandrian AS (1994) Safety profile of adenosine stress perfusion imaging: results from the Adenoscan Multicenter Trial Registry. J Am Coll Cardiol 23(2):384-389

Cherryman GR, Tranter J, Keal R, et al. (1998) Prospective comparison of contrast-enhanced MRI with thallium 201 SPECT and 2D echocardiography in the localization of acute myocardial infarction. Proceedings of International Society for Magnetic Resonance in Medicine, sixth scientific meeting and exhibition, Sydney, Australia, April 18-24, 1998

Cullen JHS, Horsfield MA, Reek CR, et al. (1999) A myocardial perfusion reserve index in humans using first-pass contrast-enhanced magnetic resonance imaging. J Am Coll Cardiol 33:1386-1394

Czernin J, Muller P, Chan S, et al. (1993) Influence of age and hemodynamics on myocardial blood flow and flow reserve. Circulation 88:62-69

Demer LL, Gould KL, Goldstein RA, et al. (1989) Assessment of coronary artery disease severity by positron emission tomography. Comparison with quantitative arteriography in 193 patients. Circulation79:825-835

Dewey M, Kaufels N, Laule M, et al. (2004) Magnetic resonance imaging of myocardial perfusion and viability using a blood pool contrast agent. Invest Radiol 39:498-505

Di Carli M, Czernin J, Hoh CK, et al. (1995) Relation among stenosis severity, myocardial blood flow, and flow reserve in patients with coronary artery disease. Circulation 91(7):1944-1951

Diesbourg LD, Prato FS, Wisenberg G, et al. (1992) Quantification of myocardial blood flow and extracellular volumes using a bolus injection of Gd-DTPA: kinetic modeling in canine ischemic disease. Magn Reson Med 23:239-253

Ding S, Wolff SD, Epstein FH (1998) Improved coverage in dynamic contrast-enhanced cardiac MRI using interleaved gradient-echo EPI. Magn Reson Med. Apr39(4):514-9

Donahue K, Burstein D, Manning W, Gary M (1994) Studies of Gd-DTPA relaxivity and proton exchange rates in tissue. Magn Reson Med 32:66-76

Donahue KM, Weiskoff RM, Burstein D (1997) Water diffusion and exchange as they influence contrast enhancement. J Magn Reson Imaging 7(1):102-110

Edelman RR, Li W (1994) Contrast-enhanced echo-planar MR imaging of myocardial perfusion: preliminary study in humans. Radiology 190:771-777

Eichenberger AC, Schuiki E, Kochli VD, et al. (1994) Ischemic heart disease: assessment with gadolinium-enhanced ultrafast MR imaging and dipyridamole stress (comments). J Magn Reson Imaging 4:425-431

Fenchel M, Helber U, Simonetti OP, et al. (2004) Multislice first-pass myocardial perfusion imaging: comparison of saturation recovery (SR)-TrueFISP-two-dimensional (2D) and SR-TurboFLASH-2D pulse sequences. J Magn Reson Imaging 19(5):555-563

Fritz-Hansen T, Rostrup E, Larsson HB, et al. (1996) Measurement of the arterial concentration of Gd-DTPA using MRI: a step toward quantitative perfusion imaging. Magn Reson Med 36(2):225-231

Fritz-Hansen T, Rostrup E, Ring P, Larsson H (1998) Quantification of gadolinium-DPTA concentrations for different inversion times using an IR-turbo flash pulse sequence: a study on optimizing multislice perfusion imgaging. Magn Reson Imaging 16(8):893-899

Galinanes M, Loubani M, Sensky PR, et al. (2004) Efficacy of transmyocardial laser revascularization and thoracic sympathectomy for the treatment of refractory angina. Ann Thorac Surg 78(1):122–128

Gallagher KP, Osakada G, Matsuzaki M, et al. (1982) Myocardial blood flow and function with critical coronary stenosis in exercising dogs. Am J Physiol 243(5):698–707

Gerber BL, Bluemke DA, Chin BB, et al. (2002) Single-vessel coronary artery stenosis: myocardial perfusion imaging with Gadomer-17 first-pass MR imaging in a swine model of comparison with gadopentetate dimeglumine. Radiology 225:104–112

Germain P, Roul G, Baruthio J, et al. (2001) Myocardial flow reserve parametric map, assessed by first-pass MRI compartmental analysis at the chronic stage of infarction. J Magn Reson Imaging 13:352–360

Giang TH, Nanz D, Coulden R, et al. (2004) Assessment of myocardial perfusion in coronary artery disease by magnetic resonance: first multicenter experience. Eur Heart J (In press)

Go RT, Marwick TH, MacIntyre WJ, et al. (1990) A prospective comparison of rubidium 82 PET and thallium 201 SPECT myocardial perfusion imaging utilizing a single dipyridamole stress in the diagnosis of coronary artery disease. J Nucl Med 31:1899-1905

Gould K (1978) Noninvasive assessment of coronary stenosis by myocardial perfusion imaging during pharmacologic coronary vasodilatation. I. Physiologic basis and experimental validation. Am J Cardiol 41:267–278

Gould KL (1990) Positron emission tomography and interventional cardiology. Am J Cardiol 66:51–58

Gould KL, Kelley KO (1982) Physiological significance of coronary flow velocity and changing stenosis geometry during coronary vasodilation in awake dogs. Circ Res 50(5):695–704

Gould KL, Kirkeeide RL, Buchi M (1990) Coronary flow reserve as a physiologic measure of stenosis severity. J Am Coll Cardiol 15:459–474

Hadjimiltiades S, Watson R, Hakki AH, Heo J, Iskandrian AS (1989) Relation between myocardial thallium-201 kinetics during exercise and quantitative coronary angiography in patients with one vessel coronary artery disease. J Am Coll Cardiol 13:1301–1308

Harris PA, Lorenz CH, Holburn GE, Overholser KA (1997) Regional measurement of the Gd-DTPA tissue partition coefficient in canine myocardium. Magn Reson Med 38(4):541–545

Harrison DG, White CW, Hiratzka LF, et al. (1984) The value of lesion cross-sectional area determined by quantitative coronary angiography in assessing the physiologic significance of proximal left anterior descending coronary arterial stenoses. Circulation 69(6):1111–1119

Hartnell G, Cerel A, Kamalesh M, et al. (1994) Detection of myocardial ischemia: value of combined myocardial perfusion and cineangiographic MR imaging. Am J Roentgenol 163:1061–1067

Heidemann RM, Ozsarlak O, Parizel PM, et al. (2003) A brief review of parallel magnetic resonance imaging. Eur Radiol 13(10):2323–2337

Henkin RE, Kalousdian S, Kikkawa RM, Kemel A (1994) 201-Thallium myocardial perfusion imaging utilizing single-photon emission computed tomography (SPECT). American Medical Association

Hunold P, Maderwald S, Eggebrecht H, Vogt FM, Barkhausen J (2004) Steady-state free precession sequences in myocar-

dial first-pass perfusion MR imaging: comparison with turboFLASH imaging. Eur Radiol 14:409–416

Ibrahim T, Nekolla SG, Schreiber K, et al. (2002) Assessment of coronary flow reserve: comparison between contrast-enhanced magnetic resonance imaging and positron emission tomography. J Am Coll Cardiol 39(5):864–870

Ishida N, Sakuma H, Motoyasu M, et al. (2003) Noninfarcted myocardium: correlation between dynamic first-pass contrast-enhanced myocardial MR imaging and quantitative coronary angiography. Radiology 229:209–216

Jerosch-Herold M, Wilke N (1997) MR first pass imaging: quantitative assessment of transmural perfusion and collateral flow. Int J Card Imaging 13:205–218

Jerosch-Herold M, Wilke N, Stillman AE (1998) Magnetic resonance quantification of the myocardial perfusion reserve with a Fermi function model for constrained deconvolution. Med Phys 25(1):73–84

Jerosch-Herold M, Swingen C, Seethamraju RT (2002) Myocardial blood flow quantification with MRI by model-independent deconvolution. Med Phys 29(5):886–897

Jerosch-Herold M, Hu X, Murthy NS, Rickers C, Stillman AE (2003) Magnetic resonance imaging of myocardial contrast enhancement with MS-325 and its relation to myocardial blood flow and the perfusion reserve. J Magn Reson Imaging 18(5):544–554

Jerosch-Herold M, Seethamraju RT, Swingen CM, Wilke NM, Stillman AE (2004) Analysis of myocardial perfusion MRI. J Magn Reson Imaging 19:758–770

Johansson LO, Akenson P, Ragnarsson A, Ahlström H (1998) Myocardial perfusion using a new ultra small paramagnetic iron oxide, enabling T2* perfusion with very short echo-times: first trials in humans. Proceedings of International Society for Magnetic Resonance in Medicine, sixth scientific meeting and exhibition, Sydney, Australia, April 18–24, 1998

Judd RM, Ataly, MK, Rottman GA, Zerhouni EA (1995a) Effects of myocardial water exchange on T1 enhancement during bolus administration of MR contrast agents. Magn Reson Med 33:215–223

Judd RM, Reeder SB, Atalar E, McVeigh ER, Zerhouni EA (1995b) A magnetization-driven gradient echo pulse sequence for the study of myocardial perfusion. Magn Reson Med 34:276–282

Judd RM, Reeder SB, May-Newman K (1999) Effects of water exchange on the measurement of myocardial perfusion using paramagnetic contrast agents. Magn Reson Med 41(2):334–342

Kantor HL, Rzedzian RR, Buxton R, et al. (1994) Contrast induced myocardial signal reduction: effect of lanthanide chelates on ultra high speed MR images. Magn Reson Imaging 12:51–59

Kaul S, Senior R, Dittrich H, et al. (1997) Detection of coronary artery disease with myocardial contrast echocardiography: comparison with ^{99m}Tc-sestamibi single-photon emission tomography. Circulation 96:785–792

Keijer JT, Rossum AC van, Eenige MJ van, et al. (1995) Semi-quantitation of regional myocardial blood flow in normal human subjects by first-pass magnetic resonance imaging. Am Heart J 130(4):893–901

Keijer JT, Rossum AC van, Eenige MJ van, et al. (2000) Magnetic resonance imaging of regional myocardial perfusion in patients with single-vessel coronary artery disease: quantitative comparison with (201)thallium-SPECT and coronary angiography. J Magn Reson Imaging 11(6):607–615

Kety SS (1951) The theory and applicatoins of the exchange of inert gas at the lungs and tissues. Pharmacol Rev 3:1

Kivelitz DE, Bis KG, Wilke NM, et al. (1997a) Quantitative MR first pass perfusion imaging demonstrates coronary artery patency post interventions (abstract). Radiology (Suppl) 205:254

Kivelitz DE, Wilke NM, Bis KG, et al. (1997b) Quantitative MR first pass versus N13-ammonia PET perfusion imaging in coronary artery disease (abstract). Radiology (Suppl) 205:253

Klein MA, Collier BD, Hellman RS, Bamrah VS (1993) Detection of chronic coronary artery disease: value of pharmacologically stressed, dynamically enhanced turbo-fast low-angle shot MR images. Am J Roentgenol 161:257–263

Klocke F (1983) Measurements of coronary blood flow and degree of stenosis: current clinical implications and continuing uncertainties. J Am Coll Cardiol 1:31–36

Klocke FJ, Simonetti OP, Judd RM (2001) Limits of detection of regional differences in vasodilated flow in viable myocardium by first-pass magnetic resonance perfusion imaging. Circulation 104:2412–2416

Kloner RA, Przyklenk K, Rahimtoola SH, Braunwald E (1992) In: Opie LH (ed) Stunning, hibernation and calcium in myocardial ischemia and reperfusion. Kluwer, Dordrecht, pp 251–280

Kraitchman DL, Wilke N, Hexeberg E, et al. (1996) Myocardial perfusion and function in dogs with moderate coronary stenosis. Mag Reson Med 35:771–780

Kraitchman DL, Chin BB, Heldman AW, Solaiyappan M, Bluemke DA (2002) MRI detection of myocardial perfusion defects due to coronary artery stenosis with MS-325. J Magn Reson Imaging 015:149–158

Kroll K, Wilke N, Jerosch-Herold M, et al. (1996) Accuracy of modeling of regional myocardial flows from residue functions of an intravascular indicator) Modeling regional myocardial flows from residue functions of an intravascular indicator., Am J Physiol Heart Circ Physiol 40:1643–1655

Kwong RY, Schussheim AE, Rekhraj S, et al. (2003) Detecting acute coronary syndrome in the emergency department with cardiac magnetic resonance imaging. Circulation 107:531–537

Laham RJ, Simons M, Pearlman JD, Ho KK, Baim DS (2002) Magnetic resonance imaging demonstrates improved regional systolic wall motion and thickening and myocardial perfusion of myocardial territories treated by laser myocardial revascularization. J Am Coll Cardiol 39(1):1–8

Landis CS, Li X, Telang FW, et al. (2000) Determination of the MRI contrast agent concentration time course in vivo following bolus injection: effect of equilibrium transcytolemmal water exchange. Magn Reson Med 44(4):563–574. Erratum: Magn Reson Med 2002 48(2):410

Larsson HB, Stubgaard M, Sondergaard L, Henriksen O (1994) In vivo quantification of the unidirectional influx constant for Gd-DTPA diffusion across the myocardial capillaries with MR imaging. J Magn Reson Imaging 4(3):433–440

Larsson HB, Fritz-Hansen T, Rostrup E, et al. (1996) Myocardial perfusion modeling using MRI. Magn Reson Med 35(5):716–726

Larsson HB, Rosenbaum S, Fritz-Hansen T (2001) Quantifica-

tion of the effect of water exchange in dynamic contrast MRI perfusion measurements in the brain and heart. Magn Reson Med 46(2):272–281

Lassen NA, Perl W (1979) Tracer kinetic methods in medical physiology. New York, Raven

Laub G, Simonetti O (1996) Assessment of myocardial perfusion with saturation-recovery Turbo FLASH sequences. ISMR, 4th Scientific Meeting, New York, p 179

Lauerma K, Virtanen KS, Sipila LM, Hekali P, Aronen HJ (1997) Multislice MRI in assessment of myocardial perfusion in patients with single vessel proximal left anterior descending coronary artery disease before and after revascularization. Circulation 96:2859–2867

Le Bihan D (1995) Diffusion and perfusion magnetic resonance imaging. Applications to functional MRI. Raven, New York

Le Bihan D, Turner R (1992) The capillary network: a link between IVIM and classical perfusion. Magn Reson Med 27:171–178

Lee DC, Simonetti OP, Harris KR, et al. (2004) Magnetic resonance versus radionuclide pharmacological stress perfusion imaging for flow-limiting stenoses of varying severity. Circulation 110:58–65

Lima JAC, Judd RM, Bazille A, et al. (1995) Regional heterogeneity of human myocardial infarcts demonstrated by contrast-enhanced MRI. Potential mechanisms. Circulation 92:1117–1125

Loghin C, Sdringola S, Gould KL (2004) Common artifacts in PET myocardial perfusion images due to attenuation-emission misregistration: clinical significance, causes, and solutions. J Nucl Med 45:1029–1039 Magn Reson Med 27(1):171–178

Manning WJ, Atkinson DJ, Grossman W, Paulin S, Edelman RR (1991) First-pass nuclear magnetic resonance imaging studies using gadolinium-DTPA in patients with coronary artery disease. J Am Coll Cardiol 18:959–965

Manning WJ, Atkinson DJ, Parker JA, Edelman RR (1992) Assessment of intracardiac shunts with gadolinium-enhanced ultrafast MR imaging. Radiology 184(2):357–361

Mansfield P (1977) Multiplanar image formation using NMR spin echoes. J Physiol (Lond) 10:55–58

Masugata H, Lafitte S, Peters B, Strachan GM, DeMaria AN (2001) Comparison of real-time and intermittent triggered myocardial contrast echocardiography for quantification of coronary stenosis severity and transmural perfusion gradient. Circulation 104(13):1550–1556

Matheijssen NA, Louwerenburg HW, Rugge FP van, et al. (1996) Comparison of ultrafast dipyridamole magnetic resonance imaging with dipyridamole SestaMIBI SPECT for detection of perfusion abnormalities in patients with one-vessel coronary artery disease: assessment by quantitative model fitting. Magn Reson Med 35:221–228

Mauss Y, Grucker D, Fornasiero D, Chambron J (1985) NMR compartmentalization of free water in the perfused rat heart. Magn Reson Med 2:187–194

Meier P, Zierler KL (1954) On the theory of the indicator-dilution method for measurement of blood flow and volume. J Appl Physiol 6(12):731–744

Meza MF, Mobarek S, Sonnemaker R, et al. (1996) Myocardial contrast echocardiography in human beings: correlation of resting defects to sestamibi single photon emission computed tomography. Am Heart J 132:528–535

Mitchell MD, Osbakken M (1991) Estimation of myocardial perfusion using deuterium nuclear magnetic resonance. Magn Reson Imaging 9:545–552

Muehling OM, Wilke NM, Panse P, et al. (2003) Reduced myocardial perfusion reserve and transmural perfusion gradient in heart transplant arteriopathy assessed by magnetic resonance imaging. J Am Coll Cardiol 42(6):1054–1060

Muzik O, Duvernoy C, Beanlands RS, et al. (1998) Assessment of diagnostic performance of quantitative flow measurements in normal subjects and patients with angiographically documented coronary artery disease by means of nitrogen 13 ammonia and positron emission tomography. J Am Coll Cardiol 31:534–540

Nagel E, Klein C, Paetsch I, et al. (2003) Magnetic resonance perfusion measurements for the noninvasive detection of coronary artery disease. Circulation 108:432–437

Nienaber CA, Spielmann RP, Salge D, et al. (1987) Noninvasive identification of collateralized myocardium by 201 thallium tomography in vasodilation and redistribution. Z Kardio 76:612–620

Panting JR, Taylor AM, Gatehouse PD, et al. (1999) First-pass myocardial perfusion imaging and equilibrium signal changes using the intravascular contrast agent NC100150 injection. J Magn Reson Imaging 10:404–410

Panting JR, Gatehouse PD, Yang GZ (2001) Echo-planar magnetic resonance myocardial perfusion imaging: parametric map analysis and comparison with Thallium SPECT. J Magn Reson Imaging 13:192–200

Panting JR, Gatehouse PD, Yang GZ, et al. (2002) Abnormal subendocardial perfusion in cardiac syndrome X detected by cardiovascular magnetic resonance imaging. N Engl J Med 346:1948–1953

Patterson RE, Horowitz SF, Eisner RL (1994) Comparison of modalities to diagnose coronary artery disease. Semin Nucl Med 24:286–310

Pearlman JD, Laham RJ, Simons M (2000) Coronary angiogenesis: detection in vivo with MR imaging sensitive to collateral neocirculation-preliminary study in pigs. Radiology 214(3):801–807

Pennell DJ (1994) Pharmacological cardiac stress: when and how? Nucl Med Commun 15:578–585

Penzkofer H, Wintersperger BJ, Knez A, Weber J, Reiser M (1999) Assessment of myocardial perfusion using multi-section first-pass MRI and color-coded parameter maps: a comparison to 99mTc Sesta MIBI SPECT and systolic myocardial wall thickening analysis. Magn Reson Imging 17:161–170

Plein S, Ridgway JP, Jones TR, Bloomer TN, Sivananthan MU (2002) Coronary artery disease: assessment with a comprehensive MR imaging protocol – initial results. Radiology 225(1):300–307

Porter TR, Xie F, Silver M, Kricsfeld D, Oleary E (2001) Real-time perfusion imaging with low mechanical index pulse inversion Doppler imaging. J Am Coll Cardiol 37(3):748–753

Reeder SB, Atalar E, Faranesh AZ, McVeigh ER (1999) Multi-echo segmented κ-space imaging: an optimized hybrid sequence for ultrafast cardiac imaging. Magn Reson Med 41(2):375–385

Reimer KA, Jennings RB (1979) The wavefront progression of myocardial ischemic cell death. II. Transmural progression of necrosis within the framework of ischemic bed size (myocardium at risk) and collateral flow. Lab Invest 40:633–644

Reimer P, Bremer C, Allkemper T, et al. (2004) Myocardial perfusion and MR angiography of chest with SHU 555C: results of placebo-controlled clinical phase I study. Radiology 231:474–481

Revel D, Canet E, Sebbag L, et al. (1996) First-pass and delayed magnetic resonance imaging studies of reperfused myocardial infarction with iron oxide particles. Acad Radiol 3:398–401

Rosen BR, Belliveau JW, Vevea JM, Brady TJ (1990) Perfusion with NMR contrast agents. Magn Reson Med 14:249–265

Rugge FP van , Boceel JJ, Wall EE van der, et al. (1991) Cardiac first-pass and myocardial perfusion in normal subjects assessed by sub-second Gd-DTPA enhanced MR Imaging J Comput Assist Tomogr 15:959–965

Saeed M, Wendland MF, Higgins CB (1994) Contrast media for MR imaging of the heart. J Magn Reson Imaging 4:269–279

Saeed M, Wendland MF, Higgins CB (1995) The developing role of magnetic resonance contrast media in the detection of ischemic heart disease. Proc Soc Exp Biol Med 208:238–254

Sambuceti G, Parodi O, Marcassa C, et al. (1993) Alteration in regulation of myocardial blood flow in one vessel coronary artery disease determined by positron emission tomography. Am J Cardiol 72:538–543

Schaefer S, Lange RA, Kulkarni PV, et al. (1989) In vivo nuclear magnetic resonance imaging of myocardial perfusion using the paramagnetic contrast agent manganese gluconate. J Am Coll Cardiol 14:472–480

Schaefer S, Tyen R van, Saloner D (1992) Evaluation of myocardial perfusion abnormalities with gadolinium-enhanced snapshot MR imaging in humans. Work in progress. Radiology 185:795–801

Schreiber WG, Schmitt M, Kalden P, et al. (2002) Dynamic contrast-enhanced myocardial perfusion imaging using saturation-prepared TrueFISP. J Magn Reson Imaging 16:641–652

Schweiger M (1994) Myocardial perfusion imaging with PET. J Nucl Med 35:693–698

Schwitter J, Debatin F (1995) MRI contrast in the assessment of myocardial perfusion. Adv MRI Contrast 3:34–47

Schwitter J, Debatin JF, Schulthess GK von, McKinnon GC (1997) Normal myocardial perfusion assessed with multi-shot echo-planar imaging. Magn Reson Med 37:140–147

Schwitter J, Nanz D, Kneifel S, et al. (2001) Assessment of myocardial perfusion in coronary artery disease by magnetic resonance. A comparison with positron emission tomography and coronary angiography. Circulation 103:2230–2235

Schwitter et al. (2004) Eur Heart J (In press)

Sensky PR, Samani NJ, Reek C, Cherryman GR (2002) Magnetic resonance perfusion imaging in patients with coronary artery disease: a qualitative approach. Int J Cardiovasc Imaging 18:373–383

Shaw LJ, Iskandrian AE (2004) Prognostic value of gated myocardial perfusion SPECT. J Nucl Cardiol 11:171–185

Siebert, JE, Eisenberg, JD, Pernicone, JR, Cooper TG (1998) Practical myocardial perfusion studies via adenosine pharmacologic stress. Proceedings of International Society for Magnetic Resonance in Medicine, sixth scientific meeting and exhibition, Sydney, Australia, April 18–24, 1998

Sigal SL, Soufer R, Fetterman RC, Mattera JA, Wackers FJ (1991) Reproducibility of quantitative planar thallium-201 scintigraphy: quantitative criteria for reversibility of myocardial perfusion defects. J Nucl Med 32:759–765

Slavin GS, Wolff SD, Gupta SN, Foo TK (2001) First-pass myocardial perfusion MR imaging with interleaved notched saturation: feasibility study. Radiology 219:258–263

Taylor AJ, Al-Saadi N, Abdel-Aty H, et al. (2004) Detection of acutely impaired microvascular reperfusion after infarct angioplasty with magnetic resonance imaging. Circulation 109:2080–2085

Taylor AM, Pennell DJ (1996) Recent advances in cardiac magnetic resonance imaging. Curr Opin Cardiol 11:635–642

Thiele H, Plein S, Ridgway JP, et al. (2003) Effects of missing dynamic images on myocardial perfusion reserve index calculation: comparison between an every heartbeat and an alternate heartbeat acquisition. J Cardiovasc Magn Reson 5(2):343–352

Tofts PS (1997) Modeling tracer kinetics in dynamic Gd-DTPA MR imaging. J Magn Reson Imaging 7:91–101

Tong CY, Prato FS, Wisenberg G, et al. (1993a) Techniques for the measurement of the local myocardial extraction efficiency for inert diffusible contrast agents such as gadopentate dimeglumine. Magn Reson Med 30:332–336

Tong CY, Prato FS, Wisenberg G, et al. (1993b) Measurement of the extraction efficiency and distribution volume for Gd DTPA in normal and diseased canine myocardium. Magn Reson Med 30:337–46

Tsekos NV, Zhang Y, Merkle H, et al. (1995) Fast anatomical imaging of the heart and assessment of myocardial perfusion with arrhythmia insensitive magnetization preparation. Magn Reson Med 34:530–536

Unger EF, Banai S, Shou M, et al. (1994) Basic fibroblast growth factor enhances myocardial collateral flow in a canine model. Am J Physiol 266:1588–1595

Uren NG, Melin JA, De Bruyne B, et al. (1994) Relation between myocardial blood flow and the severity of coronary artery stenosis. N Engl J Med 330:1782–1788

Vallee JP, Sostman HD, MacFall JR, Coleman RE (1997) Quantification of myocardial perfusion with MRI and exogenous contrast agents. Cardiology (1):90–105

Vallee JP, Sostman HD, MacFall JR, et al. (1997) MRI quantitative myocardial perfusion with compartmental analysis: a rest and stress study. Magn Reson Med 38(6):981–989

Vatner SF (1980) Correlation between acute reductions in myocardial blood flow and function in conscious dogs. Circ Res 47:201

Wacker CM, Hartlep AW, Pfleger S, et al. (2003) Susceptibility-sensitive magnetic resonance imaging detects human myocardium supplied by a stenotic coronary artery without a contrast agent. J Am Coll Cardiol 41:834–840

Wagner A, Mahrholdt H, Holly TA, et al. (2003) Contrast-enhanced MRI and routine single photon emission computed tomography (SPECT) perfusion imaging for detection of subendocardial myocardial infarcts: an imaging study. Lancet 361:374–379

Walsh EG, Doyle M, Lawson MA, Blackwell GG, Pohost GM (1995) Multislice first-pass myocardial perfusion imaging on a conventional clinical scanner. Magn Reson Med 34:39–47

Wedeking P, Sotak CH, Telser J, et al. (1992) Quantitative dependence of MR signal intensity on tissue concentration of Gd(HP-DO3A) in the nephrectomized rat. Magn Reson Imaging 10:97–108

Wei K (2002) Approaches to the detection of coronary artery disease using myocardial contrast echocardiography. Am J Cardiol 90(10A):48J–58J

Wei K, Jayaweera AR, Firoozan S, et al. (1998) Quantification of myocardial blood flow with ultrasound-induced destruction of microbubbles administered as a constant venous infusion. Circulation 97(5):473–483

Weinmann HJ, Brasch RC, Press WR, Wesbey GE (1983) Characteristics of gadolinium-DTPA complex: a potential NMR contrast agent. AJR Am J Roentgenol 142:619–624

Weiskoff RM, Chesler D, Boxerman JL, Rosen BR (1993) Pitfalls in MR measurement of tissue blood flow with intravascular tracers: which mean transit time? Magn Reson Med 29:553–558

Wendland MF, Saeed M, Masui T, et al. (1993a) Echo-planar MR imaging of normal and ischemic myocardium with gadodiamide injection. Radiology 186:535–542

Wendland MF, Saeed M, Masui T, Derugin N, Higgins CB (1993b) First pass of an MR susceptibility contrast agent through normal and ischemic heart: gradient-recalled echo-planar imaging. J Magn Reson Imaging 3:755–760

Wendland MF, Saeed M, Yu KK, et al. (1994) Inversion recovery EPI of bolus transit in rat myocardium using intravascular and extravascular gadolinium-based MR contrast media: dose effects on peak signal enhancement. Magn Reson Med 32:319–329

Wetter DR, McKinnon GC, Debatin JF, Schulthess G von (1995) Cardiac echo-planar MR imaging: comparison of single- and multiple-shot techniques. Radiology 194:765–770

Wilke N, Simm C, Zhang J, et al. (1993) Contrast-enhanced first pass myocardial perfusion imaging: correlation between myocardial blood flow in dogs at rest and during hyperemia. Magn Reson Med 29:485–497

Wilke N, Jerosch-Herold M., Stillman AE, et al. (1994) Concepts of myocardial perfusion imaging in magnetic resonance imaging. Magn Reson Q 10(4):249–286

Wilke N, Jerosch-Herold M, Wang Y, et al. (1997) Myocardial perfusion reserve: assessment with multisection, quantitative, first-pass MR imaging. Radiology 204:373–384

Williams DS, Grandis DJ, Zhang W, Koretsky AP (1993) Magnetic resonance imaging of perfusion in the isolated rat heart using spin inversion of arterial water. Magn Reson Med 30:361–365

Wilson RF, Wyche K, Christensen BV, Zimmer S, Laxson DD (1990) Effects of adenosine on human coronary arterial circulation. Circulation 82:1595–1606

Wintersperger BJ, Penzkofer H, Knez A, Reiser M (2000) Myocardial perfusion at rest and during stress. MR signal characteristics of persistent and reversible myocardial ischemia. Radiology 40:155–161

Yu K, Saeed M, Wendland M, et al. (1992) Real-time dynamics of an extravascular magnetic resonance contrast medium in acutely infarcted myocardium using inversion recovery and gradient-recalled echo-planar imaging. Invest Radiol 27:927–934

Yu KK, Saeed M, Wendland MF, et al. (1993) Comparison of T1-enhancing and magnetic-susceptibility magnetic resonance contrast agents for demarcation of the jeopardy area in experimental myocardial infarction. Invest Radiol 28:1015–1023

Zierler K (2000) Indicator dilution methods for measuring blood flow, volume, and other properties of biological systems: a brief history and memoir. Ann Biomed Eng 28(8):836–848

8 Ischemic Heart Disease

Steven Dymarkowski, Jan Bogaert, and Yicheng Ni

CONTENTS

8.1
Epidemiology of Ischemic Heart Disease

Ischemic heart disease (IHD) is the primary cause of morbidity and mortality in the industrialized countries. IHD involves a broad clinical spectrum, ranging from stable angina to sudden cardiac death.

S. Dymarkowski, MD, PhD; J. Bogaert MD, PhD;
Y. Ni MD, PhD
Department of Radiology, Gasthuisberg University Hospital, Catholic University of Leuven, Herestraat 49, 3000 Leuven, Belgium

Although the death rate from IHD has decreased in the last 3 decades, due to therapeutic improvements [e.g., thrombolytic agents, early revascularization, angiotensin-converting enzyme, (ACE) inhibitors, and beta-blockers] and prevention campaigns, the prevalence of IHD will continue to increase over the first decades of this millennium. Worldwide, IHD will be the number one cause of death by 2020 (Fuster 1999). Survivors of a first acute myocardial infarction (AMI) are thought to die of IHD at later ages due to heart failure and late cardiac deaths. Moreover, the increased lifespan will contribute to the increased incidence of cardiovascular disease and increased number of deaths from heart disease. Other contributing factors to an increased prevalence of IHD are an increasing prevalence of type II diabetes, physical inactivity, and obesity. This increasing prevalence will greatly influence the cost of health care. In the United States of America alone, it is estimated that health-care costs will increase 41% by 2010 and 54% by 2025, mainly driven by the growth in aging of the population (Beller 2001).

Application of an accurate, and cost-effective imaging technique is appealing for more accurate clinical and preclinical detection of IHD. Among other techniques, MRI has an increasing role in assessing IHD, as demonstrated by the large number of publications on this issue in radiological and cardiological journals and by the growing interest in cardiac MRI societies.

Identification of irreversibly infarcted myocardium from dysfunctional, but viable and potentially salvageable myocardium after a heart attack is of crucial importance for the management of cardiac patients. In particular, revascularization of an infarcted area by percutaneous coronary intervention (PCI) or coronary artery bypass grafting (CABG) is deemed justified only if functional recovery following the intervention is predictable, or if late outcome and patient well-being can be improved. A tremendous number of research studies, scientific papers, reviews, editorials, and books have elaborated the different aspects of this topic.

In this chapter, the different MRI strategies for the detection of viable myocardium and differentiation with nonviable myocardium in IHD will be outlined and the strengths and limitations will be discussed.

8.2
Pathophysiology of Ischemic Heart Disease

The left ventricular (LV) wall is composed of an inner, middle, and outer layer of cardiac muscle tissue, termed the endocardial, mid-wall, and epicardial layers, respectively. The specific tissue direction of and the synergistic action between these layers provide a complicated contractile phenomenon, which cannot merely be described as contraction. Other elements such as ventricular torsion and wall stress and strain are determinants of myocardial function, which are often insufficiently understood and studied (see Chap. 6). For example, it is well known that the inner layer of the myocardium (subendocardial myocardium) predominantly contributes to wall thickening during systolic contraction at rest, while the contribution of the more outward layers is dependent on increasing catecholamine stimulation (SKLENAR et al. 1994). The higher energy demand of the subendocardial myocardium plays an important role in the pathophysiology of ischemia and infarction, as will be discussed further.

The heart is provided with its own nutrient vessels (coronary arteries) that have a characteristic, high capillary-density distal vascular territory. The overall density of the microvascular bed in myocardium is 2–3 times greater than in skeletal muscle. The amount of blood passing through coronary arteries is about 250 ml/min (or about 1 ml/min per gram), i.e., approximately 5% of normal cardiac output. Coronary flow is greater during diastole than during systole, in contrast to the situation in other parts of the circulation. During maximal exercise, the myocardial blood supply is able to increase by a factor of 4–6, which is mainly obtained by a dilation of the coronary arteries.

Unfortunately, coronary arteries are particularly vulnerable to the systemic disorder of atherosclerosis, known as coronary artery disease (CAD), which is the main cause of IHD. Occlusion of the coronary artery lumen will interrupt the unique oxidative metabolism of the myocardium, characterized by a limited and short-lived capacity for anaerobic metabolism, and almost immediately lead to acute myocardial ischemia in the perfusion territory distal to the occluded coronary artery. The time course of acute myocardial ischemia has been clinically recognized and well documented in animal experiments. Myocardium ceases its aerobic metabolism within 10 s of coronary blood-flow interruption, which is soon followed by an inhibition of anaerobic metabolism due to the accumulation of lactate and other acidic metabolites (WHITEMAN et al. 1983). Regional or global myocardial ischemia triggers a cascade of events, starting with disturbed myocardial flow, followed by a decreased diastolic and later systolic function, and finally ECG changes and symptoms of angina (Fig. 8.1).

As a self-preserving mechanism, systolic contraction will cease within seconds after coronary occlusion to preserve limited high-energy phosphate or

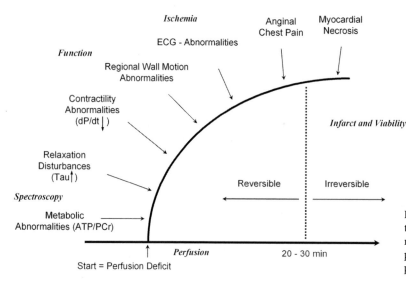

Fig. 8.1 The ischemic cascade and the role of MRI techniques. The parameters to be addressed by MRI are printed in italics. *ATP*, adenosine triphosphate; *PCr*, phosphocreatine

ATP storage, which is unavoidably depleted by the ongoing cell membrane activities (JENNINGS et al. 1978). After 20-30 min of ischemia, the transmembrane potentials can no longer be maintained and the influx of calcium and sodium causes intracellular edema, which, together with accumulation of toxic metabolites, finally leads to myocardial cell apoptosis. As systolic wall stress and the resulting oxygen consumption are greater at the endocardium than at the epicardium, the infarction will occur earlier and more prominently in subendocardial than in subepicardial tissue. As a consequence, the subendocardial lateral boundaries of a myocardial infarction are established within the first 40 min, whilst the myocardial infarction enlarges in a transmural wave front at a much slower rate over a period of 3–6 h (REIMER and JENNINGS 1970, 1979) (Fig. 8.2). The final lateral boundaries of the infarcted area closely correspond to the myocardium at risk, whereas a variable degree of transmural progression determines the final extent of necrosis (LEE et al. 1981). Islands of viable tissue, especially in the subepicardial layers, remain intermixed with necrotic cells, and, if antegrade flow in the infarct-related artery is restored, a late improvement in myocardial metabolism and function in this infarcted myocardium has been observed in humans (GROPLER et al. 1992; BOGAERT et al. 1999).

The faster the restoration of myocardial perfusion, the lesser the transmural extent, and the more ischemically jeopardized myocardium will be salvaged. Moreover, the presence of even a small fraction of perfusion to the infarct bed, for instance more than 20% of the normal coronary supply, from either antegrade or collateral flow, can significantly delay necrosis and limit infarct size (RIVAS et al. 1976). This is true especially in chronic CAD patients, because coronary collateral circulation usually takes time to become functional (PATTERSON et al. 1993). The mechanism of collateral circulation plays an important role in maintaining the viability of myocardium distal to coronary occlusion. When collateral flow is insufficient to prevent a marked fall in coronary perfusion pressure for a prolonged period, e.g., more than 1 h, infarction inevitably sets in (FUSTER et al. 1979). Although restoration of myocardial perfusion may stop the transmural progression of myocardial necrosis and salvage the jeopardized myocardium, it has been shown that the process of cell death or apoptosis may continue during the first hours of reperfusion (*myocardial reperfusion injury*) (MATSUMURA et al. 1998; BECKER et al. 1999).

Postinfarction LV remodeling is the process of changes in ventricular size, shape, and function that occur in the days, weeks, and months following the

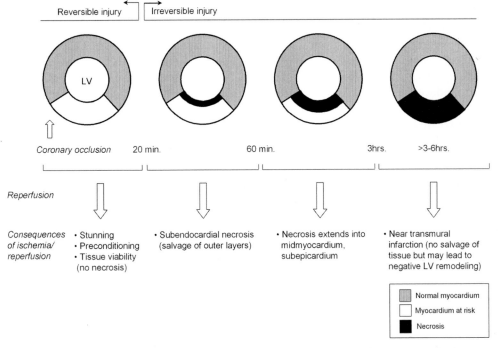

Fig. 8.2 Effects of ischemia and reperfusion on myocardial tissue viability and necrosis. Studies in anesthetized canine model of proximal coronary artery occlusion. *LV*, left ventricle. (Adapted from KLONER and JENNINGS 2001)

acute event (SUTTON and SHARPE 2000). The acute loss in myocardium results in an abrupt increase in loading conditions in the infarcted border zone and remote noninfarcted myocardium. In an early phase (within 72 h), the remodeling involves the infarct zone and is characterized by acute dilation and thinning of the necrotic wall without new tissue necrosis, and formation of a discrete collagen scar. Eventually this may result in early ventricular rupture or evolve toward aneurysm formation. The changes in the infarct zone may be associated with early LV dilatation. Especially large transmural infarctions, infarctions related to lesions in the distribution of the LAD coronary artery, and infarctions with severe microvascular obstruction (no-reflow zones), are prone to "infarct expansion." Late remodeling involves the LV globally and is associated with a time-dependent dilatation, alterations in ventricular architecture, and mural hypertrophy to distribute the increased wall stresses more evenly throughout the damaged LV. Negative LV remodeling is an important trigger for the evolution of a postinfarct ventricle toward an ischemic cardiomyopathy.

Coronary artery occlusion does not necessarily lead to myocardial infarction. Brief episodes of transient myocardial ischemia, up to 15 min, are tolerated by myocytes. Although no cell death results from the ischemia, the myocytes are reversibly damaged. This condition is known as "stunned myocardium" (BRAUNWALD and KLONER 1982), defined as "prolonged post-ischemic contractile dysfunction of myocardium salvaged by reperfusion." The clinical counterparts of brief periods of transient ischemia include angina, unstable angina, coronary vasospasm, and transient ischemia induced by inflation of an angioplasty balloon in the coronary arteries (KLONER and JENNINGS 2001). Excessive oxygen free radicals and cytosolic calcium imbalance are claimed to be the mechanisms of the impaired contraction (BOLLI 1990). Very brief episodes of ischemia, as short as 5 min, followed by reperfusion, protect the heart from a subsequent, longer coronary artery occlusion by markedly reducing the amount of necrosis that results from the test episode of ischemia. This phenomenon, called "ischemic preconditioning" is a powerful cardioprotective effect, and may be an effective means to clinically minimize the stunning phenomenon (KLONER and JENNINGS 2001).

When a certain degree of ischemia persists for weeks, months, or years, myocytes may still remain viable but become dysfunctional by downregulating their energy consumption through a lower level of aerobic and/or anaerobic metabolism (MAES et al.

1994). These dysfunctional LV areas, however, may functionally recover and eventually restore completely normal contractile function after effective reperfusion interventions with angioplasty or bypass surgery. This type of ischemia associated with a chronic and reversible LV dysfunction has been termed "hibernating myocardium" (RAHIMTOOLA 1989) and is used to describe viable myocardium in a state of persistent, but potentially reversible dysfunction secondary to chronic coronary artery stenosis (HEUSCH 1998; DI CARLI et al. 1998). It is proposed that myocardial hibernation acts as an adaptive mechanism in response to reduced coronary blood flow that preserves the structural integrity of the myocardium and prevents myocyte apoptosis. In patients with severe, chronic LV dysfunction due to CAD, it is important to distinguish dysfunctional but viable myocardium from necrotic tissue in order to determine preoperatively the benefit of a revascularization procedure (CHAUDRHY et al. 1999; VANOVERSCHELDE et al. 1997). Acute hibernation has also been observed in more recent studies (DOWNING and CHEN 1992). Increased glucose utilization and decreased free fatty acid metabolism are features of energy consumption in ischemic myocardium (LIEDTKE 1981; CAMICI et al. 1989) and have been exploited for metabolic cardiac imaging using positron emission tomography (PET). The mechanisms of contractile and metabolic "downregulation" underlying myocardial hibernation have been mainly hypothesized rather than experimentally defined (FERRARI et al. 1996; ROSS 1991).

Although the rather simplistic classification of stunned and hibernating myocardium is derived from clinical observations and imperfect animal experiments (BASHOUR and MASON 1990; NEILL et al. 1986; NIENABER et al. 1991), it is at least conceptually of clinical significance. In the light of this overlap, not in the least in clinical circumstances, it is clear that the complex, incompletely understood pathophysiology behind myocardial ischemia needs a reliable and precise diagnostic method that is able to recognize stunned and hibernating myocardium, in order to aid adjustment of therapy or to indicate a need for angioplasty or coronary bypass surgery.

8.3
Definition of Myocardial Viability

Clinically, the functional status of the left ventricle, as represented by the LV ejection fraction at rest, is known to be an important predictor of cardiac death after AMI (VOGEL 1987). However, several studies over time have shown that in itself this parameter provides a poor estimation of the severity and the extent of a myocardial infarction. The same is true for regional contractility at rest (VOGEL 1987). Gradually, understanding has developed that areas of reduced or no contractility after AMI are not always associated with necrosis. Instead they may represent areas of potentially reversible damage, which can improve spontaneously, or after reestablishment of coronary blood flow by interventional procedures (LEWIS et al. 1991). This variability between contractility and outcome provides the rationale for myocardial viability imaging studies.

From a clinical point of view, the most prominent feature of a viable heart is contractility, and cardiac management ultimately aims at restoring synergic myocardial contractility. Therefore, the following plausible interpretation based on functional recovery has been widely accepted. Jeopardized myocardium that manifests improved contractile function after appropriate therapy is considered viable, while myocardium that is persistently dysfunctional, as typically seen in completed infarction, is regarded as nonviable (GROPLER and BERGMANN 1991; LINDNER and KAUL 1996). However, this definition was formulated in the early 1990s and reflects the diagnostic capability of that time. An in vivo technique that enables clear-cut distinction between viable and nonviable myocardium was at this time not available and in fact rendered the definition of viability as "functional recovery" only of significance for retrospective diagnosis, since it relied on the eventual outcome of cardiac contractility.

Since then, the aspiration within cardiac science to noninvasively discriminate infarcted, ischemic, and normal myocardium has now been partially fulfilled due to recent advances in contrast media research, development of fast MRI techniques, and the ability to perform dobutamine-stress protocols. It is currently possible to differentiate in vivo irreversibly damaged myocardium (i.e., nonviable) from reversibly damaged (i.e., viable) myocardium, both in the setting of AMI and in CAD patients with chronic LV dysfunction, by using a combined MRI protocol assessing contractile reserve, tissue edema, perfusion, and contrast enhancement of the myocardium. The clinical application of this comprehensive MRI approach benefits coronary patients by providing near-unambiguous diagnostic information and providing relevance for optimized therapy so that the myocardium at risk may be salvaged and reperfusion damage minimized.

8.4
Imaging Strategies in Ischemic Heart Disease

Imaging has become an essential part of diagnosing IHD, in patients with acute or chronic chest pain and in patients with congestive heart failure (BELLER 2000). Imaging of IHD by means of MRI is not limited to the mere visualization of coronary artery stenoses (i.e., coronary MR angiography), but rather to the assessment of the ischemic consequences thereof. Theoretically, there are two possible strategies: (1) identification of viable myocardium or (2) exclusion of dead myocardium. The different MRI strategies used either focus on the former or the latter.

Current cardiac MRI protocols can evaluate not only regional and global ventricular function, but also the impact of a coronary stenosis on regional myocardial perfusion, detection of myocardial edema or hemorrhage, measurement of the true infarct size, and determination of the contractile reserve. In clinical practice, it is the combined information from these different elements of IHD that makes MRI currently the most appealing option to achieve a comprehensive imaging study. Although technical challenges presently limit the clinical utility of magnetic resonance spectroscopy (MRS), this technique has become a standard method in experimental cardiology for the study of many aspects of cardiac metabolism, including for instance the study of cardiac high-energy phosphate metabolites adenosine triphosphate (ATP) and phosphocreatine in IHD patients.

8.4.1
Functional Imaging in Ischemic Heart Disease

One of the major strengths of MRI in assessing cardiac diseases is definitely the accurate assessment of ventricular function (see Chap. 6). The excellent visualization of the myocardium and its endo- and epicardial borders on cine MRI allows monitoring of changes in wall thickening and wall motion throughout the cardiac cycle. Currently, the balanced steady-state free precession technique (b-SSFP; also known as: TrueFISP, b-FFE, or FIESTA) is the preferred technique for studying ventricular function. This sequence yields a high contrast between blood and myocardium, thus providing excellent visualization of small anatomical structures such as endocardial trabeculations, papillary muscles, and valve leaflets (THIELE et al. 2001; Fig. 8.3). This is especially important in IHD patients, since the image quality obtained with the older, spoiled gradient-echo techniques was often compromised in these patient populations. This could be partly attributed to the longer duration of breath-hold periods in these protocols, but, more importantly in cases of ventricular dilation (e.g., in chronic ischemic cardiomyopathy) or focal aneurysm formation, slow-flow artifacts often obscured the delineation of the endocardial border, thus resulting in errors of analysis.

For global and regional function analysis, the left ventricle is best studied in several imaging planes. Most commonly, a complete set of contiguous short-axis images is taken in successive, short breath-hold periods, allowing global ventricular volumes to be determined and regional function to be assessed. Since evaluation of the contractility of the apical and submitral regions may be troublesome on short-axis views, horizontal and vertical long-axis views are recommended. Depending on the size of the cardiac chambers, up to 14 slices (average thickness 8 mm) may be required in the short-axis view to cover the entire left ventricle (Fig. 8.4). To increase patient comfort, parallel-imaging techniques can be used to accelerate sequences by a factor of 2–4, thus allowing for the acquisition of 2 slices per breath-hold while maintaining temporal resolution. Temporal resolution should not be less than 30 ms/frame.

These images can be transferred for image processing to an off-line workstation. Delineation of endo- and epicardial contours at end-diastole and end-systole gives global functional parameters (end-diastolic volume, EDV, end-systolic volume, ESV, stroke volume, SV, ejection fraction, EF, and myocardial mass) (Chap. 6), while the impact of IHD on regional function is assessed either qualitatively (described as normal, hypokinetic, akinetic, or dys-

kinetic) or quantitatively (relative or absolute wall thickening, and wall motion). The accuracy and reproducibility of these measurements makes cine MRI appealing as the preferred imaging modality for primary diagnosis and follow-up of patients (BOGAERT et al. 1995). The cine MR images should be acquired in exactly the same views and slice positions as the other sequences of the MRI examination ("edema-weighted" images, myocardial perfusion, delayed-enhancement images) so that they can be aligned for interpretation. Furthermore, to achieve consensus between readers and between different imaging modalities, it is recommended to refer in the analysis to a model. In our center, we use a 17-segment model as proposed by the American Society for Echocardiography (SCHILLER et al. 1989; see Chap. 5). In this model, the LV myocardium is divided into 17 segments, identical to the analysis of echocardiography and FDG-PET examinations in Gasthuisberg University Hospital, Leuven, Belgium. Use of anatomical information, i.e., location of the papillary muscles, serves to define whether the short-axis cine views belong to the basal, mid, or apical segment.

Although the evaluation of cardiac function in resting conditions with cine MRI provides a substantial amount of information about myocardial contractility, it is not sufficient to provide a comprehensive assessment of the myocardial viability status and thus cannot be considered a clinically complete test. While regions displaying decreased wall motion and/or wall thickening can be clearly identified, this functional information does not elucidate in full whether the myocardium is viable or not. Cine MRI acquired at rest alone does not demonstrate the presence of an underlying myocardial infarction – subendocardial or transmural – or provide information about ischemia and potential functional recovery or contractile reserve. To com-

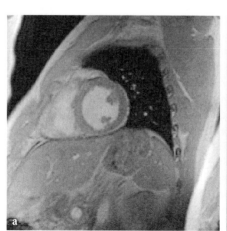
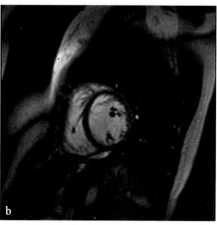

Fig. 8.3a, b Comparison between spoiled gradient-echo (a) and balanced steady-state free precession techniques (b-SSFP) (b) with regard to image quality. In the b-SSFP sequence, the blood-to-myocardium signal is higher and the spatial definition of smaller structures such as the papillary muscles is better highlighted

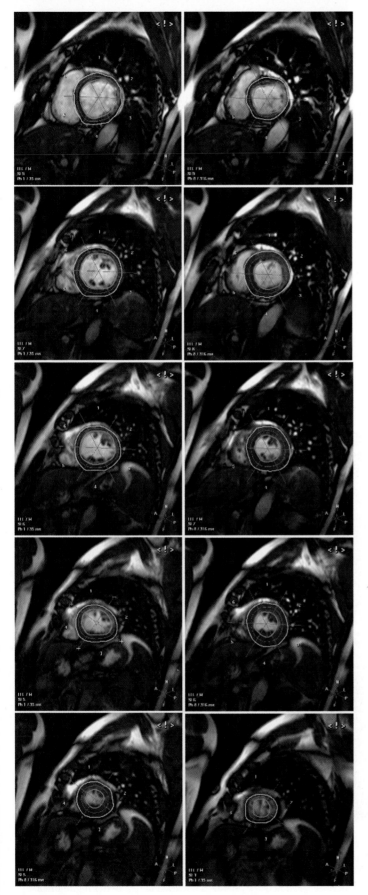

Fig. 8.4 Example of complete short-axis dataset in b-SSFP. End-diastolic (*left*) and end-systolic (*right*) frames, from base (*top*) to apex (*bottom*). The endo- and epicardial contours were delineated on a dedicated workstation for analysis of global ventricular function and myocardial mass

plete the comprehensive MRI analysis in IHD, the cine MRI findings need to be compared with other sequences, such as (stress) perfusion MRI and delayed-enhancement MRI.

Segmental wall-motion analysis of cine MRI at rest performed in conjunction with delayed-enhancement images has helped to further define myocardial viability in both acute and chronic IHD. Lack of late enhancement or mild degrees of late enhancement in the presence of normal wall motion or segmental dysfunction generally indicates that the segment is viable and will recover contractile function after revascularization (KIM et al. 1999, 2000; HILLENBRAND et al. 2000). In contrast, a segmental wall-motion abnormality in combination with extensive enhancement strongly suggests that the segment will not recover contractile function. The prognostic value of cine MRI at rest together with delayed enhancement seems clear in these cases. However, the outcome after revascularization is less clear in dysfunctional segments that show intermediate degrees of late enhancement. In these cases, it

may be necessary to perform cine MRI at rest and under stress conditions.

Another interesting and unique feature of MRI for functional analysis is the so-called myocardial tagging technique, which consists of creating a grid or tag of lines, noninvasively on the myocardium (see Chap. 6). These tag lines track the underlying myocardial deformation, either 2- or 3-dimensionally (Fig. 8.5). MR myocardial tagging can be used to noninvasively perform a myocardial strain analysis and decompose the gross wall deformation into more fundamental units of deformation such as principal strains or fiber strains (BOGAERT and RADEMAKERS 2001) This technique has been used to define the alterations in systolic LV torsion and regional loading conditions after AMI (GAROT et al. 2002; RADEMAKERS et al. 2003); to depict functional recovery after thrombolytic therapy in the infarcted myocardium (BOGAERT et al. 1999); to elucidate the mechanism of myocardial dysfunction in the remote noninfarcted regions (KRAMER et al. 1993, 1996a; BOGAERT et al. 2000); to discriminate between viable

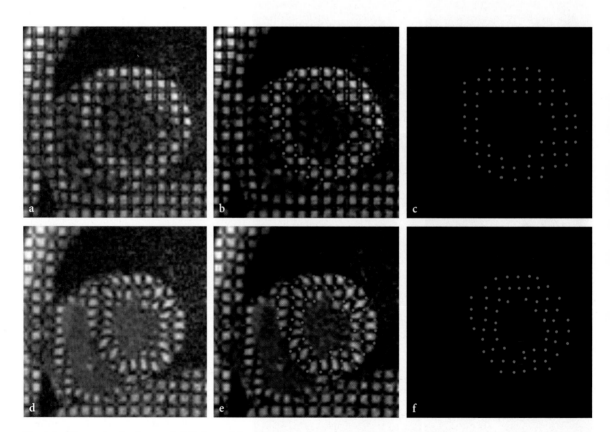

Fig. 8.5a-f Example of a short-axis MR C-spatial modulation of magnetization (SPAMM) myocardial tagging study. **a-c** End-diastolic images in native format (**a**), after tag intersection definition (**b**) and with native image subtraction (**c**), in which only the intersection points are visible. **d-f** Corresponding end-systolic images. Quantification or visual inspection of the deformation of the tag intersections allows analysis of intrinsic myocardial contractility

and nonviable myocardium using stress myocardial tagging (CROISILLE et al. 1999); and to measure the efficacy of medication on left ventricular dysfunction (KRAMER et al. 1996b). Due to the elaborative post-processing, the clinical use of MR myocardial tagging is currently still limited.

8.4.2
Stress Testing

Although multiple noninvasive modalities are currently available for the assessment of myocardial ischemia, exercise stress testing, stress SPECT imaging, and stress echocardiography are most widely used in clinical practice. For convenience most stress testing in IHD is performed by pharmacological stress, such as the β-agonist dobutamine or the vasodilators dipyridamole or adenosine. The former is preferred, since it offers the possibility of both low- and high-

dose examinations, needed for the differentiation of stunning and ischemia (CIGARROA et al. 1993; VAN RUGGE et al. 1993, 1994). Dobutamine is known to stimulate the β-receptors of myocytes and to increase regional contractility through increased ATP and oxygen consumption (BUDA et al. 1987; RUFFOLO 1987).

There are two general responses that can be detected with dobutamine-stress testing. In the presence of a hemodynamically significant coronary artery stenosis, the clinical counterpart of angina pectoris, the increase in blood flow during pharmacological (or eventually physical) stress, is insufficient to match the increased myocardial oxygen demand in the area supplied by the stenotic coronary artery, i.e., the coronary flow reserve is superseded. This in turn will cause a decrease in regional contractility in the myocardium supplied by this stenotic artery (Fig. 8.6). Several studies have shown detection of new wall-motion abnormalities using low- to high-

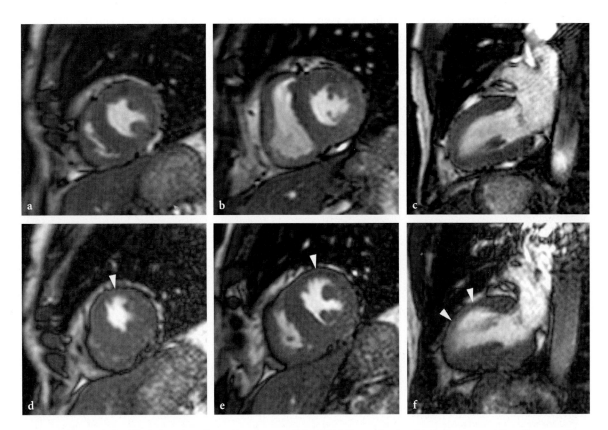

Fig. 8.6a-f Stress-inducible ischemic wall-motion abnormalities (WMA): rest (*top*) vs high-dose stress (40 µg/kg per minute + 0.25 mg atropine; *bottom*) in a 60-year old patient with recurrent ischemia after percutaneous transluminal coronary angiography (PTCA). End-systolic cine MR images, using b-SSFP technique. Stress-induced WMA in the LV anterior wall (segment 7,13) at high-dose stress, shown by focal akinesia (*arrowheads*) clearly visible on the two adjacent short-axis levels and on the vertical long-axis view. Note the increased contractility and wall thickening at end-systole in the other segments. The ischemic segment showed some postsystolic wall thickening (not shown). Cardiac catheterization confirmed the presence of a 60% stenosis in the proximal left anterior descending coronary artery (LAD)

dose dobutamine echocardiography (20–40 µg/kg per minute), with sensitivity up to 86% and specificity up to 85% for detection of IHD (NAGEL et al. 1999; HUNDLEY et al. 1999).

The second response seen with dobutamine is directly related to assessment of myocardial viability in patients with a recent AMI or chronic LV dysfunction due to CAD. Tissue that contracts normally during rest can be considered viable, whether or not it is supplied by a stenotic artery. However, if hypokinetic myocardium is observed at rest, the viability of this tissue is at least uncertain, but the key element to be investigated. In patients with chronic LV dysfunction, the dysfunctional segments will functionally improve, if viable, during low-dose (5–10 µg/kg body weight) dobutamine infusion (Fig. 8.7). As described above, the term "hibernating myocardium" is used to define viable myocardium in a state of persistent, but potentially reversible dysfunction secondary to a chronic coronary artery stenosis. Because of the limited contractility reserve, further increase in dobutamine dose results in a worsening of segmental function ("biphasic response") (SENIOR and LAHIRI 1995). From a prognostic point

of view, it is of paramount importance to detect this transient recovery of function to identify high-risk patients, who may benefit most from revascularization therapy.

In patients with a recent AMI, the dysfunctional myocardium usually exceeds the true infarct area. Stunned myocardium surrounding the infarction exhibits sustained (hours to days), reduced regional contractility after coronary reperfusion from an acute ischemic insult. However, it will respond to inotropic stimulation, and this behavior of the myocardium can be exploited to differentiate between stunned and infarcted myocardium. Although, with the advent of more sophisticated contrast-enhanced MRI techniques (see Sect. 8.4.5), detection of myocardial infarction has been greatly improved, use of low-dose dobutamine-stress cine MRI may be beneficial to better determine the myocardial area at risk.

Although such stress studies are usually performed using echocardiography, image quality is often suboptimal (>15% of studies), and the inter- and intraobserver agreement is low. In contrast, MRI offers reliable image quality with high spatial and

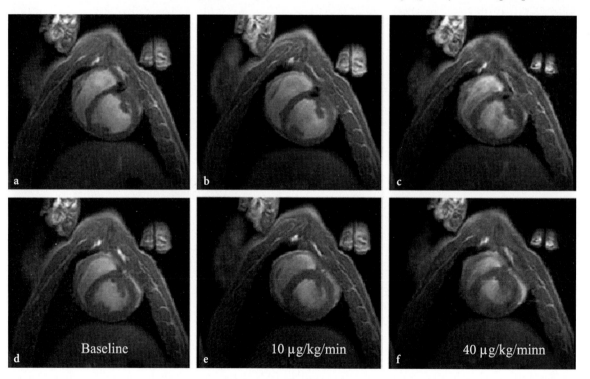

Fig. 8.7a-f. Biphasic response of chronic ischemic myocardium to inotropic stimulation in an experimental animal model of long-standing (>3 months), high-grade LAD coronary stenosis. End-diastolic (*top*) and end-systolic frames during rest (*left*), low-dose dobutamine (10 µg/kg per minute; *middle*), and high-dose (40 µg/kg per minute) dobutamine. At baseline, hypokinesia expressed decreased wall thickening is observed in the interventricular septum. During low-dose stimulation, an increase in wall thickening can be noted, which disappears during the high-dose step, expressing insufficient coronary reserve

temporal resolution, and MRI can be considered a more ideal technique to assess the myocardial contractile reserve and to visualize latent myocardial ischemia. With current fast cine MRI techniques (the b-SSFP technique in combination with parallel imaging), the entire LV can be functionally studied during the limited time period of each stress level (i.e., 3 min). A clinically useful approach is the acquisition of four short-axis views and two long-axis views (horizontal and vertical long-axis view) that can be accomplished within three successive breath-holds (Fig. 8.8).

Since the physical access to the patient in an MR scanner is much more limited than in echocardiography, and 12-lead ECG monitoring is not reliable in an MR environment, a specific approach to address the potential adverse effects is required during dobutamine-stress MRI (DSMRI) (for details see Chap. 3). Using low-dose stress protocols, side effects are minimal, but the risk for adverse effects increases at higher doses. The German Heart Institute, however, has shown that, in a large, unselected patient group of more than 1,000 patients, referred for high-dose dobutamine–atropine-stress MRI, side-effects were minimal (WAHL et al. 2003). This shows that high-dose DSMRI can be considered as safe and feasible in patients with suspected or known CAD. However, patients must be closely monitored, and

resuscitation equipment and trained personnel must be available. Typically, the patient's heart rate and blood pressure are continuously monitored, while the rate of intravenous administration of dobutamine is gradually increased from 0 to 5, 10, 20, and 40 µg/kg per minute every 3 min at each stress level. Imaging is repeated at every level and the images are immediately compared with the previous stress level according to a standardized model as discussed above (Fig. 8.9). When wall-motion abnormalities develop or worsen, or when the patient develops chest pain, the test is considered positive for hemodynamically significant coronary artery disease and the infusion is terminated. If the target heart rate of

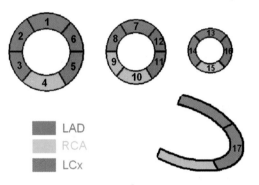

Fig. 8.9 Graphical representation of the 17-segment model as proposed by SCHILLER et al.

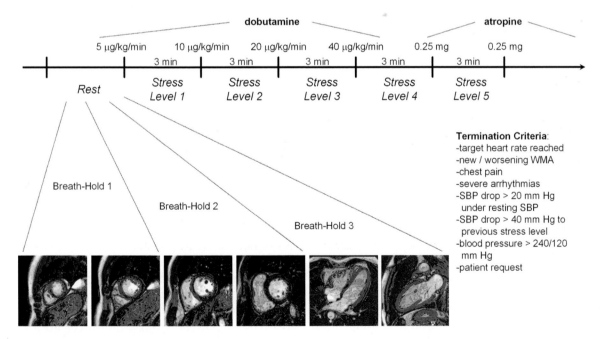

Fig. 8.8 Practical schematic for dobutamine-stress MRI (DSMRI). Four short-axis and two long-axis b-SSFP are repeated at every stress level during 3 breath-hold periods, every 3 min. If termination criteria are not met at the highest dobutamine dose, four additional levels with 0.25 mg of atropine can be performed

the patient [(220 – age)×0.85] is not reached before termination criteria are met, intravenous atropine can be administered in up to four doses of 0.25 mg as a chronotropic agent. Dobutamine administration needs to be stopped on patient request and is also discontinued: if the systolic blood pressure decreases more than 20 mmHg below the baseline systolic blood pressure; if the systolic blood pressure decreases more than 40 mmHg from a previous level; if the blood pressure increases to greater than 240/120 mmHg; or when severe arrhythmias occur.

Although Pennell et al. have attempted to assess the impact of dobutamine stress on global LV function by means of velocity-mapping MRI of the aortic flow (PENNELL et al. 1995), most DSMRI studies to date have focused on regional ventricular performance, using either regional wall motion or systolic wall thickness (relative or absolute), to give sensitivity and specificity values of 70–90% (BAER et al. 1992; PENNELL et al. 1992). These stress-test results can be enhanced by the simultaneous evaluation of regional perfusion (EICHENBERGER et al. 1994; HARTNELL et al. 1994) (see Chap. 7, Myocardial Perfusion).

Two recent studies have demonstrated the superiority of high-dose DSMRI over high-dose dobutamine-stress echocardiography in detecting patients with significant coronary heart disease (≥50% diameter stenosis) (NAGEL et al. 1999; HUNDLEY et al. 1999). Patients who are poor echocardiography subjects are ideal candidates for a DSMRI test. Nagel et al. have compared high-dose (up to 40 μg/kg per minute and atropine as needed) DSMRI with stress echocardiography in a group of 208 consecutive patients (NAGEL et al. 1999). They have found that DMRI is more sensitive (86.2% vs 74.3%) and more specific (85.7% vs 69.8%) than echocardiography in the detection of myocardial ischemia using coronary stenosis by arteriography as the gold standard. Better image quality in DSMRI is deemed responsible for the higher accuracy (86.0% vs 72.7%). HUNDLEY et al. (1999) have confirmed the safety and utility of DSMRI in assessing ventricular function and myocardial ischemia in a group of 153 patients with nondiagnostic second-harmonic echocardiographic images (83% sensitivity and 81% specificity for the detection of more than 50% stenosis in the 41 patients who underwent quantitative coronary angiography). Hundley also has reported that DSMRI provides important prognostic information. Thus, in patients with nondiagnostic stress echocardiograms, myocardial ischemia on DSMRI or an ejection fraction less than 40% at rest are independent predictors of future myocardial infarction or death in a multi-variate analysis (POHOST and BIEDERMAN 1999). In a paper by RERKPATTANAPIPAT et al. (2002), DSMRI was used to risk-stratify patients for cardiovascular events undergoing noncardiac surgery. In subjects with a positive DSMRI, the event rate was 20% (n=5/25), whereas, in subjects without ischemia on DSMRI, the event rate was 2% (n=1/59). The same group found that the presence of inducible ischemia on DSMRI or an LV ejection fraction less than 40% was associated with future AMI or cardiac death independent of risk factors for coronary arteriosclerosis (HUNDLEY et al. 2002). In a recent study by KUIJPERS et al. (2003), DSMRI combined with myocardial tagging was found more sensitive for the detection of stress-induced wall-motion abnormalities than DSMRI performed with routine (i.e., spoiled gradient-echo) cine MRI sequences in patients with CAD, and this approach more reliability separated patients at an increased risk of major adverse cardiac events from those with a normal life expectancy. Moreover, automated techniques for fast, accurate, and operator-independent analysis of tagging images, such as FastHARP, show promise as a nonsubjective method of diagnosing significant coronary lesions during DSMRI (KRAITCHMAN et al. 2003).

Use of low-dose DSMRI to detect viable myocardium in dysfunctional segments early after AMI, as well in patients with chronic IHD, has been reported by several groups (BAER et al. 1994; DENDALE et al. 1995, 1997). BAER et al. (1994) have found that viable myocardium in patients with a chronic myocardial infarction is characterized by preserved wall thickness (≥5.5 mm, i.e., mean minus 2.5 SD from a healthy group) and a dobutamine-inducible contraction reserve (using 10 μg/kg per minute). Conversely, scar formation after infarction leads to wall thinning and absence of dobutamine-inducible wall thickening. In a recent study by SHAH et al. (2004), however, it was clearly shown that a thinned (≤5.5 mm), akinetic myocardium is not a priori nonviable, but may contain enough viable tissue to recover after revascularization, a phenomenon called "reversed remodeling." Contrast-enhanced MRI, as discussed in Sect. 8.4.5, can be extremely helpful in this situation for differentiation between viable and nonviable thinned myocardium.

What is not achieved by DSMRI is the direct visualization of sustained myocardial tissue damage, albeit temporary or permanent. For this approach, MRI relies on edema-sensitive measurements and contrast-enhanced sequences to demonstrate late enhancement in akinetic or hypokinetic regions (SANDSTEDE et al. 2000).

8.4.3
Assessment of
Myocardial Perfusion in Ischemic Heart Disease

Any consideration about myocardial perfusion needs to address the pivotal relationship between myocardial oxygen requirements and coronary blood flow. In normal conditions, there is a balance between myocardial oxygen demand and oxygen supply. Since oxygen extraction in the myocardial microcirculation is already high under basal conditions, it is mandatory that changes in myocardial oxygen supply result from proportional changes in coronary flow. Therefore, imbalances between oxygen demand and supply are primarily the result of coronary atheromatosis with one or several stenoses on the coronary arteries.

In resting conditions, the myocardial perfusion is not altered until the coronary artery has an 85–90% stenosis. This is the result of the coronary vasodilator reserve, which compensates for the effects of coronary stenoses under basal conditions. However, during stress conditions the coronary reserve cannot be induced by a further vasodilatory stimulus. Under these circumstances, the myocardial distal to less severe coronary stenosis (i.e., between 50 and 85%) may become ischemic and the coronary artery stenosis can be considered as hemodynamically significant (GOULD 1978, BAER 1993). Practical guidelines on how to infuse a vasodilator agent are provided in Table 8.1.

The most frequently used approach to assess myocardial perfusion with MRI techniques is monitoring of the first-pass of contrast medium through the heart (contrast passage – systemic veins, right cavity of the heart , pulmonary vessels, left cavity of the heart , coronary arteries, myocardium). A bolus injection of MR contrast media is generally used for perfusion studies to obtain pure first-pass transit of contrast through the myocardium. Analysis of the MR perfusion images can be qualitative, semiquantitative, or quantitative. Visual (i.e., qualitative) analysis is often used clinically and is a fast but less accurate approach.

Several groups have used the myocardial perfusion reserve or myocardial perfusion reserve index to assess patients with CAD (WILKE et al. 1997; CULLEN et al. 1999; AL-SAADI et al. 2000). This reserve index is defined as the ratio of regional myocardial blood flow under hyperemic conditions to that under resting conditions. It may be a more reliable parameter than determination of coronary flow reserve, since the effects of (protective) myocardial collateral flow

Table 8.1. Myocardial perfusion protocol using adenosine (Adenocor) infusion dosage of 0.14 mg/kg body weight per minute during 6 min

Patient weight (kg)	Dose/rate (mg/min)	Vials $(n)^a$	Total volume (Adenocor + saline)	Injection rate (ml/min per 6 min)
25	3.5	4	14	2.4 (141 ml/h)
30	4.2	5	18	2.8 (168 ml/h)
35	4.9	5	20	3.3 (185 ml/h)
40	5.6	6	24	3.8 (225 ml/h)
45	6.3	7	26	4.3 (255 ml/h)
50	7.0	7	28	4.7 (282 ml/h)
55	7.7	8	32	5.1 (306 ml/h)
60	8.4	9	36	5.6 (336 ml/h)
65	9.1	10	40	6.1 (366 ml/h)
70	9.8	10	40	6.5 (390 ml/h)
75	10.5	11	44	7.0 (420 ml/h)
80	11.2	12	48	7.5 (450 ml/h)
85	11.9	12	48	7.9 (474 ml/h)
90	12.6	13	52	8.5 (510 ml/h)
95	13.3	14	56	8.9 (534 ml/h)
100	14.0	14	56	9.3 (556 ml/h)

Adenocor dose 6 mg/2 ml
[a]Patient weight determines number of vials injected: e.g., 7 vials equals 14 ml + 14 ml NaCl. Dilute with saline fluid to 1/1 (e.g., 28 ml) to obtain a dose of 1.5 mg Adenocor/ml

supply are taken into account. AL-SAADI et al. (2000) have found a significant difference in myocardial perfusion reserve between ischemic and normal myocardial segments (1.08 ± 0.23 and 2.33 ± 0.41, $p < 0.001$; Fig. 8.10). Using a cut-off value of 1.5, the diagnostic sensitivity, specificity, and diagnostic accuracy for the detection of coronary artery stenosis ($\geq 75\%$) were 90%, 83%, and 87%, respectively. In a similar study by CULLEN et al. (1999), a negative correlation has been found between the myocardial perfusion reserve index and percentage of coronary artery stenosis ($r = 0.81$, $p < 0.01$). Another potential application for MR stress perfusion studies are patients with microvascular disease ("cardiac syndrome X"). Between 10 and 20% of patients with typical anginal chest pain are found to have normal coronary angiograms. A subgroup of these patients present with classic ST-segment depression on exercise testing. PANTING et al. (2002) have reported typical subendocardial perfusion defects in patients suspected of syndrome X during adenosine-stress MRI, which was associated with chest pain in the majority of patients.

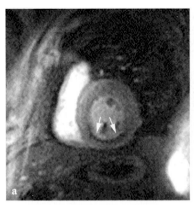 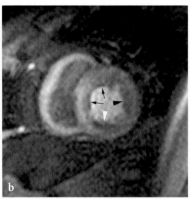

Fig. 8.10a,b Example of adenosine-stress perfusion studies. **a** Short-axis stress perfusion image demonstrating a subendocardial perfusion defect (*arrows*) in a patient with a high-grade right coronary artery (RCA) stenosis. **b** Similar image in a patient with known significant three-vessel disease, demonstrating a heterogeneous perfusion pattern in all coronary artery territories: LAD (*arrows*), RCA (*white arrowhead*) and left circumflex coronary artery (LCx; *black arrowhead*). (Images courtesy of Dr. N. Al-Saadi, La Charité, Berlin, Germany)

In patients with a recent AMI, myocardial perfusion studies at rest frequently show the infarct territory perfusion deficit. These defects are subendocardially located and the transmural extent is variable. These defects are caused by microvascular obstruction in the subendocardium (no-reflow; see Sect. 8.5.1). The extent is usually less pronounced than the extent of myocardial enhancement on late-enhancement MRI, except in cases of occlusive infarcts, where extensive perfusion defects can be found. In patients with a chronic myocardial infarction, often a faint perfusion defect or perfusion delay can be seen in the scarred region. This is related to the lower capillary density in fibrotic tissue compared with normal myocardium.

MR myocardial perfusion is an appealing technique for assessment of IHD, since it is fast and accurate, and it can be incorporated in a more global assessment of IHD, including functional stress studies and late-enhancement MR imaging. The topic of myocardial perfusion is extensively discussed in Chap. 7.

8.4.4
"Edema-weighted" MRI of the Myocardium

Since proton relaxation times are tissue specific, differences in these parameters between normal and pathological, i.e., infarcted myocardium, can be used to generate tissue contrast and thus identify myocardial necrosis (WILLIAMS et al. 1980; HIGGINS et al. 1983). Increased free water content in the infarcted myocardium prolongs the T1- and T2-relaxation times (FRANK et al. 1976). This prolongation is related to the duration of the ischemia (JOHNSTON et al. 1985). Differences in T1-relaxation are not clinically useful for infarct detection unless paramagnetic contrast agents are administered

(see below). In contrast, Higgins et al. have found a linear correlation between T2-relaxation time and the percentage water content, and, on T2-weighted MR sequences, infarcted tissues are visible as areas of increased signal intensity (HIGGINS et al. 1983; MCNAMARA et al. 1985; GOLDMAN et al. 1982). Many groups have used this approach to detect and quantify myocardial infarctions (ROKEY et al. 1986; CAPUTO et al. 1987; MATHEIJSSEN et al. 1991; DULCE et al. 1993; HOLMAN et al. 1996). However, the relation between changes in relaxation times and myocardial infarction is complex (CANBY et al. 1987; WISENBERG et al. 1988). Increased free water content does not necessarily reflect myocardial necrosis. In acute and subacute infarctions, the true infarct size may be overestimated because reversible interstitial edema and increased capillary permeability in the surrounding ischemic myocardial rim will equally show increased T2-relaxation times (WISENBERG et al. 1987; SCHAEFER et al. 1988; NI et al. 1998; PISLARU et al. 1999; CHOI et al. 2000; DYMARKOWSKI et al. 2002). In older infarcts, the noninfarct ischemic injury tends to be completely resolved, and the signal abnormalities closely mirror the extent of infarction. Furthermore, chronically infarcted regions of myocardium sometimes have decreased signal intensity compared with adjacent normal myocardium, presumably because of the lower water content of the fibrotic scar tissue (MCNAMARA et al. 1986). Due to the considerable overlap in T1 and T2 relaxation time between reperfused and nonreperfused, i.e., occluded myocardial infarcts, the success of reperfusion cannot be assessed (JOHNSTON et al. 1985; WISENBERG et al. 1987).

With conventional spin-echo sequences obtained during normal breathing, image quality, however, is often degraded due to the long echo time needed to obtain sufficient T2-weighting, and the long acquisition time, thus limiting its use in clinical practice.

Moreover, discrimination between high signal in the infarcted myocardium and high signal caused by stasis of blood adjacent to the akinetic or dyskinetic myocardial region may be difficult. Currently, segmented T2-weighted TSE sequences, equipped with inversion techniques to null the signal of fat and blood [T2-weighted, short-tau inversion-recovery (T2w-STIR) MRI], are most commonly used for this purpose and have dramatically improved image quality, which makes it an appealing technique for rapidly assessing the jeopardized myocardium (DYMARKOWSKI et al. 2002; Fig. 8.11).

8.4.5
Contrast-Enhanced MRI

8.4.5.1
History of Contrast-Enhanced MRI for Myocardial Infarction

In the past, many groups have focused on the development and use of MRI contrast agents to evalu-ate the presence or absence of myocardial infarction. Historically, the first contrast agent studied for imaging infarcted myocardium was manganese (Mn^{2+}) (LAUTERBUR et al. 1978; BRADY et al. 1982). Manganese accumulates in normal myocardial tissue and thus has characteristics similar to those of widely used thallium; however, infarcted myocardial tissue has reduced levels of manganese. The paramagnetic features of manganese shorten T1 relaxation time (and to a much lesser extent also the T2 relaxation time). Using T1-weighted sequences, normal myocardium will have a bright signal, while the signal in infarcted myocardium remains nearly unchanged and therefore appears dark relative to the viable myocardium. Mn-DPDP has the capability to define the region at jeopardy immediately after coronary artery occlusion (POMEROY et al. 1989). It may improve the detection and delineation of acute myocardial infarcts, demonstrate perfusion of the infarct, and permit discrimination between reperfused and occlusive infarcts (SAEED et al. 1989; BREMERICH et al. 2000; FLACKE et al. 2003). However, due to unacceptable cardiotoxic effects,

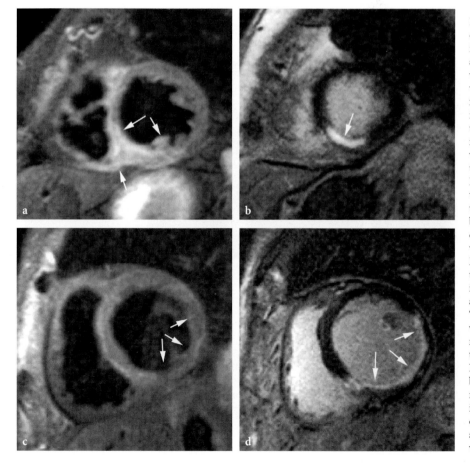

Fig. 8.11a-d Value of edema-weighted imaging of the myocardium. **a** This short-axis, T2-weighted short-tau inversion-recovery (STIR) fast SE technique (TSE) image shows hyperintense signal from the inferior and inferoseptal wall of the LV with extension to the inferior RV wall. The hyperintense signal is indicative of an acute event. **b** The corresponding contrast-enhanced inversion-recovery (CE-IR) MR image shows a small transmural myocardial infarction. **c** Short-axis, T2-weighted STIR TSE image of a patient with a known previous myocardial infarction (>3 months old). No signal increase can be noted. **d** The corresponding CE-IR MR image shows a large sub-endocardial myocardial scar in the inferolateral wall

manganese has not yet found a clinical application in detection of myocardial infarction (WOLF and BAUM 1983; BROWN and HIGGINS 1988).

Another strategy was to develop infarct-specific MRI contrast agents (WEISSLEDER et al. 1992; ADZAMLI et al. 1993). Due to their affinity for calcium-rich tissues, phosphonate-modified gadolinium (Gd)-diethylenetriamine pentaacetic acid (DTPA) complexes cause strong enhancement in the infarcted myocardium. This effect has been shown in rats with diffuse and occlusive myocardial infarction present for at least 24 h. However, these agents may result in a disorder of calcium homeostasis and subsequent impairment of ventricular contractility (ADZAMLI et al. 1993).

A third approach was to label a contrast agent with antimyosin-antibodies as infarct-selective agents. However, the possible immunogenic side-effects and the complexity in preparation and handling have excluded any clinical use to date. (WEISSLEDER et al. 1992).

Fourthly, porphyrin-based contrast agents, which were initially developed as "tumor-seeking" contrast agents, have been used (CHEN et al. 1984; VAN ZIJL et al. 1990; OGAN et al. 1997; FURMANSKI and LONGLEY 1998). Initial observations using these agents in animal models pointed toward a preferential uptake in neoplastic tissues, which were represented as areas of increased signal intensity on T1-weighted images, but were later correctly determined to be contrast enhancement in nonviable tumoral components (NI et al. 1995). This was further confirmed in studies of induced "benign" necrosis (NI et al. 1997). Eventually, an application of porphyrin-based contrast agents was developed for accurate visualization of AMI with T1-weighted MRI (NI et al. 1998; HERIJGERS et al. 1997; PISLARU et al. 1999; SAEED et al. 1999, 2001). Porphyrin-enhanced T1-weighted MR images mirror ex vivo histochemical staining specimens in all topographic features, exactly matching the degree of transmurality or subendocardial spread and providing an accurate means of detecting scattered and small infarcts such as in involvement of papillary muscles (Fig. 8.12). Unfortunately, infusion of porphyrin agents causes detectable side-effects. Due to the inherent photosensitizing properties of the agents, obvious greenish and slightly reddish discoloration appears in animals after doses greater than 50 mmol/kg, but, even more importantly, neurotoxic and hepatotoxic side-effects have been discovered, which have meant that these agents never entered the experimental arena and found clinical applications.

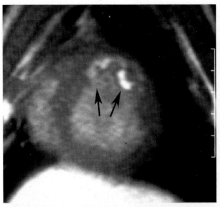

a

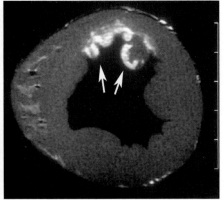

b

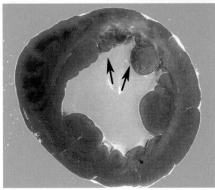

c

Fig. 8.12a-c Infarct specificity of a necrosis-avid contrast agent in an experimental animal model. In this model, the LAD coronary artery was reperfused after 90 min of occlusion. **a** In vivo T1-weighted gradient-echo image showing subendocardial enhancement in the anterior LV wall and the anterior papillary muscle after intravenous administration of 0.05 mmol/kg gadolinium-*bis*-mesoporphyrin. The corresponding ex vivo T1-weighted spin-echo image (**b**) and the postmortem TTC-stained specimen (**c**) show clear correlation toward infarct size and necrosis distribution

The most positive spin-off of these experiments has been the observation that a nonspecific MRI contrast agent such as Gd-DTPA (WEINMANN et al. 1984) could also enhance the infarcted region in animals with reperfused myocardial infarction as a result of increased distribution space and capillary permeability. It has been found, however, that there is substantial variability in the infarct size depending on the time point of imaging after injection of Gd-based contrast agents (OSHINSKI et al. 2001) (Fig. 8.13). Furthermore, it has been shown that studies performed with nonspecific agents systematically overestimated true infarct size, when compared with specific agents and with ex vivo staining methods (Fig. 8.14). Judd et al. have shown that the Gd-DTPA-enhanced areas overestimate ex vivo staining results by approximately 12%, whilst Rochitte et al. have found an overestimation of 9% (JUDD et al. 1995a; ROCHITTE et al. 1998). Similar results have been reported by Saeed and colleagues

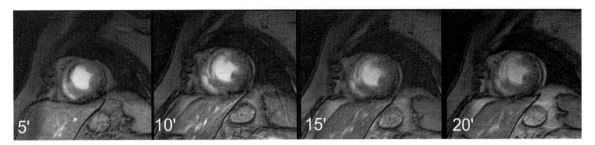

Fig. 8.13 Enhancement sequence after extracellular contrast medium administration. Short-axis CE-IR MR images taken 5, 10, 15, and 20 min (*left to right*) after intravenous injection of 0.2 mmol/kg Gd-diethylenetriamine pentaacetic acid, in a 72-year-old patient with a transmural myocardial infarction with partial microvascular obstruction. Initially, the endocardial no-reflow area can be clearly observed. The infarction enhancement is characterized by progressive fill-in from the periphery

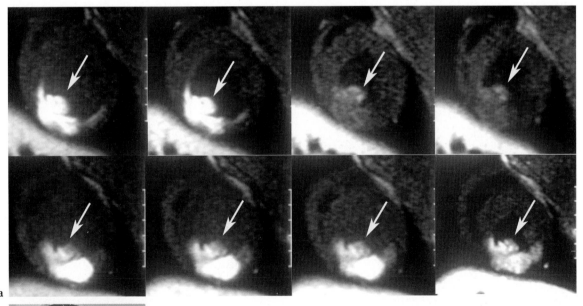

a

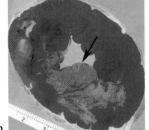

b

Fig. 8.14a,b Comparison of specific and nonspecific contrast agents in an animal model with large induced inferior wall infarction including the posterior papillary muscle. **a** *Top row from left to right*: short-axis CE-IR MR images taken 30 min, 1 h, 2 h, and 3 h after administration of Gd-DTPA (0.1 mmol/kg) shows progressive washout of the agent from the infarction. *Bottom row*: corresponding images at identical time points after injection of 0.05 mmol/kg gadolinium-bis-mesoporphyrin show constant appearance of the enhanced infarction volume

(SAEED et al. 2001). It is most likely that the enhanced region encompasses both viable and nonviable portions of the ischemically injured myocardium. It should, however, be noted that, although infarcted myocardial tissue enhances after Gd-DTPA administration, the enhancement is nonspecific and merely reflects an increased distribution volume for contrast medium and/or ultrastructural changes in myocyte organization. Abnormal enhancement can be seen in myocarditis, infiltrative cardiomyopathy, hypertrophic cardiomyopathy, and cardiac masses (BOGAERT et al. 2004), although with a different pattern from in myocardial infarction. The typical patterns of enhancement are discussed in Sect. 8.5.

The above findings lead us to the question of how to perform an accurate and reliable in vivo sizing method for myocardial infarction with nonspecific extracellular contrast agents. This in fact can only be achieved with proper knowledge of the physicochemical properties of these agents after injection, on the one hand, and by using appropriate imaging sequences on the other.

8.4.5.2
Delayed Enhancement in
Acute Myocardial Infarction

In the acute phase of a myocardial infarction, the mechanism responsible for enhancement of acutely necrotic myocardium is not clear. The enhancement is governed by several major factors such as residual blood supply to the infarcted region, distribution volume, impaired or delayed washout in the infarcted area, and size and depth of the myocardial infarction. Early after reperfusion, there is a hyperemic response both in the infarcted and in the ischemic myocardium, causing increased delivery to the reperfused myocardium as compared to normal myocardium, resulting in higher Gd-DTPA concentrations in the infarcted areas (SCHAEFER et al. 1988). The amount of Gd-DTPA supplied to the infarcted region may depend on the residual blood supply as determined by the patency of the infarct-related artery and the development of collaterals to the occluded artery. Moreover, the distribution vol-

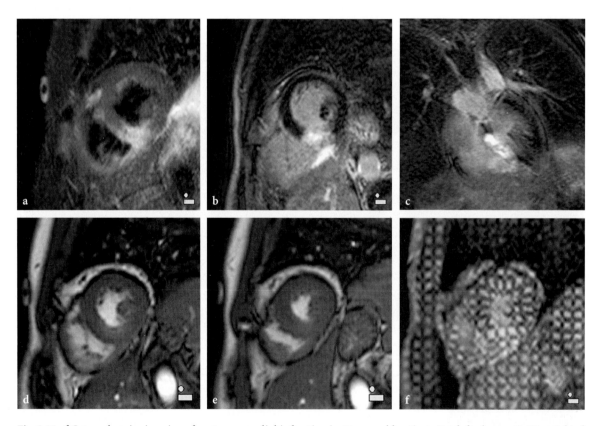

Fig. 8.15a-f Comprehensive imaging of acute myocardial infarction in 64-year-old patient. *Top left*: short-axis T2-weighted STIR TSE image with hyperintense signal in the inferoseptal region. Corresponding CE-IR MR images in short-axis (*top middle*) and vertical long-axis (*top right*) views show transmural enhancement in the inferoseptal area. Akinesia can be demonstrated with b-SSFP cine MRI and myocardial tagging (*bottom right*)

ume may increase due to interstitial edema and/or eventual disruption of the myocyte membrane after prolonged ischemia, which may allow the contrast molecule to enter the myocyte intracellular space (Fig. 8.15).

In a study of MRI contrast-enhancement mechanisms, KIM et al. (1996) have reported that, on electron microscopy, regions of enhancement systematically revealed sarcomere membrane rupture. It was argued that sarcolemmal rupture, in itself, could affect myocardial Gd-DTPA kinetics, because additional time may be required for contrast molecules to diffuse in and out of isolated breaks in the cellular membrane. Accordingly, it is possible that a physiological event specific to myocyte death, such as myocyte membrane rupture, may relate to the strong correlation between late enhancement and acute cellular necrosis.

As stated in the previous section, several authors have reported a systematic overestimation of acute infarct volume using nonspecific, extracellular agents (the only agents licensed for clinical use). This has led to the pertinent question of whether ischemically injured but potentially viable myocardium also enhances in the acute stage. And, furthermore whether ischemic myocardium without infarction can cause delayed enhancement on MRI, as it has been argued that the clearance – or washout – of contrast agents may be inhibited by the interstitial fluid accumulation and edema in ischemic myocardium surrounding the infarction.

In the hyperacute stage of myocardial infarction, many authors indeed have reported a significant overestimation of true infarct size (SCHAEFFER et al. 1988; NI et al. 1998; SAEED et al. 2000), but in general little consensus has been reached on the exact pathophysiological substrate causing this phenomenon. Interestingly, KIM et al. (1999) have demonstrated in a dog model an overestimation of infarct size when imaging 3 days after AMI, which disappeared when studies were repeated 8 weeks later. One interpretation of this is that late enhancement includes both acutely necrotic regions and surrounding reversibly injured regions at 3 days, but that, by 8 weeks, the reversibly injured regions have recovered and no longer enhance. Conversely, this data could also be explained by infarct shrinkage during the transition from myocyte necrosis to collagenous scar: REIMER and JENNINGS (1979) have reported that infarcts can shrink fourfold between 4 days and 6 weeks. MCNAMARA et al. (1985) have evaluated myocardial contrast enhancement in dogs that underwent 15 min of LAD occlusion followed

by 24 h of reperfusion. In this study, there was no evidence of delayed enhancement in the MR images or on ex vivo staining specimens.

The current general consensus is that in purely reversibly injured regions no late enhancement occurs, while in AMI there is a transient enhancement of a peripheral region surrounding the infarction representing ischemically injured myocardium that resolves during the subacute stage of the infarction. The decrease in infarct volume between the hyperacute stage and the chronic stage is currently best explained by infarct shrinkage (Fig. 8.16).

8.4.5.3
Delayed Enhancement in
Chronic Myocardial Infarction

Outside the acute phase of a myocardial infarction, several studies have reported that chronic infarcts remain enhanced (FEDELE et al. 1994; RAMANI et al. 1998), though a few, mostly older studies claimed they did not (EICHSTAEDT et al. 1986; NISHIMURA et al. 1989; VAN DIJCKMAN et al. 1991). NISHIMURA et al. have shown uptake of Gd-DTPA in AMI (5–12 days) but not in chronic myocardial infarction (30–90 days) (NISHIMURA et al. 1989). Several recent studies, however, have contradicted these studies by proving that, in patients with stable CAD, myocardial enhancement in areas of dysfunctional myocardium corresponds closely to fixed defects on thallium SPECT, and areas of flow metabolism matched necrosis on FDG-PET scans, representing scarred or fibrotic tissue (RAMINI et al. 1998; KLEIN et al. 2002; KÜHL et al. 2003; KNUESEL et al. 2003). Moreover, the clinical reproducibility of late-enhancement MRI in patients with healed myocardial infarctions is very good (MAHRHOLDT et al. 2002) (Fig. 8.17). Hypoenhanced areas in dysfunctional myocardium show a functional recovery after revascularization, whereas hyperenhanced areas do not. KIM et al. (2000) have reported on the role of late-enhancement MRI in predicting functional recovery after revascularisation in patients with chronic myocardial dysfunction.

The exact mechanism of delayed enhancement in chronic myocardial scarring remains incompletely understood. Likely mechanisms of enhancement are a combination of delayed wash-in and washout kinetics of the fibrotic scar tissue, mainly consisting of collagen, and differences in distribution volume between the viable and nonviable regions. In chronic myocardial infarction, the presence of fibrotic tissue increases the interstitial space per unit volume,

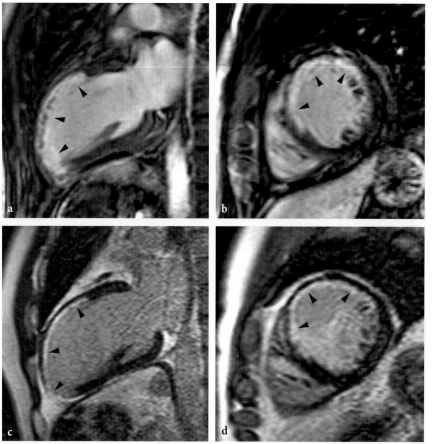

Fig. 8.16a-d Infarct shrinkage demonstrated in 54-year-old patient after LAD occlusion. *Top row*: CE-IR MRI study during the subacute phase (day 5) shows almost complete transmural enhancement in a large area located in the anteroapical wall (*arrowheads*) with several small no-reflow areas at the endocardial border. *Bottom row*: corresponding vertical long-axis (**c**) and short-axis (**d**) images taken 4 months later show significant decrease in the infarct size

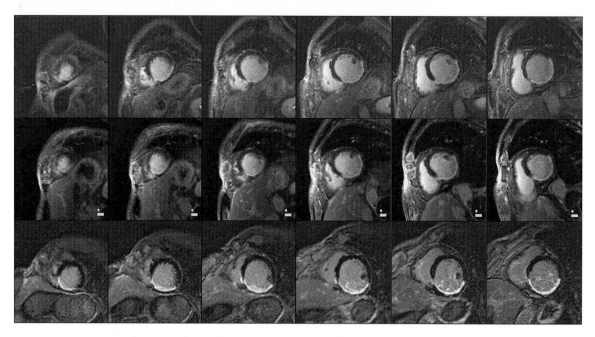

Fig. 8.17 Reproducibility of CE-IR MRI. Short-axis images of 63-year-old patient with known chronic myocardial infarction. The first study (*top row*) shows a large transmural inferior wall infarction with more subendocardial borders in the adjacent inferoseptal and inferolateral segments. Studies taken 3 and 6 months later (*middle and bottom row*, respectively) show near-identical findings

causing gadolinium agents to diffuse rapidly into the interstitial, but not the intracellular space (LIMA et al. 1995). Since myocardial viability in chronic IHD patients can be shown indirectly by using low-dose DSMRI, several groups have compared the accuracies of both techniques in predicting functional recovery after revascularization. Study results are, however, controversial. Where VAN HOE and VANDERHEIYDEN (2004) found no additional role for DSMRI over and above CE-IR MRI, WELLNHOFER et al. (2004) recently reported that low-dose DSMR is superior to CE-IR MRI in predicting functional recovery. This advantage is largest in segments with a delayed enhancement of 1–74% transmural extension. Well-controlled multicenter studies will be necessary to better determine the precise role and contribution of both techniques in assessing chronic IHD patients.

8.4.5.4
Choosing the Imaging Sequence for Delayed-Enhancement MRI

Since the initial observations that injured myocardium could be differentiated from normal myocar-dial tissue, numerous studies have been performed using a variety of pulse sequences (REHR et al. 1986; TSCHOLAKOFF et al. 1986; LIMA et al. 1995; JUDD et al. 1995b; DE ROOS et al. 1989). In these studies, significant differences in the increased signal intensities of infarcted myocardium, ranging from 70% to 123% higher than those of normal myocardium, have been reported. Apart from addressing the issue of infarct volume overestimation, it is obvious that, in a clinical setting, selection of an MR imaging technique with a favorable signal-to-noise level, and sufficient resolution and contrast level needs to be selected (Fig. 8.18).

Over the last years, the scales have tipped in favor of using gradient-echo acquisitions, a trend that was probably initiated by a paper from EDELMAN et al. (1990), describing a segmented T1-weighted gradient-echo acquisition, originally intended to be used for liver imaging without contrast agents. The sequence described in this paper produced strongly T1-weighted images owing to the use of an inversion pulse before image acquisition. Edelman demonstrated that segmentation of the acquisition can generate images that are more strongly dependent on the inversion recovery of magnetization than

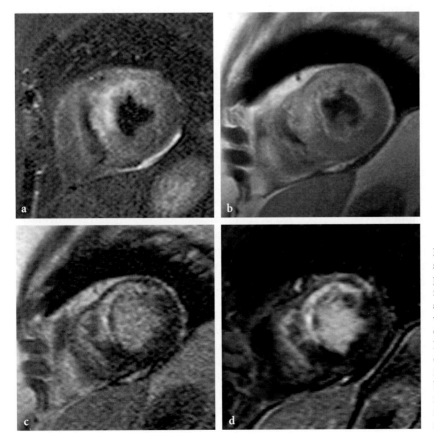

Fig. 8.18a-d Choice of imaging sequences. Fifty-nine-year-old patient with acute anteroseptal myocardial infarction imaged by **a** T2-weighted STIR TSE, **b** T1-weighted post contrast TSE, **c** 2D CE-IR MRI, and **d** 3D CE-IR MRI. Note the differential properties of the increased signal intensities in the infarct areas demonstrated by the different techniques. The main benefit of 3D over 2D techniques is the gain in signal-to-noise ratio

are single-shot sequences. This technique was further optimized by SIMONETTI et al. (2001) for use in cardiac studies: The acquisition was synchronized with diastole for motion-free imaging, and gradient-moment refocusing was used to reduce motion artifacts. More importantly, however, the inversion time (TI) of this sequence was specifically set to null the signal intensity of normal myocardium after contrast agent administration.

The value of this CE-IR MRI sequence has been demonstrated in an experimental study that compared CE-IR MRI with nine other types of sequences, both in an animal model of myocardial infarction and in patients with CAD. The main finding of this study is that the CE-IR MRI sequence, with a TI set to null normal myocardial signal intensity after contrast material administration, produces the greatest differences in regional myocardial signal intensities. The infarcted myocardium shows, on average, a 1,080% higher signal intensity than does the normal myocardium, which is a tenfold improvement in contrast in comparison to previously used techniques. Since this discovery, several groups have adopted this strategy to visualize myocardial infarcts and have demonstrated its use for imaging myocardial infarction in experimental and clinical studies (KIM et al. 1999; PISLARU et al. 1999; WAGNER et al. 2003). The spatial resolution of CE-IR MRI (e.g., 1.4×1.9×6.0 mm) is about 60-fold greater than what is currently achievable with SPECT. As a result, CE-IR MRI has been shown to be superior in detecting subendocardial infarcts that are systemically missed on SPECT (WAGNER et al. 2003).

There is some debate amongst authors as to whether two- or three-dimensional CE-IR MRI sequences are optimal for imaging (KÜHL et al. 2004). Whilst 3D volumes offer the obvious advantage of acquiring the complete cardiac volume in a single breath-hold, 2D sequences seems to suffer less from motion blurring and partial volume effects.

An equally important issue is the ideal dose of contrast agent to be used. Initial studies argued that the ideal dose should be 0.2 mmol of contrast agent/kg of body weight, but several authors have since presented comparable results with a lower total contrast dose. Too-low doses (<0.1 mmol) may result in a brief and insufficient enhancement of the infarction. It is most likely that 0.15–0.2 mmol of contrast/kg of body weight is appropriate for clinical use on a 1.5 T MR unit.

Notwithstanding the positive experiences with the CE-IR MRI technique, the approach requires the signal intensity of normal myocardium to be exactly nulled by choosing the proper inversion delay (TI), since the goal of this sequence is to maximize the signal intensity ratio between normal and abnormal enhanced myocardium (see Fig. 1.14). In practice this means that determination of the exact TI delay at which maximum nulling of normal myocardium occurs must be done iteratively for each patient and for each individual time point after injection, since renal excretion will also influence the total amount of T1-shortening induced by the agent. The total amount of contrast agent in circulation can furthermore be influenced by the patient's renal clearance, cardiac output, and other physiological phenomena. Although an experienced user can estimate the TI value reasonably well on the basis of the patient's size, the amount of contrast agent administered, and the time after contrast-agent injection, the technique still leaves quite a large margin of error. For images acquired in patients 5–20 min after the administration of 0.2 mmol of contrast agent/kg of body weight, TI values usually vary from 200–250 ms for early images to 250–300 ms for late images. An error in selecting the proper TI can lead to loss of contrast information and the introduction of specific artifacts. These artifacts are further discussed in Sect. 8.7.

To address the issue of optimization of TI, phase-sensitive inversion-recovery (PSIR) techniques have been developed to overcome this difficulty (KELLMAN et al. 2002) (Fig. 8.19). For inversion-recovery techniques, such as in sequences used for myocardial scar imaging, the inversion pulse causes a change in magnetization by 180º, in other words, the polarity of the magnetization is inverted. During the process of relaxation, this inversion will recover and, if images are acquired exactly at the TI of normal myocardium, the resulting image will show normal myocardium as dark, and hyperenhanced myocardium as bright. If TI values are chosen earlier or later than the ideal, loss of contrast will ensue. PSIR sequences acquire a background phase map during the same acquisition of the image itself. The phase map is used to make a complex pixel map of the polarities inside the image after magnetization recovery and to provide background noise reduction (KELLMAN et al. 2004). This is in fact a measure on how the different tissues regain magnetization after inversion and can be used through complex reconstruction to obtain intensity-normalized images in which the image level and window, and not the TI is used to maximize the contrast ratio. Therefore the inversion delay can be arbitrarily chosen to a default or "mean" value. In the original study by KELLMAN

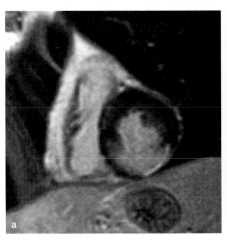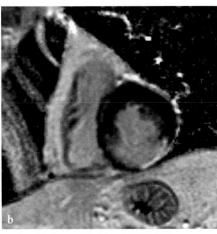

Fig. 8.19a,b Short-axis CE-IR MR images without (a) and with (b) phase-sensitive inversion recovery (PSIR) reconstruction in a 61-year-old patient with chronic inferior wall myocardial infarction. The PSIR reconstructed image can be adjusted with window and level setting to an appropriate low signal of the normal myocardium without negative effect on the infarct visualization

et al. (2004), this default value was determined as the mean of a set of patients with different contrast washout rates. This technique, although not yet available on all types of MRI scanners, obviates the need to acquire several breath-hold acquisitions to determine the optimal TI, which is very variable. This is especially important if the user chooses to acquire successive 2D measurements, thus avoiding the need to adapt the TI value every other slice.

8.5
Typical Appearance of Myocardial Infarctions on MR Images

We have previously established that use of nonspecific contrast agents in conjunction with CE-IR MRI, the so-called delayed or late-enhancement MRI technique, constitutes a valuable tool to visualize, in detail, the presence of myocardial infarction. This is mainly due to the differential and time-varying effect of the contrast agent on relaxation times of normal and infarcted myocardium and due to the high contrast ratio of the abovementioned sequence. Although the optimal time point for myocardial imaging is deemed to be 10–20 min after the injection of the contrast agent, it is important to realize what happens exactly after injection on the myocardial tissue level (Oshinski et al. 2001). Immediately after contrast administration, there is a brief enhancement of the normal myocardium, due to the rapid washout of contrast in normal myocardium, enhancement of which is already substantially less 5 min after contrast administration. An opposite phenomenon is observed in infarcted myocardium. At 5 min, T1-relaxation time is significantly shorter

than soon after contrast injection, making the infarct area bright relative to the viable myocardium, thus substantially improving the visualization of the infarct area and increasing the accuracy of infarct quantification (McNamara et al. 1986; Eichstaedt et al. 1989). Somewhere between 5 and 30 min after contrast administration, T1-relaxation of the infarcted or scarred myocardium is shortest and thus optimal for imaging with CE-IR MRI (Fig. 8.20), while, after 30 min, due to substantial washout of contrast in the infarcted myocardium, T1-relaxation times again increase, impeding visualization of the infarct area (Dymarkowski et al. 2002).

Depending on the location, depth, and the severity of the infarction, several patterns of enhancement have been described, which is important information, since analysis of these patterns helps to better understand the complex mechanism of enhancement after contrast administration (Fukuzawa et al. 1994).

8.5.1
Patterns of Enhancement Reflecting Acute Infarct Severity

In an important paper by de Roos et al. (1989), four different patterns of infarct enhancement, reflecting the depth or severity of AMI, have been described. These patterns bear a likeness to the pathophysiology of myocardial infarction, since it is well known that, during coronary artery occlusion, the infarction spreads transmurally over time, like a wave front, from the endocardium toward the epicardium. As later shown by several other groups, these enhancement patterns are proportionately linked to peak creatine kinase levels, regional functional parameters, and are prognostically important

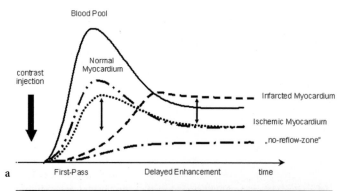

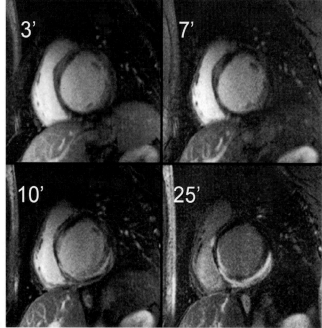

Fig. 8.20. a Schematic of the contrast kinetics in different pathophysiological states after myocardial infarction. Early wash-in similar to the blood pool (*solid line*) is observed in normal myocardium, which is dampened in ischemic areas. In infarcted myocardium, contrast wash-in is impaired and characterized by delayed signal increase. **b** Short-axis CE-IR MR images in a patient with a large transmural inferior wall infarction extending in the inferolateral and inferoseptal wall. As time after injection increases (3 min, 7 min, 10 min, 25 min), the signal intensity of normal myocardium decreases (steady washout), while the infarction enhancement gradually is augmented

(HOLMAN et al. 1993; LIMA et al. 1995; YOKOTA et al. 1995; KIM et al. 1996; ROGERS et al. 1999; GERBER et al. 2000). Subsequent investigations, in both animal and human studies, have shown the relevance of analyzing the transmural extent of enhancement on a segmental or regional basis. Assessment of this transmural extent is a critical determinant of recovery of contractile function in the postinfarction period (Fig. 8.21). HILLENBRAND et al. (2000) have evaluated, in an animal model, the relationship between the transmural extent of enhancement at 3 days and the contractile recovery at 28 days after AMI. This group found that, when the segmental transmural extent of enhancement was smaller than 25%, the majority of segments (87%) improved function, whereas, when the extent of enhancement was more than 75%, functional recovery was unlikely, with intermediate degrees of enhancement resulting

in intermediate likelihood of recovery. Similar findings have been observed in 41 patients with chronic ischemic disease undergoing revascularization. Further human studies in acute and chronic myocardial infarction have similarly demonstrated the utility of delayed-hyperenhancement MRI in predicting functional recovery (KIM et al. 2000; BEEK et al. 2003).

The first pattern of delayed MR hyperenhancement is that of subendocardial late-enhancement alone, with sparing of the subepicardial layer (Fig. 8.22). This subendocardial enhancement is related to less extensive, often non-Q-wave, infarcts that are known to have a better patient outcome. It is important to realize in this setting that, at present (2004), delayed hyperenhancement is virtually the only imaging technique that is able to demonstrate these subendocardial infarctions with sufficient

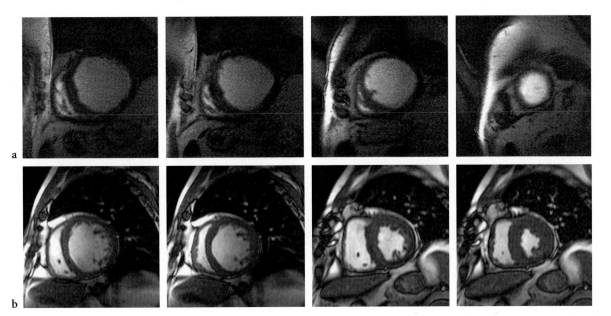

Fig. 8.21. a CE-IR MR images in a 57-year-old patient with known significant and long-standing three-vessel disease and chronic myocardial ischemia. Images show a dilated LV with absence of myocardial enhancement. **b** Corresponding end-diastolic and end-systolic cine MR images before (*left*) and 4 months after (*right*) coronary artery bypass grafting (CABG) show significant functional recovery after revascularization surgery with decrease in end-diastolic volume (EDV), increase in ejection fraction (EF) and increase in systolic wall thickening (SV). Global cardiac function values before surgery (*left*): EDV 450 ml, ESV 375 ml, SV 75 ml, EF 17%; and after surgery (*right*) EDV 200 ml, ESV 105 ml, SV 95 ml, EF 47.5%

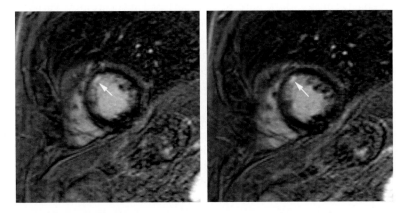

Fig. 8.22 Subendocardial myocardial infarction. Fifty-one-year-old patient with increased troponin levels and chest pain. CE-IR MR images in short-axis show a small focus of delayed enhancement in the anteroseptal apical segment, indicative for a small subendocardial myocardial infarction. The resting ECG and echocardiography were unremarkable in this patient

spatial resolution. Wu et al. (2001) have shown that delayed-enhancement MRI depicts nontransmural hyperintensity in all subjects with clinical evidence of non–Q-wave infarcts. Animal models with subacute and chronic infarct have also demonstrated remarkably close agreement between histopathological depiction of infarct and MRI findings (Kim et al. 1996; Dymarkowski et al. 2002; Wagner et al. 2003).

The second pattern shows delayed hyperenhancement extending over the full thickness of the myocardial wall, representing complete transmural but reperfused infarcts. Usually this pattern is seen in larger infarcts, and the likelihood of functional recovery of these infarcts after revascularization is very small (Fig. 8.23).

Pattern three is similar to the enhancement pattern seen in transmural infarcts, but is distinguished by the

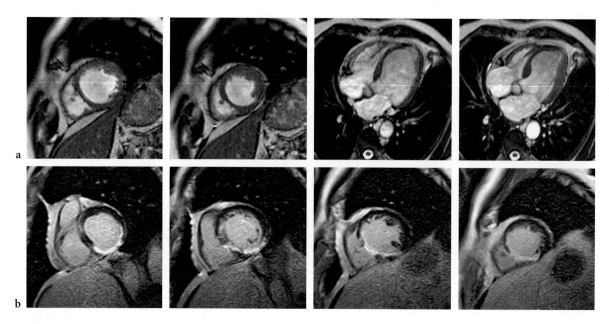

Fig. 8.23. Transmural myocardial infarction. a Cine MR images from a 68-year-old patient with previous myocardial infarction. Short-axis (*top*) and horizontal long-axis series show wall thinning and akinesia in the inferoseptal and inferobasal segments of the LV. **b** Short-axis CE-IR MR images show transmural enhancement in the corresponding dysfunctional segments

appearance of a subendocardially located hypointense area. This area is best seen on delayed-enhancement images taken early after injection, since in this phase, the contrast between this dark area and the transient myocardial enhancement, in both normal and injured myocardium, is greatest. This pattern represents transmural infarctions in which the reperfusion was only partially successful with residual lack of reperfusion at the tissue level, i.e., the *no-reflow phenomenon* (KLONER et al. 1974; ITO et al. 1992; Fig. 8.24). The area of no-reflow is associated with severe edema compressing intramural vessels or extensive myocardial necrosis and microcirculatory damage in the center of a large infarction (JUDD et al. 1995a, 1995b; ITO et al. 1996). In a recent study by ROCHITTE et al. (1998), the central hypoenhanced region in the infarct region increased threefold during the first 48 h after reperfusion. These results are consistent with progressive microvascular and myocardial injury after reperfusion. GERBER et al. (2000) have reported that the area of no-reflow is a better predictor of LV dilatation (i.e., negative LV remodeling) than the infarct size. The same group has also reported that no-reflow zones have no inotropic reserve, while the inotropic reserve in myocardium with late-enhancement MRI is mainly influenced by the transmurality of enhancement (and thus necrosis) (GERBER et al. 2001).

A fourth pattern is seen in nonreperfused, i.e., occlusive, infarcts (Fig. 8.25). These infarcts are vi-

sualized as peripheral enhancement surrounding a dark core of non-perfused myocardium. Patterns three and four reflect extensive myocardial infarction with infarct expansion, less viable myocardium, more nonischemic dysfunction, and worse outcome (YOKOTA et al. 1995; HOLMAN et al. 1993; ROGERS et al. 1999) (Fig. 8.26).

Moreover, a combination of T2w-STIR imaging ("edema-weighted" MRI) and CE-IR MRI probably enables the description of two additional patterns. A first pattern is hyperintense appearance in the area of the myocardium at risk on edema-weighted MRI without delayed enhancement, reflecting reversible ischemic injury without tissue necrosis (Fig. 8.27). Cardiac enzyme levels in these patients are often only marginally elevated. A second pattern is visible in the first days after the acute event and most likely reflects a hemorrhagic AMI. It consists of a central hypointense core with a peripheral hyperintense layer in the area of the myocardium at risk on edema-weighted MRI. Degradation of blood products in the hemorrhagic infarction strongly decreases the T2-relaxation time, causing a hypointense appearance of the core, while the hyperintense rim is caused by the surrounding periinfarct edema and inflammation. On CE-IR MR images, the infarct area is typically strongly hypoenhanced and fills in only slowly on the images acquired later (Fig. 8.28).

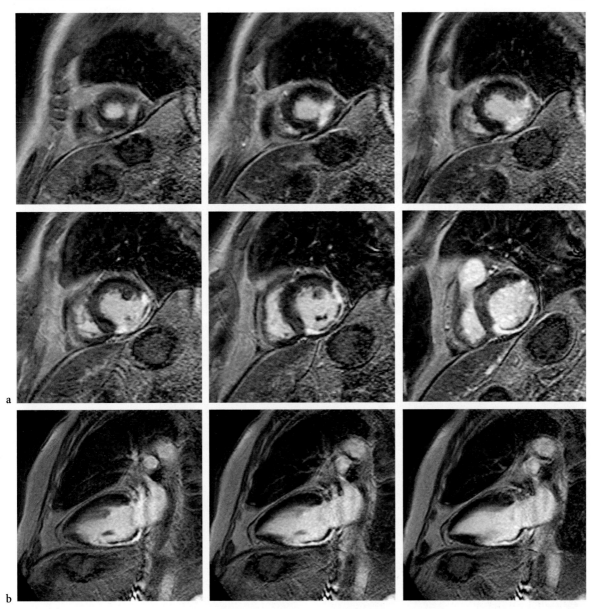

Fig. 8.24. a Transmural myocardial infarction with microvascular obstruction. Short-axis CE-IR MR images in a 65-year-old patient 8 days after acute myocardial infarction show transmural enhancement in the inferolateral wall with a strong, hypointense crescent-shaped layer located at the endocardial border. **b** The corresponding vertical long-axis images show the precise longitudinal extension of myocardial necrosis, which covers the largest part of the inferior wall

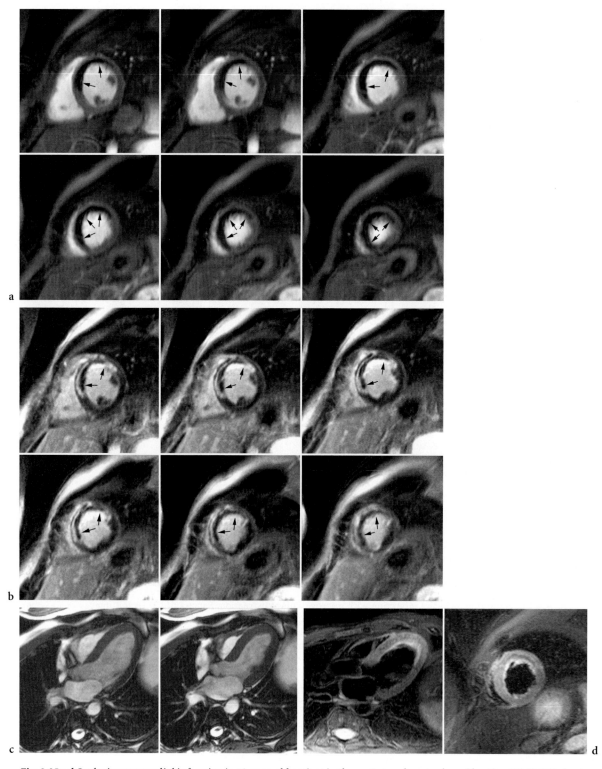

Fig. 8.25a-d Occlusive myocardial infarction in 42-year-old patient in the acute to subacute phase (day 5). **a** CE-IR MR short-axis images taken within 2 min after contrast administration show a strong intramyocardial hypointense band within the infarction area, representing complete occlusion of coronary vessels to the anteroseptal wall (*arrows*). **b** Corresponding CE-IR MR images taken 23 min after contrast injection show progressive centripetal filling in from the periphery of the infarction (*arrows*). **c** Horizontal long-axis cine MRI at end diastole (*left*) and end systole (*right*) show akinesia of the ventricular septum and LV apex. **d** T2w STIR TSE in horizontal long- axis (*left*) and short-axis (*right*) shows thickening and edema in ventricular septum and LV apex

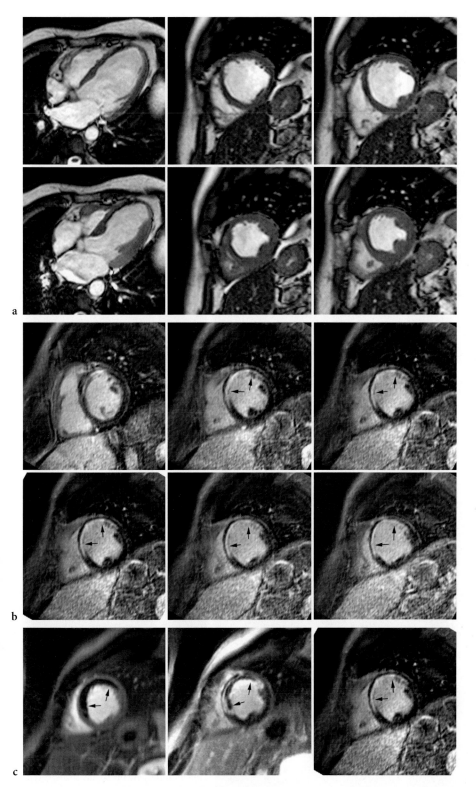

Fig. 8.26. a End-diastolic (*top* row) and end-systolic cine MR images of the previous patient (Fig. 8.25) 4 months later. Lack of functional recovery and negative ventricular remodeling is seen by ventricular dilation, extensive wall thinning in the anteroseptal segment, and complete loss of contractility. **b** CE-IR MR images show extensive wall thinning with infarct shrinkage and complete resolution of the formerly visualized obstructive enhancement pattern. **c** Comparison between CE-IR MR images in the acute phase at two points after injection: 3 min (*left*) and 23 min (*middle*). The (*right*) image shows the corresponding CE-IR MR image 4 months later, taken 20 min after injection

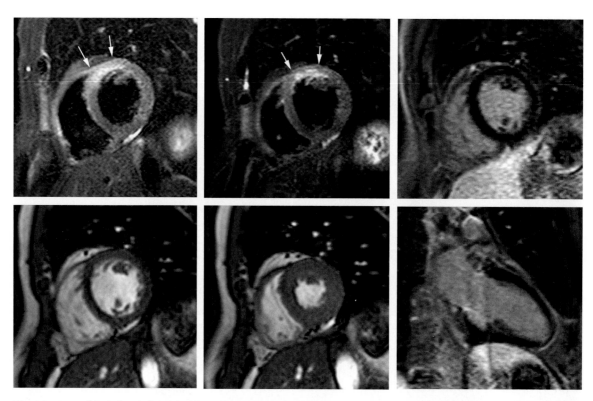

Fig. 8.27 Reversible ischemic injury without tissue necrosis in 54-year-old patient with angina-like symptoms, acute isch-emic changes on ECG, and mildly elevated troponin levels. T2-weighted STIR TSE images (*top left and middle*) show tissue edema in the anteroseptal myocardium of the LV (*arrows*). Cine MRI (*bottom left and middle*) shown regional normal wall thickening. There are no areas of delayed enhancement on CE-IR MR images (*top* and *bottom right*), ruling out macroscopic tissue infarction

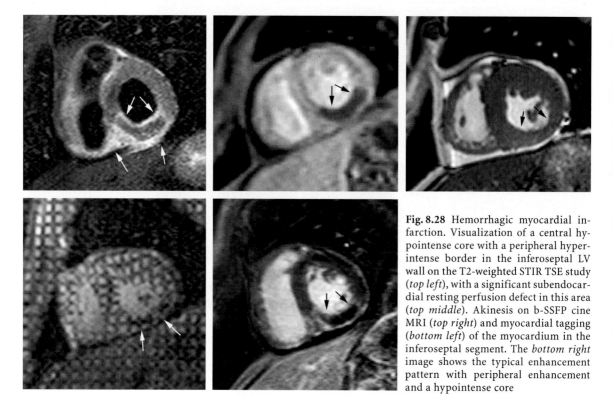

Fig. 8.28 Hemorrhagic myocardial in-farction. Visualization of a central hy-pointense core with a peripheral hyper-intense border in the inferoseptal LV wall on the T2-weighted STIR TSE study (*top left*), with a significant subendocar-dial resting perfusion defect in this area (*top middle*). Akinesis on b-SSFP cine MRI (*top right*) and myocardial tagging (*bottom left*) of the myocardium in the inferoseptal segment. The *bottom right* image shows the typical enhancement pattern with peripheral enhancement and a hypointense core

8.5.2
Patterns of Enhancement Depending on Infarct Location

As already discussed above, the tissue enhancement in myocardial infarction, albeit acute or chronic, is nonspecific and merely reflects a disturbance in local alterations of perfusion, tissue metabolism, and loss of normal myocardial matrix. Differential diagnosis in clinical circumstances may therefore be less obvious, especially in cases with atypical presentations. There are, however, a few markers by which to attribute a certain pattern of delayed enhancement with a higher degree of certainty in the IHD category.

First, regardless of the location of a myocardial infarction, the pattern of enhancement always presents as spreading outward from the endocardium. Whether the infarction itself is subendocardial or transmural, the subendocardium is always involved. Furthermore, the infarct location always can be traced back to a certain "culprit" artery, which is to say, although the supply territories of the three major coronary arteries are variable depending on coronary artery anatomy, the infarction is always located within the anatomical territory supplied by one coronary artery, and the intensity of abnormalities increases toward the distal perfusion territory of that coronary artery (Figs. 8.29–8.31).

The use of these two criteria may already allow the physician to differentiate between infarction and the enhancement seen in myocarditis, which is known to present a more diffuse multifocal enhancement pattern, often subepicardially located and not infrequently accompanied by pericardial enhancement (MAHRHOLDT et al. 2004) (see Chap. 9).

The morphology of an area of delayed enhancement in myocardial infarction is also relative to the longitudinal distribution of the blood supply of the coronary artery (BOURDILLON et al. 2003). In inferior infarctions, the area of enhancement is more pronounced in the basal and mid-ventricular myocardium (Fig. 8.29), whereas lateral wall infarctions are more oriented toward the mid-ventricular and apical portions (Fig. 8.31). Anterior infarctions are usually very large and spread out from the anterobasal wall and may include the apex (Fig. 8.30). Inferior infarctions not infrequently may extent toward the inferolateral right ventricular (RV) wall, while isolated RV infarctions seldom occur. Finally, small infarctions, often at atypical locations (e.g., mid-septum), can be seen when coronary artery side branches are involved (Fig. 8.32), and microinfarc-

tions can be seen after coronary dilations or stent placements. These are usually very small, but often transmural infarcts in the immediate vicinity of the instrumented artery (mean mass of myonecrosis 2.0 g) and are associated with mild elevations in cardiac enzymes (GERBER et al. 2003; NAGEH et al. 2003). While ECG and wall motion is often normal, CE-IR MRI can be used to provide an anatomical correlate to biochemical evidence of procedure-related myocardial injury (RICCIARDI et al. 2001).

8.6
Imaging of Complications Related to Ischemic Heart Disease

Complications of myocardial infarctions such as wall thinning, aneurysm formation, valvular regurgitation, associated pericardial effusion or postinfarction pericarditis (Dressler's syndrome) are best visualized on cardiac MR images using the comprehensive approach described above (Fig. 8.33). Due to stagnant blood flow in the infarct area, especially in transmural infarctions and postinfarction aneurysms (Fig. 8.34), these areas are at high risk of thrombus formation. Detection of these mural thrombi is of paramount importance, since their presence is an indication for strict anticoagulation therapy to avoid potential neurological and peripheral embolic symptoms (Fig. 8.35). Thrombi can be easily missed on transthoracic echocardiography, especially when located in the LV apex or when trapped within the endocardial trabeculations. Using a combination of CE-IR MRI and cine MRI, ventricular thrombi are easily demonstrated and differentiated from stagnant or slow flow (KEELEY and HILLIS 1996; MOLLET et al. 2002). Thrombi are best visualized early after the injection of contrast agent, e.g., immediately after a perfusion study, to take advantage of the high contrast of the blood pool and the hypointense signal intensity of the clot itself. Differentiation between mural thrombi and no reflow, both hypointense on CE-IR MR images, is usually straightforward, since mural thrombi have an intracavity location, whist no-reflow zones are within the myocardium. Also differences in shape are helpful to differentiate both conditions.

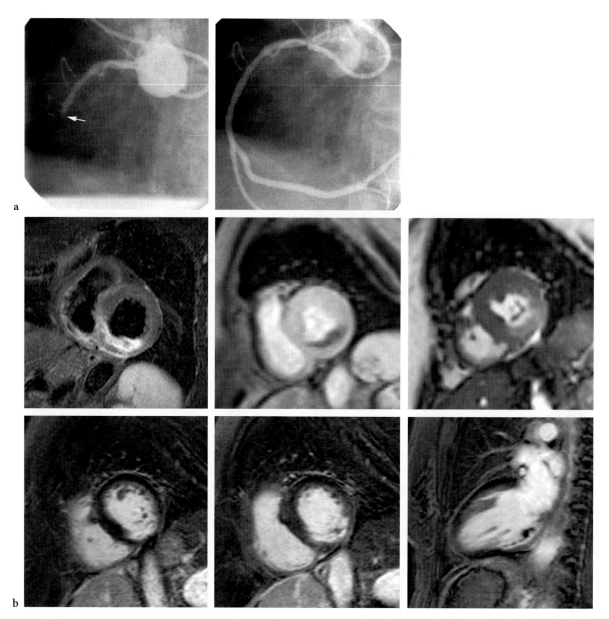

Fig. 8.29a,b Acute myocardial infarction in right coronary artery (RCA) perfusion territory. **a** Coronary angiography shows total occlusion of RCA at the middle segment (*arrow*) (*left*), with restoration of coronary artery patency after percutaneous coronary intervention (PCI) with stent placement (*right*). **b** Comprehensive MR study after PCI. Edema-weighted STIR TSE imaging in cardiac short-axis shows large area of transmural edema in inferior and inferoseptal LV wall extending to the inferior RV wall (*top left*). Resting-state perfusion MRI in cardiac short-axis (*top middle*) shows subendocardial area of non-reperfusion in inferior LV wall, while on short-axis cine MR image at end systole the inferior wall is akinetic (*top right*). CE-IR MRI with late imaging in cardiac short-axis (*bottom left* and *middle*) and vertical long-axis (*bottom right*) shows typical enhancement pattern of infarctions in the RCA territory, i.e., late enhancement of the inferobasal part of the LV wall with a variable transmural, circumferential, and longitudinal spread. Note the presence of an important subendocardial no-reflow zone in the infarct territory, representing area of microvascular obstruction

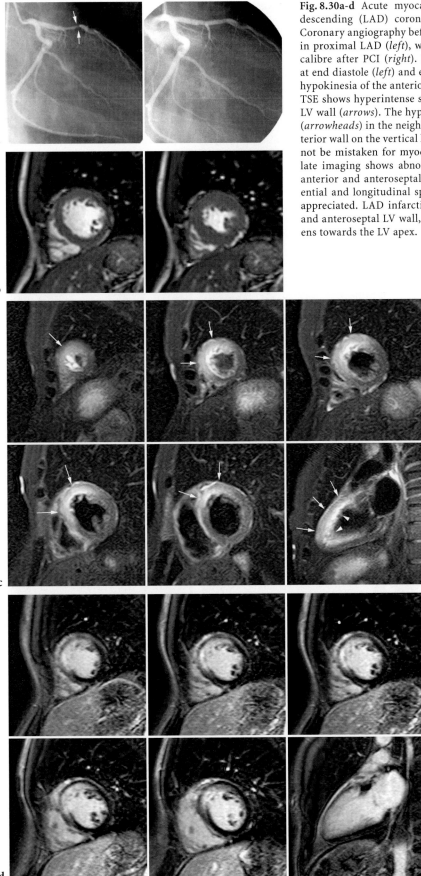

Fig. 8.30a–d Acute myocardial infarction in left anterior descending (LAD) coronary artery perfusion territory. **a** Coronary angiography before PCI shows high-grade stenosis in proximal LAD (*left*), with restoration of coronary artery calibre after PCI (*right*). **b** Cine MRI in cardiac short-axis at end diastole (*left*) and end systole (*right*) shows moderate hypokinesia of the anterior LV wall. **c** Edema-weighted STIR TSE shows hyperintense signal in anterior and anteroseptal LV wall (*arrows*). The hyperintense signal of stagnant blood (*arrowheads*) in the neighbourhood of the dysfunctional anterior wall on the vertical long-axis view (*bottom left*) should not be mistaken for myocardial edema. **d** CE-IR MRI with late imaging shows abnormal myocardial enhancement in anterior and anteroseptal wall. The transmural, circumferential and longitudinal spread of enhancement can be well appreciated. LAD infarctions typically involve the anterior and anteroseptal LV wall, and infarct severity usually worsens towards the LV apex.

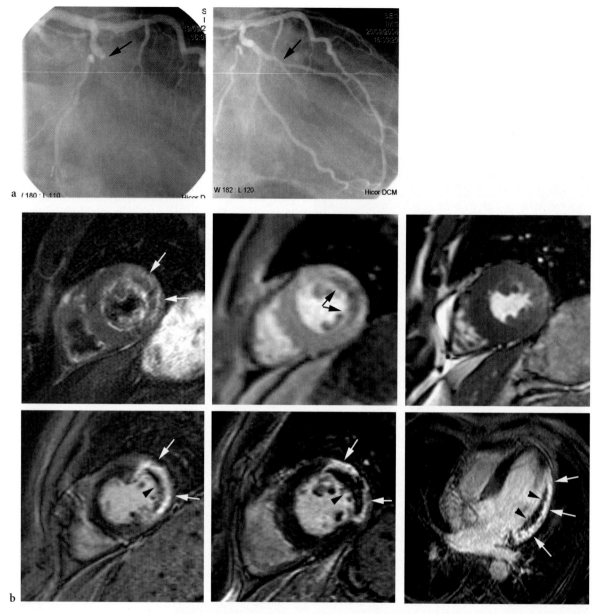

Fig. 8.31a,b Acute myocardial infarction in left circumflex (LCx) coronary artery perfusion territory. **a** Coronary angiography shows total occlusion of first lateral branch of LCx (*arrow*) (*left*), with restoration of coronary artery patency after intravenous thrombolytic therapy (*right*). **b** Comprehensive MR study shows on short-axis, edema-weighted STIR TSE (*top left*) central hypo-intense area with peripheral hyperintense rim in LV lateral wall (*arrows*). Large perfusion defect is visible on short-axis, resting-state perfusion MRI (*arrows*) (*top middle*). Short-axis, cine MR image at end systole shows akinesia of the entire lateral LV wall. CE-IR MRI with late imaging in cardiac short-axis (*bottom left* and *middle*) and horizontal long-axis (*bottom right*) shows strong enhancement of the entire lateral LV wall sparing the apical part (*arrow*). Note the presence of large non-enhancing zone with partially complete transmural extension (*arrowhead*). MRI findings are suggestive of an acute hemorrhagic myocardial infarction in lateral LV wall

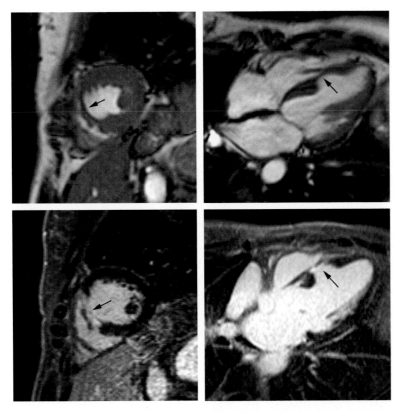

Fig. 8.32 Atypical presentation of septal infarction in 71-year-old patient. The comprehensive MR examination shows wall thinning and akinesis of the midseptal LV segment on cine MR images (*top row*), with transmural enhancement on CE-IR MR images (*bottom row*). Coronary angiography (not shown) confirmed occlusion of a septal branch of the LAD artery

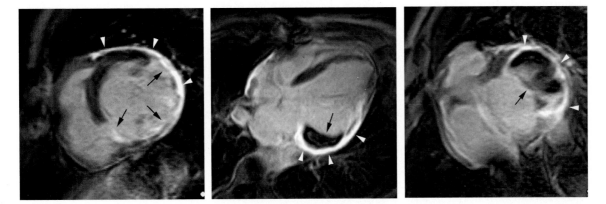

Fig. 8.33 Complications after myocardial infarction I. Chronic complicated myocardial infarction is illustrated with CE-IR MR images in short-axis (*left*), horizontal long-axis view (*middle*), and basal mitral valve view (*right*). There is transmural enhancement of the inferolateral basal segment, as well as enhancement of the overlying pericardium and aneurismal dilation of the expanded infarction (*arrowheads*). Presence of large thrombus in the ventricular aneurysm (*arrows*)

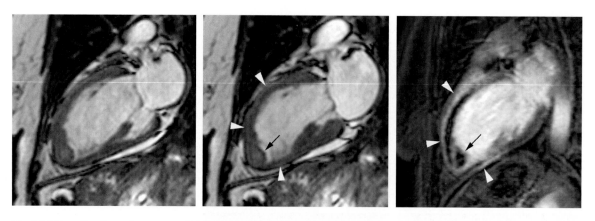

Fig. 8.34 Complications after myocardial infarction II. Study performed in a 67-year-old patient 8 days post-acute anterior wall myocardial infarction. Cine MRI (*left and middle*) shows akinesis in a large part of the anterior wall and the LV apex (*arrowheads*) and the presence of an added mass filling up the LV apex (*arrow*). The CE-IR MR image (*right*) confirms the presence of the large anteroapical infarction presenting as a large transmural enhancing wall segment overspanning the apex (*arrowheads*) with a subendocardial no-reflow area and a nonenhancing apical thrombus (*arrow*)

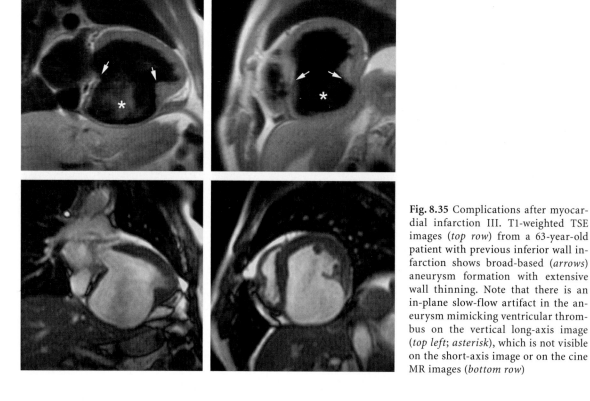

Fig. 8.35 Complications after myocardial infarction III. T1-weighted TSE images (*top row*) from a 63-year-old patient with previous inferior wall infarction shows broad-based (*arrows*) aneurysm formation with extensive wall thinning. Note that there is an in-plane slow-flow artifact in the aneurysm mimicking ventricular thrombus on the vertical long-axis image (*top left*; *asterisk*), which is not visible on the short-axis image or on the cine MR images (*bottom row*)

8.7
Artifacts in Delayed-Enhancement Images

8.7.1
Motion-Related Artifacts

In studies of patients, image quality may be compromised by several factors. First of all, most sequences are acquired in breath-hold. The duration of these multiple breath-hold periods may be at the upper limit of the patient's capability so that motion artifacts, especially at the end of an MRI study, may occur, for instance at the moment of the delayed-enhancement imaging. These artifacts may obscure interpretation; however, it is usually possible to determine whether, for example, hyperintense lines in the image are artifact or linear enhancement by following a few simple rules.

In general, MRI motion artifacts occur in the phase-encoding direction. If an artifact is noted during the acquisition, the phase-encoding direction can be changed to see if it reoccurs. Most problematic are artifacts related to motion of the heart; for example if the patient starts to breathe out at the end of the acquisition. This can create a cardiac-shaped overlay on the actual image and may hamper proper image analysis. If uncertainty exists about the nature of such an artifact, it is useful to realize that an artifact never respects anatomical borders and usually a contour can be found outside the heart, revealing the nature of this imaging finding.

Long breath-holds can be avoided by performing measurements during free breathing using navigator echoes, or by decreasing the total acquisition time. This can be performed by decreasing the rectangular field-of-view, if the patient's size permits. Another alternative is to decrease the image resolution. However, since resolution is the key element to accurate detection of abnormalities, this procedure should be avoided. A valid alternative is to use parallel imaging to decrease the total acquisition time.

Motion-related artifacts may also be caused by cardiac motion itself. If the timing of a delayed-enhancement sequence does not correspond to the diastolic diastasis, severe motion artifact of cardiac contraction can occur. This is especially true in 3D sequences, where the acquisition shot is "crammed" into diastole in order to fit the entire sequence into a single breath-hold, and in patients with higher heart rates. In these latter cases, it is advisable to use 2D sequences that have a shorter acquisition window.

8.7.2
Contrast-Related Artifacts

As previously discussed, determining the exact TI delay in a CE-IR MRI for maximum nulling of normal myocardium can be difficult. It must be done for each patient and for each time point after injection individually, since a large number of variables influence the total contrast load and inversion recovery. The normal range for TI values in patients after a contrast dose of 0.1–0.2 mmol/kg bodyweight are 280–380 ms and 200–300 ms, respectively. Errors in selecting correct inversion delays will result in loss of contrast between normal and abnormal myocardium and may introduce specific artifacts. Until the phase-sensitive image reconstruction techniques become readily available, most users may still experience problems in determining the ideal inversion time. However, some practical guidelines may be of great help in determining whether or not a late-enhancement image can be considered as adequate (Fig. 8.36).

If an appropriate TI is chosen, the signal of normal myocardium should be close to zero, or appear very dark between 10 and 20 min after contrast administration, The LV blood pool should be intermediately intense (white to gray-white) and a myocardial infarction or scar should be the most intense structure in the image. If this is not the case, the TI

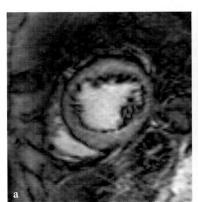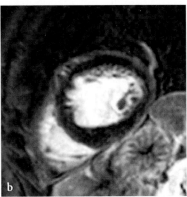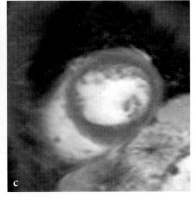

Fig. 8.36a-c Contrast alterations in CE-IR MR images. Short-axis images taken 12–14 min after injection of 0.2 mmol/kg Gd-DTPA. **a** TI=210 ms. The myocardium is gray in the mid-wall section, with hypointense bands at the epi- and endocardial borders. The inversion time is too short. **b** TI=250 ms. Normal myocardium appears hypointense with high contrast between myocardium and blood. **c** TI=300 ms. The longer TI produces prolonged recovery of magnetization with contrast loss, resulting in gray myocardium

is probably not set correctly. The following artifacts may occur:

- If the blood pool appears too dark, the TI is likely to be too short and needs to be increased significantly to allow sufficient recovery. An increase in up to 50 m may be necessary.
- If the TI is very close to the optimal inversion delay, but still too short, a speckled appearance (suppressed myocardium interspersed with nonsuppressed white spots) may occur, or the endo-and epicardial border may appear as hypointense lines with gray myocardium in between (Fig. 8.36a). If this is the case, increase the TI with small steps, e.g., of 10 ms, until the optimal suppression of normal myocardium is attained.
- If an area of delayed enhancement is gray and only slightly more intense than the myocardium or the blood, the TI is too long (Fig. 8.36c). A decrease in steps of 10 ms is advisable.
- At the other end of the spectrum, if there is no contrast between blood, myocardium, and infarcted tissue (if present) and all structures appear to be too dark, this indicates either that the contrast has washed out (e.g., >30 min after injection) or that an insufficient amount of contrast agent was injected.

An artifact that is often seen, especially in dilated ventricles, resembles subendocardial enhancement in a ring-shaped distribution, covering the entire endocardial surface. Usually "pseudo-enhancement" is not confined to a coronary artery territory and can be distant to infarction tissue elsewhere in the image. This artifact is most likely caused by trapping of contrast in between trabeculations and papillary muscles in cases of slow flow, i.e., in dilated ventricles or aneurysms. Very little can be done to avoid this artifact, although it is less pronounced the later the images are acquired, e.g., 25 min after contrast administration. One practical trick is to compare the CE-IR MR images with the corresponding cine MR images. Since the wall thickness can be easily evaluated on cine MRI, it can be easily determined whether or not the enhancement occurs in the myocardium or in the LV cavity. It is important to consider that this can only be done correctly if a similar time point during the cardiac cycle is used as the one used for acquiring the CE-IR MR image, which is normally during mid-diastole.

8.8
Clinical Imaging Strategies: Practical Recipes

An important issue is the integration of the above MRI techniques into clinical routine (BOGAERT et al. 2002). The major constraint in scanning cardiac patients is definitely the length of the scan procedure. Depending on the patient's general condition, the MRI study should be finished within 45–60 min. Besides sufficient training and experience in the field of cardiac MRI, use of standardized imaging protocols has been shown to be very helpful in improving the success rate of these kinds of demanding studies. In the last few years, several groups have reported optimized, comprehensive approaches for studying the different subgroups of IHD patients (SANDSTEDE et al. 2000; SENSKY et al. 2000; PLEIN et al. 2002; CHIU et al. 2003; KWONG et al. 2003). Sensky et al. have proposed a dual-stress MRI protocol to study patients with chronic IHD, including stress-rest perfusion, cardiac function, and low-dose DSMRI (SENSKY et al. 2000). Eventually, a late-enhancement study can be added to this protocol, offering a broad evaluation of the cardiac status of chronic IHD patients. Plein et al. have proposed, for the same subgroup of patients, a combination of rest-stress perfusion imaging, functional imaging, delayed-enhancement imaging, and coronary MR angiography of the right and left coronary artery in a scan time of less than 1 h (PLEIN et al. 2002). This approach has the advantage of depicting coronary artery stenotic lesions, evaluating the functional impact of the stenosis on coronary artery perfusion (stress perfusion), quantifying LV rest function, and depicting healed myocardial infarctions. So, when all components of the protocol are combined, MRI can thus correctly depict the presence of a previous myocardial infarction, and/or significant CAD (SANDSTEDE 2003).

Similar approaches can be used in acute IHD patients. Two groups have recently assessed the role of a comprehensive MRI approach to assess patients with non-ST segment-elevation acute coronary syndrome in the emergency department (CHIU et al. 2003; KWONG et al. 2003). The study protocols include rest or rest-stress perfusion, LV function analysis, and delayed-enhancement. MRI was shown to be the strongest predictor of acute coronary syndrome, adding diagnostic value to clinical parameters. It was concluded that MRI is helpful for triage of patients with chest pain in the emergency department. The above-used MRI protocol would most likely benefit from the addition of edema-weighted MRI, since this would enable demonstration of jeopardized myocardium without myocardial infarction in a very early stage (SCHULZ-MENGER et al. 2003) and differentiation between fresh and healed myocardial infarctions.

8.9
Key Points

- Coronary occlusion, usually caused by CAD, ensues a cascade of events in the myocardium distal to the occluded coronary artery. MRI is at present the only imaging modality that can evaluate all facets of this ischemic cascade.
- Myocardial infarction occurs soon (i.e., 20–30 min) after onset of coronary occlusion and progresses from the subendocardium, in a transmural wave front, toward the subepicardium over the next 3–6 h.
- Use of a comprehensive MRI approach, and systematic image analysis to study IHD patients.
- Edema-weighted MRI is an essential part of assessing acute IHD patients, helpful for depicting the jeopardized myocardium in vivo, as well as differentiating between acute and healed myocardial infarctions.
- In the acute stage of infarction, the nonspecific, commercially available contrast agents significantly overestimate the true size of myocardial necrosis. This is most probably related to enhancement in areas with peri-infarct edema or inflammation.
- The no-reflow phenomenon, an independent and important predictor of negative LV remodeling, can be best studied with CE-IR MRI techniques, with imaging soon after the contrast administration.
- Stress dobutamine and stress perfusion MRI have been shown to be reliable, safe and accurate procedures for studying acute and chronic IHD patients. Resuscitation material and regular training are essential to guarantee the patient's safety.
- Since the contrast mechanism of the CE-IR MRI technique is largely based on nulling of the signal of normal myocardium, appropriate choice of the inversion time is the key to success.
- The extent of infarct transmurality in both acute and chronic IHD patients is an important predictor of functional recovery.
- Be aware of complications when studying IHD patients. In particular, ventricular thrombi are

clearly seen using a combination of cine MRI and contrast-enhanced MRI techniques.

Acknowledgements

The authors wish to express gratitude to Prof. Dr. Stefan Janssens and Prof. Dr. Walter Desmet from the Department of Cardiology for their collaboration and expertise in the field of ischemic heart disease.

References

Adzamli IK, Blau M, Pfeffer MA et al (1993) Phosphonate-modified Gd-DTPA complexes. III. The detection of myocardial infarction by MRI. Magn Reson Med 29:505–511

Al-Saadi N, Nagel E, Gross M et al (2000) Noninvasive detection of myocardial ischemia from perfusion reserve based on cardiovascular magnetic resonance. Circulation 101:824–834

Baer FM, Smolarz R, Jungehulsing M (1992) Feasibility of high-dose dipyridamole MRI for the detection of coronary artery disease and comparison with coronary angiography. Am J Cardiol 69:51–56

Baer FM, Smolarz K, Theissen P et al (1993) Identification of hemodynamically significant coronary artery stenoses by dipyridamole-magnetic resonance imaging and 99mTc-methoxyisobutyl-isonitrile-SPECT. Int J Card Imaging 9:133–145

Baer FM, Voth E, Theissen P et al (1994) Gradient-echo magnetic resonance imaging during incremental dobutamine infusion for the localization of coronary artery stenoses. Eur Heart J 15:218–225

Bashour TT, Mason D (1990) Myocardial hibernation and "embalment". Am Heart J 119:706–708

Becker LC, Jeremy RW, Schaper J et al (1999) Ultrastructural assessment of myocardial necrosis occuring during ischemia and 3-h reperfusion in the dog. Am J Physiol 46: H243–H252

Beek AM, Kühl HP, Bondarenko O et al (2003) Delayed contrast-enhanced magnetic resonance imaging for the prediction of regional functional improvement after acute myocardial infarction. J Am Coll Cardiol 42:895–901

Beller GA (2000) Noninvasive assessment of myocardial viability. N Engl J Med 343:1488–1490

Beller GA (2001) Coronary heart disease in the first 30 years of the 21st Century: challenges and opportunities. Circulation 103:2428–2435

Bogaert J, Rademakers F (2001) Regional nonuniformity of the human left ventricle. A 3D MR myocardial tagging study. Am J Physiol 280:H610–H620

Bogaert J, Bosmans H, Rademakers F et al (1995) Left ventricular quantification with breath-hold MR imaging: comparison with echocardiography. Magma 3:5–12

Bogaert J, Maes A, van de Werf F et al (1999) Functional recovery of subepicardial myocardial tissue in transmural myocardial infarction after successful reperfusion. An important contribution to the improvement of regional and global left ventricular function. Circulation 99:36–43

Bogaert J, Bosmans H, Maes A et al (2000) Remote myocardial dysfunction after acute anterior myocardial infarction: impact of left ventricular shape on regional function. A magnetic resonance myocardial tagging study. J Am Coll Cardiol 35:1525–1534

Bogaert J, Dymarkowski S, Rademakers FE (2002) MRI and coronary heart disease: a review. JBR-BTR 85:57–81

Bogaert J, Taylor AM, Van Kerkhove F, Dymarkowski S (2004) Use of inversion recovery contrast-enhanced MRI for cardiac imaging: spectrum of applications. AJR Am J Roentgenol 182:609–615

Bolli R (1990) Mechanism of myocardial stunning. Circulation 82:723–738

Bourdillon PD, von der Lohe E, Lewis SJ et al (2003) Comparison of left ventriculography and coronary arteriography with positron emission tomography in assessment of myocardial viability. Clin Cardiol 26(2):60–66

Brady TJ, Goldman MR, Pykett IL et al (1982) Proton nuclear magnetic resonance imaging of regionally ischemic canine hearts: effect of paramagnetic proton signal enhancement. Radiology 144:343–347

Braunwald E, Kloner RA (1982) The stunned myocardium: prolonged, postischemic ventricular dysfunction. Circulation 66:1146–1149

Bremerich J, Saeed M, Arheden H et al (2000) Normal and infarcted myocardium: differentiation with cellular uptake of manganese at MR imaging in a rat model. Radiology 216:524–530

Brown JJ, Higgins CB (1988) Myocardial paramagnetic contrast agents for MR imaging. Am J Roentgenol 151:865–872

Buda AJ, Zotz RJ, Gallagher KP (1987) The effect of inotropic stimulation on normal and ischemic myocardium after coronary occlusion. *Circulation* 76:163–172

Camici P, Ferrannini E, Opie LH (1989) Myocardial metabolism in ischemic heart disease: basic principles and application to imaging by positron emission tomography. Prog Cardiovasc Dis 32:217–238

Canby RC, Reeves RC, Evanochko WT et al (1987) Proton nuclear magnetic resonance relaxation times in severe myocardial ischemia. J Am Coll Cardiol 10:412–420

Caputo GR, Sechtem U, Tscholakoff D et al (1987) Measurement of myocardial infarct size at early and late time intervals using MR imaging: an experimental study in dogs. AJR Am J Roentgenol 149:237–243

Chaudhry FA, Tauke JT, Alessandrini RS et al (1999) Prognostic implications of myocardial contractile reserve in patients with coronary artery disease and left ventricular dysfunction. *J Am Coll Cardiol* 34:730–738

Chen C, Cohen J, Myers C et al (1984) Paramagnetic metalloporphyrins as potential contrast agents in NMR imaging. FEBS Lett 168:70–74

Chiu CW, So NM, Lam WWM et al (2003) Combined first-pass perfusion and viability study at MR imaging in patients with non-ST segment-elevation acute coronary syndromes: feasibility study. Radiology 226:717–722

Choi SI, Choi SH, Kim ST et al (2000) Irreversibly damaged myocardium at MR imaging with a necrotic tissue-specific contrast agent in a cat model. Radiology 215:863–868

Cigarroa CG, de Filippi C, Brickner ME et al (1993) Dobutamine stress echocardiography identifies hibernating myocardium and predicts recovery of left ventricular

function after coronary revascularization. Circulation 88:430–436

Croisille P, Moore CC, Judd RM et al (1999) Differentiation of viable and nonviable myocardium by the use of three-dimensional tagged MRI in 2-day-old reperfused canine infarcts. Circulation 99:284–291

Cullen JH, Horsfield MA, Reek CR et al (1999) A myocardial perfusion reserve index in humans using first-pass contrast-enhanced magnetic resonance imaging. J Am Coll Cardiol 33:1386–1394

De Roos A, Van Rossum AC, van der Wall E et al (1989) Reperfused and nonreperfused myocardial infarction: diagnostic potential of Gd-DTPA-enhanced MR imaging. Radiology 172:717–720

Dendale PAC, Franken RP, Waldmann GJ et al (1995) Low-dosage dobutamine magnetic resonance imaging as an alternative to echocardiography in the detection of viable myocardium after acute infarction. Am Heart J 130:134–140

Dendale P, Franken PR, van der Wall EE, de Roos A (1997) Wall thickening at rest and contractile reserve early after myocardial infarction: correlation with myocardial perfusion and metabolism. Cor Art Dis 8:259–264

Di Carli MF, Maddahi J, Rokhsar S et al (1998) Long-term survival of patients with coronary artery disease and left ventricular dysfunction:implications for the role of myocardial viability assessment in management decisions. J Thorac Cardiovasc Surg 116:997–1004

Downing SE, Chen V (1992) Acute hibernation and reperfusion of the ischemic heart. Circulation 82:699–707

Dulce MC, Duerinckx AJ, Hartiala J et al (1993) MR imaging of the myocardium using nonionic contrast medium: signal-intensity changes in patients with subacute myocardial infarction. AJR Am J Roentgenol 160:963–970

Dymarkowski S, Ni Y, Miao Y et al (2002) Value of T2-weighted MRI early after myocardial infarction in dogs: comparison with bis-gadolinium-mesoporphyrin enhanced T1-weighted MRI and functional data from cine MRI. Invest Radiol 37:77–85

Edelman RR, Wallner B, Singer A et al (1990) Segmented turboFLASH: method for breath-hold MR imaging of the liver with flexible contrast. Radiology 177:515–521

Eichenberger AC, Schuiki E, Kochli VD et al (1994) Ischemic heart disease: assessment with gadolinium-enhanced ultrafast MR imaging and dipyridamole stress. J Magn Reson Imaging 4:425–431

Eichstaedt HW, Felix R, Dougherty FC, Langer M, Rutsch W, Schmutzler H (1986) Magnetic resonance imaging (MRI) in different stages of myocardial infarction using the contrast agent gadolinium-DTPA. Clin Cardiol 9:527–535

Eichstaedt HW, Felix R, Danne O et al (1989) Imaging of acute myocardial infarction by magnetic resonance tomography (MRT) using the paramagnetic relaxation substance gadolinium-DTPA. Cardiovasc Drugs Ther 3:779–788

Fedele F, Montesano T, Ferro-Luzzi M et al (1994) Identification of viable myocardium in patients with chronic coronary artery disease and left ventricular dysfunction: role of magnetic resonance imaging. Am Heart J 128:484–489

Ferrari R, Ceconi C, Curello S et al (1996) Left ventricular dysfunction due to the new ischemic outcomes: stunning and hibernation. J Cardiovasc Pharmacol 28 [Suppl 1]:18–26

Flacke S, Allen JS, Chia JM (2003) Characterization of viable and nonviable myocardium at MR imaging: comparison of gadolinium-based extracellular and blood pool contrast materials versus manganese-based contrast materials in a rat myocardial infarction model. Radiology 226:731–738

Frank JA, Feller MA, House WV et al (1976) Measurement of proton nuclear magnetic longitudinal relaxation times and water content in infarcted canine myocardium and induced pulmonary injury. Clin Res 24:217A–223A

Fukuzawa S, Watanabe H, Shimada K et al (1994) Distribution patterns of Gd-DTPA-enhanced magnetic resonance imaging after intravenous tissue plasminogen activator therapy for acute myocardial infarction. Jpn Circ J 58:199–205

Furmanski P, Longley C (1998) Metalloporphyrin enhancement of magnetic resonance imaging of human tumor xenografts in nude mice. Cancer Res 48:4604–4610

Fuster V (1999) Epidemic of cardiovascular disease and stroke: the three main challenges. Circulation 99:1132–1137

Fuster V, Frye RL, Kennedy MA et al (1979) The role of collateral circulation in the various coronary syndromes. Circulation 59:1137–1144

Garot J, Pascal O, Diéhold B et al (2002) Alterations of systolic left ventricular twist after acute myocardial infarction. Am J Physiol 282:H357–H362

Gerber BL, Rochitte CE, Melin JA et al (2000) Microvascular obstruction and left ventricular remodeling early after acute myocardial infarction. Circulation 101:2734–2741

Gerber BL, Rochitte CE, Bluemke DA et al (2001) Relation between Gd-DTPA contrast enhancement and regional inotropic response in the periphery and center of myocardial infarction. Circulation 104:998–1004

Gerber TC, Fasseas P, Lennon RJ et al (2003) Clinical safety of magnetic resonance imaging early after coronary artery stent placement. J Am Coll Cardiol 42:1295–1298

Goldman MR, Brady TJ, Pykett IL et al (1982) Quantification of experimental myocardial infarction using nuclear magnetic resonance imaging and paramagnetic ion contrast enhancement in excised canine hearts. Circulation 66:1012–1016

Gould K (1978) Noninvasive assessment of coronary stenosis by myocardial perfusion imaging during pharmacologic coronary vasodilatation I. Physiologic basis and experimental validation. Am J Cardiol 41:267–278

Gropler RJ, Bergmann SR (1991) Myocardial viability - what is the definition? J Nucl Med 32:10–12

Gropler RJ, Siegel BA, Sampathkumaran K et al (1992) Dependence of recovery of contractile function on maintenance of oxidative metabolism after myocardial infarction. J Am Coll Cardiol 19:989–997

Hartnell G, Cerel A, Kamalesh M, Finn JP, Hill T, Cohen M, Tello R, Lewis S (1994) Detection of myocardial ischemia: value of combined myocardial perfusion and cineangiographic MR imaging. AJR Am J Roentgenol 163:1061–1067

Herijgers P, Laycock SK, Ni Y et al (1997) Localization and determination of infarct size by Gd-mesoporphyrin enhanced MRI in dogs. Int J Cardiac Imaging 13:499–507

Heusch G (1998) Hibernating myocardium. Phys Rev 78:1055–1077

Higgins CB, Herfkens R, Lipton MJ et al (1983) Nuclear magnetic resonance imaging of acute myocardial infarction in dogs: alterations in magnetic relaxation times. Am J Cardiol 52:184–188

Hillenbrand HB, Kim RJ, Parker MA et al (2000) Early assessment of myocardial salvage by contrast-enhanced magnetic resonance imaging. Circulation 102:1678–1683

Holman ER, van Jonbergen HP, van Dijkman PR et al (1993) Comparison of magnetic resonance imaging studies with enzymatic indexes of myocardial necrosis for quantification of myocardial infarct size. Am J Cardiol 71:1036–1040

Holman ER, van Rossum AC, Doesburg T et al (1996) Assessment of acute myocardial infarction in man with magnetic resonance imaging and the use of a new paramagnetic contrast agent gadolinium-BOPTA. Magn Reson Imaging 14:21–29

Hundley WG, Hamilton CA, Clarke GD, Hillis LD, Herrington DM, Lange RA, Applegate RJ, Thomas MS, Payne J, Link KM, Peshock RM (1999) Visualization and functional assessment of proximal and middle left anterior descending coronary stenoses in humans with magnetic resonance imaging. Circulation 99:3248–3254

Hundley WG, Morgan TM, Neagle CM, Hamilton CA, Rerkpattanapipat P, Link KM (2002) Magnetic resonance imaging determination of cardiac prognosis. Circulation 106:2328–2333

Ito H, Tomooka T, Sakai N (1992) Lack of myocardial perfusion immediately after successful thrombolysis. A predictor of poor recovery of left ventricular function in anterior myocardial infarction. Circulation 85:1699–1705

Ito H, Maruyama A, Iwakura K (1996) Clinical implications of the 'no-reflow' phenomenon. A predictor of complications and left ventricular remodeling in reperfused anterior wall myocardial infarction. Circulation 93:223–228

Jennings RB, Hawkins HK, Lowe JE, et al (1978) Relation between high-energy phosphate and lethal injury in myocardial ischemia in the dog. Am J Pathol 92:187–214

Johnston DL, Brady TJ, Ratner AV et al (1985) Assessment of myocardial ischemia with proton magnetic resonance: effects of a three hour coronary occlusion with and without reperfusion. Circulation 71:595–601

Judd RM, Lugo-Olivieri CH, Arai M, et al (1995a) Physiological basis of myocardial contrast enhancement in fast magnetic resonance images of 2-day-old reperfused canine infarcts. Circulation 92:1902–1910

Judd RM, Atalay MK, Rottman GA et al (1995b) Effects of myocardial water exchange on T1 enhancement during bolus administration of MR contrast agents. Magn Reson Med 33:215–223

Keeley EC, Hillis LD (1996) Left ventricular mural thrombus after acute myocardial infarction. Clin Cardiol 19:83–86

Kellman P, Arai AE, McVeigh ER et al (2002) Phase-sensitive inversion recovery for detecting myocardial infarction using gadolinium-delayed hyperenhancement. Magn Reson Med 47:372–383

Kellman P, Dyke CK, Aletras AH et al (2004) Artifact suppression in imaging of myocardial infarction using B1-weighted phased-array combined phase-sensitive inversion recovery dagger. Magn Reson Med 51:408–412

Kim RJ, Chen EL, Lima JA, Judd RM (1996) Myocardial Gd-DTPA kinetics determine MRI contrast enhancement and reflect the extent and severity of myocardial injury after acute reperfused infarction. Circulation 94:3318–3326

Kim RJ, Fieno DS, Parrish TB, Harris K, Chen EL, Simonetti O, Bundy J, Finn JP, Klocke FJ, Judd RM (1999) Relationship of MRI delayed contrast enhancement to irreversible injury, infarct age, and contractile function. Circulation 100:1992–2002

Kim RJ, Wu E, Rafael A, Chen EL, Parker MA, Simonetti O, Klocke FJ, Bonow RO, Judd RM (2000) The use of contrast-enhanced magnetic resonance imaging to identify reversible myocardial dysfunction. N Engl J Med 343:1445–1453

Klein C, Nekolla SG, Bengel FM et al (2002) Assessment of myocardial viability with contrast-enhanced magnetic resonance imaging. Comparison with positron emission tomography. Circulation 105:162–167

Kloner RA, Jennings RB (2001) Consequences of brief ischemia: stunning, preconditioning and their clinical implications. Circulation 104:2981–2989

Kloner RA, Ganote CE, Jennings RB (1974) The 'no-reflow' phenomenon after temporary coronary occlusion in the dog. J Clin Invest 54:1496–1508

Knuesel PR, Nanz D, Wyss C et al (2003) Characterization of dysfunctional myocardium by positron emission tomography and magnetic resonance: relation to functional outcome after revascularization. Circulation 108:1095–1100

Kraitchman DL, Sampath S, Castillo E et al (2003) Quantitative ischemia detection during cardiac magnetic resonance stress testing by use of FastHARP. Circulation 107:2025–2030

Kramer CM, Lima JA, Reichek N et al (1993) Regional differences in function within noninfarcted myocardium during left ventricular remodeling. Circulation 88:1279–1288

Kramer CM, Rogers WJ, Theobald TM et al (1996a) Remote noninfarcted regional dysfunction soon after first anterior myocardial infarction. A magnetic resonance tagging study. Circulation 94:660–666

Kramer CM, Ferrari VA, Rogers WJ et al (1996b) Angiotensin-converting enzyme inhibition limits dysfunction in adjacent noninfarcted regions during left ventricular remodeling. J Am Coll Cardiol 27:211–217

Kühl HP, Beek AM, van der Weerdt AP et al (2003) Myocardial viability in chronic ischemic heart disease: comparison of contrast-enhanced magnetic resonance imaging with (18)F-fluorodeoxyglucose positron emission tomography. J Am Coll Cardiol 41:1341–1348

Kühl HP, Papavasilliu TS, Beek AM et al (2004) Myocardial viability: rapid assessment with delayed contrast-enhanced MR imaging with three-dimensional inversion-recovery prepared pulse sequence. Radiology 230:576–582

Kuijpers D, Yiu K, Dijkman PRM van et al (2003) Dobutamine cardiovascular magnetic resonance for the detection of myocardial ischemia with the use of myocardial tagging. Circulation 107:1592–1597

Kwong RY, Schussheim AE, Rekhraj S et al (2003) Detecting acute coronary syndrome in the emergency department with cardiac magnetic resonance imaging. Circulation 107:531–537

Lauterbur PC, Dias MM, Rudin AM (1978) Augmentation of tissue water proton spin-lattice relaxation rates by in vivo addition of paramagnetic ions. In: Dutton PL, Leigh JS, Scarpa A (eds) International symposium on frontiers of biological energetics of electrons to tissues. Academic, New York, pp 752–759

Lee JT, Ideker RE, Reimer KA (1981) Myocardial infarct size and location in relation to the coronary vascular bed at risk in man. Circulation 64:526–534

Lewis S, Sawada S, Ryan T et al (1991) Segmental wall motion abnormalities in the absence of clinically documented myocardial infarction: clinical significance and evidence of hibernating myocardium. Am Heart J 121:1088–1094

Liedtke AJ (1981) Alteration of carbohydrate and lipid metabolism in the acutely ischemic heart. Prog Cardiovasc Dis 23:321–336

Lima JA, Judd RM, Bazille A, Schulman SP, Atalar E, Zerhouni EA (1995) Regional heterogeneity of human myocardial infarcts demonstrated by contrast-enhanced MRI. Potential mechanisms. Circulation 92:1117–1125

Lindner JR, Kaul S (1996) Assessment of myocardial viability with two-dimensional echocardiography and magnetic resonance imaging. J Nucl Cardiol 3:167–182

Maes A, Flameng W, Nuyts J et al (1994) Histological alterations in chronically hypoperfused myocardium: correlation with PET findings. Circulation 90:735–745

Mahrholdt H, Wagner A, Holly TA et al (2002) Reproducibility of chronic infarct size measurement by contrast-enhanced magnetic resonance imaging. Circulation 106:2322–2327

Mahrholdt H, Goedecke C, Wagner A et al (2004) Cardiovascular magnetic resonance assessment of human myocarditis. A comparison to histology and molecular biology. Circulation 109:1250–1258

Matheijssen NA, de Roos A, van der Wall EE et al (1991) Acute myocardial infarction: comparison of T2-weighted and T1-weighted gadolinium-DTPA enhanced MR imaging. Magn Reson Med 17:460–469

Matsumura K, Jeremy RW, Schaper J et al (1998) Progression of myocardial necrosis during reperfusion of ischemic myocardium. Circulation 97:795–804

McNamara MT, Wesbey GE, Brasch RC et al (1985) Magnetic resonance imaging of acute myocardial infarction using a nitroxyl spin label (PCA). Invest Radiol 20:591–595

McNamara MT, Tscholakoff D, Revel D et al (1986) Differentiation of reversible and irreversible myocardial injury by MR imaging with and without gadolinium-DTPA. Radiology 158:765–769

Mollet NR, Dymarkowski S, Volders W et al (2002) Visualization of ventricular thrombi with contrast-enhanced magnetic resonance imaging in patients with ischemic heart disease. Circulation 106:2873–2876

Nageh T, Sherwood RA, Harris BM et al (2003) Cardiac troponin T and I and creatine kinase-MB as markers of myocardial injury and predictors of outcome following percutaneous coronary intervention. Int J Cardiol 92:285–293

Nagel E, Lehmkuhl HB, Bocksch W et al (1999) Noninvasive diagnosis of ischemia-induced wall motion abnormalities with the use of high-dose dobutamine stress MRI: comparison with dobutamine stress echocardiography. Circulation 99:763–770

Neill W, Ingwall J, Andrews E et al (1986) Stabilization of the derangement in adenosine triphosphate metabolism during sustained, partial ischemia in the dog heart. J Am Coll Cardiol 8:894–900

Ni Y, Marchal G, Yu J et al (1995) Localization of metalloporphyrin induced "specific" enhancement in experimental liver tumors: comparison of magnetic resonance imaging, microangiographic and histologic findings. Acad Radiol 2:687–699

Ni Y, Petré C, Miao Y et al (1997) Magnetic resonance imaging - histomorphologic correlation studies on paramagnetic metalloporphyrins in rat models of necrosis. Invest Radiol 32:770–779

Ni Y, Pislaru C, Bosmans H et al (1998) Validation of intracoronary delivery of metalloporphyrin as an in vivo "histochemical staining" for myocardial infarction with MR imaging. Acad Radiol 5 [Suppl 1]:537–541

Nienaber CA, Brunken RC, Sherman CT (1991) Metabolic and functional recovery of ischemic human myocardium after coronary angioplasty. J Am Coll Cardiol 18:966–978

Nishimura T, Kobayashi H, Ohara Y et al (1989) Serial assessment of myocardial infarction by using gated MR imaging and Gd-DTPA. AJR Am J Roentgenol 153:715–720

Ogan M, Revel D, Brasch R (1997) Metalloporphyrin contrast enhancement of tumors in magnetic resonance imaging. A study of human carcinoma, lymphoma, and fibrosarcoma in mice. Invest Radiol 22:822–828

Oshinski JN, Yang, Z, Jones JR et al (2001) Imaging time after Gd-DTPA injection is critical in using delayed enhancement to determine infarct size accurately with magnetic resonance imaging. Circulation 104:2838–2842

Panting JR, Gatehouse PD, Yang GZ et al (2002) Abnormal subendocardial perfusion in cardiac syndrome×detected by cardiovascular magnetic resonance imaging. N Engl J Med 346:1948–1953

Patterson RE, Jones-Collins BA, Aamodt R et al (1993) Differences in collateral myocardial blood flow following gradual vs abrupt coronary occlusion. Cardiovasc Res 17:207–213

Pennell DJ, Underwood SR, Manzara CC et al (1992) Magnetic resonance imaging during dobutamine stress in coronary artery disease. Am J Cardiol 70:34–40

Pennell DJ, Firmin DN, Burger P et al (1995) Assessment of magnetic resonance velocity mapping of global ventricular function during dobutamine infusion in coronary artery disease. Br Heart J 74:163–170

Pislaru SV, Ni Y, Pislaru C et al (1999) Noninvasive measurements of infarct size after thrombolysis with a necrosis-avid MRI contrast agent. Circulation 99:690–696

Plein S, Ridgway JP, Jones TR et al (2002) Coronary artery disease: assessment with a comprehensive MR imaging protocol - initial results. Radiology 225:300–307

Pohost GM, Biederman RW (1999) The role of cardiac MRI stress testing. Circulation 100:1676–1679

Pomeroy OH, Wendland M, Wagner S et al (1989) Magnetic resonance imaging of acute myocardial ischemia using a manganese chelate, Mn-DPDP. Invest Radiol 24:531–536

Rademakers FE, Marchal G, Mortelmans L et al (2003) Evolution of regional performance after an acute myocardial infarction in humans using magnetic resonance tagging. J Physiol (Lond) 546:777–787

Rahimtoola SH (1989) The hibernating myocardium. Am Heart J 117:211–220

Ramani K, Judd RM, Holly TA et al (1998) Contrast magnetic resonance imaging in the assessment of myocardial viability in patients with stable coronary artery disease and left ventricular dysfunction. Circulation 98:2687–2694

Rehr RB, Peshock RM, Malloy CR (1986) Improved in vivo magnetic resonance imaging of acute myocardial infarc-

tion after intravenous paramagnetic contrast agent administration. Am J Cardiol 57:864–868

Reimer KA, Jennings RB (1970) The wavefront progression of myocardial ischemic cell death. II. Transmural progression of necrosis within the framework of ischemic bed size (myocardium at risk) and collateral flow. Lab Invest 40:633–644

Reimer KA, Jennings RB (1979) The changing anatomic reference base of evolving myocardial infarction. Circulation 60:866–876

Rerkpattanapipat P, Morgan TM, Neagle CM et al (2002) Assessment of preoperative cardiac risk with magnetic resonance imaging. Am J Cardiol 90:416–419

Ricciardi MJ, Wu E, Davidson CJ (2001) Visualization of discrete microinfarction after percutaneous coronary intervention associated with mild creatine kinase-MB elevation. Circulation 103:2780–2783

Rivas F, Cobb FR, Bache RJ, Greenfield JC (1976) Relationship between blood flow to ischemic regions and extent of myocardial infarction. Circ Res 38:439–447

Rochitte CE, Lima JA, Bluemke DA et al (1998) Magnitude and time course of microvascular obstruction and tissue injury after acute myocardial infarction. Circulation 98:1006–1014

Rogers WJ, Kramer CM, Geskin G et al (1999) Early contrast-enhanced MRI predicts late functional recovery after reperfused myocardial infarction. Circulation 99:744–750

Rokey R, Verani MS, Bolli R et al (1986) Myocardial infarct size quantification by MR imaging early after coronary artery occlusion in dogs. Radiology 158:771–774

Ross J Jr (1991) Myocardial perfusion-contraction matching: implications for coronary heart disease and hibernation. Circulation 83:1076–1082

Ruffolo RR Jr (1987) The pharmacology of dobutamine. Am J Med Sci 294:244–248

Saeed M, Wagner S, Wendland MF et al (1989) Occlusive and reperfused myocardial infarcts: differentiation with Mn-DPDP-enhanced MR imaging. Radiology 172:59–64

Saeed M, Bremerich J, Wendland MF et al (1999) Reperfused myocardial infarction as seen with use of necrosis-specific versus standard extracellular MR contrast media in rats. Radiology 213:247–257

Saeed M, Wendland MF, Watzinger N et al (2000) MR contrast media for myocardial viability, microvascular integrity and perfusion. Eur J Radiol 34:179–195

Saeed M, Lund G, Wendland MF et al (2001) Magnetic resonance characterization of the peri-infarction zone of reperfused myocardial infarction with necrosis-specific and extracellular nonspecific contrast media. Circulation 10:871–876

Sandstede JJ (2003) Assessment of myocardial viability by MR imaging. Eur Radiol 13:52–61

Sandstede JJ, Lipke C, Beer M et al (2000) Analysis of first-pass and delayed contrast-enhancement patterns of dysfunctional myocardium on MR imaging: use in the prediction of myocardial viability. AJR Am J Roentgenol 174:1737–1740

Schaefer S, Malloy CR, Katz J et al (1988) Gadolinium-DTPA-enhanced nuclear magnetic resonance imaging of reperfused myocardium: identification of the myocardial bed at risk. J Am Coll Cardiol 12:1064–1072

Schiller NB, Shah PM, Crawford M et al (1989) Recommendations for quantitation of the left ventricle by two-dimensional echocardiography. American Society of Echocardiography Committee of Standards, Subcommittee on Quantitation of Two-Dimensional Echocardiograms. J Am Soc Echocardiogr 2:358–367

Schulz-Menger J, Gross M, Messroghli D et al (2003) Cardiovascular magnetic resonance of acute myocardial infarction at a very early stage. J Am Coll Cardiol 42:513–518

Senior R, Lahiri A (1995) Enhanced detection of myocardial ischemia by stress dobutamine echocardiography utilizing the "biphasic" response of wall thickening during low and high dose dobutamine infusion. J Am Coll Cardiol 26:26–32

Sensky PR, Jivan A, Hudson NM et al (2000) Coronary artery disease: combined stress MR imaging protocol - one stop evaluation of myocardial perfusion and function. Radiology 215:608–614

Shah DP, Kim HW, Elliot M et al (2004) Contrast MRI predicts reverse remodeling and contractile improvement in akinetic thinned myocardium. J Cardiovasc Magn Reson 5:66 (abstract)

Simonetti OP, Kim RJ, Fieno DS et al (2001) An improved MR imaging technique for the visualization of myocardial infarction. Radiology 218:215–223

Sklenar J, Villanueva FS, Glasheen WP et al (1994) Dobutamine echocardiography for determining the extent of myocardial salvage after reperfusion: an experimental evaluation. Circulation 90:1503–1512

Sutton MGSJ, Sharpe N (2000) Left ventricular remodeling after myocardial infarction. Pathophysiology and therapy. Circulation 101:2981–2988

Thiele H, Nagel E, Paetsch I et al (2001) Functional cardiac MR imaging with steady-state free precession (SSFP) significantly improves endocardial border delineation without contrast agents. J Magn Reson Imaging 14:362–367

Tscholakoff D, Higgins CB, Sechtem U et al (1986) Occlusive and reperfused myocardial infarcts: effect of Gd-DTPA on ECG-gated MR imaging. Radiology 160:515–519

Van Dijkman PR, van der Wall EE, de Roos A et al (1991) Acute, subacute, and chronic myocardial infarction: quantitative analysis of gadolinium-enhanced MR images. Radiology 180:147–151

Van Hoe L, Vanderheyden M (2004) Ischemic cardiomyopathy: value of different MRI techniques for prediction of functional recovery after revascularization. Am J Roentgenol 182:95–100

Vanoverschelde J-LJ, Wijns W, Borgers M et al (1997) Chronic myocardial hibernation in humans: from bedside to bench. *Circulation* 95:1961–1971

Van Rugge FP, Holman ER, van der Wall EE et al (1993) Quantitation of global and regional left ventricular function by cine magnetic resonance imaging during dobutamine stress in normal human subjects. Eur Heart J 14:456–463

Van Rugge FP, van der Wall EE, Spanjersberg SJ, et al (1994) Magnetic resonance imaging during dobutamine stress

for detection and localization of coronary artery disease. Quantitative wall motion analysis using a modification of the centerline method. Circulation 90:127–138

Van Zijl PCM, Place DA, Cohen JS et al (1990) Metalloporphyrin magnetic resonance contrast agents: feasibility of tumor-specific magnetic resonance imaging. Acta Radiol 374:75–79

Vogel JHK (1987) Determinants of improved left ventricular function after thrombolytic therapy in acute myocardial infarction. J Am Coll Cardiol 9:937–944

Wagner A, Mahrholdt H, Holly TA (2003) Contrast-enhanced MRI and routine single photon emission computed tomography (SPECT) perfusion imaging for detection of subendocardial myocardial infarcts: an imaging study. Lancet 361:374–379

Wahl A, Gollesch A, Paetsch I et al (2003) Safety and feasibility of high-dose dobutamine-atropine stress MRI for diagnosis of myocardial ischemia: experience in 1000 consecutive cases. J Cardiovasc Magn Reson 5:51 (abstract)

Weinmann HJ, Brasch RC, Press WR et al (1984) Characteristics of gadolinium-DTPA complex: a potential NMR contrast agent. Am J Roentgenol 142:619–624

Weissleder R, Lee A, Khaw B et al (1992) Antimyosin-labeled monocrystalline iron oxide allows detection of myocardial infarct: MR antibody imaging. Radiology 182:381–385

Wellnhofer E, Olariu A, Klein C et al (2004) Magnetic resonance low-dose dobutamine test is superior to scar quantification for the prediction of functional recovery. Circulation 109:2172–2174

Whiteman G, Kieval R, Wetstein L et al (1983) The relationship between global myocardial redox state and high energy phosphate profile: a phosphorous-31 nuclear magnetic resonance study. J Surg Res 35:332–339

Williams ES, Kaplan JI, Thatcher F et al (1980) Prolongation of proton spin lattice relaxation times in regionally ischemic tissue from dog hearts. J Nucl Med 21:449–453

Wilke N, Jerosch-Herold M, Wang Y et al (1997) Myocardial perfusion reserve: assessment with multisection, quantitative, first-pass MR imaging. Radiology 204:373–384

Wisenberg G, Pflugfelder PW, Kostuk WJ et al (1987) Diagnostic applicability of magnetic resonance imaging in assessing human cardiac allograft rejection. Am J Cardiol 60:130–136

Wisenberg G, Prato FS, Carroll SE et al (1988) Serial nuclear magnetic resonance imaging of acute myocardial infarction with and without reperfusion. Am Heart J 115:510–518

Wolf GL, Baum L (1983) Cardiovascular toxicity and tissue proton T1 response to manganese injection in the dog and rabbit. AJR Am J Roentgenol 141:193–197

Wu E, Judd RM, Vargas JD (2001) Visualisation of presence, location, and transmural extent of healed Q-wave and non-Q-wave myocardial infarction. Lancet 357:21–28

Yokota C, Nonogi H, Miyazaki S (1995) Gadolinium-enhanced magnetic resonance imaging in acute myocardial infarction. Am J Cardiol 75:577–581

9 Nonischemic Myocardial Disease

J. Bogaert and A.M. Taylor

CONTENTS

J. Bogaert MD, PhD
Department of Radiology, Gasthuis-berg University Hospital,
Catholic University of Leuven, Herestraat 49, 3000 Leuven,
Belgium
A.M. Taylor, MD, MRCP, FRCR
Cardiothoracic Unit, Institute of Child Health and Great
Ormond Street Hospital for Children, London, WC1N 3JH,
UK

9.1
Introduction

The heart is the central circulatory pump of the cardiovascular system. The driving force is generated by a repetitive contraction of the myocardium, which is a thick-walled layer of myocytes lying around a cavity. The myocardium may be involved in a variety of disorders in which the heart muscle is exclusively or preferentially affected (e.g. myocardial ischemia, hypertrophic cardiomyopathy, HCM) or in which the myocardial involvement is part of a multi-organ disorder (e.g. haemochromatosis, sarcoidosis); though often no underlying aetiology for myocardial dysfunction can be discovered i.e. it is idiopathic. Important causes of myocardial diseases are shown in Table 9.1. Myocardial disorders present clinically in a variety of scenarios, ranging from the asymptomatic patient to fulminant cardiac failure. Assessment of the underlying aetiology of myocardial disorders is often difficult and is usually based on patient symptoms, physical examination and a series of technical investigations (e.g. cardiac imaging, laboratory investigations, endomyocardial biopsy). MRI has become part of the investigation of patients with myocardial disorders. In this chapter the myocardial disorders unrelated to coronary artery disease (CAD) will be discussed.

9.2
MRI Strategies Used to
Study Non-ischemic Myocardial Disease

Nowadays a whole range of MRI sequences and techniques can be used to study patients with myocardial diseases. A MRI examination should include morphological analysis of the myocardium, evaluation of the functional impact of the myocardial disorder on ventricular systolic and diastolic function, and valvular function, and detection and/or characterization of pathological myocardium. Dark-blood and

Table 9.1. Aetiology and patterns of myocardial diseases (cardiomyopathies and myocarditis)

Etiology	Condition	Pattern
Idiopathic	DCM	Dilated
	HCM	Hypertrophic
	Restrictive cardiomyopathy	Restrictive
	AVRD	RV dysfunction/dilation
	Non-compaction cardiomyopathy	Dilated/restrictive
Genetic	HCM	Hypertrophic
	ARVD	RV dysfunction
	Neurodegenerative disorders (Friedreich's ataxia)	Hypertrophic/dilated
Ischemic	Coronary artery disease	Dilated
	Apical ballooning (Tako-Tsubo cardiomyopathy)	Transient apical dilation and dysfunction
Inflammatory	Infective/noninfective	Asymptomatic to fulminant cardiac failure Dilated (end-stage)
Infiltrative	Amyloidosis	Restrictive Dilated May simulate HCM
	Haemochromatosis	Restrictive Dilated (end-stage)
	Other storage diseases	Restrictive May simulate HCM
	Neoplastic	Restrictive
	Sarcoidosis	Restrictive/dilated
Fibroplastic	Endomyocardial fibrosis	Restrictive
	Endocardial fibroelastosis	
	Löffler's fibroplastic endocarditis	
	Carcinoid	
Other	Metabolic/toxic (e.g. alcohol, doxorubicin)	Dilated
	Hypersensitivity	
	Physical agents (e.g. radiation)	Restrictive
	Hematological	

ARVD, Arrhythmogenic right ventricular dysplasia; DCM, dilated cardiomyopathy; HCM, hypertrophic cardiomyopathy; RV, right ventricular

white-blood MRI techniques can be used for morphological analysis. On dark-blood spin-echo (SE) MRI, the myocardium has an intermediate signal intensity or a "grey" appearance, similar to that of skeletal muscle, and is clearly distinguishable from the surrounding bright epicardial fat and the adjacent dark intracardiac blood. The T1 relaxation time of myocardial tissue is about 800 ms, and the T2 relaxation time approximately 33 ms (at 1.5 T). Similar to diseases in other parts of the body, myocardial disorders are often characterized by changes in proton relaxation times. These changes may be helpful, since they can be used, at least to a certain degree, for tissue characterization. For instance, fatty infiltration of the free wall of the right ventricle will be visible as hyperintense intramyocardial spots on T1-weighted SE images, and these abnormalities make the diagnosis of arrhythmogenic right ventricular dysplasia likely (Fig. 9.1). Mature myocardial fibrosis or calcification, on the other hand, appears hypointense on both T1- and T2-weighted

sequences and can be found in patients with endomyocardial fibrosis. A hyperintense myocardial area on T2-weighted images in a patient with a recent myocardial infarction is suggestive of increased free-water content due to myocardial oedema and/or necrosis. The latter finding can thus be used for noninvasive localization of the myocardial infarction. However, the changes are non-specific, since other conditions such as acute rejection of a cardiac allograft or myocarditis are equally characterized by an increased water content and a subsequent rise in T2 relaxation values. Changes in relaxation times thus reflect gross morphological changes but are often non-specific.

Paramagnetic contrast agents (e.g. gadolinium chelates) can be used for improved detection of myocardial disorders (MATSUOKA et al. 1993). Differences in signal intensity changes before and after administration of contrast agent between myocardium and skeletal muscle are one way to better detect myocardial pathology such as myocardi-

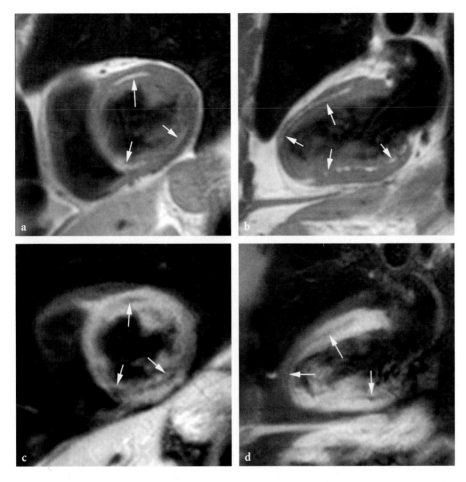

Fig. 9.1a-d.
Comprehensive use of MRI sequences for myocardial tissue characterization. T1-weighted fast spin-echo (SE)-MRI in the short-axis (**a**) and vertical long-axis (**b**). T1-weighted fast SE-MRI with fat-suppression technique in short-axis (**c**) and vertical long-axis (**d**). Fatty infiltration of myocardial left ventricular (LV) mid-wall (*arrows*) in a 60-year-old man with a history of myocardial infarction. On SE-MRI, the intramyocardial fatty infiltration has a high signal intensity, similar to that of the epicardial and mediastinal fat. Using fat-suppression techniques, the signal intensity of fat is selectively suppressed or nulled as shown in **c** and **d**. This approach can be used to confirm the presence the intramyocardial fat deposition

tis (FRIEDRICH et al. 1998). With the advent of the contrast-enhanced inversion-recovery (CE-IR) MRI with late imaging (SIMONETTI et al. 2001), superior contrast can be achieved between normal and abnormal myocardium by selectively suppressing or nulling the signal of normal myocardium (see Fig. 1.14). This revolutionary idea has led to a whole range of new applications. Nowadays this technique has become the reference technique for myocardial tissue characterization. Myocardial enhancement reflects abnormal myocardium, and the location, distribution pattern and extent of enhancement is often typical for specific myocardial disorder. For instance, in patients with myocardial infarction, the enhancement typically occurs in a coronary artery distribution territory, and involves the subendocardium, with a variable transmural spread. In patients with myocarditis, the enhancement is not related to a coronary artery territory, and usually involves the subepicardial part of the myocardium (MAHRHOLDT et al. 2004). Knowledge of the typical patterns of enhancement is helpful in the differen-

tial diagnosis of patients with myocardial diseases. Moreover, concomitant pathology, such as pericardial inflammation or ventricular thrombus formation, can be assessed with CE-IR MRI (MOLLET et al. 2002; BOGAERT et al. 2004). It should be emphasized that the current diagnostic value of the CE-IR MRI technique is not yet defined when there is a diffuse myocardial involvement, such as in diffuse myocardial fibrosis. Also, myocardial changes beyond the spatial resolution of the MRI technique may be undetected. This might explain some discrepancies between the MRI and histological findings (MAHRHOLDT et al. 2004).

Cardiac functional evaluation is another important pillar of the assessment of myocardial diseases. Cine MRI, using the new, balanced steady-state free precession (b-SSFP) techniques, allows for accurate analysis of regional function (wall motion and wall thickening), quantification of global ventricular parameters and myocardial mass, and depiction of abnormal flow patterns (e.g. flow acceleration in a narrowed left ventricular (LV) outflow tract in patients with obstructive HCM and concomitant mitral valve regurgitation). Velocity-encoded cine MRI is able to quantify flow velocities and volumes, and can therefore be applied to assess the severity of an associated valve abnormality, e.g. mitral or tricuspid regurgitation in a patient with dilated cardiomyopathy (DCM). The same MRI technique is gaining acceptance to assess diastolic function such as in patients with restrictive cardiomyopathy (RCM). Analysis of the transvalvular and venous flow patterns enables depiction of impaired myocardial relaxation and/or decreased compliance. Real-time cine MRI techniques have a large potential to assess the influence of respiration on cardiac filling and thus to differentiate patients with restrictive inflow pattern secondary to either restrictive cardiomyopathy or constrictive pericarditis. Other MRI techniques such as MRI myocardial tagging are helpful to explore wall deformation and to better understand the pathophysiology of certain myocardial disorders (ZERHOUNI et al. 1988).

In summary, the current arsenal of available MRI techniques can be used to define the many aspects of these often complex diseases, providing the clinician with a complete picture of the patients' myocardial disorder (Table 9.2). Because of the huge variety of myocardial disorders, each MRI study should be tailored towards the clinical question. MRI should also be considered as the preferred technique for follow-up of disease progression and response to treatment in patients with myocardial diseases.

9.3
Cardiac Hypertrophy

Cardiac or ventricular hypertrophy is an adaptive process induced by different physiological and pathological stimuli, which can present with a variety of geometric patterns (FREY et al. 2004). Pathological ventricular hypertrophy is an important and independent risk factor for cardiovascular complications. Ventricular hypertrophy is expressed by changes in total amount of myocardial tissue (i.e. wall mass), and relative wall thickness (RWT; ratio of wall thickness to chamber radius). Cardiac adaptation is achieved by myocardial hypertrophy characterized by an increase in volume of myocytes ("intracellular remodelling") and concomitant changes in the extracellular matrix (i.e. the amount and physical properties of collagen). It is likely that tissue properties remain normal in physiological

Table 9.2. Step-by-step approach in the assessment of non-ischemic myocardial disease

Morphology
- Ventricular size
  - Normal/increased/decreased
  - Univentricular/biventricular
- Myocardial wall thickness
  - Normal/increased/decreased/bulging
  - Homogeneous/focal
- Atrial size – atrial appendages
- Great vessels (aorta, pulmonary artery, pulmonary and caval veins)
- Associated findings (valve leaflets/thrombus/pericardial fluid, pericarditis/pleural fluid/mediastinal and hilar lymph nodes, sarcoidosis)

Function
- Systolic global (EDV/ESV/SV/EF/CO) and regional function (wall motion and contractility)
- Diastolic function (flow patterns in pulmonary/systemic veins, atrioventricular valves)
- Ventricular septal motion patterns (real-time MRI)
- Myocardial tagging

Late myocardial enhancement
- Transmural location and extent
- Distribution pattern and appearance
- Associated findings (no-reflow/thrombus/pericardial enhancement)

Myocardial perfusion imaging (rest-perfusion) (optional)

Myocardial oedema weighted MRI (T2-weighted short-tau inversion-recovery, STIR, SE-MRI) (optional)

Velocity-encoded cine MRI (optional)
- Quantification severity of concomitant valve stenosis – regurgitation
- Intraventricular gradient quantification
- Shunt calculation
- Diastolic function

Coronary MR angiography and MRI of thoracic vessels (optional)
- Exclusion of concomitant pathology

hypertrophy, while they are altered in pathological hypertrophy, leading to increased myocardial stiffness and diastolic dysfunction.

Regular and extensive physical training leads to a physiological cardiac hypertrophy, the so-called athlete's heart. The physiological cardiac adaptation is dependent on the type of sport performed. MORGANROTH et al. (1975) have postulated that three different morphological forms of athlete's heart can be distinguished: a strength-trained heart, an endurance-trained heart, and an intermediate form (MORGANROTH et al. 1975). Athletes involved in sports with a high dynamic component (e.g. long-distance running or cycling) develop predominantly increased ventricular chamber size with a proportional increase in wall thickness caused by volume overload associated with the high cardiac output of endurance training (PLUIM et al. 1999). Thus, endurance-trained athletes are considered to develop an eccentric ventricular hypertrophy, characterized by an unchanged relationship between ventricular wall thickness and chamber radius (increased wall mass, but unchanged RWT). Although most studies on the morphological changes in endurance-trained athletes are focused on the LV changes, Scharlag et al. report similar changes in LV and right ventricular (RV) mass, volumes and function in endurance-trained athletes, suggesting that the cardiac adaptation is "balanced" (SCHARLAG et al. 2002; Fig. 9.2). Athletes involved in mainly static or isometric ex-

ercise (e.g. weightlifting) develop predominantly an increased LV wall thickness with unchanged LV chamber size, which is caused by pressure overload accompanying the high systemic arterial pressure found in this type of exercise. Thus, strength-trained athletes are presumed to demonstrate concentric LV hypertrophy (increased wall mass and increased ventricular RWT). The intermediate form is found in athletes performing combined dynamic and static exercise (e.g. rowing and cycling). In a meta-analysis of cardiac structure and function in athletes' hearts, PLUIM et al. (1999) found a geometric pattern more complicated than postulated by MORGANROTH et al. (1975). In endurance-trained athletes, a significant increase in RWT was found, whilst strength-trained athletes showed an increase in LV diameter

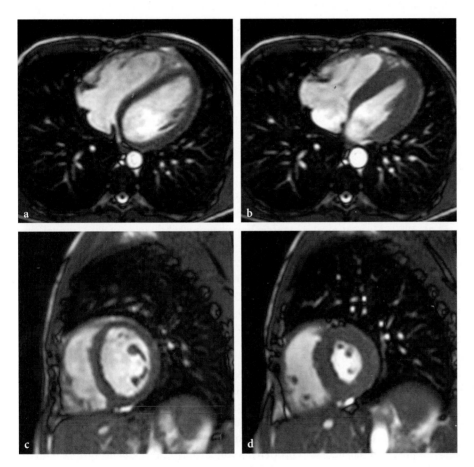

Fig. 9.2a-d. Athlete's heart in a professional cyclist with an eccentric (compensated) hypertrophy. Cine MRI, using the balanced steady-state free precession (b-SSFP) technique, in the axial view at end diastole (**a**), and end systole (**b**), and in the midventricular short-axis at end diastole (**c**) and end systole (**d**). The global LV volumes and function at rest are: end-diastolic volume, 230 ml; end-systolic volume, 102 ml; stroke volume, 128 ml; ejection fraction, 56%; LV mass, 240 g. The values for the right ventricle are 262 ml, 140 ml, 122 ml and 46%, respectively. The septal wall thickness is 12 mm at end diastole and 19 mm at end systole, and for the lateral wall the respective values are 10 and 17 mm. The functional and morphogical values show that the physiological remodelling involves both ventricles ("balanced type"). The resting EFs are lower than those obtained in untrained healthy volunteers. During exercise, the cardiac output is primarily increased by increase in stroke volume (and thus ejection fraction), less by increase in heart rate.

in addition to an increase in LV wall thickness. The combined endurance- and strength-trained athletes showed a significant increase in RWT and the highest increase in LV internal diameter. SPIRITO et al. (1994) ranked sports according to the impact on LV cavity dimensions and LV wall thickness. For example, rowing is ranked first according to the calculated effect on LV wall thickness and only seventh for the calculated effect on LV internal dimension. In general, sports associated with large cavity dimensions also have relatively high values of wall thickness. Normal LV end-diastolic septal wall thickness is 8.8 mm (8.5–9.0 mm) in control subjects, 10.5 mm (10.1–10.9 mm) in endurance-trained athletes, 11.3 mm (10.6–12.0 mm) in combined endurance and strength-trained athletes and 11.8 mm (10.9–12.7 mm) in strength-trained athletes. LV internal diameters at end-diastole are 49.6 mm (48.9–50.2 mm), 53.7 mm (52.8–54.6 mm), 56.2 mm (55.2–57.1 mm) and 52.1 mm (50.6–53.6 mm), respectively. RWT values are 0.356 (0.343–0.369), 0.389 (0.374–0.404), 0.398 (0.374–0.421), and 0.442 (0.403–0.480), respectively (PLUIM et al. 1999). All values are obtained in male athletes, with 95% confidence intervals shown in parentheses. In comparison with the pathological cardiac hypertrophy, physiological increases in wall thickness are mild, even in elite athletes. End-diastolic wall thicknesses usually do not exceed 13 mm in male and 11 mm in female athletes. Values greater than 16 mm should be regarded as abnormal (BELENKOV et al. 1992; MARON et al. 1995). Diastolic ventricular function in athletes is normal or slightly enhanced (i.e. increased E/A ratio). With the associated bradycardia, early diastolic filling is prolonged and the contribution of atrial contraction to ventricular filling reduced. Although most studies in athletes' hearts have been performed with echocardiography, MRI is definitely appealing. The morphology and function of the left and right ventricle can be quantified with a much higher accuracy and reproducibility than echocardiography, thereby reducing the sample size (SCHARLAG et al. 2002). Magnetic resonance offers other advantages such as the potential for selectively tagging the myocardium, allowing study of phenomena such as ventricular torsion in physiological and pathological ventricular hypertrophy (STUBER et al. 1999). In physiological cardiac hypertrophy (athlete's heart), torsion and twisting remain unchanged compared with normal subjects; while, in pathological cardiac hypertrophy due to increased afterload (aortic stenosis), torsion is significantly increased and diastolic apical untwisting prolonged. This delayed untwisting in pressure-overloaded hearts might contribute to the diastolic dysfunction often found is these patients.

Pathological cardiac hypertrophy is found in a variety of cardiac diseases, including cardiomyopathies, increased afterload (e.g. aortic or pulmonary stenosis, systemic or pulmonary arterial hypertension) and increased preload (e.g. volume overload), and may occur as a compensatory mechanism following myocardial infarction. Similar to physiological hypertrophy, two basic patterns are present in pathological hypertrophy: pressure overload (e.g. aortic stenosis or systemic arterial hypertension), which results in a concentric hypertrophy with increased wall thickness and unchanged cavity dimensions, stroke volume and ejection fraction (Fig. 9.3); and volume overload (e.g. aortic valve insufficiency), which leads to an eccentric hypertrophy with no or minimal increase in wall thickness, increased LV chamber volume and stroke volume, and reduced ejection fraction (RUDIN et al. 1991). In clinical practice, however, systemic arterial hypertension is associated with a spectrum of cardiac geometric adaptations, which are most likely matched to the systemic haemodynamics and ventricular load (GANAU et al. 1992). In the majority of untreated hypertensive patients (52%), LV mass (index) and regional wall thickness is normal. In 13% of patients, RWT is increased, but LV mass is normal ("concentric remodelling"); in 27% of patients there is eccentric hypertrophy, while in only 8% "typical" hypertensive concentric hypertrophy is seen. Patients with an eccentric hypertrophy may be non-dilated (or compensated) or dilated (or non-compensated). Another hypertrophy pattern found in arterial hypertension is that of asymmetric LV hypertrophy, characterized by a septal/posterior wall thickness ratio greater than 1.5 at end-diastole (CUSPIDI et al. 1997). The beneficial effects of this compensatory response to increased cardiac afterload, i.e. reduction in wall stress, are counteracted by several unwanted side-effects of the increase in LV mass, i.e. increase in myocardial oxygen consumption, reduced coronary reserve, increased cardiac fibrosis, propensity for cardiac failure due to systolic and diastolic dysfunction, and arrhythmogenesis, all contributing to an increased mortality. Consequently, determination of LV hypertrophy is mandatory to assess prognosis in arterial hypertension (GATZKA 2002). Because of its ability to measure wall thickness and to quantify ventricular volumes, function and mass in a fast, accurate and highly reproducible manner, MRI should be considered a primary im-

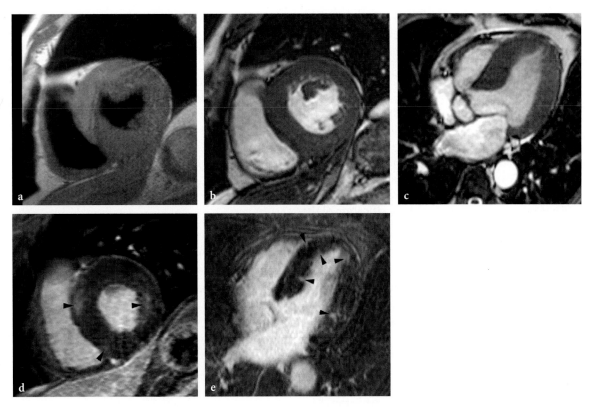

Fig. 9.3a-e. Severe pathological concentric LV hypertrophy in a 56-year-old man with a long-standing, calcified aortic stenosis, and a gradient over the stenotic valve of 125 mmHg (measured by means of velocity-encoded MRI). T1-weighted fast SE-MRI in the short-axis plane (**a**); cine MRI, using the b-SSFP technique, in the short-axis plane (**b**) and horizontal long-axis plane (**c**); contrast-enhanced inversion-recovery technique with late imaging after contrast administration, short-axis plane (**d**) and horizontal long-axis plane (**e**). Although the hypertrophy is concentric and severe (LV wall mass, 270 g), the hypertrophy is most pronounced in the ventricular septum (end-diastolic wall thickness of 25 mm). At late imaging after contrast injection (**d, e**), multiple areas of focal myocardial enhancement are shown throughout the myocardium (*arrowheads*). Although the precise nature of this focal enhancement is unknown, it may represent small micro-infarctions (ischemia-related or emboligenic) and/or areas of myocardial fibrosis.

aging modality for diagnosing patients with cardiac hypertrophy and to guide the intensity of treatment (SCHALLA et al. 2003). In a recent study by CHUANG et al. (2004), comparing echocardiography (linear approach) with MRI (volumetric approach) for studying and classifying ventricular hypertrophy in patients with arterial hypertension, the majority of patients presented with a normal pattern on MRI (63.3%). However, in contrast with the echocardiography findings, concentric remodelling was by far the second most frequent pattern (26.3% versus 9.4% on echocardiography), followed by concentric hypertrophy (7.2%), while only 3.2% had an eccentric hypertrophy (versus 23.7% on echocardiography). This pilot study suggests a prominent role for MRI for better stratification of patients with arterial hypertension and better classification of the pattern of LV hypertrophy. Moreover, CE-IR MRI with late imaging may be appealing to detect myocardial

abnormalities related to the side-effects of cardiac hypertrophy such as detection of areas of myocardial fibrosis, as well as visualization of myocardial damage caused by microvascular abnormalities and concomitant coronary heart disease (Fig. 9.3). In a small number of patients with essential hypertension, myocardial enhancement is found in the ventricular septum and lateral wall, typically within the mid-wall (MACEIRA et al. 2004a). In an experimental setting, MR spectroscopy has been used to study the myocardial high-energy phosphate metabolism in patients with hypertensive disease. LAMB et al. (1999) have found an association between altered high-energy phosphate metabolism and impaired LV diastolic function in hypertensive patients. Cardiac MRI combined with MR angiography of the thoracoabdominal aorta and renal arteries provides a comprehensive evaluation of patients with hypertension, allowing assessment of the effects of hypertension on the heart, and detection of the secondary causes of hypertension (e.g. aortic coarctation and renal artery stenosis; MACEIRA et al. 2004b).

9.4
Cardiomyopathy

Cardiomyopathies are diseases of the myocardium. The term "cardiomyopathy" was introduced by Harvey and Brigden four decades ago (BRIGDEN 1957; HARVEY et al. 1964). In the classification of the World Health Organization (WHO), the term "cardiomyopathy" is reserved for myocardial diseases of unknown aetiology, while other diseases that affect the myocardium but are of known cause or are part of a generalized systemic disorder are termed "specific heart muscle diseases". However, since the clinical presentation of a given cardiomyopathy and a specific heart muscle disease is often similar, it is preferable to use the term "secondary" cardiomyopathy to identify those patients with a specific heart muscle disease that clinically closely simulates an idiopathic or "primary" cardiomyopathy. The aetiology and pattern of the most frequent myocardial diseases causing cardiomyopathies are shown in Table 9.1. Three basic types of cardiomyopathies have been described by the WHO: *hypertrophic* cardiomyopathies (HCM), *dilated* cardiomyopathies (DCM; formerly "congestive"), and *restrictive* cardiomyopathies (RCM; FEJFAR 1968). Each type of cardiomyopathy corresponds to a basic type of functional impairment; however, overlap between the different types may exist. HCM are characterized by an inappropriate LV hypertrophy, usually with a preserved contractile function; DCM are characterized by ventricular dilatation and a contractile dysfunction; while, in restrictive forms, impaired diastolic filling is the most prominent finding. The findings of the different cardiomyopathies on cardiac imaging are shown in Table 9.3. Most forms of secondary cardiomyopathy are characterized by the DCM pattern; less frequently the restrictive pattern is present. Other conditions such as arrhythmogenic RV dysplasia or non-compaction cardiomyopathy are difficult to fit into this traditional classification scheme and are therefore discussed in separate sections.

Table 9.3. Morphological and functional abnormalities in cardiomyopathy

	Dilated	Hypertrophic	Restrictive
Morphology			
LV±RV enlargement	+++	−	−
Myocardial hypertrophy	+	+++	−/+
Atrial dilation	++	+	++
Pleural effusion	+		+
Pericardial effusion	(+)	−	+
Ventricular thrombi (apex)	+	−	−
Dilation of IVC/SVC	+	−	+++
Myocardial function			
Global dysfunction	+++	+	(+)
Segmental variation	+	+++	(+)
Diastolic dysfunction	+	+(+)	+++
Valvular function			
Mitral regurgitation	++	++	+
Tricuspid regurgitation	+	−	+

IVC, Inferior vena cava; LV, left ventricular; RV, right ventricular; SVC, superior vena cava

9.4.1
Hypertrophic Cardiomyopathy

The characteristic finding of HCM is an inappropriate myocardial hypertrophy in the absence of an obvious cause for the hypertrophy, such as systemic hypertension or aortic stenosis. Familial clustering is often observed, and the disease is genetically transmitted in about half of the cases (MARON 2002; CRILLEY et al. 2003). The natural history and clinical presentation of HCM are variable. Symptoms are caused by intraventricular, usually LV outflow tract (LVOT) obstruction, myocardial ischemia and reduced coronary vasodilator flow reserve, diastolic dysfunction and arrhythmias. Although patients might be completely asymptomatic, HCM is the most common identified cause of sudden cardiac death in young people, due to arrhythmia (MARON 2002). Histologically, HCM is characterized by a disorganization and malalignment of the myofibrils, i.e. *myofibrillar disarray*, which is not unique to HCM but is clearly more extensive in this disorder than in secondary myocardial hypertrophy from pressure overload or congenital heart disorders (BULKLEY et al. 1977; MARON et al. 1981). The combination of inappropriate myocardial hypertrophy, intimal hyperplasia of intramural coronary arteries and endothelial dysfunction causes myocardial

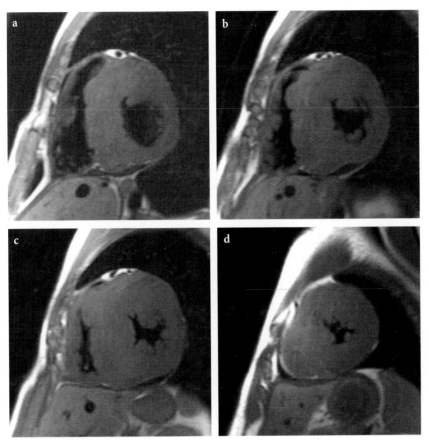

Fig. 9.4a-d. Extreme form of hypertrophic, obstructive cardiomyopathy in a young male teenager. T1-weighted fast SE-MRI in the cardiac short-axis at four different levels (**a-d**). The spread of the myocardial hypertrophy can be seen. The ventricular septum, and adjacent anterior and inferior wall are extensively thickened with end-diastolic wall thicknesses exceeding 50 mm ("asymmetrical septal" form). The total LV mass exceeds 500 g. Note the concomitant hypertrophy of the RV free wall and the presence of a small pericardial effusion.

ischemia and spontaneous myocardial infarction in the absence of abnormalities of epicardial coronary arteries. It is likely that the capillary density in the hypertrophied heart is inadequate relative to the increased myocardial mass.

Different morphological types of HCM are found. HCM typically produces marked asymmetrical hypertrophy of the left ventricle. The end-diastolic LV wall thickness is typically greater than 15 mm. In some patients, HCM might be associated with massive myocardial hypertrophy (wall thickness of 45–50 mm; Fig. 9.4). In 70% of patients, the ventricular septum and anterior LV wall are involved. Abnormalities are usually most prominent in the basal segments (previously called "idiopathic hypertrophic subaortic stenosis" and "muscular subaortic stenosis"; see also Fig. 9.7). Less frequent locations of myocardial hypertrophy include: the mid-portion of the ventricular septum, the apex, and the lower portion of the septum. Severe concentric hypertrophy may occur and papillary muscles may also be hypertrophied (Fig. 9.5). According to the definition of the WHO, HCM might also involve the right ventricle (Fig 9.4); the LV volumes are normal or might be re-

duced. Secondary, left atrial enlargement is usually found (JÄRVINEN et al. 1996).

Approximately 25% of patients with HCM have a dynamic outflow tract obstruction caused by a narrowed LVOT and abnormal systolic anterior motion of the mitral valve (BRAUNWALD et al. 1960; WIGLE et al. 1962). In nearly all patients with LVOT obstruction, the outflow tract area is smaller than 4.0 cm^2 (mean: 2.6±0.7 cm^2; SPIRITO and MARON 1983). In patients without obstruction and normal subjects, the outflow tract area is 5.9±1.6 cm^2 and 10.4±1.2 cm^2, respectively. During onset of cardiac systole, deformation and bulging of the hypertrophied septum into the LVOT contributes to the flow acceleration in the narrowed LVOT. The subsequent pressure drop leads to an anterior movement, and eventually apposition of the anterior mitral valve leaflet to the septum during systole contributes to the outflow obstruction (the "Venturi effect"; Figs. 9.6 and 9.7). The LVOT obstruction may be present at rest (resting obstructive HCM) or may be provoked by exercise, Valsalva manoeuvre, or administration of amyl nitrite (latent obstructive HCM). The anterior mitral valve leaflet motion causes a secondary mitral

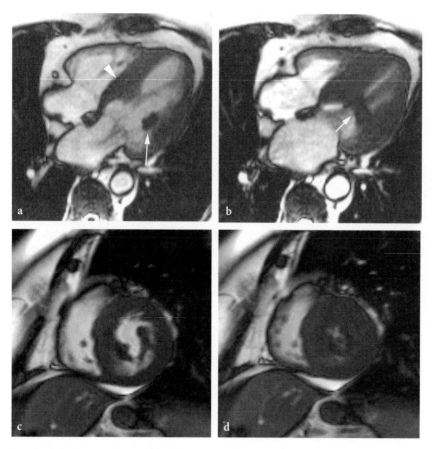

Fig. 9.5a-d. Midventricular type of hypertrophic (obstructive) cardiomyopathy in a 55-year-old woman. Cine MRI, using the b-SSFP technique in the horizontal long-axis view at end diastole (**a**) and end systole (**b**), and midventricular short-axis at end diastole (**c**) and end systole (**d**). Focal, moderate thickening of midventricular septum (end-diastolic wall thickness of 25 mm; *arrowhead*). The presence of concomitant hypertrophy of both papillary muscles (*arrow*) causes a midventricular sub-obstruction with a gradient of 55 mmHg on echo-Doppler. The low signal intensity of the papillary muscles is caused by calcification. Secondary papillary dysfunction leads to a severe mitral regurgitation (not shown).

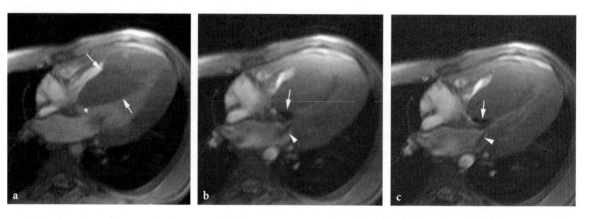

Fig. 9.6a-c. "Venturi" effect in hypertrophic (obstructive) cardiomyopathy. Cine MRI, using the spoiled gradient-echo (GE) technique, at end diastole (**a**), early systole (**b**) and mid-systole (**c**). At end diastole (**a**), an important thickening of the entire ventricular septum is visible (*arrows*), causing a narrowing the LV outflow tract (LVOT; *star*). LV contraction (**b, c**) leads to flow acceleration in the narrowed LVOT, visible as an area of signal void (*arrow*). The subsequent pressure drop causes an anterior motion of the anterior mitral valve leaflet, leading to mitral regurgitation (*arrowhead*) and left atrial enlargement

valve regurgitation, occurring in mid-late systole. In some patients, mitral regurgitation might be severe and contribute substantially to symptoms of heart failure. The pressure gradient in the LVOT is used to determine the haemodynamic relevance of the LVOT obstruction. Pressure gradients can be cal-culated by a modified Bernoulli formula, according to which maximal flow velocities across a stenosis reflect the severity of obstruction.

It is clearly recognized that not all patients have severe outflow tract pressure gradients, while ab-normalities in diastolic function are common

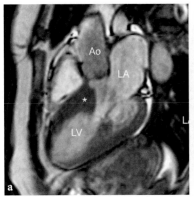 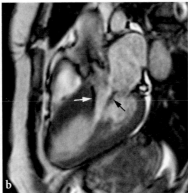 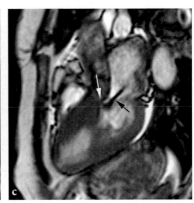

Fig. 9.7a-c. Asymmetric septal hypertrophic cardiomyopathy with complete occlusion of the LVOT in a 69-year-old woman. Cine MRI, using the b-SSFP technique, in the LV inlet-outlet view at end diastole (**a**), first half of systole (**b**) and second half of systole (**c**). Focal, important thickening of the basal ventricular septum (*star*) narrowing the LVOT. The flow acceleration in the LVOT, visible as a signal void (*white arrow*) adjacent to the hypertrophied myocardium (**b**) causes a mitral regurgitation during early systole (*black arrow*). Complete apposition of the anterior mitral leaflet to the thickened, septal myocardium (*white arrow*) causes an abrupt cessation of the forward flow in the ascending aorta in the second half of systole (**c**), leading to severe mitral regurgitation (*black arrow*). Ao, Ascending aorta; LA, left atrium; LV, left ventricle.

(STEWARD et al. 1968). At present, diastolic dysfunction is thought to be one of the major pathophysiological mechanisms present in all patients with HCM, frequently leading to diastolic heart failure. HCM patients usually present a combination of increased chamber stiffness and impaired ventricular relaxation.

The less common apical form of HCM has a high prevalence in Japan. These patients have no outflow obstruction but present with a severe apical LV hypertrophy, giant negative T-waves on their ECG, and a typical spade-shaped LV cavity (ABELMANN and LORELL 1989; Fig. 9.8). In a recent study by SOLER et al. (1997) using MRI, three types of apical HCM are described: (a) true apical form ("spadelike" configuration), (b) involvement of the apex and symmetric hypertrophy of the four ventricular wall segments, and (c) involvement of the apex with asymmetric involvement of the wall segments ("nonspade" apical HCM; SUZUKI et al. 1993). Because of near-field problems of the echo probe, apical HCM is often difficult to assess on echocardiography, and MRI should be considered the preferred imaging technique (CASOLO et al. 1989). Another form of HCM is mid-ventricular hypertrophy. These patients present with a gradient between the LV apical region and the remainder of the chamber. This may progress to a non-contractile apical aneurysm with apical thrombus formation (ABELMANN and LORELL 1989).

Although transthoracic echocardiography is the primary imaging modality in the diagnosis of HCM, MRI at present does provide the most complete de-

scription of abnormalities in HCM patients. The arsenal of MRI sequences usable in HCM includes: SE-MRI; cine MRI; velocity-encoded MRI; MRI tagging; CE-IR MRI; and MR spectroscopy. The presence, distribution and severity of the hypertrophic process can precisely be evaluated with SE MRI and cine MRI (FARMER et al. 1984; BEEN et al. 1985; HIGGINS et al. 1985; GAUDIO et al. 1992; ALLISON et al. 1993; PARK et al. 1992). An advantage of MRI over other cardiac imaging modalities is the use of angled planes, which allows accurate measurement of the myocardial wall thickness (ARRIVÉ et al. 1994). In the asymmetric septal form of HCM, the mean ratio of septal-to-free wall thickness is higher than 1.5±0.8, compared with 0.9±0.3 in normal volunteers and 0.8±0.2 in patients with LV hypertrophy (BEEN et al. 1985).

Using cine MRI sequences, obstructive forms can be differentiated from non-obstructive forms of septal HCM (PARK et al. 1992; DI CESARE et al. 1994). Flow acceleration and turbulence in the narrowed LVOT causes a dispersion of spin magnetization, generating a signal void in the LVOT during systole (PARK et al. 1992; Figs. 9.6 and 9.7). Presence of signal void in early systole is indicative of severe obstructive HCM. Mid-systolic signal voids usually represent less severe (latent) obstructions. In non-obstructive forms of HCM and in normal subjects, usually no signal voids are found. The presence and severity of signal void, however, is closely related to the length of the echo time. With the advent of the b-SSFP cine MRI techniques, the precise relation between signal void and flow acceleration needs to be reassessed. The concomitant regurgitant jet through the mitral valve is also visible as an area of signal void (Figs. 9.6 and 9.7). Velocity-encoded cine MRI can be used to quantify flow velocities in the narrowed LVOT, and to assess the mitral valve regurgitation. A combination of imaging planes is required to optimally image the LVOT and mitral valve abnormalities. These include longitudinal views through the LVOT; combined LV in- and outflow views; horizontal and vertical long-axis views through the mitral valve; views perpendicular through the LVOT (to measure the LVOT area); and views through the mitral valve plane (to quantify the mitral regurgitation).

The impact of myocardial hypertrophy on global and regional LV and RV function can be precisely assessed with cine MRI. The global functional values in HCM are often increased with high ejection fractions and low end-systolic values. During cardiac contraction, incomplete compression of the ventricular cavities may occur in patients with severe HCM. In the thickened myocardial regions, however, systolic wall thickening is markedly reduced, which is related to muscle disorganization (MARON et al. 1987; ARRIVÉ et al. 1994; BOGAERT et al. 2003). Myocardial MRI tagging techniques have been used to study the strain or deformation in HCM patients (MAIER et al. 1992; YOUNG et al. 1994; KRAMER et al. 1994; DONG et al. 1994). In the hypertrophied myocardium, the systolic myocardial strains are invariably diminished, with reduced longitudinal and circumferential shortening as well as diminished/absent systolic wall thickening (Fig. 9.9). The functional abnormalities are inversely related to the local thickness. Conversely, these studies show that the ventricular torsion significantly increases in patients with HCM. Moreover, MRI tagging techniques may be helpful to differentiate focal HCM forms from true cardiac masses (BERGEY and AXEL 2000). SUZUKI et al. (1991a) have reported assessment of diastolic dysfunction of the right ventricle in patients with HCM by means of cine MRI. Nowadays, velocity-encoded cine MRI sequences assessing the flow patterns in the caval and pulmonary veins, as well as the diastolic inflow in the tricuspid/mitral valve can be used to evaluate the cardiac diastolic function. Flow measurements in the coronary sinus at rest and after administration of vasodilating agents (e.g. dipyridamole) allow determination of the coronary flow reserve. KAWADA et al. (1999) have reported a severely depressed flow reserve ratio in patients with HCM compared with that in healthy subjects (1.72 ± 0.49 versus 3.01 ± 0.75: $p<0.01$).

Use of gadolinium (Gd)-DTPA to differentiate normal from disorganized myocardial tissue in HCM patients was reported in the mid-1990s (TSUKIHASHI et al. 1994). After Gd-DTPA administration, the hypertrophic myocardium in patients with HCM shows a higher signal intensity ratio than non-hypertrophic regions and than myocardium in normal subjects, and a delayed decay of the signal intensity is present. It has been hypothetized that the areas of abnormally high signal intensity in LV myocardium reflect myocardial ischemia and fibrosis due to small-vessel disease, or myocardial degeneration and necrosis (KOITO et al. 1995). A major limitation of the MRI techniques at this time was the insufficient contrast between normal and abnormal (e.g. infarcted) myocardium. With the advent of CE-IR MRI sequences with late imaging, the selective nulling of the signal of normal myocardium by appropriate choice of inversion time has enabled the differences in contrast between normal and abnormal myocardium to be substantially increased. For instance, infarcted myocardium can be differentiated from normal viable myocardium with differences in signal intensity of nearly 500% (KIM et al. 1999; SIMONETTI et al. 2001). Recently, several groups have reported promising results characterizing the hypertrophied regions in patients with HCM using CE-IR MRI (WU et al. 2000; CHOUDHURY et al. 2002; BOGAERT et al. 2003; MOON et al. 2003a; VAN DOCKUM et al. 2004). Abnormal late enhancement is found in the majority of HCM patients, ranging from 79%, in a selected group of patients (n=53; MOON et al. 2003a), to 81% in a non-selected group of patients (n=21; CHOUDHURY et al. 2003). Enhancement was invariably found in the hypertrophied regions (Figs. 9.8, 9.9). Mean volume of enhancement was 8–11% of LV mass. The pattern of enhancement is usually patchy with multiple foci, predominantly involving the middle third of the ventricular wall; and the junction of the ventricular septum and RV free wall is the most frequently involved area of enhancement (CHOUDHURY et al. 2002; Fig. 9.10). The extent of enhancement is positively correlated with the wall thickness, and inversely with systolic wall thickening in the hypertrophied region (CHOUDHURY et al. 2002; BOGAERT et al. 2003). Since late enhancement is a non-specific phenomenon that can reflect a variety of myocardial disorders (BOGAERT et al. 2004), the question remains: What is the histopathological correlate of late enhancement in HCM? At present, it is generally believed that enhanced regions represent scarred myocardium (KIM and JUDD 2003) or are in relation to myocardial disarray and consequent lo-

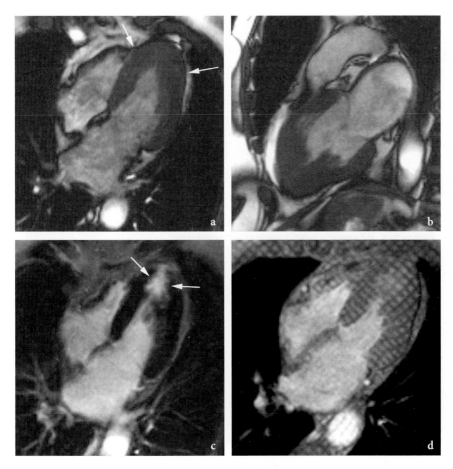

Fig. 9.8a-d. Apical form of hypertrophic cardiomyopathy in a 70-year-old woman presenting with negative Ts in anterior leads on ECG. Transthoracic echocardiography showed apical hypokinesia. Cine MRI, using the b-SSFF technique, in horizontal (**a**) and vertical (**b**) long-axis view. CE-IR MRI with late imaging in horizontal long-axis view (**c**), and SPAMM tagging in same imaging plane after contrast injection (**d**). Progressive thickening of LV walls toward the apex (*arrows*) (**a**, **b**), with a maximal end-diastolic wall thickness in the apical segments of 20 mm, causing apposition of LV walls. Strong enhancement of mainly the subendocardium in the hypertrophied myocardium (*arrows*) (**c**). Decreased deformation and contractility in the hypertrophied myocardium, as shown on SPAMM tagging (**d**).

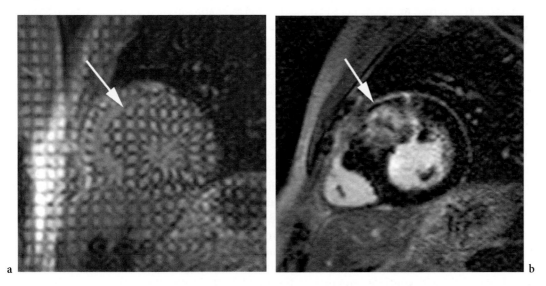

Fig. 9.9a,b. Asymmetric septal hypertrophic cardiomyopathy in a 50-year-old man. Cine MRI, using the SPAMM tagging technique, in the basal short-axis view at end-systole (**a**). CE-IR MRI with late imaging in same imaging plane (**b**). Decreased myocardial deformation of abnormally thickened wall (*arrow*), normal deformation in other wall segments (**a**). Focal, patchy enhancement in thickened myocardium (*arrow*) (**b**). (From BOGAERT et al. 2004. Reprinted with permission from the American Roentgen Ray Society.)

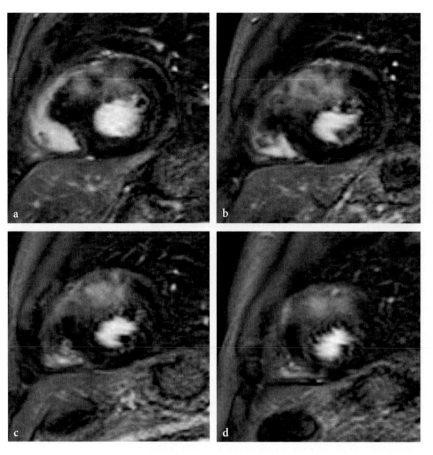

Fig. 9.10a-d. Typical late myocardial enhancement pattern in asymmetric septal hypertrophic cardiomyopathy. CE-IR MRI with late imaging in short-axis plane at four different levels. Focal, patchy to cloudy, enhancement which is limited to the hypertrophied myocardium anteroseptally. The mid-wall and subepicardium are maximally involved, while the subendocardium is relatively spared.

cal interstitial expansion (MOON et al. 2003a). The pattern of enhancement corresponds to the typical pattern of myocardial scarring found in necropsy studies. A pattern that does not correspond to any epicardial coronary artery distribution and is often limited to the mid-wall or subepicardium, with a predominant involvement of the junction of the ventricular septum and RV free wall (most prominent myocardial scarring and myocardial fibre disarray; KURIBAYASHI and ROBERTS 1992;VARNAVA et al. 2000). Moreover, it is suggested by Moon et al., studying a highly selected group of patients with HCM, that myocardial enhancement in HCM is associated with progressive disease (i.e. progressive adverse LV remodelling), and increased risk for sudden cardiac death (MOON et al. 2003a). They have found specific patterns of enhancement associations with the clinical phenotype. For instance, patients with diffuse enhancement have a higher risk of sudden cardiac death than patients with confluent enhancement. It is likely that the degree of diastolic dysfunction is linked to the extent of myocardial fibrosis, quantified by means of CE-IR MRI (MOTOYASU et al. 2004).

Cine MRI and CE-IR MRI are also useful in the evaluation of HCM patients with a dynamic LVOT obstruction after non-surgical septal reduction (NSSR), also called percutaneous transluminal septal myocardial ablation (PTSMA) (SCHULZ-MENGER et al. 2000a; WU et al. 2000; VAN DOCKUM et al. 2004). The procedure consists of selectively inducing a localized myocardial infarct by infusion of ethanol into one or several septal branches of the left anterior descending (LAD) coronary artery (SIGWART 1995; KNIGHT et al. 1997; MAZUR et al. 2001). Subsequent scarring of the induced infarct and thinning of the ventricular septum results in a widening of the LVOT, a decrease in the pressure gradient and symptomatic improvement. Ethanol causes a significant microvascular obstruction such that the penetration of Gd-DTPA is extremely slow. CE-IR MRI performed shortly (i.e. within days) after the procedure shows a large perfusion deficit with patchy enhancement on delayed imaging (Fig. 9.11). With time, the extent of microvascular obstruction decreases with a less severe first-pass perfusion defect and more pronounced delayed enhancement (WU et al. 2000). Since CE-IR MRI allows detailed evaluation of the size and location

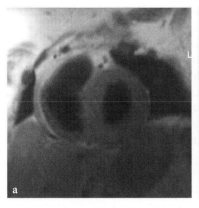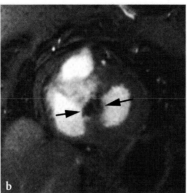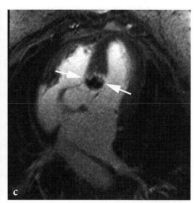

Fig. 9.11a-c. Asymmetric septal hypertrophic obstructive cardiomyopathy in a 54-year-old woman treated with alcoholization of the first septal perforator coronary artery to reduce LV outflow tract obstruction. T1-weighted fast SE-MRI in basal short-axis shows thickening of the ventricular septum with end-diastolic diameter of 23 mm (**a**). CE-IR MRI with late imaging in the basal short-axis (**b**) and horizontal long-axis view (**c**) shows a large hypointense zone surrounded by a thin hyperintense rim in thickened septum (*arrows*), corresponding to occlusive infarct caused by alcoholization. (From BOGAERT et al. (2004). Reprinted with permission from the American Roentgen Ray Society.)

of the septal infarct induced by NSSR, CE-IR MRI might be helpful in predicting the final outcome. Infarcts that are too small or are located outside the target area may not achieve the necessary reduction in LVOT gradient. Large infarcts may cause potentially hazardous conduction abnormalities or ventricular arrhythmias (VAN DOCKUM et al. 2004). Moreover, the infarct created by the septal myocardial ablation is not infrequently located exclusively on the right ventricular side of the ventricular septum (7/24 patients in the study by VAN DOCKUM et al., 2004). These patients have smaller infarction size and less reduction in LV outflow tract gradient. In some patients, no symptomatic improvement is reported. CE-IR MRI has been used recently to evaluate differences in lesion morphology and the extent of the infarct in patients treated with embolic septal infarction using micro-particles versus alcohol-induced necrosis (SCHULZ-MENGER et al. 2004). While the clinical outcome is similar (i.e. improvement in NYHA class), infarct size and infarct transmurality are smaller in the emboli group compared with the alcohol group. Cine MRI can be applied to evaluate the impact of the NSSR procedure on the improvement of the LVOT area (SCHULZ-MENGER et al. 2000a) and on changes in LV mass and volumes (VAN DOCKUM et al. 2004). At 1 month after the septal myocardial ablation, a small but significant decrease in total LV mass is found, which is most likely to reflect early regression of LV hypertrophy by decreasing LV pressure and wall stress (VAN DOCKUM et al. 2004). The LVOT area gradually increases from 1.3±0.1 cm^2 before septal myocardial ablation to 3.5±0.6 cm^2

one year after the procedure, representing a 128±12% improvement, while the LVOT gradient drops from 88±10 mmHg to 31±11 mmHg (SCHULZ-MENGER et al. 2000a).

9.4.2
Dilated Cardiomyopathy

DCM is a syndrome characterized by LV or biventricular enlargement, cardiac hypertrophy and severely depressed systolic function (DEC and FUSTER 1994). A series of morphological changes are found in the myocardial wall. At the cellular level, a combination of atrophy and hypertrophy of the myocytes is demonstrated. The myocardial hypertrophy consists of myocyte elongation with an in-series addition of newly formed sarcomeres, which is the major factor responsible for the increase in chamber size (BELTRAMI et al. 1995). The myocyte diameter also increases, although the lateral expansion of myocytes is modest and inadequate to preserve the ratio of the wall thickness to the chamber diameter at normal values. The structural correlate in the extracellular matrix is myocardial fibrosis with an excessive deposition of collagen in the ventricular wall (SCHAPER et al. 1991). Myocardial fibrosis can be divided into three groups: mild diffuse fibrosis, severe diffuse fibrosis, and segmental fibrosis. The combination of ventricular dilatation and an inadequate increase in myocardial wall thickness leads to a decompensated eccentric hypertrophy and a consequent increase in ventricular wall stress (FUJITA et al. 1993).

Although the cause of DCM is often not definable (idiopathic DCM), a variety of cytotoxic, metabolic, immunological, familial and infectious mechanisms can produce the clinical manifestations of DCM (Dec and Fuster 1994). It is likely that DCM represents the final common pathway that is the end result of myocardial damage.

The clinical presentation of DCM is variable. The most common symptom is left-sided heart failure. Many patients, however, have minimal or no symptoms and the progression of the disease in these patients is unclear (Redfield et al. 1994). Right-sided heart failure is rather uncommon and is found only in severe cases. On chest X-ray, DCM usually reveals generalized cardiomegaly and pulmonary vascular redistribution; interstitial and alveolar oedema is less common on initial presentation. However, a normal cardiac silhouette may be present in patients with DCM and can be explained on the basis of a counterclockwise transverse rotation of the heart within the thorax (Kono et al. 1992). Pleural effusions may be present, and the azygos vein and superior vena cava may be dilated when right-sided heart failure supervenes.

Cardiac imaging techniques are used to evaluate the size of the ventricular cavity and the thickness of the ventricular walls, to exclude concomitant valvular and pericardial disease, and to detect the repercussion of the LV dilatation on valvular function. They are also useful to detect LV thrombi, which are usually located in the apex (Fig. 9.12). Functional studies reveal increased end-diastolic and end-systolic LV volumes, reduced ejection fractions in one or both ventricles and wall motion abnormalities. Although segmental wall motion abnormalities are not uncommon in DCM, they are still more characteristic of ischemic heart disease, whereas diffuse global dysfunction is more typical of DCM.

MRI is able to accurately describe the morphological and functional abnormalities of DCM. At present, MRI can be considered the preferred imaging technique to quantify ventricular volumes and

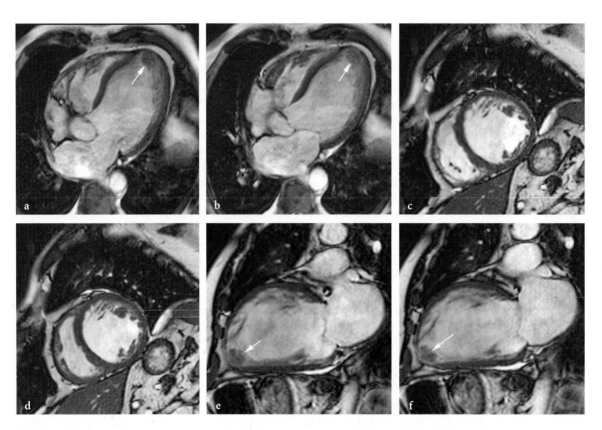

Fig. 9.12a-f. Idiopathic dilated cardiomyopathy in a 53-year-old man. Cine MRI, using the b-SSFP technique, in horizontal long-axis (**a, b**), short-axis (**c, d**), and vertical long-axis (**e, f**), at end diastole and end systole, respectively. Important LV dilation with severely diminished global and regional function (end-diastolic volume, 463 ml; end systolic volume, 417 ml; stroke volume, 46 ml; ejection fraction, 10%). Mural thrombus in LV apex (*arrow*). Note the moderate hypertrophy of the trabeculations along the lateral LV wall, and the left atrial enlargement due to mitral regurgitation secondary to the LV enlargement. CE-IR MRI shows normal myocardial signal (not shown). Normal luminal appearance of coronary arteries on coronary artery catheterization.

functional parameters, to measure the ventricular wall thickness, to calculate the ventricular (RV and LV mass, and to evaluate the presence of RV enlargement in patients with DCM (Semelka et al. 1990; Buser et al. 1990; Gaudio et al. 1991; Doherty et al. 1992a; Fig. 9.12). Buser et al. have shown a significantly more heterogeneous end-diastolic LV wall thickness in patients with DCM compared with normals. Furthermore, the normal gradient in systolic wall thickening between LV base and apex disappears in patients with DCM (Buser et al. 1990). Calculations show that the RV mass in patients with DCM is not significantly different from that in normals, whereas the LV mass is significantly greater (Doherty et al. 1992a). Imai et al. have demonstrated an enlargement of the LV trabeculae in patients with DCM (Imai et al. 1992). In normal subjects, LV trabeculae are seen at the free walls of the left ventricle, but not at the septal wall. These trabeculae are larger in patients with DCM than in normals, while in patients with old myocardial infarction the trabeculae are scarce and the inner sides of the myocardium become very smooth (Fig. 9.12).

Use of gadolinium-enhanced MRI may be helpful to characterize the myocardium and to differentiate DCM patients from LV dysfunction related to CAD (McCrohon et al. 2003). Koito et al. have previously demonstrated, in 1996, an abnormally high signal intensity on Gd-DTPA-enhanced MR images in patients with DCM. These regions may reflect areas of myocardial degeneration, necrosis and fibrosis, and the high signal intensity may predict the severity of LV dysfunction in DCM. With the introduction of the CE-IR MRI techniques with delayed imaging, contrast between normal and pathological myocar-

dium can be significantly improved. While Wu and colleagues have found no hyperenhancement in patients with non-ischemic cardiomyopathy (Fig. 9.13), in contrast to the frequent hyperenhancement in patients with healed myocardial infarction, McCrohon et al. have reported three different patterns in patients with DCM: (a) no enhancement (59%); (b) myocardial enhancement (i.e. subendocardial or transmural) indistinguishable from patients with CAD (13%); or (c) patchy or longitudinal striae of mid-wall enhancement clearly different from the distribution in patients with CAD (28%) (Wu et al. 2001; McCrohon et al. 2003). A significant number of DCM patients have normal luminal appearances by coronary angiography, but the pattern of subendocardial to transmural enhancement strongly suggests the presence of prior infarction. It is most likely that the normal coronary angiography findings can be explained by recanalization after an occlusive coronary event or embolization from minimally stenotic but unstable plaques. Therefore, these patients should be considered as having LV dysfunction related to CAD, rather than DCM patients, though a coexistence of LV dysfunction from DCM combined with CAD cannot be excluded (especially in those patients with non-extensive infarctions). The mid-wall linear and patchy enhancement probably reflects focal segmental fibrosis, though the recent findings by Mahrholdt and colleagues in patients with myocarditis suggests that these areas of enhancement may reflect sequelae of a prior, possibly subclinical myocarditis (Mahrholdt et al. 2004). Although CE-IR MRI with delayed imaging has become the standard sequence for studying focal or segmental myocardial pathology, it should be noted that diffuse myocardial involvement, such as diffuse

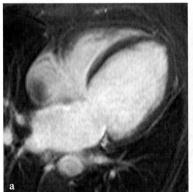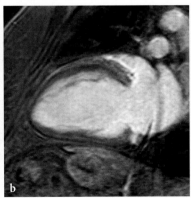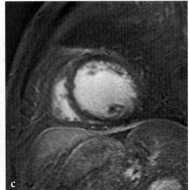

Fig. 9.13a-c. CE-IR MRI with late imaging in 59-year-old male patient with idiopathic dilated cardiomyopathy. Horizontal- (a), vertical (b) long-axis, and midventricular short-axis view (c) ten minutes after contrast administration shows no abnormal areas of signal enhancement in the myocardium of the dilated and dysfunctional left ventricle (end-diastolic volume 371 ml, ejection fraction 27%). This normal enhancement allows exclusion of previous myocardial infarction and macroscopic myocardial fibrosis.

myocardial fibrosis, will most likely not be detected with this MRI technique (BOGAERT et al. 2004).

Cine MRI can be considered the reference technique for quantifying global LV and RV function, and to evaluate segmental wall motion abnormalities in patients with DCM (STROHM et al. 2001; Fig. 9.12). Moreover, this technique can also be used to evaluate the potential beneficial effects of angiotensin-converting enzyme (ACE) inhibitor therapy on the ejection fraction in patients with DCM (DOHERTY et al. 1992b). FUJITA et al. (1993), using cine MRI, have shown an inverse relationship between regional end-systolic wall stress and regional ejection fraction in the left ventricle in patients with DCM. RADEMAKERS and colleagues (2003) have used the relation between regional wall stress and regional strain with MRI myocardial tagging to determine the intrinsic myocardial contractility (see Fig. 6.24). While in normal subjects an inverse linear relation is found between regional stress and strain; in DCM patients there is also a shift towards higher regional stresses for lower systolic strains. However, the angle of the stress-strain relation is changed in DCM patients indicative of impaired intrinsic contractility. MACGOWAN et al. have used myocardial tagging to study the impact of structural abnormalities on fibre and cross-fibre shortening in patients with DCM (MACGOWAN et al. 1997). Diastolic abnormalities, i.e. increase in the time-to-peak filling rate and impaired filling fraction, were detected in the right ventricle, showing a normal volume and normal systolic function in patients with DCM (SUZUKI et al. 1991b). It is likely that changes in LV morphology and function in patients with DCM influence the behaviour even of a normal-appearing right ventricle (DONG et al. 1995).

9.4.3
Restrictive Cardiomyopathy

RCM constitute a heterogeneous group of heart muscle disorders characterized primarily by *diastolic dysfunction*, with impairment of ventricular filling by stiffening of endocardial, subendocardial or myocardial tissue. Morphologically, especially in patients with primary RCM, ventricular chamber dimensions as well as wall thicknesses are often within normal limits, while there is a disproportionate enlargement of the cardiac atria due to increased RV and LV filling pressures, which is further enhanced by mitral and tricuspid regurgitation (Fig. 9.14). Functionally, the influence of restrictive

cardiomyopathy on LV output is variable, and the contractile function is often unimpaired. A variety of specific pathological processes may result in restrictive cardiomyopathy, although the cause often remains unknown (idiopathic or primary forms). RCM may result from myocardial fibrosis, infiltration, myocardial storage or endomyocardial scarring. Furthermore, restrictive inflow physiology may occur in patients with other myocardial disorders such HCM or hypertensive disease. In many cases, a differential diagnosis is possible only by histological analysis, and endomyocardial biopsy usually is required, because imaging techniques are of limited value in providing information about the structure of the pathological myocardium.

Functionally, RCM resembles constrictive pericarditis, which is also characterized by normal or nearly normal systolic function but abnormal ventricular filling (Fig. 9.15). Differentiation between the two can be difficult on clinical grounds, but is critical for decisions regarding the therapeutic approach, since constrictive pericarditis requires surgical resection or stripping of the pericardium, whereas non-surgical management is used for RCM (SHABETAI 1986; WENGER et al. 1986; see also Chap. 11). In both conditions, right atrial and inferior vena caval enlargement is observed, while the ventricles have a small or normal size.

The role of MRI in patients with restrictive physiology is primarily to differentiate between constrictive pericarditis and RCM (MASUI et al. 1992). MRI allows not only a detailed description of the morphological pericardial abnormalities, but also an assessment of the pericardial motion patterns as well as the impact on ventricular filling (see Chap. 11; Fig. 9.16). A combination of SE-MRI, cine MRI, VEC-MRI and CE-IR MRI with late enhancement imaging is recommended at present to study patients with RCM. Specific MRI techniques such as the calculation of the T2* relaxation times are useful in patients with cardiac haemochromatosis (see Sect. 9.4.4.3).

9.4.4
Secondary Cardiomyopathy or Specific Heart Muscle Disease

9.4.4.1
Amyloidosis

Amyloidosis frequently involves the heart and is a common cause of secondary RCM. Deposition of amyloid fibrils occurs in myocardial tissue, valve

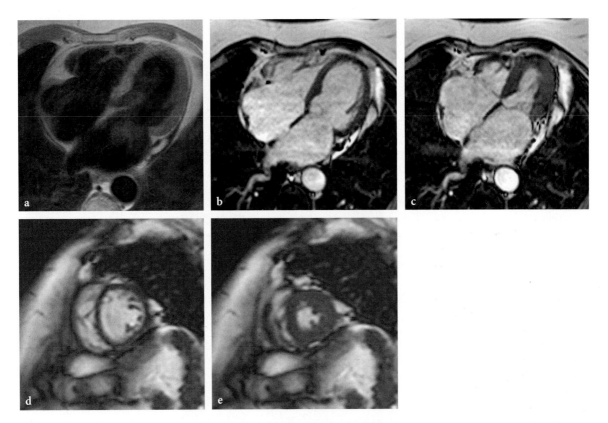

Fig. 9.14a-e. Idiopathic restrictive cardiomyopathy in a 73-year-old woman presenting with increased filling pressures. T1-weighted fast SE-MRI in the horizontal long-axis (**a**). Cine MRI, using b-SSFP technique in the same imaging position at end diastole (**b**) and end systole (**c**). Short-axis cine MRI at end diastole (**d**) and end systole (**e**). The ventricles have a normal configuration and normal systolic function. The main hallmark of RCM is increased myocardial stiffness leading to increased filling pressures, and diastolic dysfunction. As a consequence atria are markedly enlarged. Note the presence of a small pericardial effusion laterally to the left atrioventricular groove.

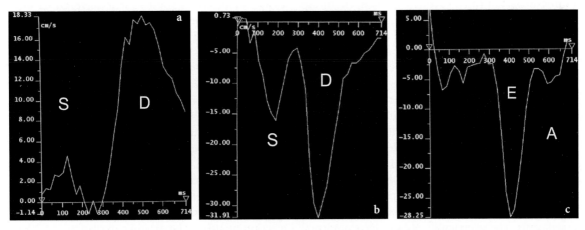

Fig. 9.15a-c. Typical flow curves in a patient with restrictive cardiomyopathy, using the velocity-encoded cine MRI technique. Flow pattern in the inferior vena cava (**a**), pulmonary vein (**b**) and mitral valve (**c**). On the *x*-axis is shown the time during the cardiac cycle (0 ms corresponds with the R-wave of the QRS complex). On the *y*-axis is shown the flow velocity (centimetres per second). The systolic forward flow (*S*) in the systemic and pulmonary veins is diminished due to the increased atrial pressures (**a**, **b**). The latter are necessary to compensate for the decreased myocardial compliance. As a consequence, early ventricular filling (*E*) is typically enhanced (**c**), while the contribution of the atrial contraction (*A*) to the ventricular filling is minimal. At the venous level, forward flow is maximal during early diastolic ventricular filling (*D*); while, later during the cardiac cycle, the forward flow may be abolished or even reversed. Without assessment of the respiratory variation of these flow curves, differentiation between restrictive cardiomyopathy and constrictive pericarditis is often not possible.

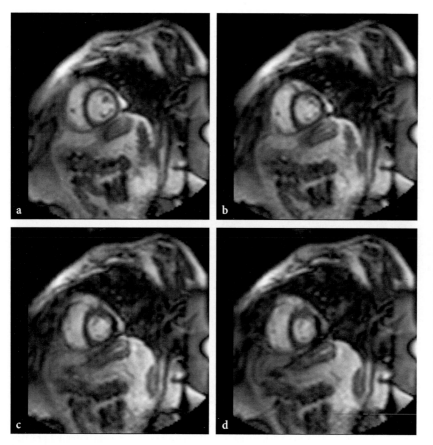

Fig. 9.16a-d. Ventricular septal motion in a patient with restrictive cardiomyopathy. Real-time MRI in cardiac short-axis, using ultrafast b-SSFP cine MRI technique (acquisition time per image 60 ms) during deep, forced in- and expiration. Four consecutive heart beats after onset of inspiration at the moment of early ventricular filling (a,b,c,d). In contrast to patients with constrictive pericarditis (see Fig. 11.25), the position and motion of the ventricular septum during early ventricular filling is minimally influenced by forced in- and expiration. In some patients, due to the increased stiffness, the respiratory variation in septal motion is even diminished compared with normals. This sign may be highly helpful in differentiating RCM patients from patients with constrictive pericarditis.

leaflets and myocardial vessels (RAHMAN et al. 2004). The clinical presentation varies and may mimic other infiltrative cardiomyopathies or storage disorders, as well as HCM (Figs. 9.17–19). Although the therapeutic means are limited and treatment is generally unsatisfactory, the diagnosis is important to exclude the potentially curable conditions that it may mimic.

Several findings have been described in cardiac amyloidosis. Although each finding alone is nonspecific, a combination of different findings makes the diagnosis of cardiac amyloidosis likely, especially in conjunction with a positive extramyocardial biopsy (SHIREY et al. 1980). Morphologically, the infiltration by amyloid protein results in a homogeneously increased thickness of ventricular and atrial walls. The ventricular cavities have a normal or reduced size. A severe concentric hypertrophy of both normal-sized ventricles in the absence of arterial hypertension or valvular heart disease is suggestive of amyloidosis (Fig. 9.19). The increase in myocardial wall thickness in cardiac amyloidosis may mimic HCM (SIQUEIRA-FILHO et al. 1981). Asymmetric septal hypertrophy is found in 15–55%

of cases of cardiac amyloidosis in combination with a systolic anterior motion of the mitral valve and early systolic closure of the aortic valve. Other morphological findings include thickening of the papillary muscles and valve leaflets (Fig. 9.18). The atria are usually enlarged owing to the diastolic dysfunction and/or valvular dysfunction due to amyloid deposition. Pleural and pericardial effusions are not infrequently seen (Fig. 9.18). The cardiac amyloid deposits generally cause severe cardiac dysfunction with a poor prognosis (SIVARAM et al. 1985), and it is generally considered that congestive heart failure is predominantly a diastolic phenomenon, with systolic dysfunction only occurring late in the disease (Fig. 9.17). Therefore, severe congestive heart failure often occurs despite a normal or mildly reduced LV ejection fraction. The diastolic dysfunction is characterized by an abnormal relaxation pattern and a restrictive pattern of transmitral valve flow in the advanced stage. However, differentiation from other restrictive cardiomyopathies is not feasible.

MRI has potential value for the diagnosis of cardiac amyloidosis (VON KEMP et al. 1989). Besides a morphological description of the cardiac abnor-

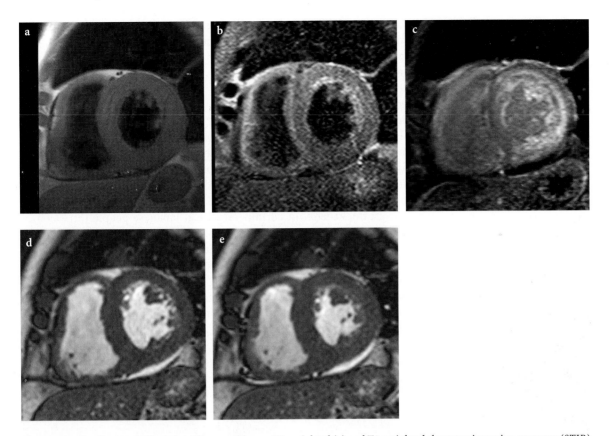

Fig. 9.17a–e. Cardiac amyloidosis in a 67-year-old man. T1-weighted (**a**) and T2-weighted short-tau inversion-recovery (STIR) (**b**) fast SE-MRI in the cardiac short-axis. CE-IR MRI with late imaging (**c**), and cine MRI, using the b-SSFP technique, at end diastole (**d**) and end systole (**e**) in the same imaging plane. Biventricular hypertrophy with moderate enlargement of both ventricles and severely reduced ventricular function (LV ejection fraction, 25%; RV ejection fraction, 26%). While the signal characteristics do not show abnormalities on T1-weighted and T2-weighted-STIR MRI (**a, b**), a strong, inhomogeneous myocardial enhancement is found on CE-IR MRI, mainly involving the anterior, lateral and inferior segments.

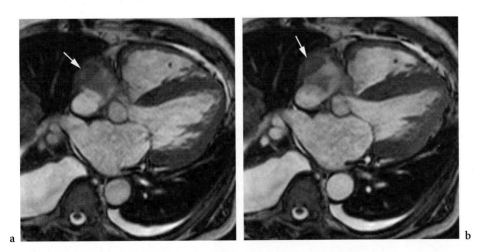

Fig. 9.18a,b. Cardiac amyloidosis in a 67-year-old man (same patient as in Fig. 9.17). Cine MRI, using the b-SSFP technique, in the horizontal long-axis plane at end diastole (**a**) and end systole (**b**). The biventricular wall thickening can be clearly seen, as well as the diminished ventricular function. The mitral valve leaflets are thickened, and there is a mild-to-moderate mitral regurgitation. Note the presence of a large thrombus in a dilated right atrial appendage (not detected on transthoracic ultrasound; *arrow*), as well as the presence of a bilateral pleural effusion and a small pericardial effusion.

malities, and assessment of systolic and diastolic dysfunction, it can provide information on the macroscopic changes of tissue composition and so can be helpful in the differential diagnosis with idiopathic RCM (CELLETTI et al. 1999). CELLETTI et al. have detected an inhomogeneously decreased signal intensity of the myocardium using SE-MRI in patients with cardiac amyloidosis, but not in patients with idiopathic RCM (CELLETTI et al. 1999), similar to the granular myocardial appearance on echocardiography. This group considers a combination of a thickened atrial septum and right atrial free wall, and depressed contractility of a thickened myocardium with inhomogeneous reduction of the signal-intensity ratio highly suggestive of cardiac amyloidosis (CELLETTI et al. 1999). A role for CE-IR MRI with delayed imaging in assessing patients with cardiac amyloidosis has not yet been established. Preliminary results in a small number of patients suggest strong, inhomogeneous enhancement with

a pattern different from that seen in patients with HCM (unpublished data; Figs. 9.17 and 9.19).

9.4.4.2
Sarcoidosis

Sarcoidosis is a multisystem granulomatous disorder of unknown aetiology. Although disease affects the hilar lymph nodes and the lungs most commonly, all parts of the body can be affected. Sarcoid myocardial involvement is present at autopsy in 20–30%, with higher incidences up to 50% in certain races, e.g. Japanese people (SILVERMAN et al. 1978; VIRMANI et al. 1980). The pathological features of cardiac sarcoidosis include patchy infiltration of the myocardium with three successive histological stages: oedema, non-caseating epitheloid granulomatous infiltration, and fibrosis leading to postinflammatory scarring (VIGNAUX et al. 2002b; Figs. 9.20–22). The clinical manifestations depend

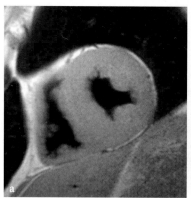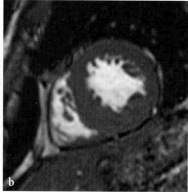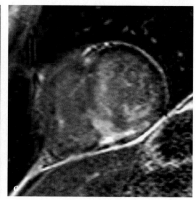

Fig. 9.19a-c. Cardiac amyloidosis in a 71-year-old man. T1-weighted fast SE-MRI (**a**), cine MRI using the b-SSFP technique (**b**) and CE-IR MRI with late imaging (**c**) in the cardiac short-axis at mid-ventricular level. Severe concentric hypertrophy, most pronounced in the septum (end-diastolic wall thickness of 26 mm). Global LV function: end-diastolic volume 134 ml, end-systolic volume 47 ml, stroke volume 87 ml, ejection fraction 65%, and LV mass 240 g. Similar to the patient in Fig. 9.17, a strong, inhomogeneous enhancement is found circumferentially involving the subendocardium, with strong enhancement in the subepicardial and mid-wall layers in the inferoseptal LV wall (**c**).

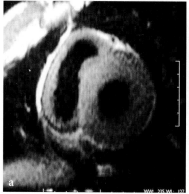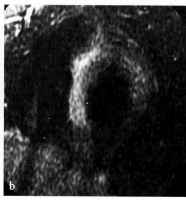

Fig. 9.20a,b. Active cardiac sarcoidosis. T1-weighted, and T2-weighted STIR SE-MRI in the cardiac short-axis. Thickening of the LV wall most pronounced in the ventricular septum, showing a hyperintense appearance (oedema) on T2-weighted STIR MRI (**b**). (Courtesy of Olivier Vignaux, Paris, France.)

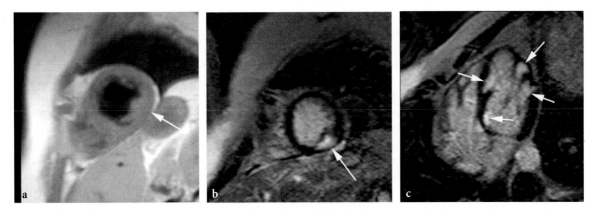

Fig. 9.21a-c. Cardiac sarcoidosis in a 41-year-old woman presenting with asymptomatic atrioventricular block. **a** T1-weighted fast SE-MRI. CE-IR MRI with late imaging in the cardiac short-axis (**b**) (same level as **a**) and horizontal long-axis (**c**). Moderate thickening of the infero-lateral LV wall is visible on SE-MRI (*arrow*) (**a**). In this area, a focal strong enhancement is found with a thin, non-enhancing subendocardial and subepicardial rim (*arrow*) (**b**). In the horizontal long-axis view, several areas of strong enhancement are found throughout the LV wall, probably representing several non-caseating granulomas. Splenic biopsy in this patient revealed non-caseating granulomas. (From BOGAERT et al. (2004). Reprinted with permission from American Roentgen Ray Society.)

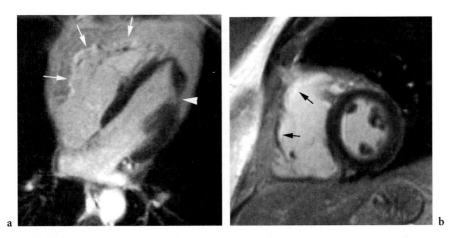

Fig. 9.22a,b. Cardiac sarcoidosis in a 48-year-old man. CE-IR MRI with late imaging in the axial plane (**a**) and short-axis plane (**b**). Strong enhancement (*arrows*) of the RV free wall showing a diffuse hypokinetic to akinetic contraction pattern on cine MRI (not shown). Reduced global RV function (ejection fraction less than 35%). Focal thinning and scarring of the apicolateral LV wall, showing enhancement on late imaging (*arrowhead*). Taking into account a history of pulmonary sarcoidosis, the above findings strongly suggest old (healed?) sarcoidosis with scarring and fibrotic replacement. The RV abnormalities are not pathognomonic for sarcoidosis but can also been in arrhythmogenic right ventricular dysplasia.

on the location and extent of granulomatous inflammation, and signs range from benign arrhythmias, heart block, intractable heart failure, intense chest pain and congestive heart failure to fatal ventricular fibrillation (SHARMA 2003). Although the incidence of myocardial infiltration at autopsy is high, only 5% of patients with cardiac sarcoidosis are symptomatic. Though most patients experience a subclinical, asymptomatic course of the disease, there is a clear increased risk of sudden cardiac death, due to ventricular arrhythmias or conduction block, accounting for 30–65% of fatalities.

Cardiac involvement may proceed, follow or occur simultaneously with the involvement of the lungs or other organs. If cardiac manifestation occurs in a patient with multi-system sarcoidosis, the diagnosis is relatively clear. However, in patients where cardiac dysfunction is the sole manifestation of sarcoidosis, the diagnosis is often challenging. Early diagnosis and effective treatment (e.g. aggressive use of corticosteroids, immunosuppressive and immune modulator therapy, automatic implantable defibrillator) in patients at risk are absolutely necessary to improve the long-term prognosis. The diagnosis of myocardial sarcoidosis is difficult and frustrating. Because of the focal myocardial involvement of cardiac sarcoidosis, endomyocardial biopsy yields low sensitivity values (as low as 20%). Most non-invasive diagnostic techniques have a low sensitivity and specificity. The findings on ECG and echocardiography, usually do not allow establishment of the diagnosis of cardiac sarcoidosis. The role of radionuclide techniques (^{201}Tl imaging, ^{67}Ga scanning and ^{123}I-meta-iodobenzyl-guanidine) is unclear and is limited by poor spatial resolution. Fibrogranulomatous lesions of the myocardium are seen as segmental areas of decreased ^{201}Tl uptake, often disappearing or decreasing in size during stress (so-called reverse distribution defects). In the presence of healthy coronary arteries, perfusion defects on ^{201}Tl imaging in a patient with known multi-system sarcoidosis strongly suggests cardiac involvement. A normal finding on ^{201}Tl imaging; however, does not exclude the presence of cardiac involvement. A combination of ^{201}Tl imaging and ^{67}Ga scanning has been reported to provide more information, but their value as a screening technique has not been established (SHARMA 2003). Recently, ^{13}N-NH$_3$/^{18}F-FDG positron-emission tomography (PET) has been used for the identification of cardiac involvement and for the assessment of cardiac sarcoidosis disease activity (YAMAGISHI et al. 2003). Myocardial abnormalities were seen as areas of decreased ^{13}N-NH$_3$ uptake (usually in the basal anteroseptal wall), or areas of increased ^{18}F-FDG uptake (usually basal-mid anteroseptal and lateral). After corticosteroid treatment, the areas of decreased ^{13}N-NH$_3$ uptake remained unchanged while the areas of increased ^{18}F-FDG uptake diminished in size and intensity or completely disappeared.

Several studies have reported promising results for MRI in the (early) diagnosis of cardiac sarcoidosis and monitoring of the disease response to treatment (DUPUIS et al. 1994; CHANDRA et al. 1996a; SCHULZ-MENGER et al. 2000b; MATSUKI and MATSUO 2000; SHIMADA et al. 2001; VIGNAUX et al. 2002a, 2002b, 2004). Although these studies are single-centre studies, often lacking correlation of MRI features with myocardial histology, the study results clearly call for a large multi-centre trial (SHARMA 2003). The imaging protocol in patients with suspected cardiac sarcoidosis should consist of a combination of T1-weighted TSE sequences before and after administration of gadolinium-DTPA, T2-(STIR)-weighted TSE sequences, CE-IR MRI with delayed imaging, and cine MRI using the new b-SSFP techniques. This approach allows depiction of the myocardial morphological abnormalities (T1-weighted TSE and cine MRI); as-

sessment of myocardial oedema (T2-STIR-weighted TSE); depiction of myocardial inflammation, necrosis and scar formation (CE-IR MRI); and assessment of the impact on regional and global function (cine MRI). Vignaux et al. have described three different MRI patterns of myocardial sarcoidosis (VIGNAUX et al. 2002a, 2002b): (1) the pure nodular pattern with a peripheral increased and a central decreased intramyocardial signal intensity on both T2-weighted and gadolinium-DTPA-enhanced T1-weighted images (representing hyaline fibrotic tissue); (2) the inflammatory focal or patchy pattern, with increased signal on gadolinium-DTPA-enhanced T1-weighted images with or without myocardial thickening; and (3) the postinflammatory pattern with focal increased signal on T2-weighted images (but no gadolinium uptake) with or without myocardial thinning. In 54% of the patients with cardiac-asymptomatic, multiple-organ sarcoidosis, cardiac abnormalities were found similar to those observed in patients with cardiac symptoms (VIGNAUX et al. 2002a). Shimada et al. have reported frequent enhancement of the anteroseptal and anterolateral LV wall following gadolinium administration (SHIMADA et al. 2001). The location of the abnormalities on cardiac MRI may be useful to guide endomyocardial biopsy (to increase sensitivity). In addition, regional and global ventricular function can be simultaneously quantified and extracardiac signs of sarcoidosis, e.g. mediastinal and hilar adenopathy, can be imaged with MRI. Regression of myocardial gadolinium-DTPA enhancement is noticed early after steroid therapy (i.e. less than 6 months), while regression of increased signal intensity on T2-weighted images is delayed (i.e. more than 6 months; VIGNAUX et al. 2004). In non-responders (i.e. stable or progressive disease), MRI abnormalities remain stable or increase in severity and extent.

At present, several issues concerning the clinical value of MRI in the diagnosis of cardiac sarcoidosis remain unanswered (MANA 2002). For instance, the myocardial abnormalities on MRI in patients with cardiac sarcoidosis are non-specific and can be found in other myocardial disorders such as myocarditis (MAHRHOLDT et al. 2004). Moreover, because of lack of a true reference standard, the predictive value of a negative cardiac MRI study remains unknown. SMEDEMA et al. (2004) have reported a poor interobserver agreement on CE-IR MRI with delayed imaging in patients with sarcoidosis. Finally, use of MRI in the follow-up of patients with cardiac sarcoidosis is often impossible, since a significant number of patients with cardiac sarcoidosis receive an automatic implantable cardioverter defibrillator (AICD).

9.4.4.3
Iron-Overload Cardiomyopathy

Iron-overload cardiomyopathy is defined as the presence of systolic or diastolic cardiac dysfunction secondary to increased deposition of iron in the heart. This cardiac dysfunction is independent from other concomitant processes such as atherosclerosis, ischemia or valvular disease (LIU and OLIVIERI 1994). It can result from primary or secondary haemochromatosis, which is classically defined as iron overload in the parenchymal cells in tissues, e.g. iron deposition in the liver cells leading to cirrhosis or in the cardiac myocytes leading to heart failure. Primary haemochromatosis is an autosomal recessive disease affecting one in 220 persons and usually presents late in life. Secondary haemochromatosis is a common cause of mortality in the young adult population in the developed world. This is the result of the large population with hereditary anaemias such as thalassaemia or sickle cell anaemia. These patients require chronic red cell transfusion starting at a young age. However, one of the complications of this transfusion therapy is iron overload. Chelation therapy may delay or prevent the occurrence of iron-induced heart failure. Other conditions in which iron overload may occur in body organs include chronic alcoholism and chronic haemodialysis.

Initially, myocardial iron overload is totally asymptomatic. There is a mild increase in LV wall thickness and end-diastolic chamber diameter. Diastolic function abnormalities usually precede systolic function abnormalities and are characterized by a restrictive filling pattern (BENSON et al. 1989; LIU et al. 1993a). Global systolic function abnormalities usually do not appear until the iron concentration reaches a critical level, but then there is often a rapid deterioration in cardiac function. More subtle wall motion abnormalities; however, may represent an early sign of cardiac disease despite preserved global function. The regional abnormalities (e.g. longitudinal shortening) are related to iron overload and easily detectable with tissue Doppler echocardiography (VOGEL et al. 2003).

MRI can be used to identify the presence of iron in the heart and to quantitate the iron levels from the image signal intensity or the calculated T2 relaxation time (CHAN et al. 1992). MRI has the potential to non-invasively evaluate myocardial iron during iron chelation therapy, since repeated endomyocardial biopsy is not feasible, due to the heterogeneity of iron distribution and the risk of complications (JENSEN et al. 2003). The availability of a non-invasive technique to quantitate myocardial iron is important because there is no significant relationship between the myocardial iron concentration and the different iron store parameters, nor with the liver iron concentration (ANDERSON et al. 2001). Imaging with MR is based on the differences in signal intensity among tissues with intrinsically different relaxation parameters in a homogeneous magnetic field. The presence of iron disturbs the magnetic field homogeneity and enhances tissue T2 relaxation. MRI techniques that are sensitive to tissue T2 changes will be able to detect a marked decrease in signal intensity on T2-weighted images (STARK et al. 1985; HARDY and HENKELMAN 1989; WESTWOOD et al. 2003a). The myocardial MRI iron concentrations demonstrate a significant positive correlation with the number of blood units given (LESNEFSKY et al. 1992; JENSEN et al. 2001). The T2 relaxation time is the best independent parameter to detect the iron content directly in the heart and so predict cardiac complications, and can be used for monitoring therapy (LIU et al. 1993b). Early intensification of iron chelation therapy, guided by this technique, should reduce mortality from this reversible cardiomyopathy (ANDERSON et al. 2001). Practically, use of a single breath-hold, multi-echo acquisition allows a reliable quantification of myocardial T2* (ANDERSON et al. 2001; WESTWOOD et al. 2003a). This fast technique has a good reproducibility (also between different MRI vendors; WESTWOOD et al. 2003a, 2003b). A single short-axis, mid-ventricular slice is acquired at nine separate echo times (5.6–18.0 ms), using a spoiled gradient-echo sequence. An alternative sequence is a T2*-weighted GRASE sequence (using a TSE factor of 7, and an echoplanar imaging, EPI, factor of 3), obtaining six echo-times (10, 20, 30, 40, 50, 60 ms) in a single breath-hold (Fig. 9.23). Myocardial signal intensities are measured in the ventricular septum for each image and then plotted against the echo time to form an exponential decay curve. To derive T2*, an exponential trend-line is fitted with an equation in the form $y=Ke^{-TE/T2^*}$, where K represents a constant (WESTWOOD et al. 2003a; Fig. 9.23). The range of echo times allows accurate quantification of T2* values in severe iron overload and provides good sensitivity at low tissue iron levels. Normal values for the T2* of myocardium at 1.5 T field strength are 33.3±7.8 ms, with lower limits (mean −2SD) 17.7 ms. In patients with myocardial iron overload, T2* values are typically below 20 ms (range of clinical interest: 5–20 ms).

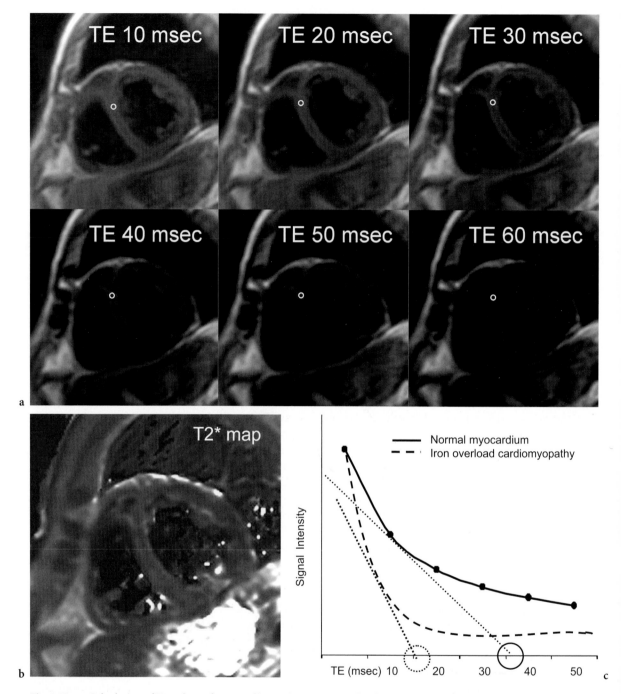

Fig. 9.23a-c. Calculation of T2-values of myocardium using a T2*-weighted GRASE sequence. Within a single breath-hold, a short-axis image is obtained with six different echo times (10–60 ms) (**a**), yielding a T2* map (**b**). The signal intensity is measured within a small area of interest in the ventricular septum and plotted against echo time. The signal decay is exponential, and the intercept with the x-axis provides the T2-value of myocardium (**c**). Normal T2-values for myocardium are greater than 20 ms.

9.4.4.4
Endomyocardial Disease
(Löffler Endocarditis and Endomyocardial Fibrosis)

Endomyocardial disease is a common form of secondary RCM and includes Löffler endocarditis and endomyocardial fibrosis (PARRILLO 1990). Although they were previously thought to be two variants of a single disease, these entities have not only a different geographical distribution but also a different clinical presentation. Löffler endocarditis occurs in temperate countries, has a more aggressive and rapidly progressive course, and is related to hypereosinophilia, while endomyocardial fibrosis occurs most commonly in equatorial Africa and is not related to hypereosinophilia. The restrictive pattern is caused by an intensive endocardial fibrotic wall thickening of the apex and subvalvular

regions of one or both ventricles, resulting in an inflow obstruction of blood (Fig. 9.24). The underlying pathogenesis of Löffler endocarditis is complex and probably related to hypereosinophilia, with a toxic effect of eosinophils on the heart causing necrosis, endomyocarditis and formation of intramyocardial thrombi (Fig. 9.25; WELLER and BUBLEY 1994). In the later phase, localized or extensive replacement fibrosis causes thickening of the ventricular wall. Atrioventricular valve regurgitation, as a result of progressive scarring of the chordae tendinae, may occur, with enlargement of the atria. The increased stiffness of the ventricles and the reduction of the ventricular cavity by organized thrombus cause a restrictive filling pattern. MRI is helpful in the diagnosis of endomyocardial disease and in the evaluation of effects of medical treatment (D'SILVA et al. 1992; LOMBARDI et al. 1995; CHANDRA et al.

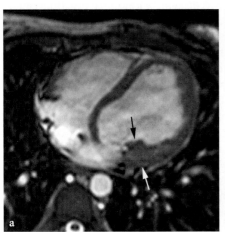
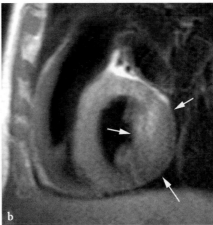

Fig. 9.24a,b. Löffler endocarditis. Cine MRI, using b-SSFP technique, in horizontal long-axis view (**a**); T1-weighted fast SE-MRI in cardiac short-axis view at basal level (**b**). Important thickening of the laterobasal part of the left ventricle extending to the posterior leaflet of the mitral valve, involving the subvalvular apparatus with secondary mitral regurgitation.

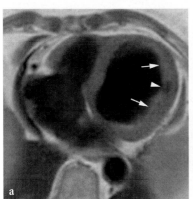
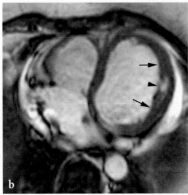
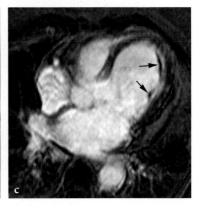

Fig. 9.25a-c. Comprehensive use of MRI sequences in Löffler endocarditis in a 71-year-old woman presenting with restrictive heart disease and hypereosinophilia. Horizontal long-axis view using T1-weighted fast SE-MRI (**a**), cine MRI (b-SSFP technique) (**b**), and CE-IR MRI technique with late imaging (**c**). Global thickening of the lateral LV wall (*arrows*) with false impression of focal abscedation (*arrowhead*) on SE-MRI and cine MRI (**a,b**). CE-IR MRI, however, allows discrimination of mural thrombus (*arrows*) from adjacent myocardium (**c**).

1996b; Pitt et al. 1996; Huong et al. 1997). Areas of myocardial fibrosis appear as areas of low signal intensity. The right, left or both ventricular walls are grossly thickened, with subsequent narrowing of the ventricular cavities. Ventricular volumes and atrioventricular regurgitation can be accurately quantified. CE-IR MRI with late imaging is recommended to differentiate mural thrombus from thickened myocardium (Fig. 9.26).

9.4.4.5
Metabolic Storage Diseases

Cardiac involvement in metabolic storage diseases such as type I or II glycogenosis, Anderson-Fabry, Gaucher and Neimann-Pick diseases, galactosialidosis and mucopolysaccharidosis is characterized by LV wall thickening, valvular involvement, and LV diastolic dysfunction, with often normal LV systolic function. The LV wall thickening may even mimic HCM with or without obstruction of the LV outflow (Fig. 9.27). In clinical practice, M-mode, two-dimensional and Doppler echocardiography are used for the determination of LV wall thickness, systolic function, anatomical derangement, valvular dysfunction and LV diastolic function; the role of MRI remains to be established (Senocak et al. 1994). CE-IR MRI with delayed imaging might have a role in further characterizing the myocardial abnormalities (Moon et al. 2003b, 2003c). In a recent paper, Moon et al. have reported abnormal enhancement in the basal infero-lateral LV wall in patients with Anderson-Fabry disease, with a distribution pattern that is not, unlike myocardial infarction, subendocardial (Fig. 9.28). This X-linked disorder of sphingolipid metabolism causes an idiopathic LV hypertrophy, but the mechanism of hypertrophy is poorly understood. While it is generally believed that the deposition of glycosphingolipid is within the myocytes, the abnormal enhancement strongly suggests concomitant presence of myocardial fibrosis.

9.4.4.6
Friedreich's Ataxia

Friedreich's ataxia is a neurodegenerative disease characterized by progressive limb and gait ataxia, areflexia, and pyramidal signs in the legs. This automosal recessive disorder is often associated with HCM (concentric or asymmetric), which may progress towards a DCM (Fig. 9.29). The underlying mechanism that triggers HCM is the production of frataxin. It is suggested that this protein, of unknown function, causes oxidative stress or respiratory chain dysfunction. It has been shown that Idebenone, a potent free-radical scavanger, may protect the myocardium against this oxidative stress and thus be effective at controlling cardiac hypertrophy in Friedreich's ataxia. Recently, a reduction in LV mass was reported in Friedreich's ataxia patients after 6 months of Idebenone treatment (Hausse et al. 2002). Though LV mass calculations in this study were performed with echocardiography, MRI has the advantage of being a more accurate and highly reproducible technique for wall mass calculations and should be recommended to perform these kind of repeat follow-up studies.

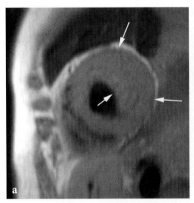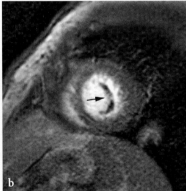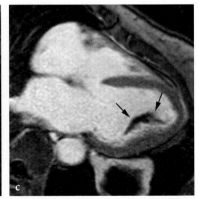

Fig. 9.26a-c. Löffler endocarditis in a 72-year-old woman with hypereosinophilia and restrictive filling pattern. Echocardiography showed extensive lateral wall thickening. **a** Short-axis, T1-weighted fast SE-MRI. CE-IR MRI with late imaging in cardiac short-axis (**b**), and horizontal long-axis view (**c**). SE-MRI shows extensive lateral wall thickening (*arrows*) with otherwise homogeneous signal. On CE-IR MRI, however, it is clearly visible that the extensive wall thickening consists of a thickened lateral wall and a mural thrombus, visible as a dark structure adjacent to the thickened myocardium (*arrow*). The long-axis views show that the abnormalities are most pronounced in the mid-third of the lateral LV wall (*arrows*). (From Bogaert et al. (2004). Reprinted with permission from the American Roentgen Ray Society.)

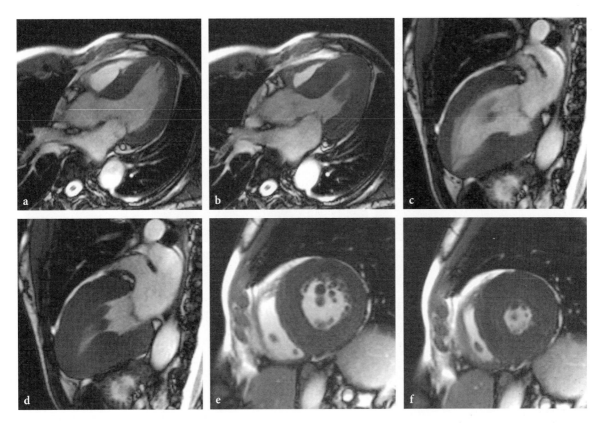

Fig. 9.27a-f. Anderson-Fabry's disease in a 46-year-old man. Cine MRI, using the b-SSFP technique, in the horizontal long-axis (**a, b**), vertical long-axis (**c, d**) and short-axis (**e, f**) at end diastole and end systole, respectively. Severe concentric LV hypertrophy (LV mass, 315 g). Although global LV function is within normal limits, the regional function (wall thickening) is clearly diminished.

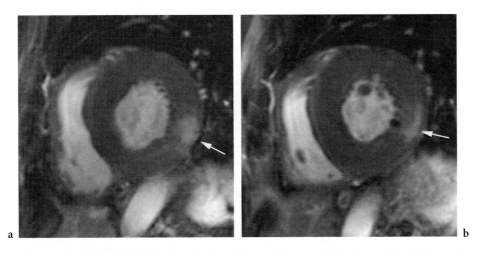

Fig. 9.28a,b. CE-IR MRI with late imaging in a 46-year-old man with Anderson-Fabry's disease (same patient as in Fig. 9.27). Two adjacent short-axis levels. Concentric LV hypertrophy with focal zone of abnormal late enhancement subepicardially in the infero-lateral LV wall (*arrow*).

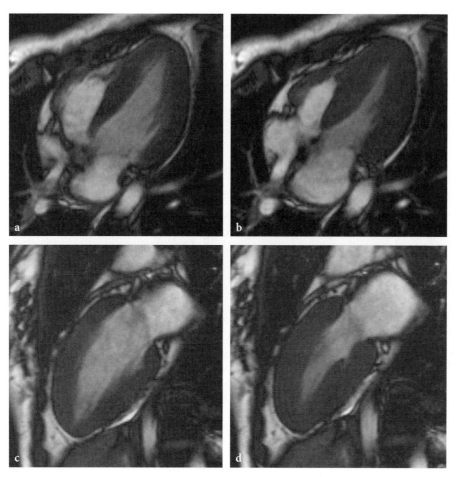

Fig. 9.29a-d. Concentric LV hypertrophy in a 22-year-old woman with Friedreichs ataxia. Cine MRI, using b-SSFP technique, in horizontal (**a, b**) and vertical long-axis (**c, d**) view at end diastole and end systole, respectively. The myocardial hypertrophy is equally spread throughout all wall segments. Maximal wall thickness at end diastole (17 mm).

9.4.5
Arrhythmogenic Right Ventricular Cardiomyopathy/Dysplasia

Arrhythmogenic right ventricular cardiomyopathy (ARVC) or dysplasia (ARVD), first described in 1977, is a heart muscle disease, characterized by structural and functional abnormalities of the right ventricle due to replacement of the myocardium by fatty and fibrous tissue, with electrical instability that precipitates ventricular arrhythmias and sudden cardiac death (BLAKE et al. 1994; FONTAINE et al. 1998; CORRADO et al. 2000; GEMAYEL et al. 2001). This disorder is often familial in origin (30–50% of cases), with both autosomal dominant and autosomal recessive (Naxos disease) inheritance patterns (FONTAINE et al. 1998; FERRARI and SCOTT 2003). The mean age of patients when symptoms arise is 30 years, and the symptoms frequently occur during exercise. This entity can result in recurrent ventricular tachyarrhythmias of RV origin (left bundle branch morphology characteristics) and must be distinguished from exercise-induced automatic ventricular tachycardias originating from the RV outflow tract in patients with normal RV anatomy. The risk of sudden cardiac death in ARVD is substantial, whereas it appears to be negligible in patients with RV outflow tract tachycardia. ARVD remains an enigmatic disease and the diagnosis of ARVD is often challenging, especially at its early stages. Minor and major diagnostic criteria for ARVD have been proposed by the Task Force of the Working Group on Cardiomyopathies (MCKENNA et al. 1994). These criteria encompass structural, histological, electrocardiographic, arrhythmic and genetic factors (Table 9.4). On the basis of this classification, diagnosis of ARVD is fulfilled in the presence of two major criteria, one major plus two minor criteria, or four minor criteria from different groups.

At histological examination, an inflammatory infiltrate with necrosis and fibroadipose replacement is found (BURKE et al. 1998). Although initially regarded as a partial or complete congenital absence of ventricular myocardium, there is convincing clini-

Table 9.4. Criteria for ARVC/D. Adapted from CORRADO et al. (2000)

1. Family History
   - Major: familial history confirmed at necropsy /surgery
   - Minor: - familial history of sudden death (<35 yr of age) due to suspected ARVD/C
            - familial history (clinical diagnosis based on present criteria)

2. ECG depolarization/conduction abnormalities
   - Major : epsilon waves or localized prolongation (> 110 ms) of QRS complex right precordial leads (V1-V3)
   - Minor: late potentials on signal averaged ECG

3. ECG repolarization abnormalities
   - Minor: inverted T-waves in right precordial leads (V2 and V3) in people > 12 years of age in absence of right bundle branch block

4. Arrhythmias (minor)
   - Sustained or nonstained left bundle branch block-type ventricular tachycardia documented on ECG or Holter monitoring or during exercise
   - Frequent ventricular extrasystoles (> 1000/24h on Holter monitoring)

5. Global or regional dysfunction and structural alterations
   - Major: - severe dilatation and reduction of RV ejection fraction with no or minor LV involvement
            - localized RV aneurysms
            - akinetic or dyskinetic areas with diastolic bulging
            - severe segmental dilatation of RV
   - Minor: - mild global RV dilatation or ejection fraction reduction with normal LV.
            - mild segmental dilatation of RV
            - regional RV hypokinesia

6. Tissue characteristics of walls
   - Major: fibrofatty replacement of myocardium on endomyocardial biopsy

cal and pathological evidence that it is an acquired disorder with a continuous, chronic process of injury and repair (ANGELINI et al. 1996). Replacement of the RV myocardium by fibrofatty tissue has been related to three different mechanisms: (1) apoptosis (or programmed cell death); (2) inflammatory heart disease; (3) myocardial dystrophy (BASSO et al. 1996; MALLAT et al. 1996; CORRADO et al. 2000). In ARVD, the fibrous-fatty replacement almost exclusively involves the RV anterolateral or free wall ("triangle of dysplasia": inflow, apical part, outflow); involvement of the septum and left ventricle is much less frequent. In a later phase, focal or diffuse thinning is noticed with bulging of the ventricular wall. Functionally, the involved regions demonstrate akinetic or dyskinetic wall motion. This fibrofatty

replacement, with a high tendency for arrhythmias, should be differentiated from for the purely fatty replacement, which has a much more benign course. Although RV endomyocardial biopsy has the potential for in vivo demonstration of fibrofatty replacement of the RV myocardium, the sensitivity of this test is low because, for reasons of safety, samples are usually taken from the ventricular septum, a region uncommonly involved in ARVD. Moreover, the test is invasive and carries a risk of perforation and tamponade.

The clinical presentation of ARVD is highly variable. It is generally considered that this disorder is a progressive disease. The natural history and presentation is a function of both cardiac electrical instability and progressive ventricular dysfunction. At present, four different clinicopathological phases should be considered:

1. A concealed phase, characterized by subtle RV structural changes, with or without minor ventricular arrhythmias, during which sudden cardiac death may occasionally be the first manifestation of the disease (mostly in young people during competitive sports or intense physical exercise)
2. An overt electrical disorder, in which symptomatic RV arrhythmias (that may cause cardiac arrest) are associated with overt RV functional and structural abnormalities
3. RV failure due to progression and extension of RV muscle disease
4. Biventricular pump failure due to significant LV involvement

The contribution of MRI to the diagnosis of AVRD relies on the demonstration of intramyocardial adipose deposits, morphological wall thickening and thinning, abnormal wall motion, detection of myocardial inflammation and fibrosis (as recently described by several groups), and abnormal global ventricular function. Whereas angiocardiography and echocardiography are able to depict only focal or diffuse ventricular bulging, MRI has the capability to relate the functional wall abnormalities directly to the underlying morphological wall changes.

A – Detection of Intramyocardial Adipose Deposits
One of the main advantages of MRI is the combination of high contrast resolution with an excellent spatial resolution. Adipose tissue has a high signal intensity on T1-weighted images and stands in clear contrast to the intermediate signal intensity of the myocardium (CASOLO et al. 1987; MENGHETTI et al.

1996; Midiri et al. 1997; see also Fig. 9.1). Detailed MR images of the RV anterolateral wall should allow detection of small, intramyocardial fatty deposits. At present, the optimal spin-echo technique to use and the way to position patients and surface coils is still matter of discussion. A generally accepted, but patient-unfriendly approach to study the free wall of the right ventricle is to position the subject in the prone position and to use a surface coil over the precordium (Blake et al. 1994; Abbara et al. 2004a). In order to maximize the spatial resolution of the RV free wall, a small field of view needs to be used, e.g. 120–140 mm. Flow signal artefact, displayed in the phase-encoding direction, can produce factitious bright signal foci in the free wall of the right ventricle. Therefore, double saturation bands placed behind the free wall will suppress flow artefacts from the ventricular blood pool. Although most studies favour the use of the double-inversion fast spin-echo MR sequence obtained in breath-hold, yielding a superior suppression of the blood signal in the cardiac cavities (Tandri et al. 2003, Castillo et al. 2004), other studies still prefer the conventional spin-echo techniques with multiple excitations obtained in free-breathing (Abbara et al. 2004a,b). Tung et al. (2004) have found better results when using a larger distance between the RV anterolateral wall and surface coil. For an optimal depiction of intramyocardial fat, a thin slice thickness, i.e. 5 mm, is recommended, with an interslice distance of 5 mm (Castillo et al. 2004). A combination of axial and cardiac short-axis images ensures optimal coverage of the right ventricle. Some groups use fat-suppression techniques in combination with spin-echo imaging to confirm fatty infiltration (Aviram et al. 2003). A combination of fat-suppressed and non-fat-suppressed techniques increases the interobserver agreement and confidence in the diagnosis (Abbara et al. 2003; see also Fig. 9.1).

Despite the theoretical superiority of MRI to other imaging techniques for detecting intramyocardial fat, detection of signal changes within the myocardium is very much dependent on image quality (Fig. 9.30). This is particularly true for patients in whom arrhythmias occur during MR examination. Neither the specificity nor sensitivity of MRI for depiction of intramyocardial fat are known. As mentioned above, endomyocardial biopsy is not reliable as a reference technique. Detection of intramyocardial fat in a thin RV free wall (2.7±0.4 mm, and only 1.9±1.1 mm at the anterior RV apex) and differentiation from the adjacent epicardial fat is challenging (Fig. 9.31). Moreover, the presence of intramyo-

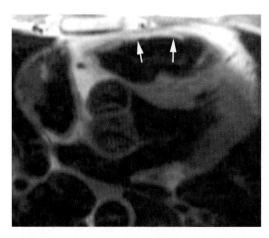

Fig. 9.30. Arrhythmogenic right ventricular dysplasia? Axial, T1-weighted fast SE-MRI obtained with the patient in prone position. Is there fatty infiltration of the RV free wall (*arrows*)? No, the (sub)epicardial fat between the thin RV free wall and the pericardial sac gives a false impression of fatty infiltration. In addition, there was no bulging or evidence of abnormal wall motion on cine MRI in this case (not shown).

cardial fat is not pathognomic for the diagnosis of ARVD. Presence of intramyocardial fat is not an infrequent feature in normal hearts, especially in the anteroapical region (Burke et al. 1998), and a benign, fatty type of RV dysplasia without inflammation and fibrosis has been described. Morphological and functional abnormalities are also found in patients with RV arrhythmia in the absence of ARVD, i.e. so-called idiopathic RV outflow tract tachycardia (Carlson et al. 1994; Globits et al. 1997; Proclemer et al. 1997; White et al. 1998). These abnormalities include fixed wall thinning, fatty myocardial infiltration and local bulging, most often limited to the RV free wall. In contrast to the regional morphological and functional abnormalities, these patients have normal RV volumes and function. It is not yet clear whether this disorder can be considered as a forme fruste of ARVD. In a recent study by Bluemke and colleagues, detection of intramyocardial fat deposits with MRI was found not to be a reliable parameter in the diagnosis of ARVD (Bluemke et al. 2003). As a rule of thumb, the presence or absence of myocardial fat and other morphological abnormalities should always be regarded and interpreted in combination with the functional studies (Aviram et al. 2003; Fig. 9.31).

B – Detection of Myocardial Inflammation and Fibrosis

Since myocardial inflammatory infiltration and fibrosis are two main features of ARVD, their detec-

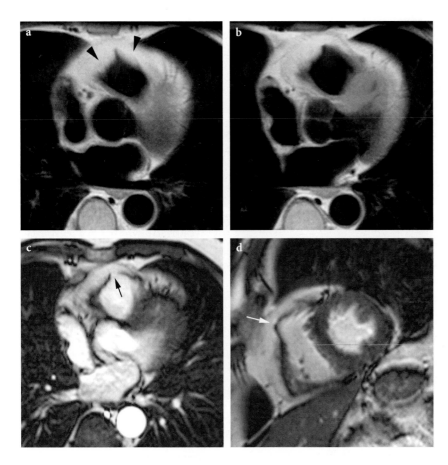

Fig. 9.31a-d. Arrhythmogenic right ventricular dysplasia in a 53-year-old man. Axial, T1-weighted, fast SE-MRI through RV outflow tract – RV free wall (**a, b**). Cine MRI, using the b-SSFP technique, in the axial (**c**) and in the short-axis plane (**d**). Complete fatty replacement of the anterolateral RV wall by fat (*arrowheads*), showing a focal bulging with akinesia to dyskinesia on cine MRI (*arrow*). The hypointense line on b-SSFP cine MRI at the anterolateral RV wall is most likely caused by chemical-shift artefacts at the fluid–fat interface.

tion might contribute to a more accurate diagnosis of ARVD. With the new CE-IR MRI sequences, superior contrast between normal and pathological myocardium can be achieved. This sequence has rapidly become the MRI sequence of choice for studying the presence and extent of myocardial necrosis and scarring in patients with previous myocardial infarction and other myocardial diseases such as myocarditis. Several groups have recently evaluated the role of CE-IR MRI in patients with suspected ARVD (HUNOLD et al. 2004; KLEM et al. 2004; PETRIZ et al. 2004; TANDRI et al. 2004; Fig. 9.32). Tandri et al. have found a good agreement between the presence of the fibrosis on histopathology and delayed enhancement on MRI in patients with ARVD (TANDRI et al. 2004). None of the patients without the diagnosis of ARVD show delayed enhancement. Similar results have been found by the other groups. Although the initial results are promising, since it has been shown that late myocardial enhancement is non-specific phenomenon, occurring in a variety of diseases (myocarditis, sarcoidosis), the precise role of CE-IR-MRI in the diagnosis of ARVD needs to be established (BOGAERT et al. 2004).

C – Detection of Wall Thickening and Thinning

The fibrofatty replacement of the RV anterolateral wall leads to a series of morphological abnormalities that can be used in the diagnosis of ARVD. Heavily fatty infiltration leads to wall hypertrophy (>8 mm wall thickness) with trabecular disarray (densely trabeculated RV with 6-11-mm-thick Y-shaped trabeculae; TANDRI et al. 2003; Fig. 9.33). Hypertrophy of the moderator band has been reported too. The later fibrotic stages with segmental loss of myocytes lead to extreme wall thinning (<2 mm wall thickness), with single or multiple aneurysm formation or outpouching of the RV wall (Fig. 9.31). Together with computed tomography (CT), MRI is the best technique to quantify exact wall thickness (HAMADA et al. 1993).

D – Assessment of Regional and Global Ventricular Function

Detailed analysis of regional ventricular function, i.e. wall motion, as well as wall thickening, and accurate quantification of global ventricular function with current b-SSFP cine MRI techniques allows evaluation of the impact of the fibrofatty myocar-

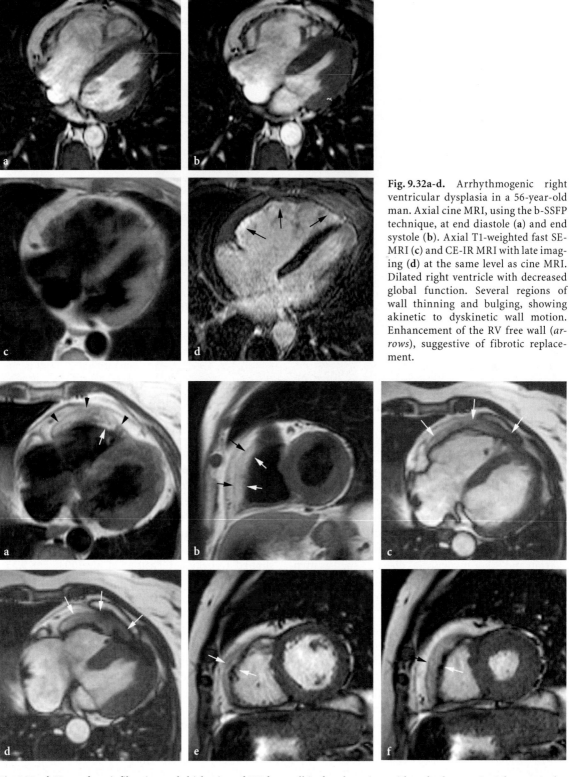

Fig. 9.32a-d. Arrhythmogenic right ventricular dysplasia in a 56-year-old man. Axial cine MRI, using the b-SSFP technique, at end diastole (a) and end systole (b). Axial T1-weighted fast SE-MRI (c) and CE-IR MRI with late imaging (d) at the same level as cine MRI. Dilated right ventricle with decreased global function. Several regions of wall thinning and bulging, showing akinetic to dyskinetic wall motion. Enhancement of the RV free wall (arrows), suggestive of fibrotic replacement.

Fig. 9.33a-f. Heavy fatty infiltration and thickening of RV free wall in female patient with arrhythmogenic right ventricular dysplasia. T1-weighted fast SE-MRI axial (a) and in short-axis (b). Cine MRI, using the b-SSFP technique, in the axial plane (c, d) and short-axis plane (e, f) at end diastole and end systole, respectively. Important thickening of the RV free wall (thickness 7–10 mm; arrows-arrowheads). The RV free wall has a mixed, hyperintense signal intensity, though clearly less hyperintense than the adjacent epicardial fat. Note that the contractility is well preserved. (Courtesy of Ilse Crevits, Roeselare, Belgium.)

dial changes on RV and, eventually also, LV function (Figs. 9.34 and 9.35). The dysfunctional areas are typically located in the RV free wall, the apex and the inflow and outflow tracts, and range from patchy areas to a more uniform and extensive involvement that correlate well with areas of abnormally low amplitude on intracardiac electrograms (BOULOS et al. 2001). Most studies report larger RV volumes and lower RV ejection fractions in patients with ARVD (FERRARI and SCOTT 2003), though it should be noted that, in the early phases of ARVD, global RV function is expected to be within normal limits. Besides, diastolic dysfunction has also been reported in patients with ARVD (KAYSER et al. 2003; MIGRINO et al. 2004).

As mentioned above, other disorders might also lead to morphological and functional abnormalities of the right ventricle (with or without involvement of the left ventricle). Uhl's anomaly of the right ventricle is an unusual, congenital cardiac disorder with almost complete absence of right ventricular myocardium, normal tricuspid valve, and preserved septal and LV myocardium (UHL 1952; GREER et al. 2000). Since structural and functional heart abnormalities quite similar to those in ARVD have been reported by several groups in patients with idiopathic RV outflow tract tachycardia, further study is warranted to better discriminate both disorders using structural and functional criteria. Other disorders that may mimic ARVD on MRI include myocarditis, idiopathic DCM and cor adiposum.

9.4.6
Non-compaction of the Myocardium (Non-compaction Cardiomyopathy)

Non-compaction of the myocardium is considered a distinct cardiomyopathy, which has been categorized as unclassified, congenital cardiomyopathy by the WHO – International Society and Federation of Cardiology task force, in 1995 (RICHARDSON et

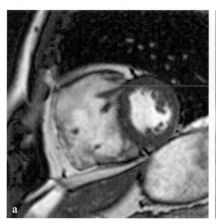
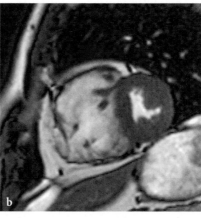

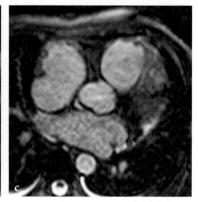

Fig. 9.34a,b. Severe RV dilation and dysfunction in a patient with arrhythmogenic right ventricular dysplasia. Mid-ventricular cine MRI, using the b-SSFP technique, at end diastole (a) and end systole (b). Important dilated RV cavity and strongly diminished global RV function. Regionally, several areas of wall thinning showing akinetic to dyskinetic wall motion. Note the normal size and function of the left ventricle.

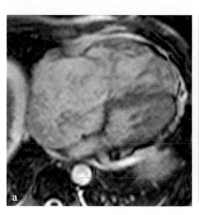
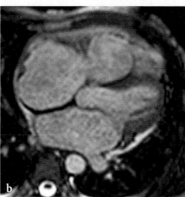

Fig. 9.35a-c. End-stage arrhythmogenic right ventricular dysplasia with severe right ventricular and atrial enlargement. Axial cine MRI, using the b-SSFP technique, at three levels (a-c). The patient received a heart transplant.

al. 1996). Previously, this entity was called "spongy myocardium", because of the spongy appearance of the non-compacted myocardium (ANGELINI et al. 1999). It is interesting to mention that the spongy mycardium pattern is found in non-mammalian vertebrates such as fish, amphibians and reptiles (these animals have no epicardial coronary arteries). It is believed that non-compaction is caused by an arrest of the endomyocardial morphogenesis, which normally occurs between 5 and 8 weeks of fetal life and is characterized by a gradual compaction of the loosely interwoven meshwork of myocardial fibres, transformation of the large intertrabecular spaces into capillaries and evolution of the coronary circulation (ELSHERSHARI et al. 2001; PIGNATELLI et al. 2003). The process of compaction typically progresses from epicardium to endocardium and from base of the heart towards the apex. As a result of this arrest of the compaction process, the non-compacted myocardium presents as a thickened wall with multiple prominent ventricular trabeculations and deep intertrabecular recesses. There is continuity between the ventricular cavity and intratrabecular recesses without evidence of communication to the epicardial coronary artery system. Because of the prominent trabeculations, this entity is sometimes called LV hypertrabeculation (FINSTERER et al. 2002; Fig. 9.36).

Non-compaction cardiomyopathy was described initially in paediatric patients, but recent studies have characterized it in adults (BORGES et al. 2003). The incidence in adults is 0.05%. Non-compaction cardiomyopathy is usually isolated and is limited to the LV myocardium ("isolated non-compaction of the left ventricle"), though occasionally the RV may

also be involved (Fig. 9.37). Most commonly, the apical and midventricular segments of both the inferior and lateral wall are affected in more than 80% of patients. Involvement of the mid-ventricular anterior wall and septum and the basal segments is much less frequent (OECHLSIN et al. 2000). Non-compaction can occasionally be associated with other congenital heart disorders ("non-isolated non-compaction of the left ventricle"), and is most likely also linked to the Barth syndrome, a rare disorder linked to chromosome Xq28, which is characterized by DCM, skeletal myopathy and neutropenia (ICHIDA et al. 2001; PIGNATELLI et al. 2003). Clinical presentations of non-compaction include depressed systolic and diastolic function, systemic embolism, ventricular tachyarrhythmias, DCM and heart failure, in both adult and paediatric populations (PIGNATELLI et al. 2003). It is a disease that is not widely known yet and, as a consequence of ignorance, its diagnosis is frequently missed. JENNI et al. have established echocardiographic criteria for isolated ventricular non-compaction, namely: (1) absence of coexisting congenital cardiac abnormalities; (2) a two-layered structure of the LV wall, with an end systolic ratio of non-compacted to compacted layer of greater than 2; (3) finding this abnormality predominantly in the apical and mid-ventricular areas; and (4) blood flow directed from the ventricular cavity into the deep intertrabecular recesses as assessed by Doppler echocardiography (JENNI et al. 1999, 2001). However, more recent literature, including findings obtained with cardiac MRI, suggest that the echocardiographic criteria might be too strict, and MRI especially may enhance the detection of more subtle forms of non-compaction (McCROHON

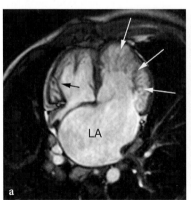 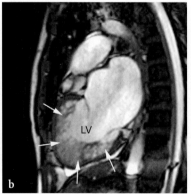 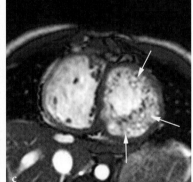

Fig. 9.36a-c. Non-compaction cardiomyopathy in a 26-year-old man. Cine MRI, using the b-SSFP technique, in the horizontal long-axis (**a**), vertical long-axis (**b**) and short-axis (**c**). Very prominent trabecular network (*white arrows*) along the entire lateral LV wall and LV apex. Thinning of the compacta of the LV lateral wall. Also in the right ventricle, a prominent network is visible (*black arrow*). Note important dilation of the left atrium (LA).

et al. 2002; Borreguero et al. 2002; Pignatelli et al. 2003; Fig. 9.38). The MRI protocol for studying patients with non-compaction of the myocardium consists of a combination of T1-weighted spin-echo MRI and b-SSFP cine MRI in different cardiac image planes (i.e. horizontal and vertical long-axis and short-axis).

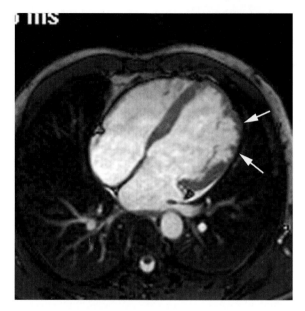

Fig. 9.37. Non-compaction cardiomyopathy. Cine MRI, using the b-SSFP technique, in the horizontal long-axis shows focal thinning of the compacta of the lateral LV wall (*arrows*) with prominent trabecular network. No evidence of prior myocardial infarction. (Courtesy of Ilse Crevits, Roeselare, Belgium)

9.4.7
Peripartum Cardiomyopathy

Peripartum cardiomyopathy is defined as LV dysfunction that develops between 1 month ante-partum to 5 months post-partum and is characterized by myocardial inflammation with or without concomitant pericarditis (Ardeholi et al. 2002). The precise aetiology of this myocardial disorder is unknown, but possible mechanisms include: myocarditis, abnormal immune response to pregnancy, maladaptive process to the haemodynamics of pregnancy and prolonged tocolysis. The patients have a high risk for venous, arterial and cardiac thrombus formation. MRI has a role in the assessment of ventricular function, to rule out myocardial damage and to detect thrombus formation (Fig. 9.39).

9.5
Myocarditis

Myocarditis is defined as an inflammatory infiltrate of the myocardium with necrosis or degeneration of adjacent myocytes, not typical of ischemic damage associated with coronary artery disease (Aretz et al. 1986). Although the aetiology is often unknown (i.e. idiopathic), myocarditis can be found in a variety of diseases affecting the myocardium and/or other parts of the heart. Though virtually any infectious agent may cause myocarditis, most cases of acute myocarditis are caused by viruses (e.g. coxsackie

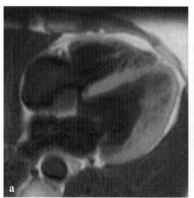
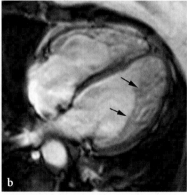
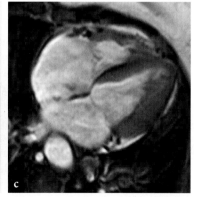

Fig. 9.38a-c. Non-compaction cardiomyopathy in a 56-year-old woman. The patient was referred for MRI because of thickened LV lateral wall on transthoracic echocardiography. Horizontal long-axis T1-weighted fast SE-MRI (**a**), cine MRI, using b-SSFP technique at end diastole (**b**) and end systole (**c**). Both SE-MRI and cine MRI at end systole suggest a thickening of the lateral LV wall. However, as shown on the end-diastolic cine MR image, the lateral LV wall has a prominent trabecular network (*arrows*) and only a thin compacta. Probably stagnant blood between these prominent trabeculations (at end systole) causes a pseudo-thickening of the lateral wall.

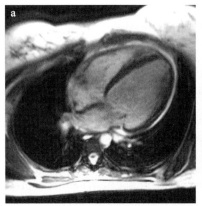
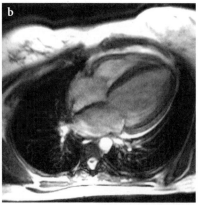

Fig. 9.39a,b. Peripartum cardiomyopathy in a 29-year-old woman, 1-month post-childbirth, presenting with cardiac failure. Horizontal long-axis cine MRI, using the b-SSFP technique, at end diastole (**a**) and end systole (**b**). Dilated left ventricle with severely compromised LV function (end diastolic volume, 193 ml; ejection fraction, 19%). No evidence of myocardial damage on CE-IR MRI (not shown).

B4 virus, adenovirus, human immunodeficiency virus; REMES et al. 1990; RAMAMURTHY et al. 1993). Myocarditis may also be caused by allergic reactions and pharmacological agents, as well as occurring during the course of some systemic diseases such as vasculitis.

The clinical features of myocarditis are varied, making the diagnosis of myocarditis often difficult at initial presentation (LIEBERMAN et al. 1991). Myocarditis is an insidious disease that is usually asymptomatic. Post-mortem studies, however, suggest that myocarditis is a major cause of sudden, unexpected death in adults less than 40 years of age (accounting for approximately 20% of cases; FELDMAN and McNAMARA 2000). Patients not infrequently present with a history of a recent, flu-like syndrome, accompanied by fever, arthralgia and malaise. Cardiac symptoms range from mild clinical cardiac failure and ventricular dilatation to fulminant cardiac failure and severe LV dysfunction with or without cardiac dilatation (McCARTHY et al. 2000; FUSE et al. 2000). Although the clinical course is usually benign with spontaneous recovery, sudden death may occasionally occur, and 5–10% of patients may progress to develop chronic DCM. Interestingly, patients with chronic persistent myocarditis usually have no ventricular dysfunction despite foci of myocyte necrosis. Laboratory tests may show leukocytosis, an elevated sedimentation rate (ESR), eosinophilia and an elevation in the cardiac fraction of creatine kinase and cardiac troponin I levels (SMITH et al. 1997). The electrocardiogram may show ventricular arrhythmias or heart block, or may mimic the findings in acute myocardial infarction or pericarditis.

Endomyocardial biopsy, using the Dallas criteria for the histological diagnosis of myocarditis, is considered the "gold standard" for diagnosis and classification of myocarditis (ARETZ et al. 1986).

Endomyocardial biopsy specimens are considered diagnostic of active myocarditis if routine light microscopy reveals infiltrating lymphocytes and myocytolysis. However, using these criteria, only 10–25% of patients in whom myocarditis is suspected on clinical grounds have positive biopsies. This suggests that endomyocardial biopsy underestimate the true incidence of myocarditis. Thus, endomyocardial biopsy has a poor negative predictive value of active myocarditis, but a high positive predictive value. The discordance between the clinical and histological features of myocarditis suggests that the diagnosis of myocarditis should not be based on histological findings alone (FELDMAN and McNAMARA 2000). Other diagnostic techniques such as myocardial scintigraphy with gallium (Ga) and monoclonal anti-myosin antibodies (AMAs) might be helpful in diagnosing myocarditis, especially in patients with a clinical presentation of myocardial infarction and normal coronary angiographic findings (LAISSY et al. 2002).

Use of MRI in the diagnosis of myocarditis was reported in the early 1990s (GALGIARDI et al. 1991; MATSOUKA et al. 1994). The lymphocyte infiltrate and myocytolysis in patients with active myocarditis increases the myocardial free-water content. As a result, the proton relaxation time, especially the T2-relaxation time, is prolonged and the diseased myocardium is visible as a hyperintense area on T2-weighted MRI sequences. GALGIARDI et al. (1991) have reported promising results regarding discrimination of infants and children with and without acute myocarditis, based on T2-weighted MRI sequences. Administration of gadolinium-based paramagnetic contrast agents is helpful in identifying the exact region of myocardial damage due to myocarditis, and to monitor the myocarditis activity (Fig. 9.40; MATSOUKA et al. 1994; FRIEDRICH et al. 1998). FRIEDRICH et al., studying 44 consecutive

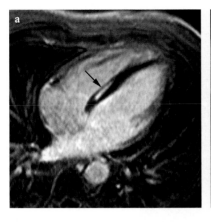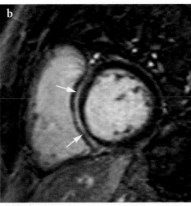

Fig. 9.40a,b. Focal myocarditis in a 32-year-old man presenting with retrosternal chest pain and slightly elevated cardiac enzymes (troponins). CE-IR MRI with late imaging in the horizontal long-axis (**a**) and basal short-axis (**b**). Strong enhancement is found in the mid-wall of the basal ventricular septum (*arrows*). Normal proximal coronary arteries were found on coronary MR angiography. Cine MRI showed mild hypocontractility of the basal ventricular septum.

patients with T1-weighted spin-echo MRI technique before and after contrast administration, found in the acute phase a focal myocardial enhancement pattern, whereas later (i.e. after 2 weeks) a more diffuse pattern was found (FRIEDRICH et al. 1998). Similar results have been reported by RODITI et al. (2000) and LAISSY et al. (2002). Increased distribution volume due to acute cell damage, with diffusion of gadolinium into the intracellular space, is the most likely mechanism to explain the enhancement in the pathological areas. In addition, a similar enhancement is shown in the pericardium if this part of the heart is involved in the inflammatory process. In patients with evidence of ongoing disease, a persistent enhancement is found. Contrast enhancement at 4 weeks after the onset of symptoms is shown to be predictive for the functional and clinical long-term outcome (WAGNER et al. 2003). The introduction of a new CE-IR gradient-echo technique by SIMONETTI et al. in 2001 has opened new avenues in non-invasively assessing myocardial damage. The selective suppression or nulling of the signal of normal myocardium allows the contrast between normal and abnormal myocardium to be significantly increased (up to 500% compared with the spin-echo protocol used by FRIEDRICH et al.). In a recent paper, MAHRHOLDT and colleagues (2004) have reported very promising results on the role of this CE-IR technique to evaluate patients who were diagnosed with myocarditis on clinical grounds. Contrast enhancement was found in 28 of 32 patients (88%). The lateral LV wall was most frequently involved, and the foci of enhancement were typically located in the outer myocardial layers, sparing the subendocardium (in contrast to the enhancement pattern found in patients with acute myocardial infarction; Figs. 9.41, 9.42). If the endocardiomyocardial biopsy was directed in the area of enhancement, histopathological analysis revealed active

myocarditis in 19 of 21 patients. Conversely, in the remaining 11 patients, in whom biopsy could not be taken from the region of contrast enhancement, active myocarditis was found in only one case. At follow-up 3 months later, a significant decrease in the area of contrast enhancement was found (9±11% to 3±4% of the LV mass), and the LV ejection fraction improved from 47±19% to 60±10%). The information on the exact localization of myocardial damage caused by the myocarditis on the CE-IR MRI can be used to guide biopsy, thus enhancing the diagnostic accuracy of endomyocardial biopsy. Increasing knowledge about the enhancement patterns of different myocardial diseases on CE-IR MRI sequences is helpful to differentiate myocarditis from other myocardial diseases such as HCM (MAHRHOLDT et al. 2004; BOGAERT et al. 2004). Moreover, cine MRI techniques, especially the new b-SSFP techniques, allow accurate assessment of the impact of the myocardial damage on regional and global ventricular function in patients with active myocarditis (RODITI et al. 2000; MAHRHOLDT et al. 2004; Fig. 9.43). In summary, it can be said that the results of the above studies suggest a prominent role of MRI in patients with a clinical suggestion of active myocarditis. In the following sections, the role of MRI in the diagnosis of Lyme disease, Chagas' heart disease, Wegener's granulomatosis and systemic lupus erythematosus is highlighted.

9.5.1
Lyme Disease

Lyme disease is caused by the spirochete *Borrelia burgdorferi* and is characterized by a multi-system disorder primarily affecting the skin, joints, heart and central nervous system (NATHWANI et al. 1990). The most common cardiac manifestation of Lyme

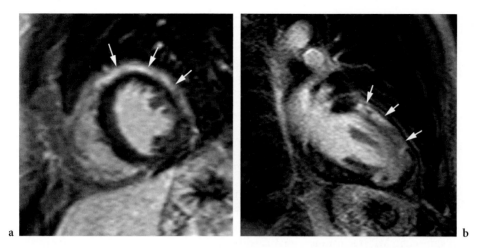

Fig. 9.41a,b. Acute myocarditis in a 36-year-old man with clinical suggestion of perimyocarditis. CE-IR MRI with late imaging in the cardiac short-axis (**a**) and vertical long-axis (**b**). Strong enhancement is seen in the subepicardial layers of the anterior wall (*arrows*). The enhancement seems to extend into the epicardial fat. Other areas of enhancement were found in the mid-lateral wall and in the apical segments. Cine MRI showed decreased contractility in the anterior LV wall (not shown).

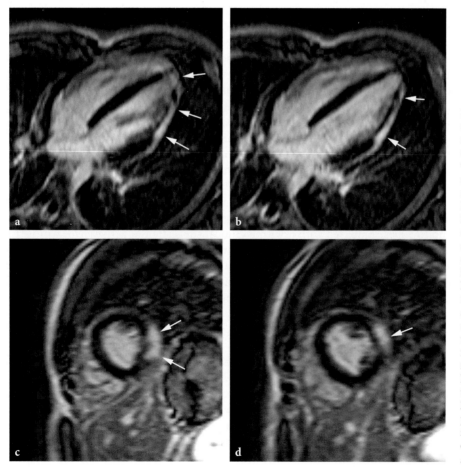

Fig. 9.42a-d. Acute myocarditis in a 16-year-old man admitted at the emergency department with a pneumomediastinum and a history of ecstasy (XTC) use. CE-IR MRI with late imaging in the horizontal long-axis (**a, b**) and cardiac short-axis (**c, d**). Strong enhancement is found in the subepicardial layers of the lateral LV (mid and apical third; *arrows*). The transmural spread is variable, but the subendocardium is not involved. Although myocardial infarction has been reported with the use of high-dose of XTC, the enhancement pattern is in favour of myocarditis. (Courtesy of Wim Volders, Antwerp, Belgium)

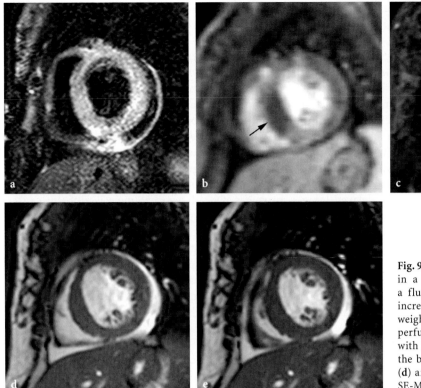

Fig. 9.43a-e. Acute perimyocarditis in a 32-week pregnant woman with a flu-like syndrome, chest pain and increased cardiac enzymes. **a** T2-weighted STIR fast SE-MRI. First-pass perfusion MRI (**b**) and CE-IR MRI with late imaging (**c**). Cine MRI, using the b-SSFP technique, at end diastole (**d**) and end systole (**e**). **a** T2-weighted SE-MRI shows inhomogeneous hyperintense appearance of the entire myocardium. On perfusion MRI, a large perfusion defect is visible in the ventricular septum (*arrow*) (**b**) and lateral wall. On late enhancement imaging (obtained 20 min after contrast administration) the myocardium appears inhomogeneously hypointense, with persistence of the hypoperfused areas (*arrows*). Cine MRI shows globally decreased LV function (end-diastolic volume, 114 ml; ejection fraction, 42%). The LV wall is inhomogeneously thickened (ventricular septum 16 mm at end diastole) and exhibits moderate to severe hypokinesia. Note the presence of a moderate pericardial effusion (100 ml). The patient's condition and cardiac status normalized soon after the start of Aspegic. The pattern of persistence of non-enhanced areas on late imaging differs from the above-described (typical) patterns of enhancement. At present the precise histological correlate of these non-enhanced area is unclear.

carditis is affection of the conduction system with transient atrioventricular block. Other manifestations such as rhythm disturbances, myopericarditis and heart failure are less common (VAN DER LINDE 1991). The cardiac manifestations are usually self-limiting, though it has been suggested that *Borrelia burgdorferi* may be associated with or even play an aetiological role in the development of DCM (STANEK et al. 1991). Abnormalities of Lyme carditis as detected by MRI include myopericarditis with myocardial wall thickening and areas of increased signal intensity within the myocardium, the presence of a subtle to moderate pericardial effusion, and ventricular dysfunction with regional or global hypokinesia (PONSONNAILLE et al. 1986; HANNEBICQUE et al. 1989; BERGLER et al. 1993; GLOBITS et al. 1994).

9.5.2
Chagas' Heart Disease

American trypanosomiasis (Chagas' disease) is a zoonosis caused by the protozoan parasite *Trypanosoma cruzi*. Chagas' disease is endemic in almost all Latin American countries, where it is one of the leading causes of death (WHO EXPERT COMMITTEE 1984). The disease is characterized by three phases: acute, indeterminate and chronic. The heart is the most commonly affected organ in chronic Chagas' disease, where lymphocytic myocarditis is often observed. It is associated with diffuse interstitial fibrosis, myocyte hypertrophy and atrophy. Patients present with severely impaired LV function and refractory heart failure, or have episodes of sustained ventricular tachycardia without severe LV dysfunction (BELLOTTI et al. 1996). MRI after gadolinium infusion may be helpful in detecting areas of intense myocardial inflammation (KALIL-FILHO and DE ALBUQUERQUE 1995). In a study by BELLOTTI et al. (1996), seven of eight patients showed a high signal intensity after gadolinium infusion in the infero-lateral free wall of the left ventricle, and in one patient in the RV septum. MRI may be helpful in guiding endomyocardial biopsy and seems a promising alternative method for the diagnosis of an inflammatory process in Chagas' heart disease. Similar results have been found by ROCHITTE et al. (2003), using the new CE-IR MRI technique with delayed imaging. Hyperenhancement, representing mycoardial fibrosis, is most frequently found in the apical and basal infero-lateral LV wall segments. Enhancement typically occurs in the mid-wall and subepicardium, in contrast to the subendocardial enhancement in myocardial infarction. A negative correlation has been found between the extent of myocardial enhancement and the LV ejection fraction.

9.5.3
Wegener's Granulomatosis

Wegener's granulomatosis is a systemic inflammatory disorder of unknown aetiology. Cardiac involvement in Wegener's granulomatosis is not as uncommon as generally thought, occurring in 6–44% of patients (GRANT et al. 1994). It may take many forms and varies from the principal clinical feature to mild or subclinical disease. Pericarditis and pericardial effusion are found in 50% of patients with cardiac involvement (FORSTOT et al. 1980). Coronary arteritis involving the proximal aorta with dilation and wall thickening is found in another 50% of patients. Myocarditis with granuloma, which may produce acute cardiac failure and progress to cardiomyopathy, is seen in 25%. Wegener's granulomatosis may also present as mass lesions within the ventricles and may result in obstruction (KOSOVSKY et al. 1991). Valve abnormalities secondary to dilation of the aorta or left ventricle and conduction abnormalities are less common findings in Wegener's granulomatosis of the heart. Non-invasive cardiac imaging modalities such as transthoracic and transoesophageal echocardiography and MRI may be helpful in identifying and delineating cardiac and proximal aortic involvement in Wegener's granulomatosis and also have a potentially important role in following the response to treatment (KOSOVSKY et al. 1991; GOODFIELD et al. 1995).

9.5.4
Systemic Lupus Erythematosus

Systemic lupus erythematosus (SLE) is a disease of unknown aetiology, thought to be autoimmune in nature (DOHERTY and SIEGEL 1985). The most common cardiac manifestations of this systemic disorder are non-bacterial "verrucous" endocarditis (Libman-Sacks endocarditis), pericardial effusion, pericardial thickening and myocarditis. Myocarditis is clinically diagnosed in 10% of patients with SLE. However, in autopsy studies the incidence approaches 40%. Myocardial injury is probably caused by immune complex deposition, but the in vivo diagnosis of myocarditis is difficult. MRI may be a valuable technique with which to detect myocardial involvement in patients with SLE, but its clinical role is unclear. In a paper by BEEN et al. (1988), the myocardial signal intensity on T1-weighted images is significantly higher in patients with SLE than in normal volunteers or patients with HCM. Furthermore, patients with active disease, indicated by the lupus activity criteria count, show significantly higher T1 values than patients with inactive disease. In addition, T1 values show a negative correlation with serum C3 in the group with SLE. The increase in T1 shows a diffuse pattern and is probably caused by a cellular (lymphocytic) infiltration. Whether SLE causes changes in T2 relaxation is as yet unknown. Myocardial involvement in SLE will also lead to an impairment of LV diastolic function in the absence of systolic abnormalities (SASSON et al. 1992).

9.6
Drug-Induced Myocardial Diseases

9.6.1
Antracycline (Doxorubicin) Cardiotoxicity

Antracyclines are highly potent cytotoxic drugs that are included in a number of polychemotherapeutic regimens for the treatment of a variety of solid tumours and haematological malignancies. Because of highly effective therapy regimens, there are an increasing number of long-term survivors of cancer who have been exposed to anthracycline chemotherapy. These long-term survivors are one of the largest and ever-increasing groups of patients at risk of premature cardiac disease (BLEYER 1990). A dose-dependent cardiotoxic effect has been described clinically and histologically, resulting in life-threatening congestive heart failure in some patients, sometimes years after completion of chemotherapy (VON HOFF et al. 1979; LIPSHULTZ et al. 1991; Fig. 9.44). There are other cardiac changes, which include: DCM and RCM, and subtler changes in cardiac function. Pre-existing heart disease, very young or advanced age, type of anthracycline, additional mediastinal radiation, high plasma concentrations after bolus injection and higher cumulative doses are accepted risk factors (SINGAL and ILISKOVIC 1998). As there is no safe threshold dose as was previously believed, anthracyclines are burdened by their cardiotoxicity. Clinical follow-up for detection of anthracycline-induced cardiotoxicity is usually performed by repeated echocardiographic studies of LV function. Interstudy and interobserver variability of this technique, however, are substantial, and early changes may be overlooked. Though some changes may be subtle, they may be of prognostic value. The role of echocardiography is therefore to detect severe early cardiotoxicity or late-stage changes of chronic disease that lack early prognostic factors. Radionuclide ventriculography is more accurate than 2D echocardiography in detecting early changes in LV performance and is used in clinical

studies. However, it is burdened by radioactivity of agents and does not allow detection of myocardial changes related to anthracyclines. Biopsy is said to be the gold standard for detecting myocardial damage after anthracycline therapy (Fig. 9.44). The ability to predict clinical outcome, however, has been questioned. Furthermore, it is limited by its invasive character, the need for serial testing, false-negative results because of sampling error and interobserver variability. MRI, in contrast, has the ability to accurately quantify and monitor ventricular function and to non-invasively detect myocardial damage (e.g. infarction, myocarditis). Therefore, it can be hypothesized that MRI has a potential to visualize subclinical myocardial changes in the early course of cardiotoxic anthracycline-containing chemotherapy and their short-term prognostic value on cardiac function. WASSMUTH et al. (2001) have studied 22 patients with normal cardiac function with MRI before, and 3 and 28 days after anthracycline chemotherapy. Although all patients remained clinically stable, the LV ejection fraction significantly decreased from 67.8±1.4% to 58.9±1.9% 28 days after treatment, while the relative myocardial enhancement significantly increased. Early (i.e. at 3 days)

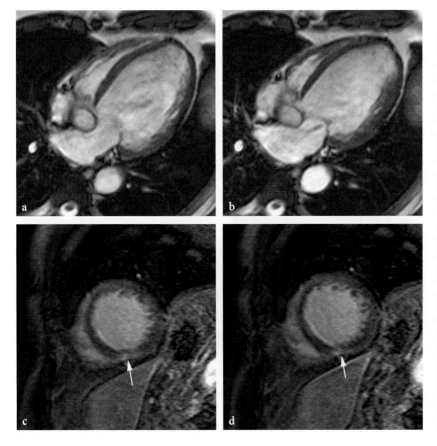

Fig. 9.44a-d. Antracycline cardiotoxicity in a 60-year-old man with previous chemotherapy for osteosarcoma, presenting with cardiac failure. Cine MRI, using the b-SSFP technique, at end diastole (**a**) and end systole (**b**), and CE-IR MRI with late imaging in two cardiac short-axis levels (**c, d**). Important dilation of the left ventricle with profound depression of global and regional function (end-diastolic volume, 269 ml; ejection fraction, 23%). Note the presence of a moderately severe mitral regurgitation secondary to the LV dilation. On late enhancement imaging, in the inferior wall an area of abnormal enhancement is visible in the subepicardium and mid-wall (*arrow*). No evidence of myocardial ischemia nor infarction (normal coronary arteries on cardiac catheterization). Though aspecific, the enhancement probably represents myocardial damage (scarring) caused by anthracycline toxicity.

pronounced increase in myocardial enhancement (>5) predicted a significant loss of ejection fraction at 28 days (mean decrease in ejection fraction of 16.1±6.6%), whereas a less pronounced increase (+5) was not associated with a significant loss of ejection fraction (mean decrease in ejection fraction of 4.1±2.6%, non-significant). The authors conclude that MRI may serve as a simple and non-invasive tool in the follow-up of patients receiving anthracycline chemotherapy.

9.6.2
Substance Abuse and Recreational Drugs

Cardiovascular complications of excessive use of ethanol, cocaine and other recreational drugs, often in combination with cigarette smoking, have become an important cause of cardiovascular-related morbidity and mortality in young adults. Although an extensive discussion of these substances and their effects on the heart is beyond the scope of this chapter, in this section a brief description is provided on cardiac side-effects of the most frequently used recreational drugs.

Substance abuse should be considered in young patients presenting with chest pain. The role of cardiac imaging, including cardiovascular MRI, is to evaluate the impact of substance abuse on cardiac morphology, ventricular and valvular function, to rule out structural myocardial damage (e.g. myocardial infarction, myocarditis), and to detect other complications such as endocarditis with abscess or pseudoaneurysm formation, and aortic dissection. The abuse of alcohol is associated with chronic cardiomyopathy, hypertension and arrhythmia. Abstinence or using alcohol in moderation can reverse these cardiovascular problems. Alcohol is also distinguished among the substances of abuse by having possible protective effects against coronary artery disease and stroke when used in moderate amounts.

Substance abuse with cocaine is associated with multiple cardiovascular conditions, including myocardial infarction, myocarditis, endocarditis, aortic dissection, LV hypertrophy, arrhythmias, sudden death and cardiomyopathy (KLONER and REZKALLA 2003; Fig. 9.45). Cocaine has effects to potentiate the physiological actions of catecholamines and has direct effects on voltage-dependent sodium ion channels

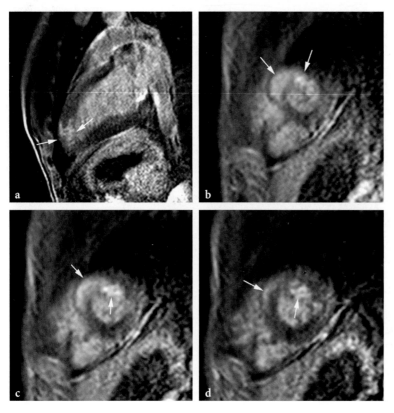

Fig. 9.45a-d. Cocaine-induced or related myocardial damage (ischemia? necrosis?) in a 20-year-old man, who was admitted with ventricular tachycardia and fibrillation. The patient showed ST-segment abnormalities on ECG and elevated cardiac troponins. CE-IR MRI with late imaging in the vertical long-axis (**a**) and three consecutive short-axis images through the apical part of the left ventricle (**b, c, d**) shows well-delineated, focal zone, with abnormal transmural enhancement clearly visible in the anterior part of the LV apex (*arrows*).

related to local anaesthetic properties. The effects of cocaine can be augmented with concomitant alcohol consumption and cigarette smoking. Acute myocardial ischemia caused by cocaine may be related to in situ thrombosis and/or coronary vasospasm.

Amphetamines (e.g. speed, ice, ecstasy) have many of the cardiovascular toxicities seen with cocaine, including acute and chronic cardiovascular diseases. Heroin and other opiates can cause arrhythmias and non-cardiac pulmonary oedema, and may reduce cardiac output. Cardiovascular problems are less common with cannabis (marijuana) than with opiates, but major cognitive disorders may be seen with its chronic use. It is still controversial whether caffeine can cause hypertension and coronary artery disease, and questions have been raised about its safety in patients with heart failure and arrhythmia (FRISHMAN et al. 2003a, 2003b).

9.7
Miscellaneous Disorders of the Myocardium

9.7.1
Tako-Tsubo Cardiomyopathy or
Transient Left Ventricular Apical Ballooning

Tako-Tsubo cardiomyopathy or transient LV apical ballooning stands for a reversible LV dysfunction with acute myocardial infarction-like ST-segment elevation without coronary artery lesions and with minimal myocardial enzymatic release (TSUCHIHASHI et al. 2001; ABE and KONDO 2002; ABE et al. 2003; DESMET et al. 2003). The dysfunction exhibits apical akinesis, causing an *apical ballooning* and basal normal wall motion to hypokinesis in the acute phase, which completely normalizes within a few weeks (Fig. 9.46). The findings on left-

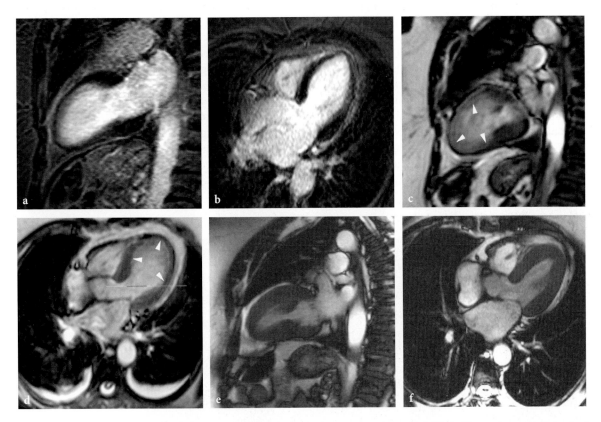

Fig. 9.46a-f. Apical ballooning in a 60-year-old woman after a (non-traumatic) car accident. The patient complained of interscapular chest pain and soon developed pulmonary oedema and severe LV dysfunction. On cardiac catheterization, coronary arteries were found to be normal. CE-IR MRI with late imaging in the vertical long-axis (**a**) and horizontal long-axis plane (**b**). Cine MRI (end-systolic frame), using the b-SSFP technique, at admission (**c, d**) and 3 weeks later (**e, f**) using similar imaging planes to the CE-IR MRI study. No abnormal late myocardial enhancement is found during the acute phase (**a, b**), nor during the repeat study (not shown). Cine MRI at admission shows bulging and akinesia of the apical half of the left ventricle (*arrowheads*), with profound reduction in global LV function (end-diastolic volume, 110 ml; ejection fraction, 32%). Note also the presence of bilateral pleural effusion. Three weeks later, the LV has regained its normal configuration, and regional and global function are completely normalized. The pleural effusion has disappeared. Acute stress related to the car accident was the probable trigger to develop transient apical ballooning.

sided ventriculography in the acute phase corresponds to a *tako-tsubo*, which in Japanese means an octopus fishing pot with a round bottom and a narrow neck. Another name for this entity is *ampulla cardiomyopathy*. The clinical course of this dysfunction is very distinct from acute myocardial infarction and acute myocarditis. Emotional and physical stresses are the most frequent precipitating factors; and this disorder preferentially affects elderly woman (DESMET et al. 2003; ABE et al. 2003). At present, the causal relation between stress and this syndrome has not been clarified. Several hypotheses have been presented, ranging from spasms of the epicardial coronary arteries, through stress-related impairment of the coronary microcirculation, to catecholamine-related cardiotoxicity with activation of cardiac adrenoceptors (AKASHI et al. 2002; AKO et al. 2002; TSUCHIHASHI et al. 2001; UEYAMA et al. 2002). This reversible LV dysfunction can be considered as an atypical presentation of myocardial stunning. Although myocardial stunning is usually observed in ischemic heart disease (BRAUNWALD and KLONER 1982), and is accompanied by a coronary event with segmental dysfunction, the reversible dysfunction in tako-tsubo cardiomyopathy is not limited to a specific coronary artery territory, but involves the apical part of the left ventricle. Although most cases of tako-tsubo cardiomyopathy are described on left-sided ventriculography, MRI is appealing in the

diagnosis and follow-up of this infrequent myocardial disorder. The apical ballooning and dysfunction, as well as the functional recovery, can be perfectly demonstrated on cine MRI using the horizontal and vertical long-axis imaging planes (Fig. 9.46). The absence of myocardial necrosis can be confirmed on CE-IR MRI with delayed imaging.

9.7.2
Congenital Myocardial Disorders in the Adult Population

When performing cardiac MRI studies on a regular basis, a series of myocardial disorders may be encountered, usually in adults, that do not fit with one of the above-mentioned, non-ischemic myocardial abnormalities nor with ischemic heart disease. Knowledge of cardiac anatomy (see Chap. 4) and congenital heart disorders (see Chap. 15) may be helpful to recognize these entities that often can be considered as congenital. For instance, congenitally corrected transposition of the great arteries may be asymptomatic until adult life. Ventricular diverticula, congenital aneurysms or spontaneously closed ventricular septal defects are rare entities, but can be easily recognized using a comprehensive MRI approach (Figs. 9.47–48).

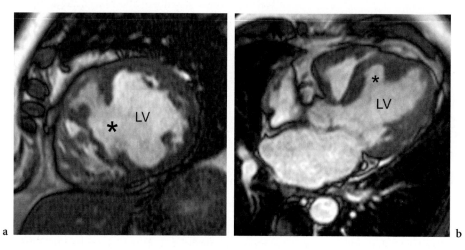

a   b

Fig. 9.47a,b. Spontaneously closed muscular ventricular septal defect in a 65-year-old male suspected of ischemic myocardial disease. Cine MRI, using the b-SSFP technique, in the short-axis (**a**) and horizontal long-axis view (**b**). A large defect (*star*) is visible in the middle third of the ventricular septum. However, the patient had no symptoms of interventricular shunt and flow measurements through the great vessels revealed similar flow volumes. Hypertrophy of the RV muscular trabeculations has spontaneously sealed the defect. This phenomenon is not infrequent in muscular, even large, ventricular septal defects

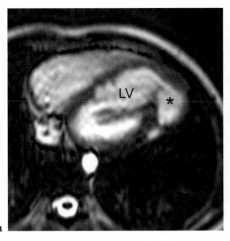
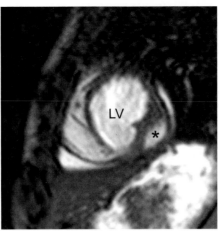

Fig. 9.48a,b. Congenital LV diverticulum in an 8-year-old girl. Cine MRI, using the b-SSFP technique, in the horizontal long-axis (**a**) and short-axis direction (**b**). The apicolateral LV wall is interrupted, with presence of a well-delineated outpouching (*star*) in communication with the LV cavity by a rather small neck. In contrast to an LV aneurysm, usually the result of an infarction, this diverticulum shows contraction during systole, because it contains a muscular wall.

9.8
Key Points

- At present, MRI is probably the best technique for studying non-ischemic myocardial disease.
- Contrast-enhanced inversion-recovery MRI with late imaging enables visualization of myocardial damage in a variety of diseases. Better knowledge about typical appearances of myocardial enhancement will further expand the role of MRI.
- MRI is better than echocardiography in determining the type of cardiac hypertrophy (e.g. in patients with arterial hypertension).
- Delayed enhancement in HCM is limited to the hypertrophied area and probably represents myocardial fibrosis.
- Apical HCM is not infrequently missed on transthoracic ultrasound. If clinically suspected, these patients should undergo an MRI study. Make sure to scan along the true intrinsic cardiac axes (i.e. vertical and horizontal long-axis), so that the LV apex can be optimally visualized.
- Thrombus formation in DCM is a frequent finding. Similar to ischemic heart disease, use a combination of cine MRI and CE-IR-MRI in different imaging planes.
- Morphological abnormalities in RCM are often limited. The main hallmark is decreased myocardial compliance, leading to diastolic dysfunction.

- Myocardial hypertrophy (concentric, asymmetric) can be the result of a variety of disorders. A combination of SE-MRI, cine MRI, CE-IR MRI may be extremely helpful in the differential diagnosis.
- Although promising, the role of MRI in the diagnosis of cardiac sarcoidosis is not yet established.
- Fibrofatty, not fatty replacement is the pathological substrate of ARVD. A comprehensive MRI approach is probably helpful in the diagnosis of ARVD, though the precise role is not yet defined.
- Non-compaction cardiomyopathy can be easily visualized with MRI.
- Myocardial damage in myocarditis is often subepicardially located.

References

Abelmann WH, Lorell BH (1989) The challenge of cardiomyopathy. J Am Coll Cardiol 13:1219–1239

Abarra S, Migrino RQ, Sosnovik D, et al (2004a) Value of fat suppression in the MRI evaluation of suspected arrhythmogenic right ventricular dysplasia. Am J Roentgenol 182:587–591

Abarra S, Migrino RQ, Sosnovik D et al (2004)b Conventional spin echo magnetic resonance imaging is superior to fast spin echo in detection of intramyocardial fatty infiltration (abstract). J Cardiovasc Magn Reson 6:233–234

Abe Y, Kondo M (2002) Apical ballooning of the left ventricle: a distinct entity? Heart 89:974–976

Abe Y, Kondo M, Matsuoka R, et al (2003) Assessment of clinical features in transient left ventricular apical ballooning. J Am Coll Cardiol 41:737–742

Akashi Y, Nakazawa K, Sakakibara M, Miyake F, Sasaka K (2002) Reversible left ventricular dysfunction "Takotsubo" cardiomyopathy related to catecholamine cardiotoxicity. J Electrocardiol 35:351–356

Ako J, Kozaki K, Yoshizumi M, Ouchi Y (2002) Transient left ventricular apical ballooning without coronary artery stenosis: a form of stunning-like phenomenon? J Am Coll Cardiol 39:741–742

Allison JD, Flickinger FW, Wright JC et al (1993) Measurement of left ventricular mass in hypertrophic cardiomyopathy using MRI: comparison with echocardiography. Magn Reson Imaging 11:329–334

Anderson LJ, Holden S, Davis B et al (2001) Cardiovascular T2-star (T2*) magnetic resonance for the early diagnosis of myocardial iron overload. Eur Heart J 22:2171–2179

Angelini A, Basso C, Nava A, Thiene G (1996) Endomyocardial biopsy in arrhythmogenic right ventricular cardiomyopathy (editorial). Am Heart J 132:203–206

Angelini A, Melacini P, Barbero F, Thiene G (1999) Evolutionary persistence of spongy myocardium in humans. Circulation 99:2475

Ardeholi H, Kasper EK, Baughman KL (2002) Peripartum cardiomyopathy. Minerva Cardioangiol 51:41–48

Aretz HT, Billingham ME, Edwards WD et al (1986) Myocarditis: a histopathologic definition and classification. Am J Cardiovasc Pathol 1:3–14

Arrivé L, Assayag P, Russ G, et al (1994) MRI and cine MRI of asymmetric septal hypertrophic cardiomyopathy. J Comput Assist Tomogr 18:376–382

Aviram G, Fishman JE, Young M-L, et al (2003) MR evaluation of arrhythmogenic right ventricular cardiomyopathy in pediatric patients. Am J Roentgenol AJR 180:1135–1141

et al Basso C, Thienne G, Corrado D, et al (1996) Arrhythmogenic right ventricular cardiomyopathy. Dyplasia, dystrophy, or myocarditis? Circulation 94:983–991

Been M, Kean D, Smith MA, et al (1985) Nuclear magnetic resonance in hypertrophic cardiomyopathy. Br Heart J 54:48–52

Been M, Thomson BJ, Smith MA et al (1988) Myocardial involvement in systemic lupus erythematosus detected by magnetic resonance imaging. Eur Heart J 9:1250–1256

Belenkov Y, Vikhert OA, Belichenko OI, Arabidze GG (1992) Magnetic resonance imaging of cardiac hypertrophy in malignant arterial hypertension. Am J Hypertens 5:195S–199S

Bellotti G, Bocchi EA, Moreas A de et al (1996) In vivo detection of Trypanosoma cruzi antigens in hearts of patients with chronic Chagas' heart disease. Am Heart J 131:301–317

Beltrami CA, Finato N, Rocco M et al (1995) The cellular basis of dilated cardiomyopathy in humans. J Mol Cell Cardiol 27:291–305

Benson L, Liu P, Olivieri N, Rose V, Freedom R (1989) Left ventricular function in young adults with thalassemia. Circulation 80:274

Bergey PD, Axel L (2000) Focal hypertrophic cardiomyopathy simulating a mass: MR tagging for correct diagnosis. Am J Roentgenol 174:242–244

Bergler KJ, Sochor H, Stanek G, et al (1993) Indium-111 monoclonal antimyosin antibody and magnetic resonance imaging in the diagnosis of acute Lyme myopericarditis. Arch Intern Med 153:2696–2700

Blake LM, Scheinman MM, Higgins CB (1994) MR features of arrhythmogenic right ventricular dysplasia. Am J Roentgenol 162:809–812

Bleyer WA (1990) The impact of childhood cancer on the United States and the world. CA Cancer J Clin 40:355–367

Bluemke DA, Krupinski EA, Ovitt T et al (2003) MR imaging of arrhythmogenic right ventricular cardiomyopathy: morphological findings and interobserver reliability. Cardiology 99:153–162

Bogaert J, Goldstein M, Tannouri F, Golzarian J, Dymarkowski S (2003) Late myocardial enhancement in hypertrophic cardiomyopathy using contrast-enhanced magnetic resonance imaging. Am J Roentgenol AJR 180:981–985

Bogaert J, Taylor AM, Van Kerckhove F, Dymarkowski S (2004) Use of inversion-recovery contrast-enhanced MRI technique for cardiac imaging: spectrum of diseases. Am J Roentgenol AJR 182:609–615

Borges AC, Kivelitz D, Baumann G (2003) Isolated left ventricular non-compaction: cardiomyopathy with homogeneous transmural and heterogeneous segmental perfusion. Heart 89:e21–e23

Borreguero LJJ, Corti R, Soria RF de, et al (2004) Diagnosis of isolated noncompaction of the myocardium by magnetic resonance imaging. Circulation 105:e177–e178

Boulos M, Lashevsky I, Reisner S, Gepstein L (2001) Electroanatomic mapping of arrhytmogenic right ventricular dyplasia. J Am Coll Cardiol 38:2020–2027

Braunwald E, Morrow AG, Cornwell WP, Aygen MM, Hillbish TF (1960) Idiopathic hypertrophic subaortic stenosis. Clinical, hemodynamic, and angiographic manifestations. Am J Med 29:924–945

Braunwald E, Kloner RA (1982) The stunned myocardium: prolonged, postischemic ventricular dysfunction. Circulation 66:1146–1156

Brigden W (1957) The noncoronary cardiomyopathies. Lancet II:1179–1243

Bulkley BH, Weisfeldt ML, Hutchins GM (1977) Asymmetric septal hypertrophy and myocardial fiber disarray. Features of normal, developing and malformed hearts. Circulation 56:292–298

Burke AP, Farb, A, Tashko G, Virmani R (1998) Arrhythmogenic right ventricular cardiomyopathy and fatty replacement of the right ventricular myocardium. Are they different diseases? Circulation 97:1571–1580

Buser PT, Wagner S, Auffermann W et al (1990) Three-dimensional analysis of the regional contractility of the normal and the cardiomyopathic left ventricle using cine-magnetic resonance imaging (in German). Z Kardiol 79:573–579

Carlson MD, White RD, Trohman RG et al (1994) Right ventricular outflow tract ventricular tachycardia: detection of previously unrecognized anatomic abnormalities using cine magnetic resonance imaging. J Am Coll Cardiol 24:720–727

Casolo GC, Poggesi L, Boddi M et al (1987) ECG-gated magnetic resonance imaging in right ventricular dysplasia. Am Heart J 113:1245–1248

Casolo GC, Trotta F, Rostagno C et al (1989) Detection of

apical hypertrophic cardiomyopathy by magnetic resonance imaging. Am Heart J 117:468–472

Castillo E, Tandri H, Rodriguez R et al (2004) Arrhythmogenic right ventricular dysplasia: ex vivo and in vivo fat detection with black-blood MR imaging.Radiology 232:38–48

Celletti F, Fattori R, Napoli G et al (1999) Assessment of restrictive cardiomyopathy of amyloid or idiopathic etiology by magnetic resonance imaging. Am J Cardiol 83:798–801

Chan PCK, Liu P, Cronin C, Heathcote J, Uldall R (1992) The use of nuclear magnetic resonance imaging in monitoring total body iron in hemodialysis patients with hemosiderosis treated with erythropoietin and phlebotomy. Am J Kidney Dis 19:484–489

Chandra M, Silverman ME, Oshinski J, Pettigrew R (1996a) Diagnosis of cardiac sarcoidosis aided by MRI. Chest 110:562–565

Chandra M, Pettigrew RI, Eley JW, Oshinski JN, Guyton RA (1996b) Cine-MRI-aided endomyocardectomy in idiopathic hypereosinophilic syndrome. Ann Thorac Surg 62:1856–1858

Choudhury L, Mahrholdt H, Wagner A et al (2002) Myocardial scarring in asymptomatic or mildly symptomatic patients with hypertrophic cardiomyopathy. J Am Coll Cardiol 40:2156–2164

Chuang ML, Levy D, Salton CL, et al (2004) Effect of volumetric imaging and characterization of geometry on prevalence and patterns of left ventricular hypertrophy in the Framingham Pilot MRI Study (abstract). J Cardiovasc Magn Reson 6:239–240

Corrado D, Fontaine G, Marcus FI et al (2000) Arrhythmogenic right ventricular dysplasia/cardiomyopathy. Need for an international registry. Circulation 101:101–106

Crilley JG, Boehm EA, Blair E et al (2003) Hypertrophic cardiomyopathy due to sarcomeric gene mutations is characterized by impaired energy metabolism irrespective of the degree of hypertrophy. J Am Coll Cardiol 41:1776–1782

Cuspidi C, Lonati L, Sampieri L, Leonetti G, Zanchetti A (1997) Physiological versus pathological hypertrophy. The athlete and the hypertensive. Adv Exp Med Biol 432:145–158 et al

Dec GW, Fuster V (1994) Idiopathic dilated cardiomyopathy. N Engl J Med 331:1564–1574

Desmet WJR, Adriaenssens BFM, Dens JAY (2003) Apical ballooning of the left ventricle: first series in white patients. Eur Heart J 89:1027–1031

Di Cesare E, Marsili L, Chichiarelli A, et al (1994) Characterization of hypertrophic cardiomyopathy with magnetic resonance (in Italian). Radiol Med (Torino) 87:614–619

Doherty NE, Siegel RJ (1985) Cardiovascular manifestations of systemic lupus erythematosus. Am Heart J 110:1257–1265

Doherty N III, Fujita N, Caputo GR, Higgins CB (1992a) Measurement of right ventricular mass in normal and dilated cardiomyopathic ventricles using cine magnetic resonance imaging. Am J Cardiol 69:1223–1228

Doherty N III, Seelos KC, Suzuki J et al (1992b) Application of cine nuclear magnetic resonance imaging for sequential evaluation of response to angiotensin-converting enzyme inhibitor therapy in dilated cardiomyopathy. J Am Coll Cardiol 19:1294–1302

Dong SJ, MacGregor JH, Crawley AP et al (1994) Left ventricular wall thickness and regional systolic function in patients with hypertrophic cardiomyopathy. Circulation 90:1200–1209

Dong SJ, Crawley AP, MacGregor JH et al (1995) Regional left ventricular systolic function in relation to the cavity geometry in patients with chronic right ventricular pressure overload. A three-dimensional tagged magnetic resonance study. Circulation 91:2359–2370

D'Silva SA, Kohli A, Dalvi BV, Kale PA (1992) MRI in right ventricular endomyocardial fibrosis. Am Heart J 123:1390–1392

Dupuis JM, Victor J, Furber A, et al (1994) Value of magnetic resonance imaging in cardiac sarcoidosis. Apropos of a case (in French). Arch Mal Coeur Vaiss 87:105–110

Elshershari H, Okutan V, Celiker A (2001) Isolated noncompaction of the ventricular myocardium. Cardiol Young 11:472–475

Farmer D, Higgins CB, Yee E, et al (1984) Tissue characterization by magnetic resonance imaging in hypertrophic cardiomyopathy. Am J Cardiol 55:230–232

Fejfar Z (1968) Accounts of international meetings: idiopathic cardiomegaly. Bull WHO 38:979–992

Feldman AM, McNamara D (2000) Myocarditis. N Engl J Med 343:1388–1398

Ferrari VA, Scott CH (2003) Arrhythmogenic right ventricular dysplasia. Time for a new look. J Cardiovasc Electrophysiol 14:483–484

Finsterer J, Stöllberger C, Feichtinger H (2002) Histological appearance of left ventricular hypertrabeculation/noncompaction. Cardiology 98:162–164

Fontaine G, Fontaliran F, Frank R (1998) Arrhythmogenic right ventricular cardiomyopathies. Clinical forms and main differential diagnoses. Circulation 97:1532–1535

Forstot JZ, Overlie PA, Neufeld GK, Harmon CE, Forstot SL (1980) Cardiac complications of Wegener's granulomatosis: a case report of complete heart block and review of the literature. Semin Arthritis Rheum 10:148–154

Frey N, Katus HA, Olson EN, Hill JA (2004) Hypertrophy of the heart. A new therapeutic target? Circulation 109:1580–1589

Friedrich MG, Strohm O, Schulz-Menger J, et al (1998) Contrast-enhanced magnetic resonance imaging visualizes changes in the course of viral myocarditis. Circulation 97:1802–1809

Frishman WH, Vecchio A del, Sanal S, Ismail A (2003a) Cardiovascular manifestations of substance abuse part 1: cocaine. Heart 5:187–201

Frishman WH, Vecchio A del, Sanal S, Ismail A (2003b) Cardiovascular manifestations of substance abuse part 2: alcohol, amphetamines, heroin, cannibas, and caffeine. Heart 5:253–271

Fujita N, Duerinckx AJ, Higgins CB (1993) Variation in left ventricular regional wall stress with cine magnetic resonance imaging: normal subjects versus dilated cardiomyopathy. Am Heart J 125:1337–1345

Fuse K, Kodama M, Okura Y (2000) Predictors of disease course in patients with acute myocarditis. Circulation 102:2829–2835

Gagliardi MG, Bevilacqua M, Di Renzi P, et al (1991) Usefulness of magnetic resonance imaging for diagnosis of acute myocarditis in infants and children, and comparison with endomyocardial biopsy. Am J Cardiol 68:1089–1091

Ganau A, Devereux RB, Roman MJ (1992) Patterns of left ventricular hypertrophy and geometric remodeling in essential hypertension. J Am Coll Cardiol 19:1550–1558

Gatzka CD (2002) Left ventricular hypertrophy, cardiac imaging and cardiac electric activity. J Hypertens 20:2153–2156

Gaudio C, Tanzilli G, Mazzarotto P et al (1991) Comparison of left ventricular ejection fraction by magnetic resonance imaging and radionuclide ventriculography in idiopathic dilated cardiomyopathy. Am J Cardiol 67:411–415

Gaudio C, Pelliccia F, Tanzilli G, et al (1992) Magnetic resonance imaging for assessment of apical hypertrophy in hypertrophic cardiomyopathy. Clin Cardiol 15:164–168

Gemayel C, Pelliccia A, Thompson PD (2001) Arrhythmogenic right ventricular cardiomyopathy. J Am Coll Cardiol 38:1773–1781

Globits S, Bergler KJ, Stanek G, Ullrich R, Glogar D (1994) Magnetic resonance imaging in the diagnosis of acute Lyme carditis. Cardiology 85:415–417

Globits S, Kreiner G, Frank H et al (1997) Significance of morphological abnormalities detected by MRI in patients undergoing successful ablation of right ventricular outflow tract tachycardia. Circulation 96:2633–2640

Goodfield NER, Bhandari S, Plant WD, Morley-Davies A, Sutherland GR (1995) Cardiac involvement in Wegener's granulomatosis. Br Heart J 73:110–115

Grant SCD, Levy RD, Venning MC, Ward C, Brooks NH (1994) Wegener's granulomatosis and the heart. Br Heart J 71:82–86

Greer ML, MacDonald C, Adatia I (2000) MRI of Uhl's anomaly. Circulation 101:230

Hamada S, Takmiya M, Ohe T, Ueda H (1993) Arrhythmogenic right ventricular dysplasia: evaluation with electron-beam CT. Radiology 187:723–727

Hannebicque G, Becquart J, Gommeaux A et al (1989) Cardiac manifestations of Lyme disease. Apropos of a case (in French). Ann Cardiol Angeiol Paris 38:87–90

Hardy P, Henkelman RM (1989) Transverse relaxation rate enhancement caused by magnetic particles. Magn Reson Imaging 7:265–275

Harvey WP, Segal JP, Gurel T (1964) The spectrum of primary myocardial disease. Prog Cardiovasc Dis 7:17–42

Hausse AO, Aggoun Y, Bonnet D et al (2002) Idebenone and reduced cardiac hypertrophy in Friedreich's ataxia. Heart 87:346–349

Higgins CB, Byrd B 3rd, Stark D et al (1985) Magnetic resonance imaging in hypertrophic cardiomyopathy. Am J Cardiol 55:1121–1126

Hunold P, Wieneke H, Bruder O, et al (2004) Late enhancement in MR imaging of arrhythmogenic right ventricular cardiomyopathy (abstract). J Cardiovasc Magn Reson 6:85–86

Huong DL, Wechsler B, Papo T et al (1997) Endomyocardial fibrosis in Behçet's disease. Ann Rheum Dis 56:205–208

Ichida F, Tsubata S, Bowles KR (2001) Novel gene mutations in patients with left ventricular noncompaction or Barth syndrome. Circulation 103:1256–1263

Imai H, Kumai T, Sekiya M et al (1992) Left ventricular trabeculae evaluated with MRI in dilated cardiomyopathy and old myocardial infarction. J Cardiol 22:83–90

Järvinen VM, Kupari MM, Poutanen V-P, Hekali PE (1996) Right and left atrial phasic volumetric function in mildly symptomatic dilated and hypertrophic cardiomyopathy: cine MR imaging assessment. Radiology 198:487–495

Jenni R, Rojas J, Oechslin E (1999) Isolated noncompaction of the myocardium. N Engl J Med 340:966–967

Jenni R, Oechslin E, Schneider J et al (2001) Echocardiographic and pathoanatomical characteristics of isolated left ventricular non-compaction: a step towards classification as a distinct cardiomyopathy. Heart 86:666–671

Jensen PD, Jensen FT, Christensen T, et al (2001) Indirect evidence for the potential ability of magnetic resonance imaging to evaluate the myocardial iron content in patients with transfusional iron overload. MAGMA 12:153–166

Jensen PD, Jensen FT, Christensen T, et al (2003) Evaluation of myocardial iron by magnetic resonance imaging during iron chelation therapy with deferrioxamine: indication of close relation between myocardial iron content and chelatable iron pool. Blood 101:4632–4639

Kalil-Filho R, Albuquerque CP de (1995) Magnetic resonance imaging in Chagas' heart disease. Rev Paul Med 113:880–883

Kawada N, Sakuma H, Yamakado T et al (1999) Hypertrophic cardiomyopathy: MR measurement of coronary blood flow and vasodilator flow reserve in patients and healthy subjects. Radiology 21:129–135

Kayser HWM, Roos A de, Schalij MJ et al (2003) Usefulness of magnetic resonance imaging in diagnosis of arrhythmogenic right ventricular dysplasia and agreement with electrocardiographic criteria. Am J Cardiol 91:365–367

Kim RJ, Judd RM (2003) Gadolinium-enhanced magnetic resonance imaging in hypertrophic cardiomyopathy. In vivo imaging of the pathologic substrate for premature cardiac death? (editorial comment). J Am Coll Cardiol 41:1568–1572

Kim RJ, Fieno DS, Parrish TB et al (1999) Relationship of MRI delayed contrast enhancement to irreversible injury, infarct age, and contractile function. Circulation 100:1992–2002

Klem I, Weinsaft J, Heitner JF et al (2004) The utility of contrast enhanced MRI for screening patients at risk for malignant ventricular tachyarrythmias. J Cardiovasc Magn Reson 6: 84–85 (abstract)

Kloner RA, Rezkalla SH (2003) Cocaine and the heart. N Engl J Med 348:487–488

Knight C, Kurbaan AS, Seggewiss H et al (1997) Nonsurgical septal reduction for hypertrophic obstructive cardiomyopathy: outcome in the first series of patients. Circulation 95:2075–2081

Koito H, Suzuki J, Nakamori H et al (1995) Clinical significance of abnormal high signal intensity of left ventricular myocardium by gadolinium-diethylenetriaminepentaacetic acid enhanced magnetic resonance imaging in hypertrophic cardiomyopathy. J Cardiol 25:163–170

Koito H, Suzuki J, Ohkubo N, et al (1996) Gadolinium-diethylenetriamine pentaacetic acid enhanced magnetic resonance imaging of dilated cardiomyopathy: clinical significance of abnormally high signal intensity of left ventricular myocardium. J Cardiol 28:41–49

Kono T, Suwa M, Hanada H, Hirota Y, Kawamura K (1992) Clinical significance of normal cardiac silhouette in dilated cardiomyopathy – evaluation based upon echocardiography and magnetic resonance imaging. Jpn Circ J 56:359–365

Kosovsky PA, Ehlers KH, Rafal RB, et al (1991) MR imaging of cardiac mass in Wegener granulomatosis. J Comput Assist Tomogr 15:1028–1030

Kramer CM, Reichek N, Ferrari VA, et al (1994) Regional heterogeneity of function in hypertrophic cardiomyopathy. Circulation 90:186–194

Kuribayashi T, Roberts WC (1992) Myocardial disarray at the junction of ventricular septum and left an right ventricular free wall in hypertrophic cardiomyopathy. Am J Cardiol 70:1333–1340

Kurland RJ, West J, Kelley S et al (1989) Magnetic resonance imaging to detect heart transplant rejection: sensitivity and specificity. Transplant Proc 21:2537–2543

Laissy JP, Messin B, Varenne O et al (2002) MRI of acute myocarditis. A comprehensive approach based on various imaging sequences. Chest 122:1638–1648

Lamb HJ, Beyerbacht HP, Laarse A van der et al (1999) Diastolic dysfunction in hypertensive heart disease is associated with altered myocardial metabolism. Circulation 99:2261–2267

Lesnefsky EJ, Allen KG, Carrea FP, Horwitz LD (1992) Iron-catalyzed reactions cause lipid peroxidation in the intact heart. J Mol Cell Cardiol 24:1031–1038

Lieberman EB, Hutchins GM, Herskowitz A, Rose NR, Baughman KL (1991) Clinicopathologic description of myocarditis. J Am Coll Cardiol 18:1616–1626

Lipshultz SE, Colan SD, Gelber RD et al (1991) Late cardiac effects of doxorubicin therapy for acute lymphoblastic leukemia in childhood. N Engl J Med 324:808–815

Liu P, Olivieri N (1994) Iron overload cardiomyopathies: new insights into an old disease. Cardiovasc Drugs Ther 8:101–110

Liu P, Stone J, Collins A, Olivieri N (1993a) Is there a predictable relationship between ventricular function and myocardial iron levels in patients with hemochromatosis. Circulation 88:183

Liu P, Olivieri N, Sullivan H, Henkelman M (1993b) Magnetic resonance imaging in beta-thalassemia: detection of iron content and association with cardiac complications. J Am Coll Cardiol 21:491

Lombardi C, Rusconi C, Faggiano P, et al (1995) Successful reduction of endomyocardial fibrosis in a patient with idiopathic hypereosinophilic syndrome. A case report. Angiology 46:345–351

Maceira AM, Moon JCC, Prasad SK, Mohiaddin R (2004a) Detection of myocardial fibrosis in systemic hypertension using delayed-enhancement magnetic resonance imaging (abstract). J Cardiovasc Magn Reson 6:222–223

Maceira AM, Prasad SK, Mohiaddin R (2004b) Integrated approach to the evaluation of the hypertensive patient using cardiac MRI (abstract). J Cardiovasc Magn Reson 6:218–219

MacGowan GA, Shapiro EP, Azhari H et al (1997) Shortening in the fiber and cross-fiber directions in the normal human left ventricle and in idiopathic dilated cardiomyopathy. Circulation 96:535–541

Mahrholdt H, Goedecke C, Wagner A et al (2004) Cardiovascular magnetic resonance assessment of human myocarditis. A comparison to histology and molecular biology. Circulation 109:1250–1258

Maier SE, Fischer SE, McKinnon GC, et al (1992) Evaluation of left ventricular segmental wall motion in hypertrophic cardiomyopathy with myocardial tagging. Circulation 86:1919–1928

Mallat Z, Tedgui A, Fontaliran F, et al (1996) Evidence of apoptosis in arrhythmogenic right ventricular dysplasia. N Engl J Med 335:1190–1196

Mana J (2002) Magnetic resonance imaging and nuclear imaging in sarcoidosis. Curr Opin Pulm Med 8:457–463

Maron BJ (2002) Hypertrophic cardiomyopathy. Circulation 106:2419–2421

Maron BJ, Anan TJ, Roberts WC (1981) Quantitative analysis of the distribution of cardiac muscle cell disorganization in the left ventricular wall of patients with hypertrophic cardiomyopathy. Circulation 63:882–894

Maron BJ, Bonow RO, Cannon ROI, Leon MB (1987) Hypertrophic cardiomyopathy: interrelations of clinical manifestations, pathophysiology, and therapy. N Engl J Med 316:780–789

Maron BJ, Pelliccia A, Spirito P (1995) Cardiac disease in young trained athletes. Insight into methods for distinguishing athlete's heart from structural heart disease, with particular emphasis on hypertrophic cardiomyopathy. Circulation 91:1596–1602

Masui T, Finck S, Higgins CB (1992) Constrictive pericarditis and restrictive cardiomyopathy: evaluation with MR imaging. Radiology 182:369–373

Matsuoka H, Hamada M, Honda T et al (1993) Precise assessment of myocardial damage associated with secondary cardiomyopathies by use of Gd-DTPA-enhanced magnetic resonance imaging. Angiology 44:945–950

Matsuoka H, Hamada M, Honda T et al (1994) Evaluation of acute myocarditis and pericarditis by Gd-DTPA enhanced magnetic resonance imaging. Eur Heart J 15:283–284

Matsuki M, Matsuo M (2000) MR findings of myocardial sarcoidosis. Clin Radiol 55:323–325

Mazur W, Nagueh SF, Lakkis NM et al (2001) Regression of left ventricular hypertrophy after nonsurgical septal reduction therapy for hypertrophic obstructive cardiomyopathy. Circulation 103:1492–1496

McCarthy RE III, Boehmer JP, Hruban RH et al (2000) Long-term outcome of fulminant myocarditis as compared with acute nonfulminant myocarditis. N Engl J Med 342:690–695

McCrohon JA, Richmond DR, Pennell DJ, Mohiaddin RH (2002) Isolated noncompaction of the myocardium. A rarity or missed diagnosis? Circulation 106:e22–e23

McCrohon JA, Moon JCC, Prasad SK et al (2003) Differentiation of heart failure related to dilated cardiomyopathy and coronary artery disease using gadolinium-enhanced cardiovascular magnetic resonance. Circulation 108:54–59

McKenna WJ, Thiene G, Nava A et al (1994) Diagnosis of arrhythmogenic right ventricular dysplasia/cardiomyopathy. Br Heart J 71:215–218

Menghetti L, Basso C, Nava A, Angelini A, Thiene G (1996) Spin-echo nuclear magnetic resonance for tissue characterisation in arrhythmogenic right ventricular cardiomyopathy. Heart 76:467–470

Midiri M, Finazzo M, Brancato M et al (1997) Arrhythmogenic right ventricular dysplasia: MR features. Eur Radiol 7:307–312

Migrino R, Abbara S, Cury R, et al (2004) Right ventricular intramyocardial fatty infiltration is associated with diastolic dysfunction (abstract). J Cardiovasc Magn Reson 6:219–220

Morganroth J, Maron BJ, Henry WL, Epstein SE (1975) Comparative left ventricular dimensions in trained athletes. Ann Intern Med 82:521–524

Mollet NR, Dymarkowski S, Volders W et al (2002) Visualization of ventricular thrombi with contrast-enhanced MRI in patients with ischemic heart disease. Circulation 106:2873–2876

Moon JCC, McKenna WJ, McCrohon JA, et al (2003a) Toward clinical risk assessment in hypertrophic cardiomyopathy with gadolinium cardiovascular magnetic resonance. J Am Coll Cardiol 41:1561–1567

Moon JCC, Mundy HR, Lee PJ, Mohiaddin RH, Pennell DJ (2003b) Myocardial fibrosis in glycogen storage disease type III. Circulation 107:e47

Moon JCC, Sachdev B, Elkington AG et al (2003c) Gadolinium enhanced cardiovascular magnetic resonance in Anderson-Fabry disease. Evidence for a disease specific abnormality of the myocardial interstitium. Eur Heart J 24:2151–2155

Motoyasu M, Sukuma H, Uemura S et al (2004) Correlation between hyperenhancement on delayed contrast enhanced MRI and diastolic function in hypertrophic cardiomyopathy (abstract). J Cardiovasc Magn Reson 6:246

Nathwani D, Hamlet N, Walker E (1990) Lyme disease: a review (see comments). Br J Gen Pract 40:72–74

Oechslin EN, Attenhofer Jost CH, Rojas JR et al (2000) Long-term follow-up of 34 adults with isolated left ventricular noncompaction: a distinct cardiomyopathy with poor prognosis. J Am Coll Cardiol 36:493–500

Park JH, Kim YM, Chung JW, et al (1992) MR imaging of hypertrophic cardiomyopathy. Radiology 185:441–446

Parrillo JE (1990) Heart disease and the eosinophil. N Engl J Med 323:1560–1561

Petriz JLF, Hadlich M, Mendonça A et al (2004) Identification of fibrotic form of arrhythmogenic right ventricular dysplasia/cardiomyopathy using gadolinium-enhanced cardiovascular magnetic resonance (abstract). J Cardiovasc Magn Reson 6:224–225

Pignatelli RH, McMahon CJ, Dreyer WJ et al (2003) Clinical characterization of left ventricular noncompaction in children. A relatively common form of cardiomyopathy. Circulation 108:2672–2678

Pitt M, Davies MK, Brady AJ (1996) Hypereosinophilic syndrome: endomyocardial fibrosis. Heart 76:377–378

Pluim BM, Zwinderman AH, van der Laarse A van der, Wall EE van der (1999) The athlete's heart. A meta-analysis of cardiac structure and function. Circulation 100:336–344

Ponsonnaille J, Citron B, Karsenty B et al (1986) Myocardite aiguë au cours d'un syndrome de Lyme. Intérêt de la scintagraphie myocardique au gallium 67. Arch Mal Coeur 13:1946–1950

Proclemer A, Basadonna PT, Slavich GA, et al (1997) Cardiac magnetic resonance imaging findings in patients with right ventricular outflow tract premature contractions. Eur Heart J 18:2002–2010

Rademakers FE, Marchal G, Mortelmans L, Werf F van de, Bogaert J (2003) Evolution of regional performance after an acute anterior myocardial infarction in humans using magnetic resonance tagging. J Physiol (Lond) 546:777–787

Rahman JE, Helou EF, Gelzer-Bell R (2004) Noninvasive diagnosis of biopsy-proven cardiac amyloidosis. J Am Coll Cardiol 43:410–415

Ramamurthy S, Talwar KK, Goswani KC et al (1993) Clinical profile of biopsy proven idiopathic myocarditis. Int J Cardiol 41:225–232

Redfield MM, Gersh BJ, Bailey KR, Rodeheffer RJ (1994) Natural history of incidentally discovered, asymptomatic idiopathic dilated cardiomyopathy. Am J Cardiol 74:737–742

Remes J, Helin M, Vaino P, Rautio P (1990) Clinical outcome and left ventricular function 23 years after acute Coxsackie virus perimyocarditis. Eur Heart J 11:182–188

Richardson P, McKenna W, Bristow M et al (1996) Report of the 1995 World Health Organization/International Society and Federation of Cardiology Task Force on the definition and classification of cardiomyopathies. Circulation 93:841–842

Rochitte CE, Oliveria PF, Andrade JM et al (2003) Chagas disease is characterized by specific pattern and location of myocardial delayed enhanced MRI (abstract). J Cardiovasc Magn Reson 5:13

Roditi GH, Hartnell GG, Cohen MC (2000) MRI changes in myocarditis - evaluation with spin echo, cine MR angiography and contrast enhanced spin echo imaging. Clin Radiol 55:752–758

Rudin M, Pedersen B, Umemura K, Zierhut W (1991) Determination of rat heart morphology and function in vivo in two models of cardiac hypertrophy by means of magnetic resonance imaging. Basic Res Cardiol 86:165–174

Sasson Z, Rasooly Y, Chow CW, Marshall S, Urowitz MB (1992) Impairment of left ventricular diastolic function in systemic lupus erythematosus. Am J Cardiol 69:1629–1634

Schalla S, Higgins CB, Chujo M, Saeed M (2003) Value of nicorandil therapy in preventing myocardial hypertrophy and preserving viability: quantitative MRI study (abstract). J Cardiovasc Magn Reson 5:205

Schaper J, Froede R, Hein S et al (1991) Impairment of the myocardial ultrastructure and changes of the cytoskeleton in dilated cardiomyopathy. Circulation 83:504–514

Scharlag J, Schneider G, Urhausen A, et al (2002) Athlete's heart. Right and left ventricular mass and function in male endurance athletes and untrained individuals determined by magnetic resonance imaging. J Am Coll Cardiol 40:1856–1863

Schulz-Menger J, Strohm O, Waigand J, et al (2000a) The value of magnetic resonance imaging of the left ventricular outflow tract in patients with hypertrophic obstructive cardiomyopathy after septal artery embolization. Circulation 101:1764–1766

Schulz-Menger J, Strohm O, Dietz R, Friedrich MG (2000b) Visualization of cardiac involvement in patients with systemic sarcoidosis applying contrast-enhanced magnetic resonance imaging. MAGMA 11:82–83

Schulz-Menger J, Abdel-Aty H, Goos H, Dietz R, Friedrich MG (2004) Lesion patterns after septal ablation in hypertrophic cardiomyopathy-relation to interventional approach (abstract). J Cardiovasc Magn Reson 6:220

Semelka RC, Tomei E, Wagner S et al (1990) Interstudy reproducibility of dimensional and functional measurements between cine magnetic resonance studies in the morphologically abnormal left ventricle. Am Heart J 119:1367–1373

Senocak F, Sarclar M, Ozkutlu S (1994) Echocardiographic

findings in some metabolic storage diseases. Jpn Heart J 35:635–643

Shabetai R (1986) The pericardium and its diseases. McGraw-Hill, New York, pp 1249–1275

Sharma OP (2003) Diagnosis of cardiac sarcoidosis. An imperfect science, a hesitant art. Chest 123:18–19

Shimada T, Shimada K, Sakane T et al (2001) Diagnosis of cardiac sarcoidosis and evaluation of the effects of steroid therapy by gadolinium-DTPA-enhanced magnetic resonance imaging. Am J Med 110:520–527

Shirey EK, Proudfit WL, Hawk WA (1980) Primary myocardial disease. Correlation with clinical findings, angiographic and biopsy diagnosis. Am Heart J 99:198–207

Sigwart U (1995) Non-surgical reduction for hypertrophic obstructive cardiomyopathy. Lancet 346:211–214

Silverman KJ, Hutchins GM, Bulkley BH (1978) Cardiac sarcoid: a clinicopathologic study of 84 unselected patients with systemic sarcoidosis. Circulation 58:1204–1211

Simonetti OP, Kim RJ, Fieno DS et al (2001) An improved MR imaging technique for the visualization of myocardial infarction. Radiology 218:215–223

Singal PK, Iliskovic N (1998) Doxorubicin-induced cardiomyopathy. N Engl J Med 339:900–905

Siqueira-Filho AG, Cunha CLP, Tajik AJ, et al (1981) M-mode and two-dimensional echocardiographic features in cardiac amyloidosis. Circulation 63:188–196

Sivaram CA, Jugdutt BI, Amy RWM, et al (1985) Cardiac amyloidosis: combined use of two-dimensional echocardiography and electrocardiography in non-invasive screening before biopsy. Clin Cardiol 8:511–588

Smedema JP, Snoep G, Kroonenburgh M van, Gorgels AP (2004) Interobserver agreement of delayed gadolinium enhanced cardiac magnetic resonance imaging in sarcoidosis (abstract). J Cardiovasc Magn Reson 6:242

Smith SC, Ladenson JH, Mason JW, Jaffe AS (1997) Elevations of cardiac troponin I associated with myocarditis. Experimental and clinical correlates. Circulation 95:163–168

Soler R, Rodriguez E, Rodriguez JA, Perez ML, Penas M (1997) Magnetic resonance imaging of apical hypertrophic cardiomyopathy. J Thorac Imaging 12:221–225

Spirito P, Maron BJ (1983) Significance of left ventricular outflow tract cross-sectional area in hypertrophic cardiomyopathy: a two-dimensional echocardiographic assessment. Circulation 67:1100–1108

Spirito P, Pellicia A, Proschan MA et al (1994) Morphology of the "athlete's heart" assesses by echocardiography in 947 elite athletes representing 27 sports. Am J Cardiol 74:802–806

Stanek G, Klein J, Bittner R, Glogar D (1991) *Borrelia burgdorferi* as an etiologic agent in chronic heart failure? Scand J Infect Dis [Suppl] 77:85–87

Stark DD, Mosely ME, Bacon BR et al (1985) Magnetic resonance imaging and spectroscopy of hepatic iron overload. Radiology 154:137–142

Steward S, Mason D, Braunwald E (1968) Impaired rate of left ventricular filling in idiopathic hypertrophic subaortic stenosis and valvular aortic stenosis. Circulation 37:8–14

Strohm O, Schulz-Menger J, Pilz B, et al (2001) Measurement of left ventricular dimensions and function in patients with dilated cardiomyopathy. J Magn Reson Imaging 13:367–371

Stuber M, Scheidegger MB, Fischer SE et al (1999) Alterations in the local myocardial motion pattern in patients suffering from pressure overload due to aortic stenosis. Circulation 100:361–368

Suzuki J, Chang JM, Caputo GR, Higgins CB (1991a) Evaluation of right ventricular early diastolic filling by cine nuclear magnetic resonance imaging in patients with hypertrophic cardiomyopathy. J Am Coll Cardiol 18:120–126

Suzuki J, Caputo GR, Masui T, et al (1991b) Assessment of right ventricular diastolic and systolic function in patients with dilated cardiomyopathy using cine magnetic resonance imaging. Am Heart J 122:1035–1040

Suzuki J, Watanabe F, Takenaka K et al (1993) New subtype of apical hypertrophic cardiomyopathy identified with nuclear magnetic resonance imaging as an underlying cause of markedly inverted T waves. J Am Coll Cardiol 22:1175–1181

Tandri H, Calkins H, Nasier K et al (2003) Magnetic resonance imaging findings in patients meeting task force criteria for arrhythmogenic right ventricular dysplasia. J Cardiovasc Electrophysiol 14:476–482

Tandri H, Martinez C, Saranathan M et al (2004) Non-invasive detection of myocardial fibrosis in arrhythmogenic right ventricular dysplasia by delayed-enhancement magnetic resonance imaging – correlation with histopathology (abstract). J Cardiovasc Magn Reson 6:44–45

Tsukihashi H, Ishibashi Y, Shimada T et al (1994) Changes in gadolinium-DTPA enhanced magnetic resonance signal intensity ratio in hypertrophic cardiomyopathy. J Cardiol 24:185–191

Tsukihashi K, Ueshima K, Uchida T et al (2001) Transient left ventricular apical ballooning without coronary artery stenosis: a novel heart syndrome mimicking acute myocardial infarction. J Am Coll Cardiol 38:11–18

Tung K, DePhilip RM, King MA, Raman SV (2004) Exploring a novel coil position in the magnetic resonance imaging of arrhythmogenic right ventricular dysplasia/cardiomyopathy (abstract). J Cardiovasc Magn Reson 6:247

Ueyama T, Kasamatsu K, Hano T, et al (2002) Emotional stress induces transient left ventricular hypocontraction in the rat via activation of cardiac adrenoceptors. A possible animal of "Tako-Tsubo" cardiomyopathy. Circ J 66:712–713

Uhl HSM (1952) A previously undescribed congenital malformation of the heart: almost total absence of the myocardium of the right ventricle. Bull Johns Hopkins Hosp 91:197–205

Van der Linde MR (1991) Lyme carditis: clinical characteristics of 105 cases. Scand J Infect Dis [Suppl] 77:81–84

Van Dockum WG, Gate FJ ten, Berg JM ten et al (2004) Myocardial infarction after percutaneous transluminal septal myocardial ablation in hypertrophic obstructive cardiomyopathy: evaluation by contrast-enhanced magnetic resonance imaging. J Am Coll Cardiol 43:27–34

Varnava AM, Elliot PM, Sharma S, McKenna WJ, Davies MJ (2000) Hypertrophic cardiomyopathy: the interrelation of disarray, fibrosis, and small vessel disease. Heart 84:476–482

Vignaux O, Dhote R, Duboc D et al (2002a) Detection of myocardial involvement in patients with sarcoidosis applying T2-weighted, contrast-enhanced, and cine magnetic resonance imaging: initial results of a prospective study. J Comput Assist Tomogr 26:762–767

Vignaux O, Dhote R, Duboc D et al (2002b) Clinical significance of myocardial magnetic resonance abnormalities in patients with sarcoidosis. A 1-year follow-up study. Chest 122:1895–1901

Vignaux O, Dhote R, Blanche P, et al (2004) Myocardial MRI in sarcoidosis: 3-years follow-up and evaluation of the effects of steroid therapy (abstract). J Cardiovasc Magn Reson 6:44

Virmani R, Bures JC, Roberts WC (1980) Cardiac sarcoidosis: a major cause of sudden death in young individuals. Chest 77:423–428

Vogel M, Anderson LJ, Holden S, et al (2003) Tissue Doppler echocardiography in patients with thalassaemia detects early myocardial dysfunction related to myocardial iron overload. Eur Heart J 24:113–119

Von Hoff D, Layard M, Basa P (1979) Risk factors for doxorubicin-induced congestive heart failure. Ann Intern Med 91:710–717

Von Kemp K, Beckers R, Vandenweghe J, et al (1989) Echocardiography and magnetic resonance imaging in cardiac amyloidosis. Acta Cardiol 44:29–36

Wagner A, Schulz-Menger J, Dietz R, Friedrich MG (2003) Long-term follow-up of patients with acute myocarditis by magnetic resonance imaging. MAGMA 16:17–20

Walpoth BH, Lazeyras F, Tschopp A et al (1995) Assessment of cardiac rejection and immunosuppression by magnetic resonance imaging and spectroscopy. Transplant Proc 27:2088–2091

Wassmuth R, Lentzsch S, Erbruegger U et al (2001) Subclinical cardiotoxic effects of anthracyclines as assessed by magnetic resonance imaging - a pilot study. Am Heart J 141:1007–1013

Weller PF, Bubley GJ (1994) The idiopathic hypereosinophilic syndrome. Blood 83:2759–2779

Wenger NK, Goodwin JF, Roberts WC (1986) Cardiomyopathy and myocardial involvement in systemic disease. McGraw-Hill, New York, pp 1181–1248

Westwood M, Anderson LJ, Firmin DN et al (2003a) A single breath-hold multi-echo T2* cardiovascular magnetic resonance technique for diagnosis of myocardial iron overload. J Magn Reson Imaging 18:33–39

Westwood M, Anderson LJ, Firmin DN et al (2003b) Interscanner reproducibility of cardiovascular magnetic resonance T2* measurements of tissue iron in thalassemia. J Magn Reson Imaging 18:616–620

White RD, Trohman RG, Flamm SD et al (1998). Right ventricular arrhythmia in the absence of arrhythmogenic dysplasia: MR imaging of myocardial abnormalities. Radiology 207:743–751

Wigle ED, Heimbecker RO, Gunton RW (1962) Idiopathic ventricular septal hypertrophy causing muscular subaortic stenosis. Circulation 26:325–340

World Health Organization Expert Committee (1984) Chagas' disease. World Health Organization technical report series 697. WHO, Geneva, pp 50–55

Wu K, Heldman AW, Brinker JA, Hare JM, Lima JAC (2000) Microvascular obstruction after nonsurgical septal reduction for the treatment of hypertrophic cardiomyopathy. Circulation 104:1868

Wu E, Judd RM, Vargas JD et al (2001) Visualisation of the presence, location and transmural extent of healed Q-wave and non-Q-wave myocardial infarction. Lancet 357:21–28

Yamagishi H, Shirai N, Takagi M et al (2003) Identification of cardiac sarcoidosis with 13N-NH3/18F-FDG PET. J Nucl Med 44:1030–1036

Young AA, Kramer CM, Ferrari VA, Axel L, Reichek N (1994) Three-dimensional left ventricular deformation in hypertrophic cardiomyopathy. Circulation 90:854–867

Zerhouni EA, Parish DM, Rogers WJ, Yang A, Shapiro EP (1988) Human heart: tagging with MR imaging - a new method for noninvasive assessment of myocardial motion. Radiology 169:59–63

10 Heart Failure, Pulmonary Hypertension, and Heart Transplantation

Steven Dymarkowski and Jan Bogaert

CONTENTS

10.1
Heart Failure

10.1.1
Rationale for MRI in Heart Failure

Despite huge efforts by the pharmaceutical industry focused on conservative therapy of patients with heart failure, morbidity and mortality remain unacceptably high (SCHOCKEN et al. 1992). Key elements for detecting the presence of ventricular dysfunction, defining prognosis, and for following therapy are accurate and reproducible measurements of ventricular dimensions, mass, and function (WHITE et al. 1987; DUNN and PRINGLE 1993; LEVY et al. 1990). Under clinical circumstances, evaluation of ventricular systolic function alone most often forms the basis for decision-making, because it can be easily assessed in most patients by echocardiography or radionuclide ventriculography. Nevertheless, absolute quantifica-

S. DYMARKOWSKI, MD, PhD
J. BOGAERT MD, PhD
Department of Radiology, Gasthuisberg University Hospital, Catholic University of Leuven, Herestraat 49, 3000 Leuven, Belgium

tion of ventricular volumes or mass is not routinely performed in daily clinical practice, because the methods used are relatively time-consuming and have unfortunately been limited to clinical trials. From the limited number of trials, however, analysis of serial changes in ventricular volumes, mass, and shape has provided substantial insight into clinically relevant aspects of the remodeling process in heart failure. Studies of the effect of drug interventions on the process of remodeling by noninvasive imaging techniques have unraveled potential mechanisms by which particular pharmacological therapies improve morbidity and mortality in patients with heart failure and after myocardial infarction (KOBER et al. 1995; SOLOMON et al. 2001).

Much of the current knowledge about left ventricle (LV) remodeling in heart failure originates from clinical trials in which serial echocardiography studies have been performed in large patient groups to assess changes in the size and shape of the heart in the context of specific drug therapies (OLDROYD et al. 1991; GAUDRON et al. 1993; PFEFFER et al. 1997). The contributions of these trials to the understanding of the remodeling process are important, as they have guided pharmacological therapy of myocardial infarction or heart failure and stressed the value of echocardiography for the assessment of left ventricular changes over time. Definite advantages of echocardiography are the low cost, availability, and its use to perform a bedside examination. Currently, echocardiography offers additional information about cardiac valvular function and diastolic function that is currently unsurpassed by other imaging modalities. Nevertheless, this technique suffers from unpredictable variation in image quality and a number of studies are not interpretable due to patient-related echogenicity. Therefore, the reproducibility and overall accuracy of echocardiography may not be as high as some of the other available techniques.

Cardiac magnetic resonance imaging (MRI) does not have these limitations and is currently the only imaging technique which provides a comprehensive study of the heart, including anatomical evaluation, functional data, and information about myocardial perfusion and viability. An MRI examination is independent of slice orientation or acoustic window, and postprocessing requires no geometric assumptions as in echocardiography to determine ventricular dimensions, which is particularly important in evaluating ventricles of patients with heart failure who may have severely altered morphology as a result of chronic hibernation or infarction and have regional heterogeneity in wall thickness and contractility. Particularly interesting in patients with severe LV dysfunction is the use of balanced steady-state free precession (b-SSFP) cine MRI techniques, which eliminate the troublesome edge detection between blood and myocardium in the presence of ventricular dilation and slow flow, compared with conventional gradient-echo cine acquisitions. Using this technique in combination with parallel imaging, the breath-hold period in cardiac failure patients can be reduced down to 6 s per slice while maintaining sufficient spatial resolution. Using the latest generation of ultrafast acquisition strategies, cine MRI can even be performed in a single three-dimensional breath-hold of approximately 12 s, covering the entire ventricle, and real-time sequences during free breathing are also becoming more available (YANG et al. 1998; NAGEL et al. 2000).

The highly reproducible results have turned MRI into the reference technique for the noninvasive assessment of LV dimensions, mass, and function (BOGAERT et al. 1995; HOLMAN et al. 1997) and offer an ideal means of serial assessment of disease progression or response to treatment in an individual patient, as well as allowing smaller sample sizes for studies of changes in ventricular function with pharmacological treatment (BELLENGER et al. 2000).

10.1.2
Outcome Studies in Heart Failure

Because of the proven accuracy of quantitative results derived from cardiac MRI studies and due to the recent technical advances that increase feasibility in heart failure patients, several large scale clinical trials are currently including MRI substudies in the research protocol. The Endothelin A Receptor Antagonist Trial in Heart Failure (EARTH study; LUSCHER 2001) was the first study to assess changes in LV dimensions and function over time by serial MRI in all patients. Data from MRI were used to assess the effects of the tested drug on ventricular remodeling before initiating a larger mor-

tality trial. In another smaller study (Metoprolol Randomized Interventional Trial in Heart Failure, MERIT-HF, – 41 patients with chronic heart failure; METOPROLOL 1999), the antiremodeling effects of metoprolol CR/XL on the LV were proven. Other randomized clinical trials, including the Valsartan Heart Failure Trial (Val-HeFT; COHN et al. 1999; WONG et al. 2002) and the Randomized Etanercept North American Strategy to Study Antagonism of Cytokines (RENAISSANCE) trial, have had MRI substudies (Fig. 10.1), with the results pending (ANAND et al. 2004). Even though this method may be more expensive than two-dimensional (2D) echocardiography, in the future we will probably see its greater reproducibility exploited as the imaging modality of choice for similar trials, thereby compensating the greater cost by the savings from recruiting and studying fewer patients.

10.2
Pulmonary Hypertension

10.2.1
Pathophysiology

Pulmonary arterial hypertension is defined by the World Health Organization as a spectrum of conditions which include primary pulmonary hypertension and several diseases with different pathogenesis and high risk factors to develop pulmonary arterial hypertension (secondary forms). Pulmonary arterial hypertension can occur on an idiopathic or hereditary basis or can be drug induced. Pulmonary venous hypertension is often caused by left-sided heart disease or by compression of lung veins, e.g., due to compression by a lung tumor. Furthermore pulmonary hypertension can be associated with disorders of the respiratory system (chronic obstructive pulmonary disease, interstitial lung disease) or from chronic thrombotic and/or embolic disease (obstruction of pulmonary arteries).

Pulmonary hypertension is diagnosed when mean and systolic pulmonary arterial pressures exceed 20 and 30 mmHg, respectively (FOWLER et al. 1953). If the increased pressure persists, right-sided heart insufficiency and cor pulmonale may develop. This condition is associated with a poor prognosis. It should be remarked that in patients, but also in asymptomatic people, pulmonary arterial pressure increases with age, due to decreased compliance of the pulmonary artery and increased pulmonary vascular resistance.

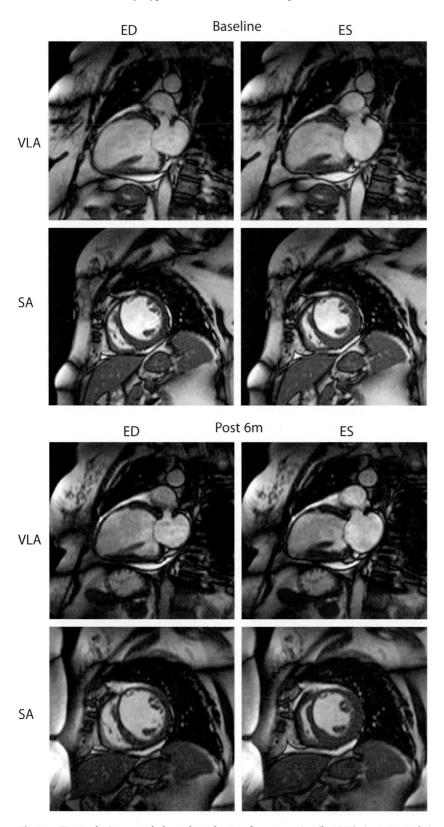

Fig. 10.1. *Top*: Inclusion-stage balanced steady-state free precession (b-SSFP) cine MRI study in vertical long-axis (*upper row*) and short-axis (*lower row*) orientation of a 69-year-old heart failure patient included in the Valsartan Heart Failure Trial (Val-HeFT). Wall thinning in the anterior LV wall is observed. The ventricle appears dilated and globally hypokinetic. *Bottom*: Corresponding images of the follow-up study 6 months later show comparable morphological and functional features. No additional negative remodeling effects can be observed. *ED*, end-diastole; *ES*, end-systole; *VLA*, vertical long-axis; *SA*, short axis

Symptoms of pulmonary hypertension are nonspecific: dyspnea, exercise intolerance, chronic fatigue, and chest pains. Diagnosis can therefore be delayed until in an advanced stage of disease, leading to poor prognosis and lack of therapeutic options.

The incidence of idiopathic pulmonary hypertension is approximately two to three persons per one million per year, with a male predominance of 3.1:1.7 (CHATTERJEE et al. 2002).

The secondary forms of pulmonary hypertension should be conceived as a complication of other pathological entities. About half of patients with chronic obstructive lung disease develop pulmonary hypertension, and 40% of patients with scleroderma develop pulmonary hypertension. In the USA, more than 5,000 patients a year develop chronic thromboembolic pulmonary hypertension as a delayed complication following acute pulmonary embolism (1% of all cases of acute pulmonary embolism).

10.2.2
Role of Imaging in Pulmonary Hypertension

As discussed above, many pathological entities can be deemed responsible for pulmonary hypertension. Therefore, the result of the workup in these patients needs to provide a clear, differential diagnosis beyond reasonable doubt in order to select the correct treatment option. Beside the patient's (family) history and laboratory findings, cardiac and pulmonary function analysis needs to be performed next to imaging of the pulmonary vasculature. Traditionally, imaging for pulmonary hypertension principally includes echocardiography, catheterization of the right side of the heart, and ventilation/perfusion scintigraphy (McLAUGHLIN 2002). However, there is reasonable ground to assume that recent evolutions both in computed tomography (CT) and MRI have more to offer than most experienced clinicians are aware of.

10.2.2.1
Role of CT

The strength of computed tomography (CT) in the workup of pulmonary hypertension has been mainly expressed by the new multi-slice CT scanner technology.

With conventional single-slice scanning techniques, thick-slice (5 mm) imaging of the entire thorax can take up to 30 s, which is almost impossible for patients with dyspnea. Recent technological advances in multi-slice CT (4–64 simultaneous slices) have made it possible to image the complete lung parenchyma with high resolution in less than 10 s with a slice thickness of approximately 1 mm. Due to the high and isotropic spatial resolution, parenchymal changes at the level of the secondary lobule can now be visualized in any plane. The role of CT is to demonstrate imaging features of secondary forms of pulmonary hypertension: emphysema is visualized as a decrease in mean lung density, whereas fibrosis leads to an increased mean lung density. Both changes accompany chronic, progressive hypoxia leading to hypoxic vasoconstriction of the peripheral pulmonary arteries. Parenchymal changes resulting from acute or chronic pulmonary embolism are mainly effusion- or pleural-based (hemorrhagic) lung infarcts (Thickened septal lines, poorly defined nodular opacities, and enlarged lymph nodes are suggestive of veno-occlusive disease or pulmonary capillary hemangiomatosis (GLUECKER et al. 1999). Cystic fibrosis is another disease which accompanies hypoxemia and subsequent development of pulmonary hypertension (FRASER et al. 1999).

The second benefit of the increased image acquisition speed of multi-slice CT technology is the ability to perform CT angiography. The central pulmonary vessels can be imaged with thinner slices in a shorter time (5–8 s). The increased speed greatly reduces respiratory motion artifacts, and the thin collimation improves the depiction of subsegmental arteries.

As multislice CT is widely accepted and available, CT is often considered as the first-line cross-sectional imaging modality for evaluation of acute pulmonary embolism (REMY-JARDIN et al. 2003). Thrombi within the pulmonary arteries are detected as wall-adherent filling defects surrounded by contrast material. Especially during the acute phase, complete triangular perfusion defects can be visualized within the pulmonary parenchyma. Parenchymal changes resulting from acute or chronic pulmonary embolism are mainly effusion- or pleural-based (hemorrhagic) lung infarcts (ROBERTS et al. 1997).

In spite of the different obvious advantages of CT, it is nevertheless under discussion whether CT is going to be the modality of choice for pulmonary hypertension. TRABOLD et al. (2003) have compared the radiation expose of a 16-row detector CT examination with conventional angiography and concluded that radiation exposure is comparable with a scan of the thorax or abdomen (4.3 mSv). This might become an important drawback in the future, especially if close follow-up examinations are being considered.

10.2.2.2
Role of MRI

Depending on the severity of pulmonary hypertension, patients develop progressive right ventricular myocardial hypertrophy, dilatation of the right ventricle (RV) and atrium, and a global and regional reduction in right ventricular contractility (NAKAMURA et al. 1995; CASO et al. 2001). There is progressive increase in right ventricular pressure, which is exerted on the interventricular septum as an abnormal curvature and paradoxical motion during the early filling phase of diastole. In an echocardiography study of right and left ventricular dysfunction in 434 patients with severe pulmonary disease, right ventricular dysfunction (right ventricular ejection fraction less than 45%) was found to be more severe in patients with pulmonary hypertension than in the patients with parenchymal or airway disease (VIZZA et al. 1998).

However, any physician experienced in echocardiography knows that evaluation of the RV is difficult for a number of reasons. First, the spatial position of the RV within the chest makes a complete evaluation nearly impossible, due in part to the near position of the ultrasound probe. A second disadvantage is the absence of standardized model equations for calculation of end-diastolic and end-systolic volumes and ejection fraction. A third problem is that several patients presenting with pulmonary hypertension have coexisting advanced obstructive pulmonary disease, which presents the echocardiographer with poor acoustic windows (ARCASOY et al. 2003).

Therefore the main role for MRI in pulmonary hypertension should be quantification of ventricular volumes and contractility (Fig. 10.2). The accuracy and reproducibility of MRI in evaluation of the RV has been extensively researched and equals the results of studies performed for the LV (ROMINGER et al. 1999; ALFAKIH et al. 2003). The reproducibility certainly encourages follow-up examinations to monitor drug therapy, evaluate invasive options, or to evaluate functional recovery after surgery (e.g., pulmonary thromboendarterectomy for chronic thromboembolic pulmonary hypertension; Fig. 10.3). A combination of transversal and ventricular short-axis cine MRI series provides a solid base for contour delineation for the RV and LV, respectively, since the increased trabeculations of the RV may be difficult to assess on one single orientation.

Furthermore, the process of pathological ventricular coupling (abnormal septal flattening or inversion during the filling phase of diastole) can be studied using real-time untriggered cine MRI and can be useful to discriminate pulmonary hypertension from constrictive pericarditis or restrictive heart disease. Using phase-contrast flow measurements, flow profiles through the major pulmonary artery branches can be performed, correlating well to both echocardiography (ROMINGER et al. 2002) and invasive pulmonary artery pressure measurements (LAFFON et al. 2001).

The MRI examination of patients who are suspected of having pulmonary hypertension can be further completed by performing a 3D MR angiography of the pulmonary arteries using ultrafast gradient-echo sequences. Although results of initial studies are promising (VOGT et al. 2003), even with the application of parallel imaging technology to increase imaging speed, MR angiography is currently inferior to CT angiography in the evaluation of pulmonary embolism due to lower spatial and temporal resolution (OHNO et al. 2003). MR angiography is therefore mainly used

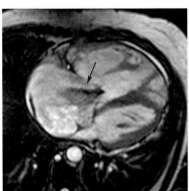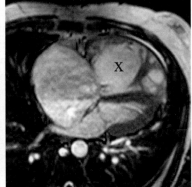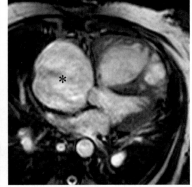

Fig. 10.2. Transverse b-SSFP cine MR images in a 73-year-old patient with pronounced pulmonary arterial hypertension. The right atrium (*asterisk*) and right ventricle (*X*) appear dilated and, due to dilation of the tricuspid valve ring, there is tricuspid regurgitation (*arrow*). Functional analysis: RV EDV 512 ml, ESV 402 ml, SV 115 ml, EF 23%

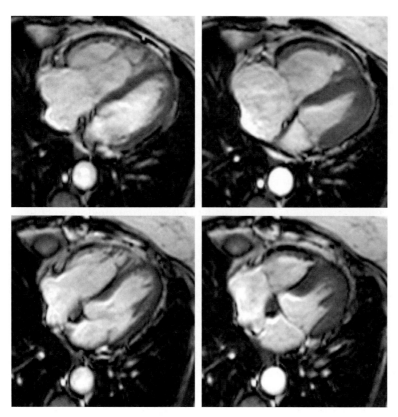

Fig. 10.3. Cine MRI study in a 68-year-old-patient with thromboembolic pulmonary hypertension acquired before (*top*) and 3 months after (*bottom*) pulmonary thromboendarterectomy. End-diastolic (*left*) and end-systolic (*right*) frames. The control study confirms decrease in the right ventricular and atrial volumes, regression of the flattening of the interventricular septum, and increase in regional right ventricular contractility

for detection of acute or chronic thromboembolic pulmonary hypertension. Oudkerk et al. have examined 141 patients with suspected pulmonary embolism and found a sensitivity of MR angiography for isolated subsegmental, segmental, and central pulmonary emboli of 40%, 84%, and 100%, respectively, compared with conventional X-ray angiography (OUDKERK et al. 2002). Future improvements will certainly again raise the question of whether to perform CT of MR angiography for this indication if the issue of radiation exposure is to be addressed.

10.3
Heart Transplantation

10.3.1
Detection of Allograft Rejection

Since Christiaan Barnard performed the first procedure on 3 December 1967, the technique of orthotopic heart transplantation has been perfected and has become an established treatment for selected patients with refractory heart failure. Long-term survival rates are superior to those resulting from other forms

of therapy for that patient population. In addition, an improved quality of life has been reported by many patients. A vigilant eye remains necessary to detect acute allograft rejection, which remains one of the major causes of death during the 1st year posttransplantation. Thus, a crucial factor in improving results is accurate evaluation of the severity and extent of cardiac rejection, with differentiation of rejection from other conditions such as infection (WALPOTH et al. 1995).

In the early phase, myocardial rejection consists of interstitial edema and mononuclear cell infiltration, which progresses toward myocytolysis or myocyte necrosis (SASAKI et al. 1987). Therefore, early diagnosis and adequate treatment before the occurrence of myocardial necrosis are mandatory. However, the clinical presentation of acute cardiac rejection may be silent in patients receiving cyclosporine treatment. Right endomyocardial biopsy and histological grading is the gold standard for the detection of myocardial rejection (CAVES et al. 1973; BILLINGHAM 1982). However, endomyocardial biopsy has several drawbacks: it is invasive and costly, 6–12 h is required before the diagnostic results become available, experienced pathologists are required for the histological diagnosis, and it is prone to sampling error (NISHIMURA et al. 1988; SMART et al. 1993). Therefore, a noninvasive modality that would guide the timing of endomyocardial biopsy and assess the response to changes in immunosuppressive therapy would be advantageous. Several pathways to use MRI as such a monitoring tool have been explored.

Since one of the early findings in cardiac rejection is an increase in the myocardial water content, principally due to myocardial edema, assessment of relaxation times theoretically provides a sensitive measure of rejection (SCOTT et al. 1983). Although animal studies have consistently shown increases in T2 relaxation times in cardiac transplants as early as 2 days after transplantation (SASAGURI et al. 1985; AHERNE et al. 1986; NISHIMURA et al. 1987, 1988), studies in patients, however, have proved to be more contradictory. While some investigators have shown an increase in T2 relaxation times in patients with cardiac rejection (SMART et al. 1993; MARIE et al. 2001), others could not confirm these results (DOORNBOS et al. 1990). There is a large degree of overlap between the T2 values of normal volunteers, patients without signs of cardiac rejection, and patients with such signs. In other words, the absence of a demarcation value between normal or nonrejected and rejected myocardium precludes the clinical application of T2 relaxation times for assessment of cardiac rejection.

The contradictory results between these animal and patient studies can be explained in several ways. First, the signal intensity on T2-weighted images of supposedly abnormal myocardium may be influenced by the presence of varying degrees of necrosis, edema, and fibrosis, making measurement of T2 relaxation times difficult with present spatial resolution. Second, animal studies represent optimized conditions, while the clinical situation is far more complex. Factors such as variable ischemia time of the donor heart or effects of cyclosporine therapy may contribute to changes in T2 relaxation time.

Several investigators have evaluated the role of contrast agents for the assessment of cardiac transplant rejection. Animal studies using extracellular gadolinium-diethylene triamine penta-acetic acid (Gd-DTPA) have shown that, in the absence of rejection, Gd-DTPA induces mild homogeneous myocardial enhancement (NISHIMURA et al. 1987; KURLAND et al. 1989), while moderate and severe allograft rejection are characterized by one or more areas of intense myocardial enhancement. The extent and distribution of intense myocardial enhancement corresponds to the severity and extent of histological rejection. Studies using blood-pool agents have found statistically significant contrast-enhancement differences between acutely rejecting heart transplants and nonrejecting ones at 4 min after injection of the contrast agent, and these increase with increasing time after injection, with relative contrast enhancement reflecting the histologically determined degree of rejection (JOHANSSON et al. 2002).

In patients, these results have not been reproduced. Mousseaux et al. have reported myocardial enhancement not to be significantly different in patients with mild histological rejection compared with those with moderate or severe rejection (MOUSSEAUX et al. 1993) In a more recent paper using 3D contrast-enhanced inversion-recovery (CE-IR) MRI techniques (ALMENAR et al. 2003), beside a trend toward increased myocardial uptake in patients with acute necrosis, analysis of myocardial perfusion and CE-IR MRI sequences do not reflect any significant changes.

Bearing in mind these often contradictory results, the large overlap between patients and control groups on the one hand, and the overlap between the different degrees of acute rejection on the other hand, the role for MRI in diagnosing allograft rejection remains questionable. Nevertheless, the increased capability of MRI to visualize even small areas of focal necrosis, using newer CE-IR MRI techniques, and the advent of interventional cardiac MRI should inspire investigators to continue research. A potential role of MRI could be to serve as an interactive imaging modality, helpful in guiding endomyocardial biopsy as the current undisputed gold standard, and thus reducing the sampling error.

10.3.2
Long-Term Allograft Surveillance

It is important to realize that the transplanted heart does not provide the recipient with normal cardiac function. Cardiac physiology after heart transplantation is unique. When the native heart is removed, sympathetic and parasympathetic innervation is severed, causing resting hemodynamics to differ significantly, acutely and chronically, from those seen in healthy subjects. In addition, the renin–angiotensin–aldosterone regulation mechanism undergoes changes as a result of surgical denervation. Afferent control mechanisms and efferent responses both are altered, leading to important clinical abnormalities. The heart rate does not vary according to respiration and does not respond to Valsalva maneuvers or carotid massage. Other examples include altered cardiovascular responses to exercise, altered cardiac electrophysiology, and altered responses to cardiac pharmacological agents (COTTS and OREN 1997). Finally, most patients do not experience angina after cardiac transplant, because of denervation, although there are reports of angina during myocardial ischemia. Several authors have noted limited sympathetic reinnervation in some cardiac transplant recipients (WILSON et al. 1991; BENGEL et al. 2001). This finding suggests that reinnervation may include a return of sympathetic neural mediation of heart rate, ventricular contractility, and modulation of artery vasomotor tone. An improved understanding of the changes in cardiac physiology, which occur after heart transplant, may allow the care of these patients to be optimized.

It is known that patients develop high ejection fractions and present with concentric hypertrophy in the later stages after transplantation (Fig. 10.4). In a recent study by Wilhelmi et al. in a patient cohort 12.5±1.4 years after heart transplantation, it was shown with Doppler echocardiography that ejection

fraction increased to 71±11.7%, left ventricular mass increased to 263.8±111.4 g in men and 373.0±181.1 g in women. Focused on right ventricular morphology, enlargement of both the right atrium and the RV was observed in the majority of the patients (WILHELMI et al. 2002).

MRI has a definite role in the long-term follow up of patients after cardiac transplantation to assess cardiac morphology and function, since one of the major strengths of MRI in assessing cardiac diseases is the accurate assessment of ventricular function and mass (Fig. 10.5). The excellent visualization of the myocardium on cine MRI and its endo- and epicardial surfaces enables tracking of changes in wall thickening and wall motion over time and has undisputed benefits in terms of accuracy over echocardiography (BOGAERT et al. 1995). Cardiac MRI with b-SSFP cine studies can offer increased sensitivity of long-term follow-up studies and also allows evaluation of changes in time which otherwise would be missed (BARKHAUSEN et al. 2001).

Furthermore, a comprehensive MRI examination may be used to noninvasively detect transplant arteriopathy. Due to the denervation of the allograft as

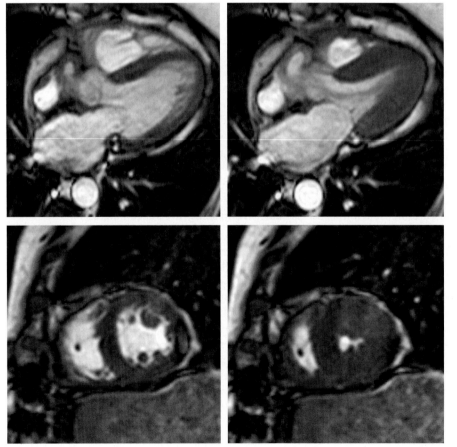

Fig. 10.4. Long-axis (*top*) and short-axis (*bottom*) cine MRI series in a 66-year-old patient, 7 years after cardiac transplantation. The images emphasize the long-term effects of cardiac denervation. Note the very small end-systolic left ventricular cavity volume (*right*) with normal end-diastolic wall thickness. The ejection fraction is increased to 84%, end-diastolic volume 101 ml, myocardial mass 134 g

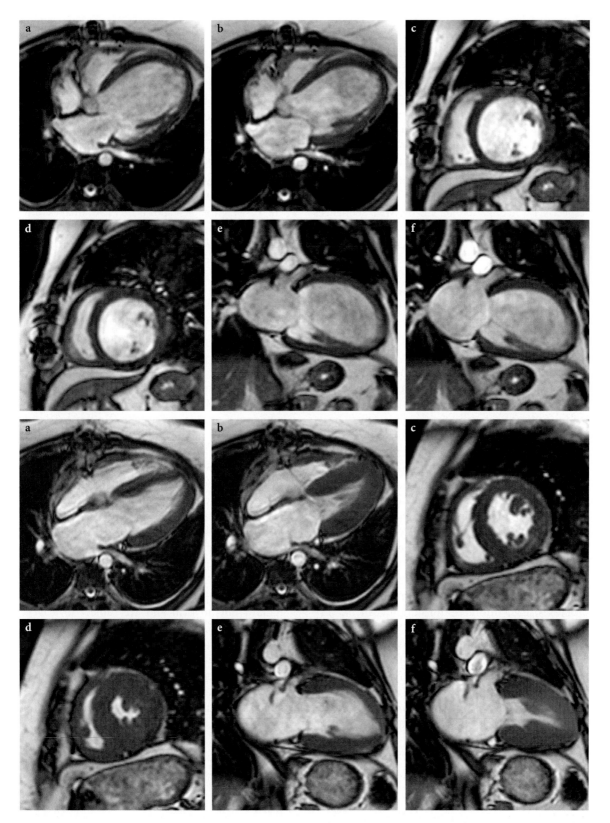

Fig. 10.5a-f. Comparison of pre- and posttransplant MRI studies. *Upper two rows*: Cine MRI images from a 38-year-old patient with idiopathic dilated cardiomyopathy. The LV is dilated and severely hypokinetic (EDV 344 ml, ESV 290 ml, SV 54 ml, EF 23%). *Lower two rows*: Corresponding cine MRI series 3 years after transplantation. Horizontal long-axis (**a,b**), midventricular short-axis (**c,d**) and ventricular long-axis (**e,f**) at end diastole (**a,c,e**) and end systole (**b,d,f**). Note the surgically altered atrial anatomy (part donor and receptor atrium) and the good systolic function of the allograft (EDV 117 ml, ESV 44 ml, SV 73 ml, EF 62%). Measurement of the end-diastolic wall thickness (average 16 mm) and the total myocardial mass (235 g) indicates the patient has developed concentric hypertrophy

mentioned above, transplant arteriopathy often lacks clinical symptoms and is the reason for frequent surveillance angiography in heart transplant recipients. By performing resting state and hyperemic MR perfusion measurements, myocardial perfusion reserve (MPR) and endomyocardial to epimyocardial perfusion ratio can be assessed. In a study by MUELING et al. (2003), transplant arteriopathy was detected, expressed as a decreased myocardial perfusion reserve with sensitivity and specificity of 100% and 85%, respectively. Acquisition of CE-IR MRI sequences and coronary MR angiography will certainly in the near future further increase the specificity of this approach.

10.3.3
Detection of Complications

After transplantation both sections of the recipient and donor atria are intact but do not contract synergistically. The decreased atrial input results in a lower net stroke volume than that in a native heart. In the immediate postoperative period, a "stiff" heart develops, causing a restrictive hemodynamic pattern that results in low cardiac output. Low cardiac output may be caused by one or more of the following: vasopressors used in the donor, ischemic injury at the time of donor procurement, denervation, high peripheral vascular resistance, edema, and allograft rejection (COTTS and OREN 1997). Next to complications associated with restrictive heart disease and the difficult differential diagnosis with constrictive pericarditis, other complications such as pleural or pericardial effusion, hemorrhage, and endocavitary processes, e.g., thrombus formation, can be very well assessed with MRI.

Pericardial effusions appear as high-intensity, crescent-shaped structures within the myocardium and can contain linear densities, representing hemorrhagic content of fibrotic strands. Thrombus formation occurs most currently in the morphologically abnormal atria and is usually broad based on the atrial

wall. Thrombi appear on cine MR images as a heterogeneously intense, soft tissue mass, easily detectable if large, but smaller thrombi may be masked on b-SSFP cine images, due to the intrinsic contrast mechanism of these sequences. Because the T2 and T1 values of the blood itself contribute more to the hyperintense signal than does intracardiac flow, a thrombus – or blood clot – can be nearly invisible in an abnormally shaped atrium with sluggish blood flow near the borders. Therefore it is recommended to acquire either T1- or T2-weighted fast spin-echo (TSE) images or to inject intravenous contrast and to acquire CE-IR MRI series to improve visualization (MOLLET et al. 2002). Thrombi will appear as intermediate to high signal intensity on TSE images and as nonenhancing structures on CE-MRI images (Fig. 10.6).

Key Points

- Noninvasive serial MRI assessment of LV remodeling provides important information regarding outcome and therapy response in patients with LV dysfunction and heart failure. The limited measurement variability and reproducibility maximizes the value of the data obtained.

- In pulmonary hypertension, CT is valuable in depiction of parenchymal changes and visualization of vascular abnormalities. MRI should be considered as a diagnostic tool to monitor therapeutic effects on right-sided heart performance and to noninvasively assess hemodynamic parameters.

- Results of MRI studies in acute allograft rejection remain unequivocal and are subject to a large standard deviation over different study populations. MRI after cardiac transplantation is especially well suited to monitor long-term effects of cardiac denervation and the corresponding cardiovascular adaptation. MRI offers a comprehensive evaluation of complications following transplantation surgery.

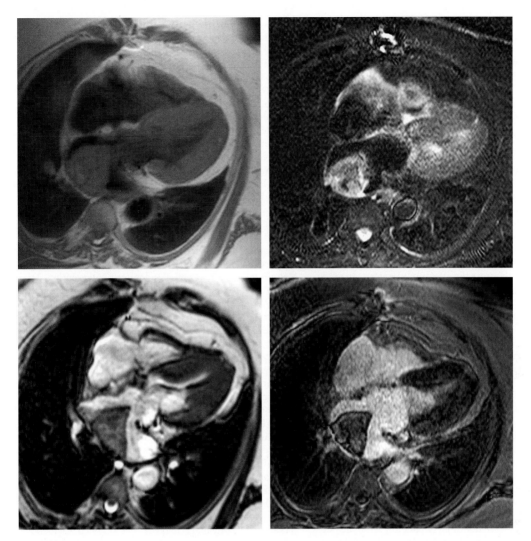

Fig. 10.6. Atrial thrombus formation. A large soft-tissue mass is located on the posterior wall of the left atrium in a 59-year-old transplant patient. *Top row:* T1-weighted TSE (*left*) and T2-weighted TSE-STIR image (*right*). *Bottom row:* The mass does not contain any internal flow on cine MRI (*left*) and does not enhance on CE-IR MR images (*right*). Findings consistent with thrombus formation. Note the increased left ventricular wall thickness (20 mm), indicating concentric hypertrophy

References

Aherne T, Tscholakoff D, Finkbeiner W et al (1986) Magnetic resonance imaging of cardiac transplants: the evaluation of rejection of cardiac allografts with and without immunosuppression. Circulation 74:145–156

Alfakih K, Plein S, Thiele H et al (2003) Normal human left and right ventricular dimensions for MRI as assessed by turbo gradient echo and steady-state free precession imaging sequences. J Magn Reson Imaging 17:323–329

Almenar L, Iguala B, Martínez-Dolza L et al (2003) Utility of cardiac magnetic resonance imaging for the diagnosis of heart transplant rejection. Transplant Proc 35:1962–1964

Anand I, McMurray JJ, Whitmore J et al (2004) Anemia and its relationship to clinical outcome in heart failure. Circulation (Electronic version)

Arcasoy SM, Christie JD, Ferrari VA et al (2003) Echocardiographic assessment of pulmonary hypertension in patients with advanced lung disease. Am J Respir Crit Care Med 167:735–740

Barkhausen J, Ruehm SG, Goyen M et al (2001) MR evaluation of ventricular function: true fast imaging with steady-state precession versus fast low-angle shot cine MR imaging: feasibility study. Radiology 219:264–269

Bellenger NG, Davies LC, Francis JM et al (2000) Reduction in sample size for studies of remodelling in heart failure by the use of cardiovascular magnetic resonance. J Cardiovasc Magn Reson 2:271–278

Bengel FM, Ueberfuhr P, Schiepel N et al (2001) Effect of

sympathetic reinnervation on cardiac performance after heart transplantation. N Engl J Med 345:731–738

Billingham ME (1982) Diagnosis of cardiac rejection by endomyocardial biopsy. Heart Transpl 1:25–30

Bogaert J, Bosmans H, Rademakers FE et al (1995) Left ventricular quantification with breath-hold MR imaging: comparison with echocardiography. Magma 3:5–12

Caso P, Galderisi M, Cicala S et al (2001) Association between myocardial right ventricular relaxation time and pulmonary arterial pressure in chronic obstructive lung disease: analysis by pulsed Doppler tissue imaging. J Am Soc Echocardiogr 14:970–977

Caves PK, Stinson EB, Graham AF, et al (1973) Percutaneous transvenous endomyocardial biopsy. JAMA 225:288–291

Chatterjee K, Marco T de, Alpert JS (2002) Pulmonary hypertension: hemodynamic diagnosis and management. Arch Int Med 162:1925–1933

Cohn JN, Tognoni G, Glazer RD et al (1999) Rationale and design of the Valsartan Heart Failure Trial: a large multinational trial to assess the effects of valsartan, an angiotensin-receptor blocker, on morbidity and mortality in chronic congestive heart failure. J Card Fail 5:155–160

Cotts WG, Oren RM (1997) Function of the transplanted heart: unique physiology and therapeutic implications. Am J Med Sci 314:164–172

Doornbos J, Verwey H, Essed CE, Balk AH, Roos A de (1990) MR imaging in assessment of cardiac transplant rejection in humans. J Comput Assist Tomogr 14:77–81

Dunn FG, Pringle SD (1993) Sudden cardiac death, ventricular arrhythmias and hypertensive left ventricular hypertrophy J Hypertens 11:1003–1010

Fowler NO, Wescott RN, Scott RC (1953) Normal pressure in right heart and pulmonary artery. Am Heart J 46:264–270

Fraser KL, Tullis DE, Sasson Z et al (1999) Pulmonary hypertension and cardiac function in adult cystic fibrosis: role of hypoxemia. Chest 115:1321–1328

Gaudron P, Eilles C, Kugler I, Ertl G (1993) Progressive left ventricular dysfunction and remodeling after myocardial infarction. Potential mechanisms and early predictors. Circulation 87:755–763

Gluecker T, Capasso P, Schnyder P et al (1999) Clinical and radiologic features of pulmonary edema. Radiographics 19:1507–1531

Groenning BA, Nilsson JC, Sondergaard L et al (2000) Anti-remodeling effects on the left ventricle during beta-blockade with metoprolol in the treatment of chronic heart failure. J Am Coll Cardiol 36:2072–2080

Holman ER, Buller VG, Roos A de et al (1997) Detection and quantification of dysfunctional myocardium by magnetic resonance imaging. A new three-dimensional method for quantitative wall-thickening analysis. Circulation 95:924–931

Johansson L, Johnsson C, Penno E et al (2002) Acute cardiac transplant rejection: detection and grading with MR imaging with a blood pool contrast agent – experimental study in the rat. Radiology 225:97–103

Kober L, Torp-Pedersen C, Carlsen JE et al (1995) A clinical trial of the angiotensin-converting-enzyme inhibitor trandolapril in patients with left ventricular dysfunction after myocardial infarction. Trandolapril Cardiac Evaluation (TRACE) Study Group. N Engl J Med 333:1670–1676

Kurland RJ, West J, Kelley S et al (1989) Magnetic resonance imaging to detect heart transplant rejection: sensitivity and specificity. Transplant Proc 21:2537–2543

Laffon E, Laurent F, Bernard V et al (2001) Noninvasive assessment of pulmonary arterial hypertension by MR phase-mapping method. J Appl Physiol 90:2197–2202

Levy D, Garrison RJ, Savage DD et al (1990) Prognostic implications of echocardiographically determined left ventricular mass in the Framingham Heart Study. N Engl J Med 322:1561–1566

Luscher TF, Ruschitzka F, Anand I et al (2001) Endothelin A receptor antagonist trial in heart failure. Heart Drug 1:294–298

Marie PY, Angioi M, Carteaux JP et al (2001) Detection and prediction of acute heart transplant rejection with the myocardial T2 determination provided by a black-blood magnetic resonance imaging sequence. J Am Coll Cardiol 37:825–831

McLaughlin VV (2002) Primary pulmonary hypertension. Hospital Physician Board Review Manual 9:1–11

Metoprolol CR/XL (1999) Randomised Intervention Trial in Congestive Heart Failure Group: effect of metoprolol CR/XL in chronic heart failure: Metoprolol CR/XL Randomised Intervention Trial in Congestive Heart Failure (MERIT-HF). Lancet 353:2001–2007

Mollet NR, Dymarkowski S, Volders W et al (2002) Visualization of ventricular thrombi with contrast-enhanced magnetic resonance imaging in patients with ischemic heart disease. Circulation 106:2873–2876

Mousseaux E, Farge D, Guillemain R et al (1993) Assessing human cardiac allograft rejection using MRI with Gd-DOTA. J Comput Assist Tomogr 17:237–244

Muehling OM, Wilke NM, Panse P et al (2003) Reduced myocardial perfusion reserve and transmural perfusion gradient in heart transplant arteriopathy assessed by magnetic resonance imaging. J Am Coll Cardiol 42:1054–1060

Nagel E, Schneider U, Schalla S (2000) Magnetic resonance real-time imaging for the evaluation of left ventricular function. J Cardiovasc Magn Reson 2:7–14

Nakamura K, Miyahara Y, Ikeda S et al (1995) Assessment of right ventricular diastolic function by pulsed Doppler echocardiography in chronic pulmonary disease and pulmonary thromboembolism. Respiration 62:237–243

Nishimura T, Sada M, Sasaki H et al (1987) Cardiac transplantation in dogs: evaluation with gated MRI and Gd-DTPA contrast enhancement. Heart Vessels 3:141–145

Nishimura T, Sada M, Sasaki H et al (1988) Assessment of severity of cardiac rejection in heterotopic heart transplantation using indium-111 antimyosin and magnetic resonance imaging. Cardiovasc Res 22:108–112

Ohno Y, Kawamitsu H, Higashino T et al (2003) Time-resolved contrast-enhanced pulmonary MR angiography using sensitivity encoding (SENSE). J Magn Reson Imaging 17:330–336

Oldroyd KG, Pye MP, Ray SG et al (1991) Effects of early captopril administration on infarct expansion, left ventricular remodeling and exercise capacity after acute myocardial infarction. Am J Cardiol 68:713–718

Oudkerk M, van Beek EJ, Wielopolski et al (2002) Comparison of contrast-enhanced magnetic resonance angiography and conventional pulmonary angiography for the diagnosis of pulmonary embolism: a prospective study. Lancet 359:1643–1647

Pfeffer MA, Greaves SC, Arnold JM et al (1997) Early versus

delayed angiotensin-converting enzyme inhibition therapy in acute myocardial infarction. The healing and early afterload reducing therapy trial. Circulation 95:2643-2651

Remy-Jardin M, Mastora I, Remy J (2003) Pulmonary embolus imaging with multislice CT. Radiol Clin North Am 41:507-519

Roberts HC, Kauczor H-U, Schweden F, Thelen M (1997) Spiral CT of pulmonary hypertension and chronic thromboembolism. J Thorac Imaging 12:118-127

Rominger MB, Bachmann GF, Pabst W et al (1999) Right ventricular volumes and ejection fraction with fast cine MR imaging in breath-hold technique: applicability, normal values from 52 volunteers, and evaluation of 325 adult cardiac patients. J Magn Reson Imaging 10:908-918

Rominger MB, Dinkel HP, Bachmann et al (2002) Comparison between fast MR flow quantification in breathhold technique in ascending aorta and pulmonary trunk with right and left ventricular cine-MRI for the assessment of stroke volumes in healthy volunteers. Fortschr Röntgenstr 174:196-201

Sasaguri S, LaRaia PJ, Fabri BM et al (1985) Early detection of cardiac allograft rejection with proton nuclear magnetic resonance. Circulation [Suppl II] 72:231-236

Sasaki H, Sada M, Nishimura T et al (1987) The expanded scope of effectiveness of nuclear magnetic resonance imaging to determine cardiac allograft rejection. Transplant Proc 19:1062-1064

Schocken DD, Arrieta MI, Leaverton PE et al (1992) Prevalence and mortality rate of congestive heart failure in the United States. J Am Coll Cardiol 20:301-306

Scott GE, Nath RL, Friedlich JA, Fallon JT, Erdmann AJ (1983) Usefulness of myocardial edema to assess heterotopic allograft rejection in dogs. Heart Transplant 2:232-237

Smart FW, Young JB, Weilbaecher D, et al (1993) Magnetic resonance imaging for assessment of tissue rejection after heterotopic heart transplantation. J Heart Lung Transplant 12:403-410

Solomon SD, Glynn RJ, Greaves S et al (2001) Recovery of ventricular function after myocardial infarction in the reperfusion era: the healing and early afterload reducing therapy study. Ann Intern Med 134:451-458

Trabold T, Buchgeister M, Kuttner A et al (2003) Estimation of radiation exposure in 16-detector row computed tomography of the heart with retrospective ECG-gating. Fortschr Röntgenstr 175:1051-1055

Vizza CD, Lynch JP, Ochoa LL et al (1998) Right and left ventricular dysfunction in patients with severe pulmonary disease. Chest 113:576-583

Vogt FM, Goyen M, Debatin JF (2003) MR angiography of the chest.Radiol Clin North Am 41:29-41

Walpoth BH, Lazeyras F, Tschopp A et al (1995) Assessment of cardiac rejection and immunosuppression by magnetic resonance imaging and spectroscopy. Transplant Proc 27:2088-2091

White HD, Norris RM, Brown MA et al (1987) Left ventricular end-systolic volume as the major determinant of survival after recovery from myocardial infarction. Circulation 76:44-51

Wilhelmi M, Pethig K, Wilhelmi M et al (2002) Heart transplantation: echocardiographic assessment of morphology and function after more than 10 years of follow-up. Ann Thorac Surg 74:1075-1079

Wilson RF, Christiansen BV, Olivari MT et al (1991) Evidence for structural reinnervation after orthotopic cardiac transplantation in humans. Circulation 83:1210-1220

Wong M, Staszewsky L, Latini R et al (2002) Valsartan benefits left ventricular structure and function in heart failure: Val-HeFT echocardiographic study. J Am Coll Cardiol 40:970-975

Yang PC, Kerr AB, Liu AC et al (1998) New real-time interactive cardiac magnetic resonance imaging system complements echocardiography. J Am Coll Cardiol 32:2049-2056

11 Pericardial Disease

Jan Bogaert, Andrew M. Taylor, and Steven Dymarkowski

CONTENTS

11.1
Introduction

With the advent of modern non-invasive cardiac imaging modalities such as echocardiography, cardiac computed tomography (CT) and cardiac magnetic resonance imaging (MRI), direct visualization of the pericardium and related pathology has become a reality. Although echocardiography is still the first-line modality used to explore the pericardium, imaging of the pericardium is often suboptimal especially in "non-echogenic" patients such as patients with lung emphysema or chest wall deformities. Moreover, differentiation between the pericardium

J. Bogaert MD, PhD; S. Dymarkowski MD, PhD
Department of Radiology, Gasthuisberg University Hospital, Catholic University of Leuven, 3000 Leuven, Belgium
A.M. Taylor, MD, MRCP, FRCR
Cardiothoracic Unit, Institute of Child Health and Great Ormond Street Hospital for Children, London, WC1N 3JH, UK

and adjacent pleural fluid, and between paracardiac fat and fluid is often not feasible. Computed tomography and MRI are second-line imaging modalities that have the ability to overcome, by and large, the limitations of echocardiography. Both are tomographic techniques with excellent spatial and contrast resolution. Since the pericardium, a fibro-fluid structure, is surrounded on both sides by fat (mediastinal and epicardial fat layer), excellent contrast is created, and thus the pericardium is a priori ideally suited for evaluation on CT and MRI (Smith et al. 2001). On routine chest CT examinations, the pericardium and pericardial pathology (fluid, inflammation, calcification or masses) are very well depicted. The coupling of CT data acquisition with ECG gating enables reduction in cardiac-related motion artefacts and optimal visualization of the pericardium.

However, the study of the pericardium goes beyond morphological imaging and includes assessment of the impact of pericardial pathology on cardiac function, mainly diastolic heart function and cardiac filling. Often, the severity of pericardial abnormalities is not closely linked to the severity of the patient's symptoms and vice versa. Hence, as a rule of thumb, the morphological and functional parameters should be assessed together. MRI is ideally suited to this role, since accurate information can be obtained not only on the pericardial morphology, but also on cardiac function (Francone et al. 2004). This chapter focuses on MRI of the pericardium and the pathologies that affect the pericardium and presents an MRI approach for assessing patients with suspected pericardial disease using the current arsenal of MRI techniques.

11.2
Pericardial Anatomy and Physiology

The pericardium is a relatively inelastic, thin, flask-shaped sac (Fig. 11.1) that envelops the heart, extends

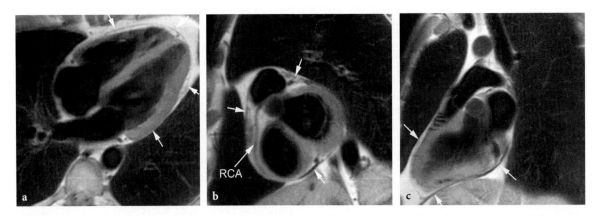

Fig. 11.1a-c. Normal pericardium on SE-MRI. T1-weighted fast SE-MRI in the horizontal long-axis (**a**), short-axis (**b**), and vertical long-axis (**c**). The normal pericardium is visible as a thin curvilinear structure (*arrows*) with low signal intensity surrounded by the bright epicardial and mediastinal fat. Visualization of the pericardium is often hampered along the lateral wall of the LV because of the sparsity of surrounding fat. Parts of the coronary artery tree can be seen in the epicardial fat, such as the right coronary artery (*RCA*) in Fig. 11.1.b

to the origin of the great vessels and is attached to the sternum, the dorsal spine and the diaphragm (HOIT 1990). It is composed of two layers, an inner serous membrane consisting of a monolayer of mesothelial cells and an outer fibrocollagenous layer. The inner serosal layer, termed the visceral pericardium, is closely attached to the epicardial surface of the heart and covers a subepicardial layer of conjunctive tissue containing fat and coronary vessels. The serosal layer reflects back on itself to become the inner lining of the outer fibrous layer. Together, these layers form the parietal pericardium.

Besides the pericardial sac, the pericardium contains two major pericardial sinuses which are composed of different recesses (GROELL et al. 1999). The transverse sinus is the connection between the two tubes of pericardium that envelop the great vessels (Fig. 11.2). The aorta and pulmonary artery are enclosed in one anterosuperior tube, and the vena cava and pulmonary veins are enclosed in a more posterior tube. Pericardial effusion located in the superior recess should not be mistaken for an intimal flap of an aortic dissection. The oblique sinus lies behind the left atrium so that the posterior wall of the left atrium is actually separated from the pericardial space (Fig. 11.3). This explains why a posterior pericardial effusion is seen behind the left atrium only when it is very large.

The pericardial virtual cavity normally contains between 10 and 50 ml of an ultrafiltrate of plasma (ROBERTS and SPRAY 1976). The fluid is produced by the visceral pericardium and drainage of the cavity is towards both the thoracic duct and the right lymphatic duct.

It is important to emphasize the essential role of the pericardium in maintaining normal cardiac function. An extensive description of all its functions is beyond the scope of this chapter, but, to summarize, the function of the pericardium is threefold: (a) *mechanical function* – improvement of cardiac efficiency, (b) *membranous function* – reduction of friction from cardiac motion, and (c) *ligamentous function* – limitation of cardiac displacement (SPODICK 1997). The pericardial sac has a subatmospheric pressure and should be regarded as a compartment between the pleural space and heart chambers. There is a physiological interaction between the pleural space and pericardium, and between the pericardium and ventricles. The latter interaction is more pronounced for the right ventricle (RV) than the left ventricle (LV), because of the thin anterior RV wall. The *myocardial transmural pressure* is the difference between the pressure in the ventricular cavity and the pericardial pressure, measuring ±3 mmHg at end diastole, and should be regarded as a measure of preload because it expresses the true filling pressure. The pericardium, furthermore, is involved in the interaction between left and right ventricular function, a phenomenon called *ventricular dependence* or *coupling*. This phenomenon is explained in the section on constrictive pericarditis (11.6.3).

11.3
MRI Techniques

For many years, the spin-echo (SE)-MRI technique has been advocated for pericardial imaging

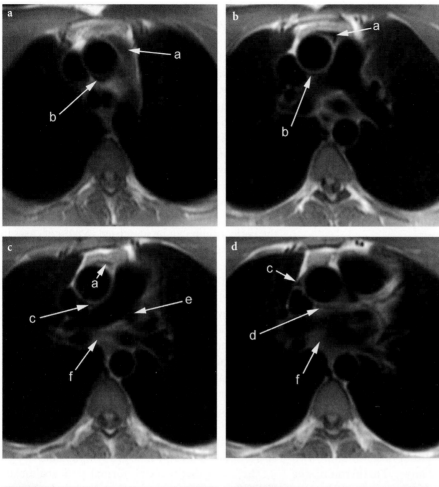

Fig. 11.2 a-d. Pericardial recesses on SE-MRI. T1-weighted fast SE-MRI in the transverse plane at four different levels through the origin of the great vessels. Transverse sinus: superior aortic recess, anterior portion (*a*), posterior portion (*b*), right lateral portion (*c*); transverse sinus: inferior aortic recess (*d*) and the left pulmonic recess (*e*). The oblique sinus (*f*) lies behind the left atrium

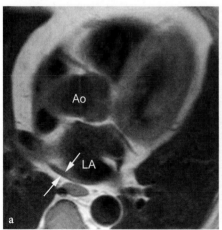
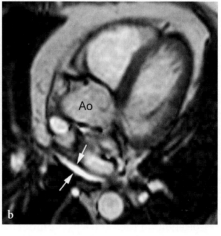

Fig. 11.3 a-b. Oblique sinus. T1-weighted fast SE-MRI (**a**) and balanced-SSFP cine MRI (**b**) in the horizontal long-axis plane. The oblique sinus, containing a small amount of pericardial fluid, is visible as a curvilinear structure (*arrows*) behind the left atrium (*LA*). Ao, aorta

(LANZER et al. 1984). However, currently a variety of MRI sequences are available and should be used to study the pericardium. These sequences can be applied for morphological imaging of the pericardium and other cardiac structures, for the differentiation between pericardial fluid and the pericardial layers, for characterization of this fluid and the layers, for studying ventricular function and for assessing cardiac filling (Table 11.1). T1-weighted SE-MRI, using a fast, segmented approach, is the preferred sequence for morphological imaging of the heart and pericardium. Use of small fields-of-view and a saturation block on the frontal chest wall may improve the visualization of the pericardium. A va-

- Pericardial width (*normal or increased*), position, and extent (*focal, multiloculated or diffuse*)
- Pericardial delineation (*smooth or irregular*)
- Signal characteristics (T1- & T2-weighted MRI/gradient-echo; signal void – *low, inhomogeneous or high*)
- Thickness and enhancement pattern of pericardial layers (SE-MRI/cine MRI/CE-IR MRI)
- Pericardial motion (cine MRI; *normal, rigid or immobile*)
- Ventricular septal shape and motion during early diastolic filling (short-axis view, using real-time cine MRI; *convex to RV, flattened or inverted*)
- RV Morphology (*normal, compressed or enlarged*)
- Right atrial and inferior vena caval size (*normal or enlarged*)
- Pleural fluid
- Inflow patterns (pulmonary/caval veins and atrioventricular valves; *normal or restrictive physiology*)

riety of imaging planes can be chosen to image all parts of the pericardium. In practice, imaging can be started with axial views, followed by views in other direction, such as the coronal or cardiac short-axis view. Administration of paramagnetic contrast agents can be recommended in cases of pericardial masses or inflammatory pericarditis. T2-weighted SE-MRI, preferably using a short-tau inversion-recovery (STIR) sequence, is useful for detecting pericardial fluid and/or pericardial inflammation with oedema of the pericardial layers. Furthermore, the contrast-enhanced inversion-recovery MRI technique (CE-IR MRI) with delayed enhancement, a similar MRI sequence to that used for imaging of myocardial infarction (see Chap. 8), can be applied to enhance tissue contrast in the pericardium and thus to better detect pericardial inflammation and oedema (KLEIN et al. 2003; BOGAERT et al. 2004).

Cine MRI, using balanced steady-state free precession (SSFP) gradient-echo sequences, can be used to evaluate both cardiac function and pericardial motion. The assessment of pericardial motion is useful to differentiate normally mobile pericardium from stiffened immobile pericardium in patients with constrictive pericarditis. Real-time MRI can also be used to evaluate the effects of respiration on the ventricular septal motion in patients with clinical suspicion of constrictive pericarditis (see Sect. 11.6.3). MRI tagging can be applied to detect fibrotic adhesion between both pericardial layers (KOJIMA et al. 1999), and velocity-encoded or phase-encoded MRI (velocity mapping) can be used to study diastolic function by analysing the inflow patterns in the systemic and pulmonary veins and through the atrioventricular valves.

11.4
Normal Pericardium

On SE-MRI, the normal pericardium appears as a low-intensity line that is surrounded by the high-intensity mediastinal and epicardial fat, or medium-intensity myocardium (SECHTEM et al. 1986b; STARCK et al. 1984; ; Fig. 11.1). In the vicinity of the lung, the pericardium is more difficult to visualize due to the low intensity of the adjacent lung parenchyma. Therefore, the sensitivity of SE-MRI for visualizing the pericardium varies from only 61% for the pericardium over the free wall of the LV to 100% over the region of the RV (SECHTEM et al. 1986b). The transverse sinus of the pericardium can be identified in 80% of cases in the transverse or sagittal plane, and in 70% of cases in the coronal plane, and the preaortic and retroaortic recesses of the pericardium in 67–100% of the cases (IM et al. 1988; Fig. 11.2). Similar results have been reported by GROELL et al. (1999) using electron-beam CT. Knowledge of the normal anatomy and appearance of the pericardial recesses (especially the superior pericardial recesses) is important in order to avoid misdiagnosis of aortic dissection or confusion with lymph nodes or mediastinal vessels (McMURDO et al. 1985; SOLOMON et al. 1990; GROELL et al. 1999). Additional cine MRI studies can be very helpful in further differentiating pericardial recesses from the aortic dissection of an enlarged lymph node.

The mean thickness of normal pericardium on SE-MRI varies from 1.2 mm in diastole to 1.7 mm in systole, with similar results reported by BOGAERT and DUERINCKX (1995) on 2D-coronary MR angiograms. The MRI values are larger than those found in anatomical studies of the heart (0.4–1 mm thickness; see Sect. 4.4.5). The small increase in pericardial thickness during systole is probably related to the volume reduction of the heart during contraction. Although some authors have mentioned an improved visualization of the pericardium during systole (CHAKO et al. 1995; SECHTEM et al. 1986b), images acquired using current fast SE-MRI techniques during breath-holding obtained during mid-diastole provide the best depiction of the pericardium and other structures of the heart. It should be emphasized that perpendicular slices through the pericardium are necessary to obtain reliable measurements of the exact pericardial thickness.

It is important to be familiar with the presentation of the normal pericardium on other MRI sequences. On T2-weighted SE-MRI, the normal pericardium has low signal intensity. On balanced-SSFP (b-SSFP) cine MRI, the pericardial layers have low signal intensity, while pericardial fluid has a high signal intensity (Fig. 11.4). However, one should be careful not to overestimate the true pericardial thickness, since chemical-shift artefacts can be present at the fat–fluid interface, creating a low-intensity zone. On coronary MR angiograms, large portions of the pericardium are visible as intermediately high-signal intensity zones, with thicknesses in the same range as those measured on SE-MRI (BOGAERT and DUERINCKX 1995). Knowledge of the pericardial appearance on coronary MR angiography is necessary to differentiate pericardium from epicardial coronary arteries. Using the newer 3D coronary MR angiography techniques with balanced gradients, pericardial fluid is visible with a much higher signal than the coronary blood (GIORGI et al. 2002; Fig. 11.5).

11.5
Congenital Anomalies

11.5.1
Pericardial Cyst

Pericardial cysts (congenital encapsulated cysts) are most frequently found in the cardiophrenic sulcus (90%), most often located on the right side (70%; Fig. 11.6). They are implanted on the pericardium and should not communicate with the pericardial cavity. Pericardial cysts are usually found as incidental findings on the chest radiograph, visible as well-defined outpouchings on the lateral heart border. On MRI, they appear as a paracardial liquid mass, which may be surrounded by a line of low intensity consistent with pericardium (SECHTEM et al. 1986a). The diagnosis of pericardial cysts on MRI is usually easy, because of their location and consistency (homogeneous high signal on T2-weighted images). Pericardial cysts are usually asymptomatic, though rarely they may become symptomatic when compressing other cardiac structures (Fig. 11.7). Pericardial cysts should be differentiated from other cystic structures such as bronchogenic cysts (preferentially located around the central bronchial structures, often with a fluid/fluid level) and thymic cysts (located in the upper, anterior mediastinum).

11.5.2
Pericardial Defect

Pericardial defect or agenesis is an uncommon entity and results from an abnormal embryonic development that may be secondary to abnormalities in

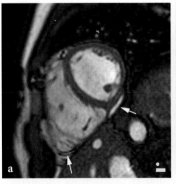
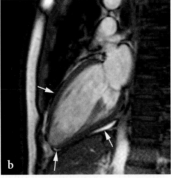

Fig. 11.4a,b. Normal pericardium on balanced-SSFP cine MRI in cardiac short-axis (**a**) and vertical long-axis plane (**b**). The pericardial sac is visible as low signal-intensity line while pericardial fluid demonstrates a high-signal (*arrows*)

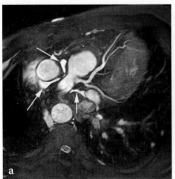
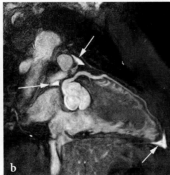

Fig. 11.5a,b. Pericardium and pericardial recesses on 3D- MR coronary angiography. Tangential view through left coronary artery tree (**a**), perpendicular view through left main stem and left anterior descending coronary artery (**b**). Parts of the pericardium and pericardial recesses are visible as well-defined high-signal areas (*arrows*). The signal intensity is higher than of the blood in the coronary arteries

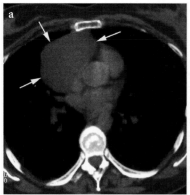

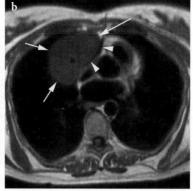

Fig. 11.6a,b. Pericardial cyst. Axial non-enhanced CT (**a**) and T1-weighted SE-MRI (**b**). The pericardial cyst is visible as a well-delineated, homogeneous low-density (0 HU) and low signal-intensity soft-tissue structure visible along the right paracardiac border (*arrows*), implanted on a normal pericardium (*arrowhead*)

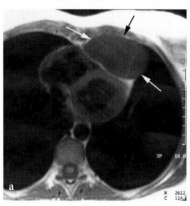

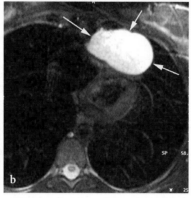

Fig. 11.7a,b. Symptomatic pericardial cyst. Axial T1-weighted (**a**) and T2-STIR weighted (**b**) fast SE-MRI. A well-delineated homogeneous soft-tissue structure with low signal on T1-weighted and high signal on T2-weighted SE-MRI, corresponding with a pericardial cyst. The pericardial cyst located ventrally to the cardiac apex compresses the left and right ventricle. The cardiac compression can be well appreciated on cine MRI

the vascular supply of the pericardium. Pericardial defects occur in a spectrum ranging from a small defect to total absence of the pericardium. They are more common on the left side (70%) than on the right side (4%) or inferiorly (17%) (AMPLATZ and MOLLER 1993; SECHTEM et al. 1986a). Partial defects (large partial defects more common than small) are far more common than total defects. This congenital abnormality may be associated, in at least one-third of cases, with other malformations, particularly malformations of the heart (tetralogy of Fallot, atrial septal defect, patent ductus arteriosus) or other types of abnormalities (bronchogenic cyst or hiatus hernia; LORELL and BRAUNWALD 1988; LETANCHE et al. 1988).

As a consequence of the defect, cardiac structures or portions of the lung can herniate through the defect. The clinical presentation is variable. Patients are often asymptomatic, and the disease is detected on a routine chest radiograph as an abnormal left cardiac contour (GLOVER et al. 1969). Symptoms occur when cardiac structures are transiently entrapped or incarcerated in the defect. Herniation of the left atrial appendage through a small defect may lead to infarction of the appendage or the left

coronary artery might be compressed leading to ischemia especially during exercise (AMPLATZ and MOLLER 1993).

Contrary to some reports in the literature, the diagnosis of a pericardial defect on MRI is not always straightforward, since in normal conditions the pericardium over the lateral side of the LV is usually not well depicted; corresponding to the most frequent location of pericardial defects (GUTIERREZ et al. 1985). So, the diagnosis usually relies on other signs such as an abnormal location of cardiac structures. Since herniation is often intermittent in time, positional changes such as positioning the patient in left lateral decubitus position, can be helpful in diagnosing pericardial defects.

11.5.3
Pericardial Diverticulum

Pericardial diverticulum is exceedingly rare, and can be congenital or acquired. This entity corresponds to a herniation through a defect in the parietal pericardium that communicates with the pericardial cavity (SECHTEM et al. 1986a).

11.6
Acquired Diseases

11.6.1
Effusive Pericardial Disease

Imaging of pericardial effusions is used to confirm the presence, severity and extent of fluid; to characterize the nature of the pericardial effusion; and to determine the impact of the effusion on cardiac function and filling. Although the diagnosis of pericardial effusion is usually accomplished by echocardiography, the accuracy of echocardiography can be limited in some circumstances: (1) false-positive cases may occur in the presence of atelectasis, or pleural effusion or mediastinal lesions that mimic pericardial effusion; (2) false-negative cases may occur in the presence of loculated fluid collections, such as in cases of inflammatory adhesions or haemopericardium; and (3) there may be difficulties in differentiating fluid from epicardial fat in the anterior or posterior recesses or from pericardial thickening (WALINSKY 1978). MRI is of value compared with echocardiography because of its ability to better identify anatomical structures and interfaces, which reduces the false-positive rate. MRI will provide valuable information regarding the distribution of pericardial fluid, which may vary considerably, even though, in 70% of the cases, fluid collection is observed posterolateral to the LV due to the gravitational dependency of the fluid (SECHTEM et al. 1986a; Figs. 11 8 and 11.9). Another common location for fluid collection is the superior recess, as witnessed in cases of abundant pericardial effusion.

Although MRI can detect pericardial effusions as small as 30 ml, a relationship between the measured width of the pericardial space and total fluid volume cannot be established because of focal fluid accumulations. Regions in which pericardial width is greater than 4 mm can be regarded as abnormal. Moderate effusions (between 100 and 500 ml of fluid) are associated with a greater than 5-mm pericardial space anterior to the RV (SECHTEM et al. 1986a). If needed, the exact amount of the pericardial effusion can be quantified by delineating the pericardial sac on contiguous slices through the entire heart, similar to the approach used to calculate ventricular volumes or myocardial masses.

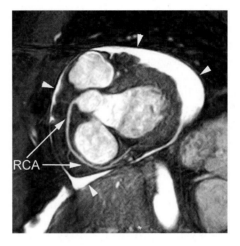

Fig 11.9. Moderate pericardial effusion using 3D MR coronary angiography (balanced-SSFP sequence). The inhomogeneous spread of the pericardial effusion on this short-axis view through the right coronary artery (*RCA*) is well visible (*arrowheads*). Most of the fluid (high-signal) in this patient is located along the left side of the heart. The patient has also a small pleural effusion

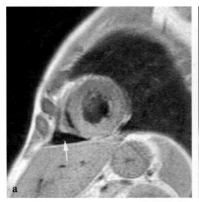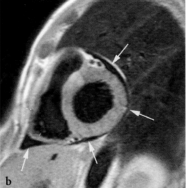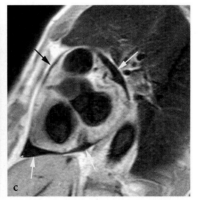

Fig 11.8a-c. Small pericardial effusion. T1-weighted fast SE-MRI at three cardiac short-axis levels. The pericardial effusion (*arrows*) is homogeneously spread within the pericardial sac. Most of the pericardial fluid is located infero-laterally of the right ventricle and supero-laterally of the left ventricle

MULVAGH et al. (1989) have shown that MRI is more sensitive than echocardiography for the detection of small pericardial effusions; this improved sensitivity is even more pronounced in the presence of loculated effusions when adhesions occur between the visceral and parietal pericardium. In such cases, it is common to observe a heterogeneous and high signal intensity that can be attributed to a reduction of fluid motion and cellular content.

Although a pericardial effusion usually has no or only limited impact on cardiac filling, acute accumulation of pericardial contents (e.g. fluid, blood, air) can lead to a *pericardial tamponade* with decreased cardiac filling and impaired stroke volume, a phenomenon that might be lethal within minutes after onset. The symptomatology is linked to the increase in pericardial pressure determined by the absolute volume of fluid, rate of fluid accumulation and the physical characteristics of the pericardium (degree of stretching). The diagnosis of pericardial tamponade is a clinical one that is confirmed by echocardiography. The role of MRI is limited in the acute phase. Hallmarks of cardiac tamponade are: the diastolic inversion or collapse of the RV free wall (intrapericardial pressure greater than interventricular pressure); right atrial compression during early systole; exaggerated respiratory variation in cardiac inflow; and abnormal flow patterns in the caval veins (Fig. 11.10).

Attempts to characterize the nature of the effusion based on the signal intensity have been disappointing. Pericardial effusions, either transudative or exudative, usually show up on T1-weighted SE-MRI as hypointense owing to the flow-void effects (fluid motion during cardiac contraction). Higher signal intensity might be related to a high proteinaceous or haemorrhagic content. With gradient-echo techniques, especially with the b-SSFP technique, often a better characterization of the pericardial fluid content can be achieved, such as the visualization of fibrinous strands or presence of coagulated blood (Fig. 11.11). Associated abnormalities helpful in the diagnosis are depiction of thickened pericardial blades with assessment of the degree of inflammation (Fig. 11.12; see Sect. 11.6.2).

11.6.2
Pericardial Inflammation

Inflammation of the pericardium (*inflammatory pericarditis*) can be caused by: infectious diseases (viral/bacterial/tuberculosis/fungal); can be a manifestation of various systemic diseases (e.g. rheumatoid arthritis, lupus erythematosus, scleroderma); can be found in patients with uremia or following an acute myocardial infarction (Fig. 11.13); or can be the result of irradiation (e.g. breast cancer, mediastinal lymphoma). However, often no underlying pathology is found (idiopathic). The symptoms are mainly related to the severity of pericardial inflammation. In the acute phase, inflammation of the pericardial layers is characterized by formation of young, highly vascularized granulation tissue with fibrin deposition. Usually, a variable amount of pericardial fluid is present, and the fibrin deposition may lead to a fibrinous adhesion of the pericardial layers. Chronic inflammation is characterized by a progressive sclerosing pericarditis with fibroblasts, collagen and a lesser amount of fibrin deposition. This may progress towards an end-stage, chronic fibrosing pericarditis with fibroblasts and collagen. The main feature of this end stage is a stiff pericardium with constriction of the heart (*constrictive pericarditis*; see Sect. 11.6.3).

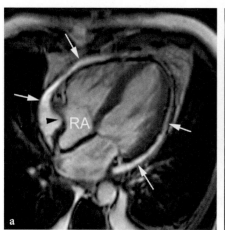
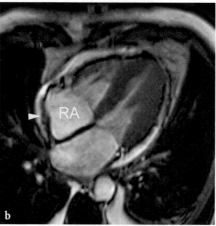

Fig 11.10a,b. Collapse of the right atrial wall (*arrowhead*) in a patient with pericardial effusion (*arrows*). Horizontal long-axis view using balanced-SSFP technique. Collapse of the right atrial wall occurs when the intrapericardial pressure exceeds the right atrial pressure. Abbreviations: right atrium, RA

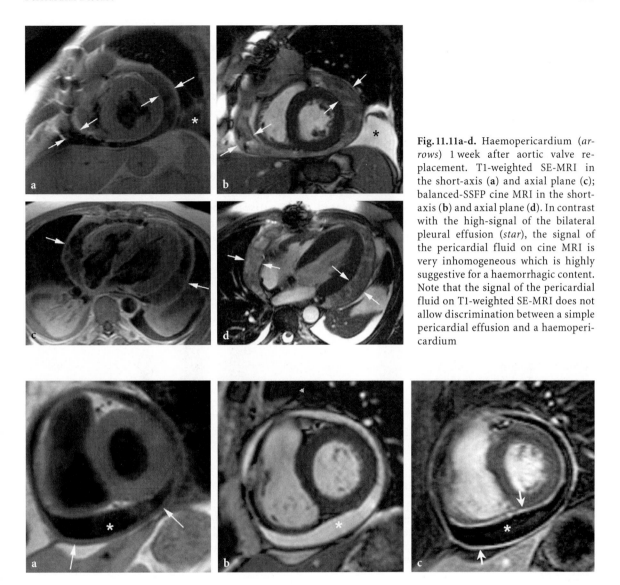

Fig. 11.11a-d. Haemopericardium (*arrows*) 1 week after aortic valve replacement. T1-weighted SE-MRI in the short-axis (**a**) and axial plane (**c**); balanced-SSFP cine MRI in the short-axis (**b**) and axial plane (**d**). In contrast with the high-signal of the bilateral pleural effusion (*star*), the signal of the pericardial fluid on cine MRI is very inhomogeneous which is highly suggestive for a haemorrhagic content. Note that the signal of the pericardial fluid on T1-weighted SE-MRI does not allow discrimination between a simple pericardial effusion and a haemopericardium

Fig. 11.12a-c. Chronic inflammatory pericarditis in a patient presenting with pericardial effusion and fever of underdetermined origin. On short-axis SE-MRI (**a**), balanced-SSFP cine MRI (**b**) a moderate pericardial effusion (*star*) and thickened pericardial layers (*arrows*) are clearly seen. On CE-MRI (**c**), strong enhancement of both thickened pericardial layers is shown, allowing better differentiation between pericardial layers and fluid than on SE-MRI

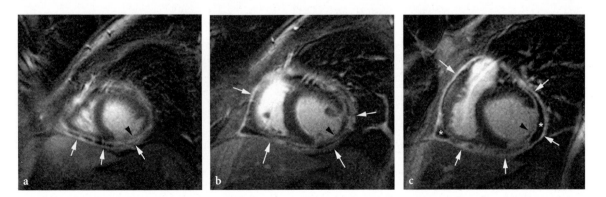

Fig. 11.13a-c. Chronic inflammatory pericarditis in a patient with history of proximal occluded left circumflex artery and transmural myocardial infarction. CE-IR MRI in cardiac short-axis shows the infarct as a strongly enhancing thinned lateral LV wall (*arrowhead*). A diffusely thickened, strongly enhancing pericardium (*arrows*) is clearly visible with a small pericardial effusion along the left ventricle and inferolaterally of the right ventricle (*star*)

Diagnosis of inflammatory pericarditis remains challenging. The thickening of the pericardial layers can be depicted on SE-MRI, and cine MRI (SECHTEM et al. 1986a; Fig. 11.14). Presence of an inflammatory component can be best seen on T2-weighted STIR SE-MRI, and after contrast administration using the CE-IR MRI or SE-MRI technique (Fig. 11.15). Differentiation between pericardial layers and pericardial effusion is achieved using CE-IR MRI or cine MRI (Figs. 11.12–11.15). Pericardial calcifications, which may be associated with chronic fibrosing pericarditis, will appear as focal regions of decreased signal intensity with irregular shapes (SOULEN et al. 1985), but are much better demonstrated by CT.

11.6.3
Constrictive Pericarditis

The main hallmark of constrictive pericarditis is a thickened, fibrotic and/or calcified pericardium, constricting the heart and impairing cardiac filling (MYERS and SPODICK 1999). Today the majority of cases of constrictive pericarditis are late sequelae of viral pericarditis, whereas formerly tuberculous pericarditis accounted for most cases. Other aetiologies include infectious pericarditis, connective tissue disease, neoplasm and trauma. Constriction may also be a complication of long-term renal dialysis, cardiac surgery and radiation therapy. An

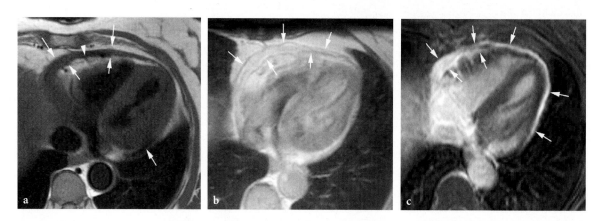

Fig. 11.14a-c. Acute relapsing pericarditis. Axial T1-weighted fast SE-MRI before (**a**) and after (**b**) adminstration of Gadolinium-dimeglumine, CE-IR MRI (**c**). An irregular thickened pericardium is found, mainly over the right heart with strong enhancement of the entire pericardium. The CE-IR MRI allows better depiction of the inflammatory thickened pericardium over the left heart than contrast-enhanced SE-MRI

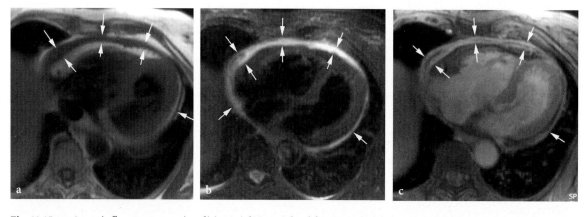

Fig. 11.15a-c. Acute inflammatory pericarditis. Axial T1-weighted fast SE-MRI (**a**) shows slightly irregular thickening of the pericardium, mainly over the right side of the heart (*arrows*). On axial T2-weighted STIR fast SE-MRI (**b**) the pericardium shows hyperintense appearance with cloudy appearance (*arrows*). Strong enhancement of the pericardium (*arrows*) on CE-IR MRI (**c**). On the contrast-enhanced images, only a minimal amount is visible between the inflamed pericardial layers

often unrecognized (subclinical) acute (viral) pericarditis may evolve into a subacute and later chronic inflammatory pericarditis, leading to progressive pericardial fibrosis and constriction of the heart. Pathological findings include calcium deposition in a scarred and fibrotic pericardium that is adherent to the myocardium.

A major dilemma in the diagnosis of constrictive pericarditis is that diseases decreasing the myocardial compliance, such as restrictive cardiomyopathy, are also characterized by an impaired ventricular filling and their clinical presentation can be very similar to constrictive pericarditis. Distinction between the two entities is crucial, since constrictive pericarditis is successfully treated by early pericardiectomy while, for restrictive cardiomyopathy, medical treatment is recommended (KUSHWAHA et al. 1997; MYERS and SPODICK 1999). The current diagnosis of constrictive pericarditis and differentiation from restrictive cardiomyopathy is based on a combination of: (a) clinical presentation, (b) visualization of pericardial abnormalities and its impact of the other cardiac structures, (c) assessment of cardiac diastolic function and ventricular filling patterns, (d) measurement of cardiac pressures, and (e) less frequently endomyocardial biopsy to rule out specific myocardial disorders (HANCOCK 2001). Even with current accurate non-invasive cardiac imaging techniques, the diagnosis of constrictive pericarditis often remains challenging.

11.6.3.1
Morphological Abnormalities in Constrictive Pericarditis

Morphological abnormalities of the pericardium on MRI in constrictive pericarditis are: (a) thickened pericardium, usually with irregular margins, (b) low signal of the thickened pericardium on T1- and T2-weighted SE-MRI due to the presence of extensive fibrosis or calcification (Figs. 11.16 and 11.17). It is commonly accepted that a normal pericardial thickness is 2 mm or less, a thickness greater than 4 mm suggests pericardial constriction, and one greater than 5–6 mm has a high specificity for constriction (SOULEN et al. 1985; SPODICK 1997). It should be emphasized, however, that the diagnosis of constrictive pericarditis cannot be based on morphological abnormalities of the pericardium alone.

First, other indirect morphological signs associated with constrictive pericarditis may be helpful in the diagnosis of constrictive pericarditis. These are: (a) narrowing (tubular-shaped) of the ventricles,

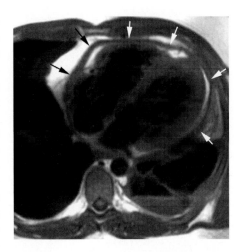

Fig. 11.16. Constrictive pericarditis (chronic fibrosing pericarditis). Transverse SE-MR image. Diffusely thickened, and irregularly defined pericardium surrounding the entire heart (*arrows*). Note the presence of the left-sided pleural effusion

(b) narrowing of one or both of the atrioventricular grooves, (c) enlargement of one or both atria, (d) dilatation of the vena cava and hepatic vein, and (e) presence of pleural effusion (Figs. 11.17, 11.18). The ventricular narrowing is usually more pronounced on the right side because of the larger incidence of pericardial thickening over the RV and the thinner right ventricular free wall. The absence of these associated findings, however, does not exclude constrictive pericarditis.

Second, it may be difficult to differentiate a pericardial effusion from constrictive pericarditis on T1-weighted SE-MRI: both pathologies present as a pericardial broadening with low signal intensity. How to differentiate both conditions? (a) A pericardial effusion typically has a signal void (i.e. black signal), while the thickened, fused pericardial blades have a low (grey) signal (Fig. 11.16), except when heavily calcified (Fig. 11.18); (b) the delineation of a pericardial effusion is usually smooth, while irregular in constrictive pericarditis; (c) cine MRI is often useful to differentiate both conditions, since fluid has a high signal intensity on gradient-echo sequences, while thickened pericardium exhibits a low (or very low) signal. Other MRI techniques may be helpful in the differentiation. KOJIMA et al. (1999) have used MRI tagging to demonstrate fibrotic adhesions between the visceral and parietal pericardial layers. Persistence of the pericardial tag line integrity throughout the cardiac cycle can only occur if there is a fusion of the pericardial layers. To complicate matters, pericardial effusions may be constrictive (*effusive-constrictive*

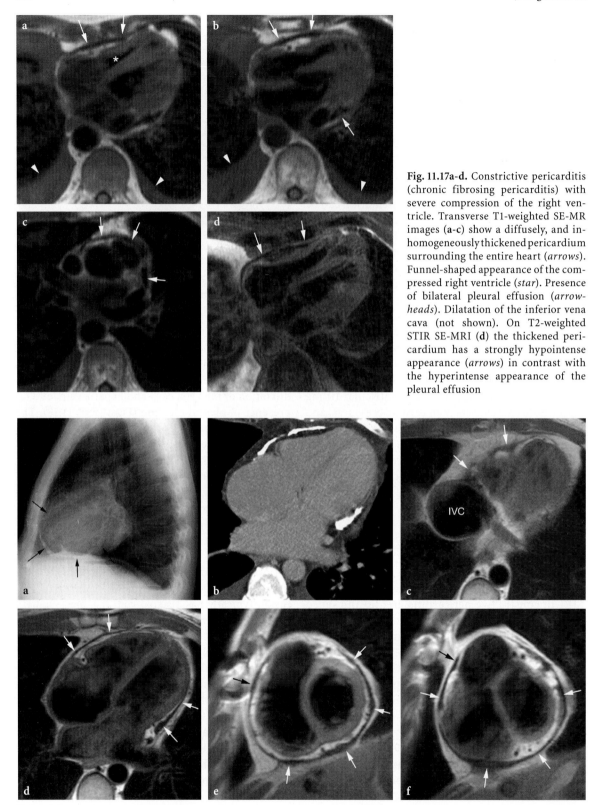

Fig. 11.17a-d. Constrictive pericarditis (chronic fibrosing pericarditis) with severe compression of the right ventricle. Transverse T1-weighted SE-MR images (**a-c**) show a diffusely, and inhomogeneously thickened pericardium surrounding the entire heart (*arrows*). Funnel-shaped appearance of the compressed right ventricle (*star*). Presence of bilateral pleural effusion (*arrowheads*). Dilatation of the inferior vena cava (not shown). On T2-weighted STIR SE-MRI (**d**) the thickened pericardium has a strongly hypointense appearance (*arrows*) in contrast with the hyperintense appearance of the pleural effusion

Fig. 11.18 a-f. Calcified constrictive pericarditis. Lateral (**a**) chest radiograph shows irregular defined, curvilinear pericardial calcifications (*arrows*). The pericardial calcifications are much better depicted on CT (**b**). Axial (**c, d**) and short-axis (**d, e**) T1-weighted fast SE-MRI show irregular thickened, strongly hypo-intense appearance of the pericardium (*arrows*). Note the impressive enlargement of the inferior vena cava (*IVC*), and the slow flow in the left atrium and right atrial appendage

pericarditis; SAGISTRA-SAULEDA 2004; SAGISTRA-SAULEDA et al. 2004; Fig. 11.19). The inflamed, thickened pericardial layers (with a variable amount of pericardial fluid) may have a constrictive effect on the cardiac filling. While most cases of effusive constrictive pericarditis will eventually evolve to persistent constriction requiring pericardiectomy, some may be transient and resolve spontaneously (*transient constrictive pericarditis;* HALEY et al. 2004; Fig. 11.20). CE-IR MRI with delayed imaging may be useful to differentiate between inflammatory and fibrosing forms of constrictive pericarditis (Fig. 11.21; KLEIN et al. 2003; BOGAERT et al. 2004).

Third, except when pericardial calcifications are extensive, MRI is definitely not well suited to differentiate pericardial fibrosis from calcification, be-cause of a lack in signal intensity difference between both tissues. CT should be considered as the most sensitive technique.

Fourth, pericardial thickening in constrictive pericarditis is often not generalized. This requires a detailed analysis of the entire pericardium, using a combination of different imaging planes (e.g. horizontal long-axis and short-axis images). It is important to understand that focal pericardial thickening, if located at strategic places such as over the atrio-ventricular grooves, can give raise to a full clinical picture of constrictive pericarditis even when the morphological abnormalities are not that impressive (Fig. 11.22). Less strategically located but otherwise morphologically important pericardial abnormalities can be clinically silent.

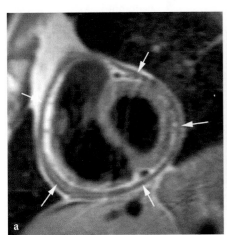
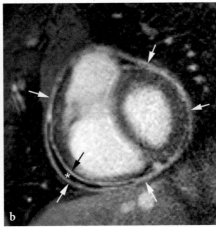

Fig. 11.19a,b. Effusive-constrictive form of constrictive pericarditis. Short-axis SE-MRI (**a**) and CE-IR MRI (**b**). Diffusely thickened pericardium, with strong enhancement of the pericardial layers after contrast administration. Presence of a small pericardial effusion (*star*) along the inferolateral side of the right ventricle. At surgery, a heavily thickened and inflamed pericardium was found

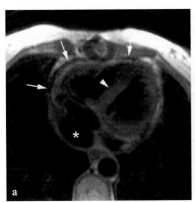
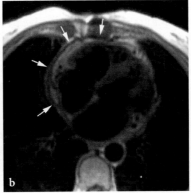
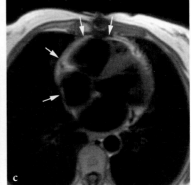

Fig. 11.20a-c. Transient constrictive pericarditis in a patient with a history of cardiac surgery (replacement of three cardiac valves). After surgery the patient developed pulmonary oedema and cardiac failure. Axial T1-weighted SE-MRI three weeks after cardiac surgery (**a, b**), and control study 6 months later (**c**). The first MRI study (**a, b**) shows an irregularly thickened, hypointense pericardium, mainly over the right heart (*arrows*) with a straight interventricular septum (*arrowhead*) and a dilated inferior vena cava (*star*). Abnormal motion and flattening of the interventricular septum during early diastolic filling. Six months later (**c**) the pericardial thickness (*arrows*), ventricular septal shape and motion have normalized.

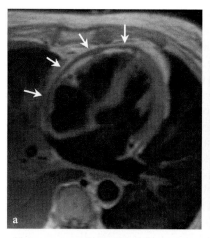

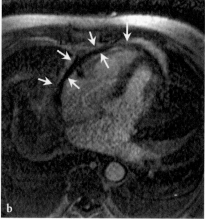

Fig. 11.21a,b. Constrictive pericarditis. Axial T1-weighted SE-MRI (a), and CE-IR MRI (b). Irregularly thickened pericardium (*arrows*) over the right heart without enhancement after contrast administration (b). On cine MRI, the thickened pericardium is rigid and immobile (not shown). Histology of the pericardiectomy specimen shows chronic fibrosing pericarditis with mainly fibroblasts and collagen

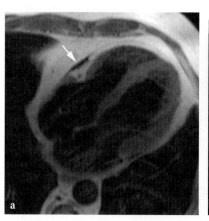

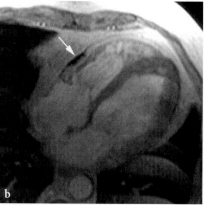

Fig. 11.22 a-b. Focal constrictive pericarditis. Axial T1-weighted SE-MRI (a) and axial cine-MRI (b) show focal pericardial thickening (*arrow*) at the level of the right atrioventricular groove and basal part of the free wall of the right ventricle with focal compression of the heart. The very low signal of the focal pericardial thickening is caused by pericardial calcification. (Partially reprinted from B. Giorgi et al. Radiology 2003, 228:417-424, with permission.)

Fifth, the presence of increased pericardial thickness is not an essential feature of constrictive pericarditis. It might even create a diagnostic dilemma in patients with haemodynamic findings suggestive of constriction without increased pericardial thickness. It has recently been shown by TALREJA et al. (2003) that a significant number (up to 18%) of patients with histologically proven constrictive pericarditis have a normal or near-normal pericardial thickness (i.e. less than 2 mm; TALREJA et al. 2003; Fig. 11.23). Pericardiectomy is equally effective in relieving symptoms regardless of the presence or absence of increased thickness. Symptoms in constrictive pericarditis are caused by the stiffness and the degree of constriction, and not by the thickness of the pericardium as such. A pericardium may be extensively thickened but, if not very constrictive, symptoms might be minimal or even absent. On the other hand, a pericardium with a normal or near-normal thickness can be very rigid and, if tightly constricting the cardiac chambers, give rise to a full-blown clinical picture of constrictive pericardi-

tis. In a similar way, the degree of ventricular filling (pre-load) will contribute to the degree of constriction. Assessment of the inflow characteristics and septal motion under fluid challenge (increased pre-load) sometimes can be helpful in the diagnosis of constrictive pericarditis (see Sect. 11.6.3.2).

11.6.3.2
Functional and Haemodynamic Abnormalities in Constrictive Pericarditis

At least equally important in the diagnosis of constrictive pericarditis is the analysis of the impact of pericardial changes on ventricular function and cardiac filling (the constriction factor). MRI is not able to measure ventricular filling pressures, but can be applied to study the indirect effects of the increase and equalization of ventricular pressures on ventricular filling. This can be done by velocity or phase-encoded MRI, analysis of inflow patterns through the atrioventricular valves and venous return in the caval and pulmonary veins.

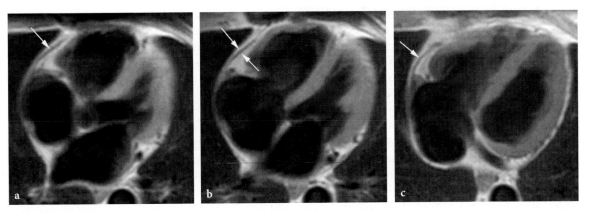

Fig. 11.23a-c. Non-thickened constrictive pericarditis in a patient with previous CABG surgery, presenting with increased right heart filling pressures, dyspnea and peripheral oedema. Transthoracic echocardiography shows restrictive physiology. Axial T1-weighted SE-MRI at three levels through the heart. The pericardium is visible as a thin curvilinear line with a maximal thickness 1.7 mm (*arrows*). Real-time cine MRI of the ventricular septal motion shows diastolic septal inversion at the onset of inspiration, and an increased total septal excursion ("pathologic ventricular coupling"; see Fig. 11.25). During the pericardiectomy, a non-thickened but very stiff pericardium was found, and the cardiac output increased spectacularly from 1.7 to 7.5 l/min

The increased filling pressures lead to an enhancement of early, diastolic filling (pseudonormalization pattern). Depending on the degree of pericardial constriction, ventricular filling in late diastole is impaired, with an abrupt stop in filling once the fixed cardiac volume is reached (Fig. 11.24). As a result, the atrial filling peak is decreased or absent. Flow analysis of the venous return shows a diminished, absent or even a reversed systolic forward flow due to the increased atrial filling pressure, an increased diastolic forward flow and an increased

atrial backflow (Fig. 11.24). Unfortunately, a very similar pattern is found in patients with restrictive cardiomyopathy. To discriminate both conditions, the influence of respiration on right and left ventricular cardiac filling patterns should be assessed. In normal conditions, inspiration decreases the intrathoracic pressure, leading to an enhancement of RV filling (increased systemic venous return) and decreased LV filling (pooling of blood in the pulmonary veins); an opposite phenomenon is found during expiration. In patients with constrictive peri-

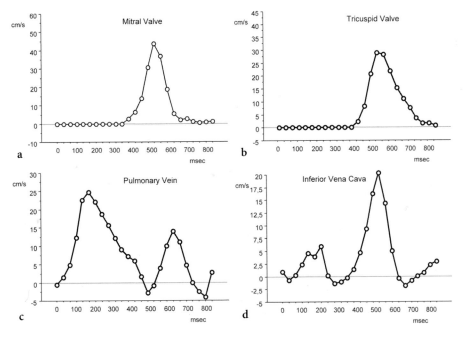

Fig. 11.24a-d. Inflow curves, using velocity-mapping MRI, through the mitral valve (**a**), tricuspid valve (**b**), pulmonary vein (**c**) and inferior vena cava (**d**) in a patient with constrictive pericarditis (same patient as in Fig. 11.18). Inflow curves show a severe restrictive inflow physiology with absent A-waves through the atrioventricular valves (**a, b**), and absent systolic forward in the inferior vena cava (**d**)

carditis, this pattern is enhanced owing to the presence of a stiff pericardium, while in patients with restrictive cardiomyopathy this pattern is normal or diminished (HATLE et al. 1989). Although real-time velocity mapping is feasible, accurate assessment of the transvalvular or venous flow patterns might be hampered by problems of through-plane motion caused by the respiration.

Alternatively, analysis of the position and configuration of the interventricular septum with MRI is of interest in patients with clinical suggestion of constrictive pericarditis. The position and configuration of the septum is primarily determined by the transseptal pressure gradient. In the unloaded or unstressed human heart, the septal configuration is flat, while it becomes concave in shape towards the LV, during normal loading conditions owing to a left-to-right positive transseptal pressure gradient. The phenomenon whereby the function of one ventricle is altered by changes in the filling of the other is called *ventricular interdependence* or *ventricular coupling* (TAYLOR et al. 1967; JANICKI and WEBER 1980). In patients with constrictive pericarditis, the pericardial inflexibility leads to an increased ventricular interdependence or pathological ventricular coupling, characterized by septal flattening or inversion during early ventricular filling. Since RV filling starts just before LV filling, the presence of a non-compliant pericardium impedes the RV free wall outward motion during filling. As a consequence, the instantaneous diastolic transseptal gradient will change and lead to a septal reconfiguration and paradoxical motion during filling. Because of the thin nature of the RV free wall, the influence of pericardial thickening is more pronounced on the right than on the left side of the heart. Moreover, this pattern is typically enhanced by respiration, leading to a pronounced leftward shift during inspiration and an opposite shift during expiration. Besides the physiological effects of respiration on ventricular filling, the thickened, fibrotic pericardium acts as a barrier, creating a pressure gradient between ventricles and supplying veins. This will contribute to the observed septal abnormalities.

In a recent paper by GIORGI et al. (2003) using a breath-hold cine MRI technique, septal flattening during early diastolic filling was found in the majority of patients with constrictive pericarditis. This pattern was not seen in normal subjects or in patients with restrictive cardiomyopathy or pericardial effusion. The septal abnormalities are typically most evident in the basal part of the interventricular septum. Taking into account the pathophysiology of

abnormal septal motion in constrictive pericarditis, septal flattening may be absent if the constrictive pericardium does not impede the ventricular expansion but restricts the ventricular filling by constricting the atrioventricular groove(s), or when the constrictive pericardium compresses parts of the heart other than the RV (HASUDA et al. 1999). Moreover, it should be stressed that even in obvious pericardial thickening, septal flattening may be minimal or absent if the ventricular constriction is minimal. However, since the breath-hold acquisition takes several heartbeats, the effects of respiration on cardiac dynamics, an essential feature to differentiate between constrictive pericarditis and restrictive cardiomyopathy, cannot be evaluated. With the advent of real-time MRI techniques, the septal dynamics can be evaluated during free breathing. The preliminary results from a study by FRANCONE et al. (in press) show in patients with constrictive pericarditis abnormal septal motion with septal flattening/inversion during early ventricular filling. The septal abnormalities are most pronounced in the first heartbeat after the onset of inspiration and rapidly decrease in magnitude during subsequent heartbeats (Fig. 11.25). During expiration an opposite pattern with increased right-sided septal motion is found. Total respiratory septal excursion, obtained by measuring the maximal distance in septal position between inspiration and expiration divided by the transverse biventricular diameter, is significantly larger in constrictive pericarditis patients (18.7±1.2%) than normal subjects (7.1±2.4 %) and restrictive cardiomyopathy patients (5.8±2.1%). A cut-off value of 11.9% (mean normal value +2 SD) can be used to discriminate constrictive pericarditis patients from non-constrictive pericarditis patients (see also Chap. 9).

Cine MRI can also be applied to evaluate the motion of the pericardium throughout the cardiac cycle, and thus to get a direct idea about the rigidity of the pericardium. A normal pericardium moves in synchronization with the in- and outward motion of the heart throughout the cardiac cycle, while a fixed pericardium shows a reduced or eventually an absent motion during the cardiac cycle. Moreover, cine MRI allows the demonstration of the restricted ventricular expansion during cardiac filling, abutted towards the thickened, rigid pericardium. Assessment of systolic function is normally also part of an MRI study in patients with constrictive pericarditis. The intrinsic myocardial contractility is normally preserved (except in cases where the fibrotic/calcified process involves the myocardium or in long-stand-

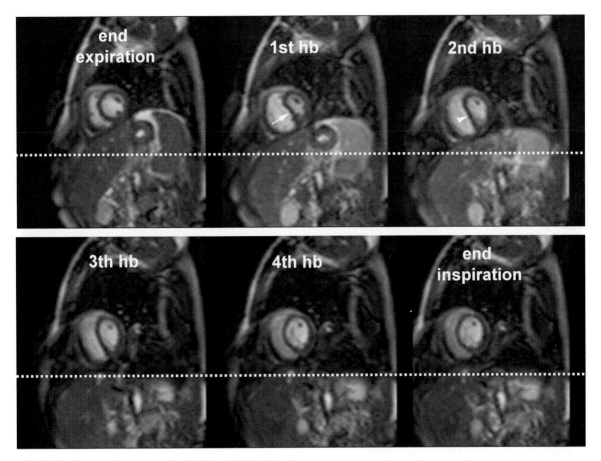

Fig. 11.25. Abnormal respiratory variation of ventricular septal shape and motion in a patient with constrictive pericarditis ("pathologic ventricular coupling"). At the onset of inspiration (1st heartbeat, *hb*), a sudden left-sided septal shift with septal inversion is found (*arrow*). The intensity of septal abnormalities rapidly decreases the next heartbeats. The septum is flattened by the second heartbeat (*arrowhead*) and becomes convex to the right later during inspiration. During expiration (not shown) the opposite phenomenon is found with increased right-sided septal shift. The respiratory variation in septal position is increased in patients with constrictive pericarditis

ing cases of constrictive pericarditis). As a consequence of impaired ventricular filling, however, stroke volumes and cardiac output are decreased.

11.6.4
Pericardial Masses

Primary tumours of the pericardium are rare entities, occurring much less frequently than pericardial metastasis (see also Chap. 12). The most common primary malignant tumour of the pericardium is the mesothelioma, which is often associated with haemorrhagic pericardial effusion. Other primary tumours include malignant fibrosarcoma, angiosarcoma, and benign and malignant teratoma (GOMES et al. 1987).

Pericardial metastases are relatively common (having a frequency of up to 22% in autopsy series of cancer patients) and are, in most cases, secondary to lung or breast carcinoma, leukaemia or lymphoma (HANOCK 1982). They are frequently associated with a large and haemorrhagic effusion that is disproportionate in size to the amount of tumour present. The metastatic pericardial implants are often small and difficult to visualize on MR images.

MRI has advantages over other techniques for the assessment of pericardial tumours, because it better delineates the implantation of the tumour outlined by either pericardial fat or pericardial fluid, and provides additional information on the contiguous anatomical structures (myocardial wall or great vessels). In the assessment of mediastinal and lung tumours, MRI is also the imaging modality of choice for detecting tumour invasion of the pericardium, which can be inferred when there is focal absence of the pericardial line. In cases where malignancy is adjacent to cardiac structures, visualization of the pericardial line indicates that pericardial invasion has not occurred (LUND et al. 1989). Characterization of the pericardial tumour is usually not possible, exceptions being lipoma and liposarcoma, which appear with high signal intensity owing to their fatty content.

11.7
Key Points

- Consider the pericardium as a functional rather than a purely morphological structure
- Pericardial pathology may be focal, and imaging in different (preferably perpendicularly oriented) imaging planes guaranties assessment of the entire pericardium, including the pericardial recesses
- Use a combination of MRI techniques to morphologically describe pericardial abnormalities and to assess their impact on cardiac function
- A simple pericardial effusion has smooth contours and no visible pericardial layers
- Contrast-enhanced MRI is helpful for depicting pericardial inflammation, and for better differentiation between pericardial layers and fluid
- The main hallmark in constrictive pericarditis is not a thickened pericardium but a stiff pericardium
- A normal or near-normal thickness of the pericardium does not rule out constrictive pericarditis
- Pathological ventricular coupling is frequently found in constrictive pericarditis and is very helpful in the differentiation with restrictive cardiomyopathy

References

Amplatz K, Moller JH (1993) Radiology of congenital heart disease. Mosby Year Book, St Louis, MO, USA

Beghetti M, Prieditis M, Rebeyka IM, Mawson J (1998) Intrapericardial teratoma. Images in cardiovascular medicine. Circulation 97:1523–1524

Bogaert J, Duerinckx AJ (1995) Appearance of the normal pericardium on coronary MR angiograms. J Magn Reson Imaging 5:579–587

Bogaert J, Taylor AM, Kerkhove F van, Dymarkowski S (2004) Use of the inversion-recovery contrast-enhanced MRI technique for cardiac imaging: spectrum of diseases. Am J Roentgenol 182:609–615

Chako AC, Tempany CM, Zerhouni EA (1995) Effect of slice acquisition direction on image quality in thoracic MRI. J Comput Assist Tomogr 19:936–940

Francone M, Dymarkowski S, Kalantzi M, Bogaert J (in press) Real-time cine MRI of ventricular septal motion. A novel approach to assess ventricular coupling.

Francone M, Dymarkowski S, Kalantzi M, Bogaert J (2004) La risonanza magnetica nello studio del pericardio: tecnica di studio, anatomia e principali quadri patologici. Radiol Med (In press)

Giorgi B, Dymarkowski S, Maes F, Kouwenhoven M, Bogaert J (2002) Improved visualization of coronary arteries using a new three-dimensional submillimeter MR coronary angiography sequence with balanced gradients. Am J Roentgenol 179:901–910

Giorgi B, Mollet NRA, Dymarkowski S, Rademakers FA, Bogaert J (2003) Assessment of ventricular septal motion in patients clinically suspected of constrictive pericarditis, using magnetic resonance imaging. Radiology 228:417–424

Glover LB, Barcia A, Reeves TJ (1969) Congenital absence of the pericardium. Am J Radiol 106:542–548

Gomes AS, Lois JF, Child JS et al (1987) Cardiac tumours and thrombus: evaluation with MR imaging. Am J Roentgenol 149:895–899

Groell R, Schaffler G.J., Rienmueller R (1999) Pericardial sinuses and recesses: findings at electrocardiographically triggered electron-beam CT. Radiology 212:69–73

Gutierrez FR, Shackelford GD, McKnight RC, Levitt RG, Hartmann A (1985) Diagnosis of congenital absence of left pericardium by MR imaging. J Comput Assist Tomogr 9:551–553

Haley JH, Tajik J, Danielson GK, et al (2004) Transient constrictive pericarditis: causes and natural history. J Am Coll Cardiol 43:271–275

Hanock EW (1982) Pericardial disease in patients with neoplasm. In: Reddy PS, Leon DF, Shaver JA (eds) Pericardial disease. Raven, New York

Hancock EW (2001) Differential diagnosis of restrictive cardiomyopathy and constrictive pericarditis. Heart 86:343–349

Hasuda T, Satoh T, Yamada N et al (1999) A case of constrictive pericarditis with local thickening of the pericardium without manifest ventricular interdependence. Cardiology 92:214–216

Hoit BD (1990) Imaging the pericardium. Cardiol Clin 8:587–600

Hatle LK, Appleton CP, Popp RL (1989) Differentiation of constrictive pericarditis and restrictive cardiomyopathy by Doppler echocardiography. Circulation 79:357–370

Janicki JS, Weber KT (1980) The pericardium and ventricular interaction, distensibility, and function. Am J Physiol Heart Circ Physiol 238:494–503

Im JG, Rosen A, Webb WR, Gamsu G (1988) MR imaging of the transverse sinus of the pericardium. Am J Roentgenol 150:79–84

Klein C, Graf K, Fleck E, Nagel E (2003) Acute fibrinous pericarditis assessed with magnetic resonance imaging. Images in cardiovascular medicine. Circulation 107:e82

Kojima S, Yamada N, Goto Y (1999) Diagnosis of constrictive pericarditis by tagged cine magnetic resonance imaging. N Engl J Med 341:373–374

Kushwaha SS, Fallon JT, Fuster V (1997) Restrictive cardiomyopathy. N Engl J Med 336:267–276

Lanzer BH, Botvinick EH, Schiller NB et al (1984) Cardiac imaging using gated magnetic resonance. Radiology 150:121–127

Letanche G, Gayer C, Souquet PJ et al (1988) Agenesis of the pericardium: clinical, echocardiographic and MRI aspects. Rev Pneumol Clin 44:105–109

Lorell BH, Braunwald E (1988) Pericardial disease. In: Braunwald E (ed) Heart disease, a textbook of cardiovascular medicine. Saunders, Philadelphia, pp 1484–1485

Lund JT, Ehman RL, Julsrud PR, Sinak LJ, Tajik AJ (1989) Cardiac masses: assessment by MR imaging. AJR Am J Roentgenol 152:469–473

McMurdo KK, Webb WR, Schulthess GK von, Gamsu G (1985) Magnetic resonance imaging of the superior pericardial recesses. AJR Am J Roentgenol 145:985–988

Mulvagh SL, Rokey R, Vick GWD, Johnston DL (1989) Usefulness of nuclear magnetic resonance imaging for evaluation of pericardial effusions, and comparison with two-dimensional echocardiography. Am J Cardiol 64:1002–1009

Myers RBH, Spodick DH (1999) Constrictive pericarditis: clinical and pathophysiologic chararcteristics. Am Heart J 138:219–232

Roberts WC, Spray TL (1976) Pericardial heart disease: a study of its causes, consequences, and morphologic features. Cardiovasc Clin 7:11–65

Sagrista-Sauleda J (2004) Pericardial constriction: uncommon patterns. Heart 90:257–258

Sagrista-Sauleda J, Angel J, Sanchez A, Permanyer-Miralda G, Soler-Soler J (2004) Effusive-constrictive pericarditis. N Engl J Med 350:469–475

Sechtem U, Tscholakoff D, Higgins CB (1986a) MRI of the abnormal pericardium. AJR Am J Roentgenol 147:245–252

Sechtem U, Tscholakoff D, Higgins CB (1986b) MRI of the normal pericardium. AJR Am J Roentgenol 147:239–244

Smith WHT, Beacock DJ, Goddard AJP, et al (2001) Magnetic resonance evaluation of the pericardium: a pictorial review. Br J Radiol 74:384–392

Solomon SL, Brown JJ, Glazer HS, Mirowitz SA, Lee JKT (1990) Thoracic aortic dissection: pitfalls and artifacts in MR imaging. Radiology 177:223–228

Soulen RL, Stark DD, Higgins CB (1985) Magnetic resonance imaging of constrictive pericardial disease. Am J Cardiol 55:480–484

Spodick DH (1997) The pericardium: a comprehensive textbook. Dekker, New York

Starck DD, Higgins CB, Lanzer P et al (1984) Magnetic resonance imaging of the pericardium: normal and pathologic findings. Radiology 150:469–474

Talreja DR, Edwards WD, Danielson GK et al (2003) Constrictive pericarditis in 26 patients with histologically normal pericardial thickness. Circulation 108:1852–1857

12 Cardiac Masses

JAN BOGAERT and STEVEN DYMARKOWSKI

CONTENTS

J. BOGAERT MD, PhD
S. DYMARKOWSKI MD, PhD
Department of Radiology, Gasthuisberg University Hospital,
Catholic University of Leuven, Herestraat 49, 3000 Leuven,
Belgium

12.1
Introduction

Before the era of modern cardiac imaging techniques, the diagnosis of cardiac tumors was extremely difficult and often not made antemortem. Nowadays, the availability of transthoracic (TTE) and transesophageal echocardiography (TEE), cardiac computed tomography (CT), and magnetic resonance imaging (MRI) has greatly facilitated their detection. However, because of their rarity and the nonspecific, often misleading symptomatology that causes them to be placed at the bottom of the differential diagnostic list, their diagnosis may be considerably delayed. Therefore, a great deal of suspicion is required to direct the clinician toward the proper diagnosis.

The title to this chapter, "Cardiac Masses," was preferred to "Cardiac Tumors" for more than one reason. First, not only are nontumoral cardiac masses much more frequent than true cardiac tumors, but also nontumoral masses usually require a medical (or no) treatment, whereas cardiac surgery is still the preferred therapeutic approach for cardiac tumors. Thus, accurate differentiation between the two conditions is a first requirement for each imaging technique dealing with the diagnosis of cardiac masses. Second, precise knowledge of the normal cardiac anatomy and its variants is required, since, with the advent of modern cardiac imaging techniques, not only are abnormal masses much more easily and frequently detected, but normal cardiac structures may be interpreted as abnormal by inexperienced people. Therefore the major aims of this chapter are to guide the reader in recognizing the diversity of cardiac tumors, nontumoral masses, and normal variants, to discuss their appearance on MRI, and to highlight the role of MRI in the detection and differentiation of cardiac masses, comparing this technique with the other cardiac imaging techniques.

12.2
Clinical Presentation

The clinical presentation of tumors originating in the heart is often atypical, suggestive more of a systemic illness than a cardiovascular problem (SALCEDO et al. 1992). Therefore, a high index of suspicion and a goal-directed diagnostic approach are required. Cardiac tumors can manifest in one of several ways (Table 12.1). They can be an incidental finding on chest radiography, echocardiography, or another cardiovascular diagnostic test. The first symptoms can be constitutional, particularly in patients with myxomas, and a high index of suspicion is needed to make the proper diagnosis. Cardiovascular symptoms, specifically congestive heart failure and thromboembolism, can be the presenting manifestations. Since these are rather nonspecific, a great deal of suspicion is required to direct the clinician toward the proper diagnosis. Finally, patients with noncardiac malignancies can have cardiac involvement with or without cardiovascular symptoms.

Table 12.1. Presentation of cardiac tumors

Systemic illness

Cardiovascular symptoms

  Congestive heart failure

  Thromboembolism

  Arrhythmias/interventricular conduction disturbances

Incidental finding

History of noncardiac malignancy

In patients with cardiac tumors, the history and clinical findings are determined primarily by the anatomical location of the tumor rather than by the histopathology. It can be said that cardiac tumors can be clinically and pathologically benign, but have a "malignant" and fatal outcome, or they can be clinically and pathologically malignant. Generally, tumors manifest symptomatology and clinical signs by virtue of tumor growth that impedes cardiac hemodynamics. Thus, large infiltrative tumors may be clinically silent, while smaller, yet strategically located tumors can produce dramatic symptomatology due to transient obstruction of flow across the valve. Arrhythmias and interventricular conduction defects may also be encountered as a consequence of tumor infiltrating the conduction system.

12.3
Conventional Imaging Modalities

Whether a cardiac imaging modality is useful in the diagnosis of patients with suspected cardiac masses depends on following requirements: high accuracy (i.e., low rate of false-negative and false-positive results); accurate evaluation of tumor extent and tumor composition (i.e., tissue characterization); and detection of complications (e.g., valvular obstruction). At present, several cardiac imaging techniques are available. Although this chapter is focused on the role of MRI, the advantages and limitations of the other currently available imaging techniques are briefly discussed and summarized in Table 12.2.

12.3.1
X-ray Angiography

In many cases, the noninvasive imaging modalities (i.e., echocardiography, CT, and MRI) will provide adequate preoperative information on the location and extent of the cardiac tumor, so that no further cardiac catheterization and selective angiocardiography is required. However, in special circumstances information can be needed: (a) when inadequate information on the tumor location, attachment, or extent is obtained by the noninvasive imaging methods; (b) when a malignant tumor is considered likely; and (c) when other cardiac lesions (e.g., coronary artery or valvular lesions) may coexist with a cardiac tumor and possibly dictate a different surgical approach (FUEREDI et al. 1989). Cardiac tumors can be seen on X-ray angiograms as: (a) intracavitary filling defects; (b) compression, displacement, or deformation of the cardiac chambers; (c) increased myocardial wall thickness; or (d) local alteration in wall motion. Furthermore, coronary arteriography may provide information on the vascular pattern of the tumor, its vascular supply, and its relation to the coronary arteries (SINGH et al. 1984). Differentiation with nontumoral conditions such as thrombus, intramuscular hydatid cyst, and aneurysm may not be possible, which yields a high number of false-positive results. Furthermore, X-ray angiocardiography may be false-negative in patients not suspected of having cardiac tumor prior to the catheterization. Finally, the invasiveness of this procedure entails the risk of peripheral embolization due to dislodgement of tumor fragments.

Table 12.2. Advantages and limitations of current cardiac imaging techniques in the detection of cardiac masses

	Advantages	Limitations
X-ray	Tumor size/shape/mobility/location	Radiation/cost
Angiography	Tumor vascularity Nutritive supply	Invasive Dislodgement of tumor fragments Only indirect information on – Myocardial masses or invasion – Pericardial effusions/masses False-positive/-negative results
TTE	Widely available/portable Accurate/real-time imaging Relatively inexpensive Tumor size/shape/mobility/location	Poor echogenicity in 30% of patients No tissue characterization Poor evaluation of pericardium/extracardiac structures
TEE	Advantages = those of TTE Better than TTE in: – Defining tumor attachment and tumor extension – Detecting cardiac thrombi – Evaluation of pericardium and extracardiac structures	Semi-invasive procedure Evaluation of pericardium/extracardiac structures may be insufficient No tissue characterization
CT	Noninvasive High spatial resolution High temporal resolution (ultrafast mode) Possibility of multiplanar reconstruction Tumor size/shape/mobility/location Tissue characterization to a limited extent	Radiation Iodinated contrast material required No real multiplanar imaging capability
MRI	Noninvasive High spatial and temporal resolution Multiplanar imaging capability Large field of view Tumor size/shape/mobility/location Accurate information on tumor extent and tumor vascularity Tissue characterization to a certain extent	Absolute and relative contraindications (such as pacemaker, intracranial vascular clips) Claustrophobia

12.3.2
Echocardiography

Echocardiography is considered the procedure of choice for the diagnosis of intracardiac tumors. This technique may provide information on the size, mobility, shape, and location of cardiac masses, but it cannot describe histological features. The transthoracic approach is totally noninvasive and often sufficient for a complete evaluation. However, when TTE provides inadequate images, as in obese patients and patients with obstructive pulmonary disease, TEE or MRI offers a diagnostic alternative. TEE is superior to TTE in the diagnosis of intracardial and peri- or paracardial tumors (HERRERA et al. 1992). Details such as the attachment point of myxomas, compression of cardiac structures, or infiltration of the great vessels by a malignant disease in close contact with the heart can be better identified by TEE (ENGBERDING et al. 1993). TEE is also superior to

TTE in the detection of left atrial thrombi, especially when located in the left atrial appendage (MUGGE et al. 1991). After surgery, TEE can detect an early recurrence of a tumor or, if a patient receives chemotherapy, the result can be more easily quantified.

While cardiac masses can be very well depicted with echocardiography, additional imaging modalities such as multislice computed tomography (MSCT) or MRI may be required to define the extent of pericardial and extracardiac masses (TESORO TESS et al. 1993; KUPFERWASSER et al. 1994). Absolute contraindications to the performance of TEE include a history of or current pathological conditions of the esophagus, and recent esophageal operations. In patients with relative contraindications, such as unstable angina, esophageal varices, or active upper gastrointestinal bleeding, an individual assessment must be made before TEE is performed. Complications associated with TEE can be related to the probe, to the procedure, or to drugs used during the examination.

12.3.3
Computed Tomography

Electron beam CT and MSCT are probably the closest competitors to MRI for morphological evaluation of the heart, including assessment of cardiac masses. These techniques have a very high spatial resolution and a sufficiently high temporal resolution. In combination with cardiac triggering, artifacts related to cardiac motion can be substantially reduced. Injection of iodinated contrast medium enhances the contrast between the heart chambers and vessels and surrounding myocardium and vessel walls. Both intra- and extracardiac masses can be very clearly depicted, as well as their degree of myocardial or pericardial involvement (STANFORD et al. 1991; BLEIWEIS et al. 1994; KEMP et al. 1996; ARAOZ et al. 2000). High radiation doses of cardiac CT, especially with the multislice technique, limit at present a more routine use of this technique, e.g., detection of coronary artery stenosis in patients with coronary artery disease.

12.3.4
Magnetic Resonance Imaging

At present, MRI is definitely one of the preferred imaging modalities in the evaluation of patients with suspected cardiac masses. Major advantages of this technique are: the excellent spatial resolution; the large field of view; the inherent natural contrast between flowing blood and the surrounding heart chambers, vessel walls, and tumor masses, without the need for contrast agents; the multiplanar imaging capability; and the ability to administer paramagnetic contrast agents in order to obtain a better detection of the tumor borders and the degree of tumor vascularization. These advantages are important in planning the patient's therapy, particularly if surgical intervention is being considered. Using MRI, cardiac tumors can be depicted with a very high accuracy. Not only are abnormal masses easily detected, but tumor mimics, e.g., normal anatomical variants, not infrequently misinterpreted as tumor masses by other imaging modalities, are easily recognized by means of MRI. A distinct advantage over echocardiography is the large field of view, which allows perfect assessment not only of the intracardiac but also of the extracardiac extent of the tumor. Also, masses originating in the pericardium or in the neighboring lung parenchyma or mediastinum can be much better evaluated. For instance,

frequently misinterpreted paracardiac tumors using TEE include diaphragmatic hernias and aneurysmal dilatation of the descending thoracic aorta. MRI may be particularly useful in detecting recurrence in the postoperative period, since echocardiography may not be suitable if surgery has decreased the echo window (KAMINAGA et al. 1993). A relative advantage over cardiac CT is still the multiplanar imaging capability by which directly tomographic images in any desired plane can be obtained, which aids in the determination of the location, size, and anatomical relationships of normal and abnormal cardiac structures. Furthermore, MRI can provide contiguous image slices of known thickness and accurately measure cardiac and tissue volumes, and can be used to quantify tumor volume. The availability of new, ultrafast sequences enabling study of the heart in real time has made MRI more competitive with the real-time cardiac imaging modality by excellence, i.e., echocardiography (SPUENTRUP et al. 2003).

Historically speaking, the ECG-triggered spin-echo (SE) technique was the first sequence used for the evaluation and tissue characterization of cardiac masses. Though still important, nowadays this sequence has become part of a more broader approach to investigate patients with suspected cardiac masses. Using a set of different cardiac MRI sequences, important information is obtained on the cardiac mass, i.e., morphology and tissue characterization, perfusion and enhancement patterns, mobility and deformation, as well as on the impact of a cardiac mass on the cardiac dynamics and integrity (Fig. 12.1). Currently used dark-blood-prepared SE-MRI techniques allow excellent anatomical evaluation of the heart. A combination of T1- and T2-weighted measurements allows a better description of the composition of cardiac masses, although the initial hope that the pattern of signal intensity would allow differentiation between benign and malignant neoplasms has not been fulfilled. Cystic fluid, e.g., (pleuro)pericardial cyst, has a very low signal on T1-weighted images, but a very high signal on T2-weighted images. Masses with a lipomatous composition, e.g., lipomas and lipomatous hypertrophy of the interatrial septum, have a signal intensity that resembles that of epicardial or subcutaneous fat. They have a relatively high signal on T1-weighted sequences and a moderate signal on T2-weighted sequences (AMPARO et al. 1984; SECHTEM et al. 1986; BROWN et al. 1989). Fat-suppression techniques, as applied, for instance, in coronary MR angiography, will selectively saturate the signal coming from fat

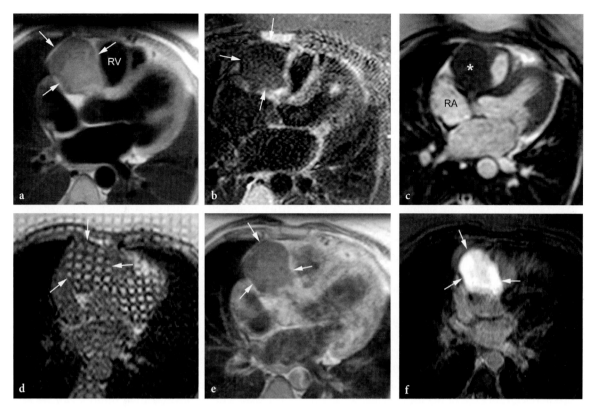

Fig. 12.1a-f. Contribution of different MRI sequences in the description and characterization of a cardiac mass located in the right atrioventricular groove (*arrows. star*) in a 27-year-old woman with neurofibromatosis. All images are obtained in the axial image plane. T1-weighted turbo spin-echo (TSE)-MRI shows a well-defined mass in the right atrioventricular groove, with minor compression of the RV cavity (**a**). The mass is isointense to the signal of myocardial tissue on T1-weighted sequences, and hypointense on T2-weighted short-tau inversion-recovery (STIR) TSE sequences (**b**). Cine MRI using the balanced steady-state free precession (b-SSFP) technique (**c**) and MRI myocardial tagging using the spatial modulation of magnetization (SPAMM) technique (**d**) are very helpful in evaluating the mobility and absence of deformation of the cardiac mass. Although after administration of paramagnetic contrast agents (gadopentetate dimeglumine) the mass is slightly hypointense compared with the myocardium (**e**), it appears strongly hyperintense on the contrast-enhanced inversion-recovery (CE-IR) MR images (inversion time of 250 ms) (**f**). The *star* and *arrows* indicate the cardiac mass in the right atrioventricular groove. Abbreviations: *RA*, right atrium; *RV*, right ventricle

and can be used to prove the fatty composition of cardiac masses. Most soft tissue tumors have relaxation times shorter than fluid, but long enough to produce a relatively low signal on T1-weighted images and a relatively high signal on T2-weighted images (GAMSU et al. 1984). Some cardiac tumors may have a prolongation of T1 and T2 relaxation times as a result of an increased water content (WILLIAMS et al. 1980). Especially the newer, short-tau inversion-recovery (STIR) SE techniques with strong T2 weighting, used to detect the presence and extent of myocardial edema in patients with a recent myocardial infarction, can be applied to estimate the water content of a cardiac mass. Mineral-rich tissues, containing cortical bone and calcifications, and mature fibrotic tissue have few mobile protons, resulting in low signal regardless of the repetition time and echo

time used. Subacute and chronic hemorrhage will show a high signal intensity on both T1-weighted and T2-weighted MRI (MITCHELL et al. 1987).

The distinction of intramural tumors from normal myocardium may be equivocal because of the similarity of signal intensity between tumor and normal myocardium on SE images (FUNARI et al. 1991). Paramagnetic contrast agents such as gadolinium-diethylene triamine penta-acetic acid (Gd-DTPA), may be administered for improved visualization of cardiac tumors. Differences in perfusion and washout of these contrast agents between normal and tumoral tissue may facilitate demonstration of the extent of pathology. Gd-DTPA usually accumulates in higher concentrations in tissues which contain augmented vascularization or a substantial proportion of interstitial space (BRASCH et al. 1984).

Paramagnetic contrast agents can also provide information about the internal architecture, i.e., nonvascularized, necrotic, or cystic areas of a tumor, because they do not accumulate contrast medium (Neuerburg et al. 1989). This may be of clinical importance, since the presence of such regions inside a mass may help to formulate the differential diagnosis or to assess the efficacy of radiotherapeutic or chemotherapeutic treatment on follow-up MRI studies (Funari et al. 1991). Gd-DTPA may also be helpful to differentiate tumor from acute and subacute thrombus, since the latter does not have vascularization and therefore cannot be enhanced by contrast media. However, on rare occasions chronic thrombi do acquire vascularization, so potentially they can enhance after administration of contrast medium (Johnson et al. 1988). Two new MRI techniques, nowadays routinely used to study patients with ischemic heart disease, i.e., first-pass myocardial perfusion sequences and the contrast-enhanced inversion-recovery MRI (CE-IR MRI) technique, are probably very helpful too in a more accurate assessment of cardiac masses (Barkhausen et al. 2002; Mollet et al. 2002; Bogaert et al. 2004).

Dynamic evaluation of the heart using fast gradient-echo techniques (e.g., balanced steady-state-free-precession technique, b-SSFP) has a central place in the assessment of cardiac masses. Cine MRI allows evaluation of the mobility of cardiac masses, to detect the site of implantation, to detect atrioventricular obstruction, to differentiate slow flow from thrombus, and to evaluate the effects of cardiac masses on myocardial contractility. Calcifications which are "invisible" on SE MRI because they cannot be differentiated from the surrounding black blood can be very easily detected on cine MRI as areas devoid of signal surrounded by bright blood (Glazer et al. 1985; de Roos et al. 1989). Other MRI techniques such as MR myocardial tagging and MR phase imaging can be applied to improve the differentiation between tumor and, respectively, myocardium and intracavitary blood. MR myocardial tagging allows a selective saturation of myocardial tissue, in this fashion creating tag lines or a grid pattern on the myocardium (Zerhouni et al. 1988). This technique has been applied to differentiate normal contractile myocardium from noncontractile tumor in a neonate with a cardiac rhabdomyoma (Bouton et al. 1991). Phase-imaging techniques can be used to distinguish cardiac masses, e.g., tumor tissue or thrombus, from moving blood adjacent to the cardiac mass (Rumancik et al. 1988; Kaminaga et al. 1993). SE magnitude images alone are not an accurate indicator in differentiating intracavitary tumor

or thrombus from flow-related enhancement. Phase images, however, are sensitive for identifying flow, and this technique is complementary to conventional SE magnitude images in helping to distinguish flow-related signal from intraluminal pathological conditions (Rumancik et al. 1988; Hatabu et al. 1994).

In a recent study, Hoffmann et al. (2003) have compared MRI with histology to evaluate the usefulness of this technique to distinguish malignant from benign cardiac and paracardiac masses. The study results have identified tumor location, tissue composition, and the presence of pericardial or pleural effusion as key predictors of lesion type. MRI was accurate in the prediction of the lesion type (area under the receiver operating characteristic, ROC, curve of 0.88 and 0.92), and a good interobserver agreement was found (kappa-score 0.64).

12.4
Classification

Cardiac masses are divided into neoplasms and nonneoplastic conditions. Cardiac tumors can be primary or secondary. Primary cardiac tumors may be benign or malignant, while secondary tumors may involve the heart by direct extension, venous extension, lymphatic extension, or metastatic spread. The heterogeneous group of nonneoplastic conditions includes all nontumoral cardiac masses and other abnormalities which may present as cardiac masses on cardiac imaging. This group also includes normal anatomical variants which may mimic cardiac masses. The MRI characteristics of the most common cardiac masses are shown in Table 12.3.

12.4.1
Primary Cardiac Tumors

Primary tumors of the heart and pericardium are extremely rare, with an incidence of between 0.0017% and 0.28% in unselected patients at autopsy, while metastatic tumors to the heart are 20–40 times more common than primary tumors (Heath 1968; McAllister and Fenoglio 1978). Three-quarters of the primary tumors are benign; nearly half the benign tumors are myxomas, and the majority of the rest are lipomas, papillary fibroelastomas, and rhabdomyomas (Grebenc et al. 2000). Whereas myxomas are the most common primary tumors in adults, rhabdomyomas clearly predominate in children.

Table 12.3. MRI characteristics of the most common cardiac masses

	Preferential location	SE (T1)	SE (T2)	GE	Contrast enhancement	Appearance
Benign cardiac tumors						
Myxoma	Left atrium (IAS)	Variable	Variable	Low	Yes	Heterogeneous sharp border
Lipoma	No	High	High	Medium	No	Homogeneous, sharp border
Papillary fibroelastoma	Cardiac valves	Medium	Medium	Low	?	Small (less than 1 cm)
Rhabdomyoma	Atrium	Medium/high	Medium	Low	Similar to myocardium	Multiple
	Intramural/intracavitary					
Fibroma	Ventricles	Medium	Medium	Low	Variable	Usually single
	Intramural					
Pheochromocytoma	Intrapercardial (roof of left atrium)		High		Yes	
Hemangioma	Ventricles	Medium	Very high	Variable	Yes	Heterogeneous
	Intramural/intracavitary				Variable	Sharp border
Malignant cardiac tumors						
Angiosarcoma	Right atrium	Variable (mixed)	Variable (mixed)	Low	Yes	Heterogeneous
	Pericardial and myocardial invasion					"Cauliflower" appearance
Rhabdomyosarcoma	No	Medium	High	?	Yes	
Malignant fibrous histiocytoma	Left atrium (posterior wall)	Medium	High	?	?	Slightly heterogeneous
Lymphoma	Pericardial effusion	Medium	Medium	Low	Yes	Variable
	Intracardiac masses					
Malignant pericardial mesothelioma	Pericardium	Medium	High	Low	Yes	Heterogeneous (no myocardial invasion)
Nontumoral cardiac masses and mimics						
Thrombus	Atrium / Appendage (valve disease / AF)	Medium to high	Medium to high	Low	No (possible if chronic)	Appearance related to age of thrombus
	Ventricles (if diseased)					
Valvular vegetations	Cardiac valves	Not visible	Not visible	Low	No	
Lipomatous hypertrophy of the interatrial septum	Interatrial septum	High	High	Medium	Low	"Camel hump" or "dumbbell"-shaped, sparing the fossa ovalis
Hydatid cyst	Left ventricle (IVS)	Low	Very high		No	Low signal intensity peripheral border (pericyst)
Pleuropericardial cyst	Right cardiophrenic angle	Low	Very high		No	Sharply defined

The signal intensity of the cardiac masses on SE sequences is compared with the signal intensity of myocardium. The signal intensity of the cardiac masses on GE sequences is compared with the signal intensity of blood flow
AF: atrial fibrillation, IAS, Interatrial septum; IVS, interventricular septum; GE, gradient-echo; SE, spin-echo

12.4.1.1
Benign Cardiac Tumors

12.4.1.1.1
Myxoma

Cardiac myxoma, the most frequent primary cardiac tumor, is an intracavitary neoplasm that can occur anywhere in the heart. Seventy-five percent of myxomas occur in the left atrium and 75% of these have a pedunculated attachment to the atrial septum near the fossa ovalis (Hanson 1992; Grebenc et al. 2000, 2002). Twenty percent of myxomas occur in the right atrium, without the predilection for the fossa ovalis (McAllister 1979). Five percent of myxomas are found in either the right or the left ventricle.

The typical patient diagnosed with this condition is a middle-aged woman presenting to her physician or referred to a cardiologist with vague complaints such as atypical chest pains, palpitations, or intermittent shortness of breath, with few if any clinical findings. Before the widespread use of modern diagnostic imaging, the majority of patients were diagnosed late and were moderately or severely symptomatic. Today, myxomas are frequently discovered in the asymptomatic or nearly asymptomatic patient who is essentially free of clinical findings.

Depending on their size and mobility, myxomas commonly give rise to signs of obstructed filling of the left and right ventricle, with subsequent dyspnea, recurrent pulmonary edema, and right-sided heart failure. These signs mimic the clinical picture of mitral or tricuspid valve stenosis. Embolism occurs in 30–40% of patients with myxomas. It is suggested that myxomas with high mobility or gelatinous consistency might present a higher incidence of embolization (Engberding et al. 1993; Grebenc et al. 2002). Since most myxomas are located in the left atrium, systemic embolism is particularly frequent. In the majority of cases, the cerebral arteries, including the retinal arteries, are affected. The differential diagnosis of peripheral embolism should therefore include myxoma. The rate of growth of myxomas is unknown but they generally appear to grow rather quickly. Myxomas have a malignant counterpart, "myxosarcomas," which also arise in the left atrium (Klima et al. 1986; Burke et al. 1992).

The signal characteristics of cardiac myxomas on MRI depend on the tumor composition. Areas of high signal in the myxoma correspond to subacute intratumoral hemorrhage, while areas with low signal intensity correspond to calcification or deposition of hemosiderin (i.e., chronic hemorrhage; De Roos et al. 1989; Watanabe et al. 1994; Fig. 12.2). Additionally, the surface of the tumor is often covered by thrombus (Semelka et al. 1992). Massive hemosiderin deposition in a cardiac myxoma has been reported by Lie and Watanabe (Lie 1989; Watanabe et al. 1994). Its presence may lead to an apparent enlargement of the tumor volume on cine MRI compared with the tumor volume on SE-MRI (Fig. 12.2). Though calcification of myxomas is reported to be rare, occurring more commonly in myxomas of the right atrium, in a paper by Fueridi et al. (1989), up to one-third of all myxomas in the left atrium were

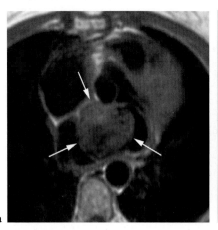

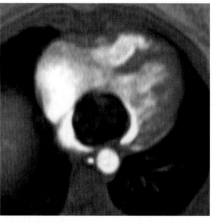

a   b

Fig. 12.2a,b. Left atrial myxoma in a 67-year-old woman. **a** A large, well-defined inhomogeneous mass is visible in the left atrium on an axial T1-weighted SE MR image (*arrows*). Due to its large size, the tumor attachment to the atrial septum is difficult to assess. The tumor demonstrates an inhomogeneous enhancement pattern after contrast administration (not shown). **b** On cine MRI, using the spoiled gradient-echo (GE) technique, the myxoma is strongly hypointense due to the presence of hemosiderin and appears somewhat larger than on the SE-MRI ("blooming artifact")

calcified. After administration of paramagnetic contrast agents, myxomas may exhibit a homogeneous or heterogeneous enhancement pattern depending on the histological characteristics of the tumor (MATSUOKA et al. 1996). Areas of enhancement correspond with histological myxoma or inflammation, while unenhanced regions reflect necrosis of cystic changes. In addition, myxomas are highly vascular, showing tortuosity of the vessels within the tumor; this may explain the significant enhancement after Gd-DTPA administration (FUEREDI et al. 1989). On cine MRI, myxomas have a low signal intensity and this technique may be used to depict atrioventricular tumor entrapment and to detect tumor attachment (Fig. 12.3–12.5).

Differential diagnosis of myxoma primarily encompasses other benign and malignant primary tumors, metastatic tumors, and organized atrial thrombi (Fig. 12.6). Valvular vegetations are also an important part of the differential diagnosis. In cases of right atrial masses, a prominent eustachian valve and an aneurysm of the interatrial septum must be considered, in addition to tumors, sessile or mobile, and vegetations on the tricuspid valve. As mentioned later in this chapter, normal variants which may mimic cardiac masses can be easily recognized with MRI.

12.4.1.1.2
Lipoma

Cardiac lipomas account for approximately 10% of all cardiac neoplasms and about 14% of benign cardiac tumors (HANANOUCHI and GOFF 1990). True lipomas are less frequent than lipomatous hypertrophy of the interatrial septum (see Sect. 12.4.4.4). Lipomas are benign tumors of encapsulated mature adipose cells. Lipomas can be intracavitary, intra-

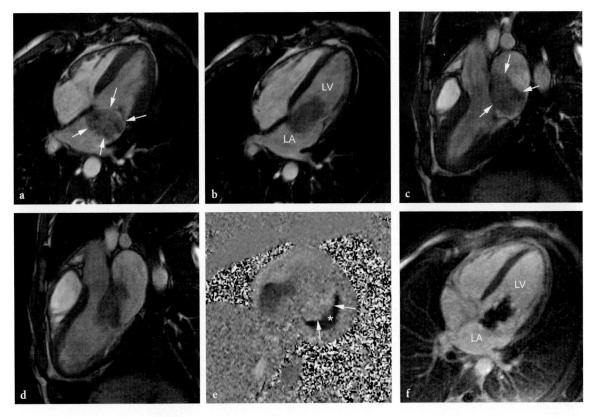

Fig. 12.3a-f. Mobile left atrial myxoma in a 26-year-old man, partially obstructing the mitral valve orifice during ventricular filling. The b-SSFP cine MR image at mid-systole, obtained in the horizontal long-axis (**a**) and LV in- and outflow tract view (**c**) shows an inhomogeneous and irregular defined mass (*arrows*) attached to the base of the atrial septum. During ventricular filling this mass is displaced in the LV cavity (**b-d**) and partially occludes the mitral valve orifice, as shown on a short-axis phase-contrast image (**e**). The *arrows* indicate the myxoma, while the semilunar black area indicated by the *star* shows the nonobstructed part of the mitral valve (**e**). After administration of gadolinium dimeglumine (0.1 mmol/kg body weight), the myxoma has a dark appearance on CE-IR MRI (**f**). CE-IR MRI obtained at 10 min after contrast administration using an inversion time of 340 ms. Abbreviations: *LA*, left atrium; *LV*, left ventricle

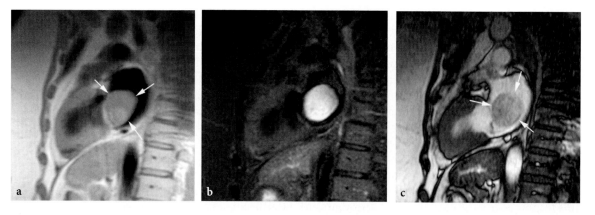

Fig. 12.4a-c. Left atrial myxoma in 72-year-old woman. All images are obtained in the vertical long-axis image plane through the middle of the left ventricle. On the T1-weighted TSE-MR image (**a**), the myxoma is visible as a well-defined homogeneous mass (*arrows*) with a signal intensity slightly superior to that of myocardial tissue. On T2-weighted STIR TSE, the myxoma exhibits a uniform, very high signal, probably corresponding with an abundant extracellular matrix (**b**). On cine MRI, using the b-SSFP sequence, the myxoma (*arrows*) is mobile and shows atrioventricular entrapment (**c**)

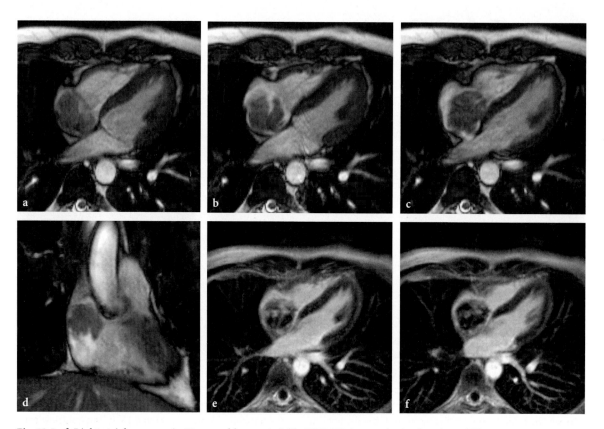

Fig. 12.5a-f. Right atrial myxoma in 35-year-old man. Axial b-SSFP MR image obtained at three different time-points during the cardiac cycle (**a-c**). Coronal b-SSFP image through the right atrium (**d**). Axial CE-IR MR images obtained after administration of gadopentetate dimeglumine (**e, f**). The RA myxoma appears as an irregularly defined, highly deformable, mobile mass attached to the atrial septum, with entrapment in the tricuspid valve during diastole. The coronal view (**d**) shows the extension of the myxoma into the right atrial appendage. A strong, but highly inhomogeneous enhancement is found following administration of gadopentetate dimeglumine

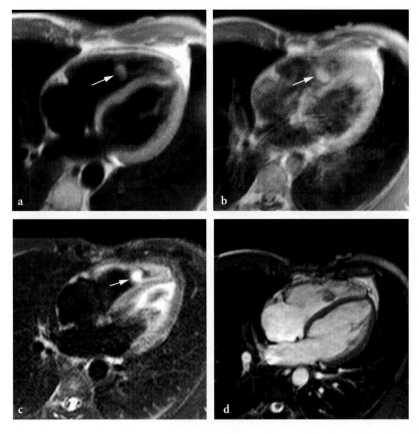

Fig. 12.6a-d. Benign tumor of mesenchymal origin (*arrows*) in the right ventricle in a 27-year-old man. Axial T1-weighted TSE before (**a**) and after (**b**) administration of gadopentetate dimeglumine, axial T2-weighted STIR-TSE (**c**), and axial cine MRI using the b-SSFP technique (**d**). A well-defined, nodular mobile mass is visible in the RV cavity attached to the papillary muscle. This mass enhances after contrast-administration and is hyperintense on strong T2-weighted images. Based on signal characteristics and overall appearance, this mass is most likely a benign tumor. Differentiation between myxoma and other benign tumors, such as benign mesenchymoma in this patient, is usually not possible

myocardial, or intrapericardial (WOLF et al. 1987) and are most frequently located in the left ventricle and right atrium. Lipomas are usually asymptomatic and in most cases require no treatment or surgical intervention. Symptoms may be produced depending on the size and the location of the tumor. Characteristic is the very low density (average –100 Hounsfield units) on CT (GREBENC et al. 2000; ARAOZ et al. 2002; GAERTE et al. 2002; OYAMA et al. 2003). MRI is the most informative imaging technique in that it reveals the nature, size, location, and blood flow pattern of the tumor. T1- and T2-weighted MRI can be compared with clearly differentiated fat from other surrounding tissue. Differential diagnosis includes subacute hemorrhage. Both entities have a high signal intensity on T1-weighted MRI. On T2-weighted MRI, lipomas have an intermediate signal intensity, whereas subacute hemorrhage has a high signal intensity. The use of fat-suppression techniques may be useful to further differentiate fatty tissue from subacute hemorrhage.

12.4.1.1.3
Papillary Fibroelastoma

Papillary fibroelastomas are rare cardiac benign tumors, but they are the most common primary tumor of the cardiac valves (EDWARDS et al. 1991; ARAOZ et al. 2002). The lesions occur on any of the cardiac valves or endothelial surfaces of the heart, such as the apex of the left ventricle, the chordae tendineae, or the outflow tract (UCHIDA et al. 1992; SHAHIAN et al. 1995; COLUCCI et al. 1995). They are discovered accidentally or when neurological or cardiological complications occur owing to emboli with stroke or coronary artery occlusion and myocardial infarction (MCFADDEN and LACY 1987; KASARSKIS et al. 1988; PINELLI et al. 1995). They do not cause valvular dysfunction (KLARICH et al. 1997). Papillary fibroelastomas are small tumors, with a mean diameter of 12±9 mm, that are usually pedunculated and mobile (KLARICH et al. 1997; Fig. 12.7). TTE and TEE are the preferred imaging modalities for detection. In addition, MRI can also be used (GROTE et al. 1995; PINELLI et al. 1995). The embolic risks justify the surgical treatment of these lesions, while

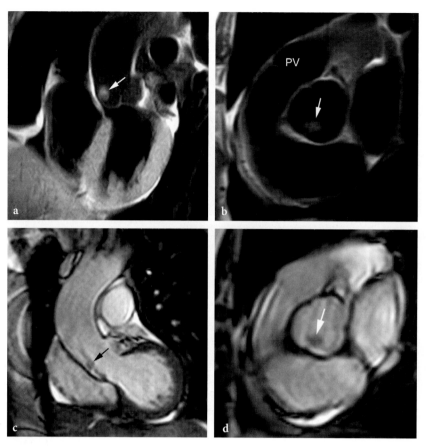

Fig. 12.7a-d. Papillary fibroelastoma attached on the right coronary cusp of the aortic valve in a 69-year-old woman presenting with systemic emboli. T1-weighted TSE MR image in the LV outflow tract view (**a**) and a perpendicular view through the aortic root just above the aortic valve (**b**). **c, d** Cine MRI, using the b-SSFP technique, obtained in similar planes. A small (8 mm) nodular structure (*arrow*) is clearly visible. Because of the small size, assessment of enhancement after administration of contrast agents is often not possible

anticoagulation therapy can be suggested as a substitute for surgery in high-risk patients (KLARICH et al. 1997).

12.4.1.1.4
Rhabdomyoma

Rhabdomyoma is the commonest cardiac tumor in early childhood, representing 75% of all primary cardiac tumors arising in the neonatal period (YANAGISAWA 1991; AGGOUN et al. 1992; KIAFFAS et al. 2002). Rhabdomyoma is not infrequently considered as a hamartoma rather than a true tumor, since it may regress spontaneously by the age of 2 years (MATTEUCCI et al. 1997). This tumor may have similar clinical features to a fibroma. However, rhabdomyomas are frequently multiple, involve both atria and ventricles, and, while usually located intramurally, can have an intracavitary location. Fibromas, in contrast, are infrequently multiple or located in the atria. Rhabdomyomas rarely calcify. A most important differential feature is the association of rhabdomyomas with tuberous sclerosis (Bourneville's tuberous sclerosis), and the tendency

to completely disappear with aging (BADER et al. 2003). MRI is very helpful in locating and determining the extent of the tumor. Cardiac rhabdomyomas have an intermediate to high signal intensity on T1-weighted MRI and an intermediate signal intensity on T2-weighted images. The postcontrast enhancement of the tumor is similar to the surrounding myocardium (SEMELKA et al. 1992). BOUTON et al. (1991) have used MRI tagging to differentiate viable myocardium from tumor in a pediatric patient with intramyocardially located rhabdomyoma.

12.4.1.1.5
Fibroma

In the large series of 533 cases of primary cardiac tumors reported by the Armed Forces Institute of Pathology, fibromas constitute only 3.2% of the total (MCALLISTER and FENOGLIO 1978; PARMLEY et al. 1988). Fibromas are predominantly found in the pediatric age group, though they may be detected in adolescents and adults (BURKE et al. 1994). Very probably cardiac fibroma is a congenital tumor, since it is usually manifest at birth or in early infancy or childhood. Fibromas primarily arise in the ventricles and are commonly located intramurally, i.e., in the anterior wall and intraventricular septum (Fig. 12.8, 12.9 and 12.10). These tumors not infrequently calcify. The high frequency of sudden death and the potential for preventing this occurrence emphasize the need for early diagnosis and appropriate surgical and medical therapy (PARMLEY et al. 1988). The major tumors requiring differentiation are myxoma, lipoma, and rhabdomyoma. Echocardiography and MRI are very sensitive in the diagnosis and preoperative assessment (PARMLEY et al. 1988; BURKE et al. 1994). The signal characteristics on SE sequences are similar to the surrounding myocardium, while after contrast administration fibromas demonstrate a heterogeneous enhancement with a lower-intensity central area surrounded by a peripheral hyperintense rim (FUNARI et al. 1991).

The central area probably corresponds to a poorly vascularized fibrous region (Fig. 12.8).

12.4.1.1.6
Intrapericardial Paraganglioma (Pheochromocytoma)

Intrapericardial paraganglioma (pheochromocytoma) is a catecholamine-secreting tumor causing persistent or paroxysmal hypertension. The incidence of pheochromocytoma is less than 1% of the hypertensive population. Ninety percent of pheochromocytomas arise from the chromaffin cells of the adrenal medulla and about 10% of the tumors originate from other parts of the adrenal glands, retroperitoneally in the para-aortic region, the urinary bladder, or rarely the chest (less than 2% of tumors) or neck (less than 0.1% of tumors; MANGER

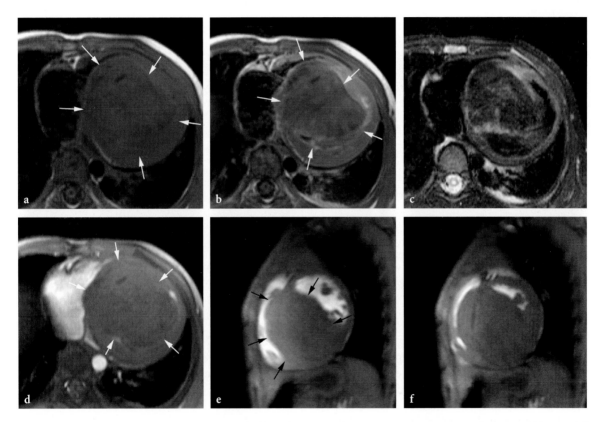

Fig. 12.8a-f. Huge cardiac fibroma (*arrows*) arising from the ventricular septum in an asymptomatic 7-year-old boy. Axial T1-weighted TSE MR image before (**a**) and after (**b**) administration of gadopentetate dimeglumine. Axial T2-weighted TSE MR image (**c**). **d** Axial cine MR image using the segmented spoiled GE-technique. Midventricular short-axis cine MR image, using the the spoiled GE-technique at end diastole (**e**) and end systole (**f**). On the axial image, both ventricular cavities are nearly completely obliterated by a large soft-tissue mass, whose origin and exact location are difficult discernible. The mass, slightly hypointense on T1-weighted TSE-MRI, does not enhance following contrast administration (except a small peripheral rim of enhancement), and it has a heterogeneous hypointense appearance on T2-weighted TSE. The short-axis cine MR images are helpful to locate the mass, i.e., in the ventricular septum, and to depict the compression of the ventricular cavities during mainly during systole. It is worth mentioning that this boy was asymptomatic, and the presence of a cardiac fibroma was detected because of an abnormal murmur during a medical school exam

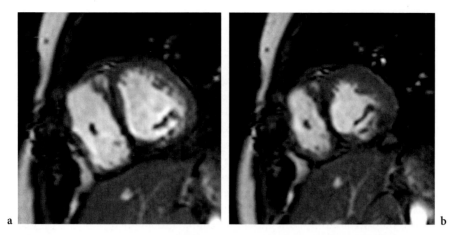

Fig. 12.9a,b. Same patient as in Fig. 12.8 after surgical resection of the cardiac fibroma. Short-axis cine MR image at end diastole (**a**) and end systole (**b**), using the b-SSFP technique. The ventricular septum has regained a near-normal thickness, while the contractility of the septum is slightly diminished. This patient was closely followed for 3 years. Because of onset of arrhythmias and increase in volume, a surgical resection of the fibroma was performed

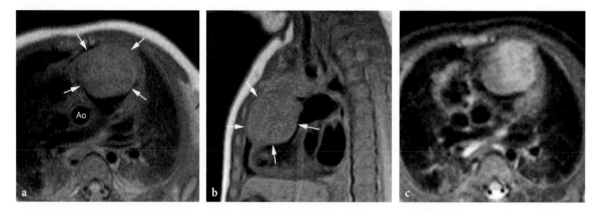

Fig. 12.10a-c. Cardiac fibroma arising from the anterior RV wall in a 2-month-old boy. Axial (**a**) and sagittal (**b**) T1-weighted TSE-MRI, axial T2-weighted TSE (**c**). A well-circumscribed mass (*arrows*) is found in the RVOT arising from the anterior wall. This mass is subtotally obstructing the RVOT. On T2-weighted TSE, the fibroma appears slightly hyperintense

and GIFFORD 1990). The majority of tumors in the chest occur in the posterior mediastinum and originate from the paravertebral sympathetic ganglia. Cardiac pheochromocytomas are exceedingly rare and are usually found intrapericardially, most often in relation to the roof of the left atrium, and less frequently arise in the interatrial septum (HAOUZI et al. 1989; KAWASUJI et al. 1989; GOMI et al. 1994; Fig. 12.11). For initial detection, regional location of these extra-adrenal tumors and detection of distant metastases by means of metaiodobenzylguanidine (MIBG) scintigraphy is recommended. MRI can then provide detailed anatomical delineation before surgical resection (FISHER et al. 1985; HAMILTON et al. 1997). Pheochromocytomas usually have a high

signal intensity on T2-weighted pulse sequences (VARGHESE et al. 1997; Fig. 12.11). They usually reveal a marked enhancement after administration of paramagnetic contrast agents (ICHIKAWA et al. 1995).

12.4.1.1.7
Hemangioma

Hemangiomas are vascular tumors composed of blood vessels that can be either capillaries, i.e., capillary hemangioma, or large cavernous vascular channels, i.e., cavernous hemangioma. Hemangiomas are most frequently localized in the skin and subcutaneous muscles, and their localization in the heart is

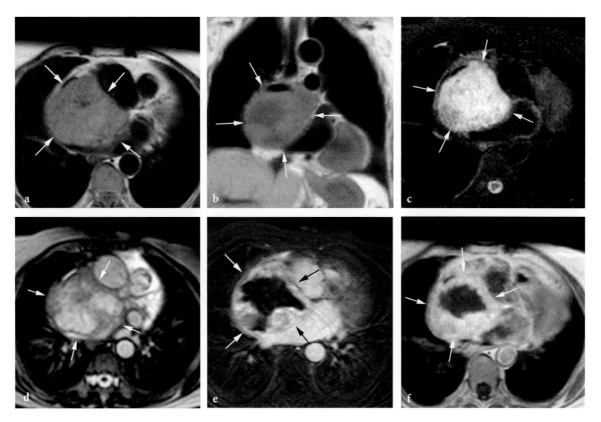

Fig. 12.11a-f. Cardiac paraganglioma (or pheochromocytoma; *arrows*) in a 72-year-old woman. This patient had a history of systemic arterial hypertension and flushing for more than 2 decades. Axial (**a**) and coronal (**b**) T1-weighted TSE. **c** Axial T2-weighted STIR TSE. **d** Cine MRI using the b-SSFP technique. CE-IR MRI (**e**) and axial T1-weighted TSE (**f**) and following administration of gadopentetate dimeglumine. A large, well-circumscribed mass is shown at the roof of the atrial septum compressing the surrounding structures, e.g., superior vena cava, left atrium. The mass is fairly homogeneous, isointense on T1-weighted sequences, homogeneous hyperintense on images with strong T2-weighting. On cine MRI, the mass has a heterogeneous consistence. Following contrast administration, a strong peripheral enhancement is found in combination with a large, central nonperfused region (**e-f**). (Reprinted in part from BOGAERT et al. 2004, with permission.)

extremely rare (MOSTHAF et al. 1991; BRIZARD et al. 1993). The most common localizations are the lateral walls of the left ventricle, the anterior wall of the right ventricle, and the septum, while in 30% of cases multiple locations are found. Half of these tumors grow intramurally, while the other 50% have an intracavitary localization. On coronary angiography, these tumors have a typical vascular blush. MRI may be helpful in demonstrating the vascular nature of the tumor and in evaluating the surgical resectability (BRIZARD et al. 1993). Hemangiomas generally show up on MR images as heterogeneous masses (OSHIMA et al. 2003). They have an intermediate signal intensity on T1-weighted images and a high signal intensity on T2-weighted images (Fig. 12.12). After contrast administration, the increase in signal intensity depends on the blood flow through the tumor. High-flow angiomas demonstrate a much

lower increase in signal intensity than low-flow angiomas (KAPLAN and WILLIAMS 1987; KONERMANN et al. 1989). Newer MRI modalities such as perfusion MRI and CE-IR MRI are helpful to discriminate a hemangioma from other cardiac masses. As shown in Figure 12.12, due to the highly vascular nature of a hemangioma, on CE-IR MR images the tumor is not discernible from the surrounding blood pool.

12.4.1.1.8
Teratoma

Teratomas are generally benign tumors typically occurring in infancy. These tumors are not infrequently detected during intrauterine life by means of fetal ultrasonography. Teratomas are intrapericardially located pedunculated tumors, arising from the root of the ascending aorta, and may cause large pericar-

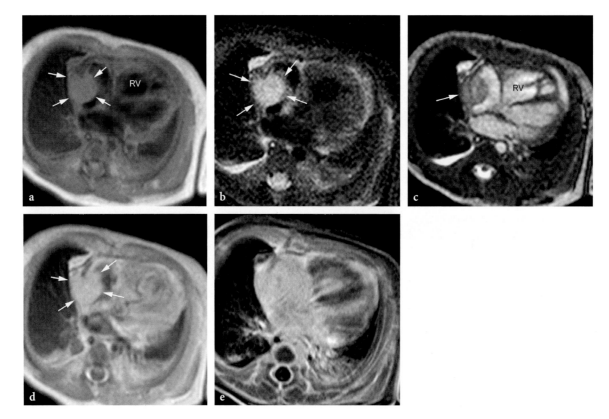

Fig. 12.12a-e. Cardiac hemangioma (*arrows*) in a 1-day-old girl. On fetal echocardiography (27 weeks of gestation), a pericardial effusion and a right atrial mass were detected. At 37 weeks, an urgent delivery was performed because of cardiac tamponade due to an important pericardial effusion. After pericardiocenthesis, the baby was referred for further evaluation of the RA mass to MRI. All images are obtained in the axial plane. T1-weighted (**a**) and T2-weighted STIR (**b**) TSE-MRI. Cine MRI, using the b-SSFP technique (**c**). T1-weighted TSE (**d**) and CE-IR MRI (**e**) after administration of gadopentetate dimeglumine. A well-defined mass is visible in the RA attached to the lateral wall. The mass is isointense on T1-weighted TSE, hyperintense on T2-weighted STIR TSE. Following contrast administration, the mass strongly enhances. Remarkably, due to its high vascularity, the mass is no longer discernible from the RA cavity on CE-IR MRI. Besides a small amount of residual pericardial fluid, no pericardial abnormalities are found. Although a combination of a cardiac mass and a pericardial effusion is suspected of cardiac malignancy, it may occur in benign tumors too

dial effusion with cardiac tamponade (ARCINIEGAS et al. 1980; BENETAR et al. 1992). They consist of the three germ layers (i.e., endodermic, mesodermic, and neuroectodermic germinal layers) and may be cystic as well as solid. Early surgical removal is usually curative. Echocardiography generally suggests the diagnosis by showing a heterogeneous intrapericardial mass associated with a pericardial effusion compressing the heart. MRI is advantageous to better define the relationship of large tumorous masses to adjacent structures, in visualizing echocardiographic "blind" spots, and in defining tissue characteristics (BARAKOS et al. 1989a; BEGHETTI et al. 1998; KIAFFAS et al. 2002).

12.4.1.2
Malignant Cardiac Tumors

Primary malignant cardiac tumors can be divided into three major groups, i.e., sarcomas, lymphomas, and mesotheliomas (GREBENC et al. 2000).

12.4.1.2.1
Sarcomas

Soft tissue sarcoma is the most common malignant neoplasm of the heart, pericardium, and great vessels. Its presentation is infrequent, nonspecific, and subtle, and may mimic other diseases. New noninvasive techniques such as echocardiography and MRI aid in the diagnosis and preoperative assessment (RAAF and RAAF 1994). Overall survival is poor; at this time (2004), aggressive and complete surgical resection seems to offer the best hope for palliation and survival in an otherwise fatal disease.

Angiosarcoma. In adults approximately 25% of all primary cardiac tumors are malignant. One-third of these tumors are angiosarcomas (HERRMANN et al. 1992; BURKE et al. 1992). This highly aggressive malignant tumor can develop from the endothelium of lymphatics, i.e., lymphangiosarcoma, or blood vessels, i.e., hemangiosarcoma. In a review study by NAKA et al. (1995), 12 of 99 angiosarcomas arose in the heart. Most cardiac angiosarcomas arise in the right atrium (75%), although the reasons for this remain unclear (JANIGAN et al. 1986). They present as single or multiple nodules, filling the right atrium and/or infiltrating the myocardium and pericardium (MCALLISTER and FENOGLIO 1978; URBA and LONGO 1986). The pericardial sac is filled with blood. Since the presentation is often nonspecific, diagnosis is delayed and at the time of the diagnosis cardiac angiosarcomas have usually metastasized, most frequently to the lung (URBA and LONGO 1986; AOUATE et al. 1988). The pulmonary metastases most frequently have irregular margins due to peripheral hemorrhages. Calcified and cavitary metas-

tases have been reported but are seldom and have to be differentiated from calcified pulmonary metastases arising from the colon, breast, ovary, and thyroid gland. Cardiac angiosarcomas have a dismal prognosis, with a mean survival of 6 months after presentation.

Angiosarcomas usually show on MR images as heterogeneous masses (BEST et al. 2003; Figs. 12.13–12.15). A characteristic presentation of angiosarcomas is the mosaic pattern, consisting of nodular areas of increased signal intensity interspersed with areas of intermediate signal intensity on T1-weighted images. The high-signal areas result from intratumoral hemorrhage. T2-weighted images usually show a clear demarcation of the tumor from the normal myocardium (SATO et al. 1995). Angiosarcomas may have a "cauliflower" appearance on MRI, with focal areas of increased signal intensity probably related to thrombosis or hemorrhage (KIM et al. 1989). Probably the most typical finding of an angiosarcoma on MRI is that of an ill-defined mass arising from the right atrial wall extending into the pericardium, usually in combination with a pericardial effusion. Not infrequently one or more pericardial metastases may be visible. Hemangiopericytomas,

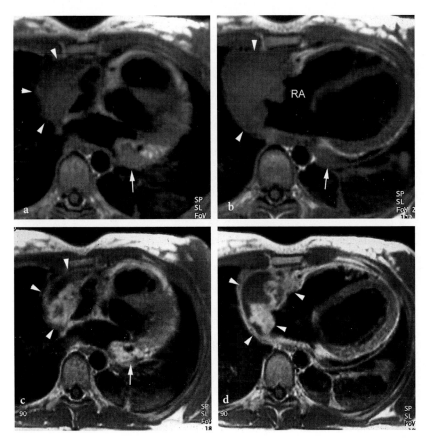

Fig. 12.13a–d. Cardiac angiosarcoma (*arrowheads*) of the right atrium with massive pericardial invasion in 21-year-old woman. Axial T1-weighted SE images before (**a, b**) and after (**c, d**) administration of gadopentetate dimeglumine. A large mass originating in the lateral right atrial wall is invading the pericardium. Pericardial effusion and malignant pericardial seeding (*arrow*) are present. After contrast administration the tumor borders can be better delineated and the tumor better differentiated from the adjacent pericardial effusion. The angiosarcoma shows a strong, but inhomogeneous enhancement

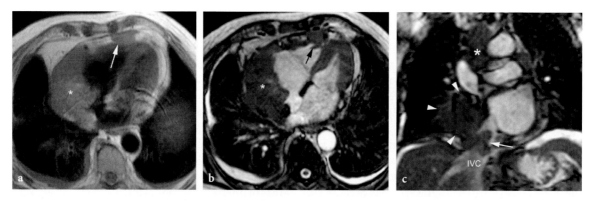

Fig. 12.14a-c. Cardiac angiosarcoma arising from the RA lateral wall in an 83-year-old man. Axial T1-weighted TSE image (**a**), axial (**b**) and coronal (**c**) cine MRI using the b-SSFP technique. A large, irregularly defined mass (*star*) is visible in the right atrium extending in the pericardium. On the axial views a pericardial metastasis is visible ventrally to the right ventricle (*arrow*). A second metastatic deposit is visible above the left atrium on the coronal view (*star*). The (poly)lobulated tumor appearance (*arrowheads*) with incomplete obstruction of the inferior vena cava (*arrow*) is clearly visible on the coronal image (**c**). Note the presence of a small amount of pleural fluid bilaterally

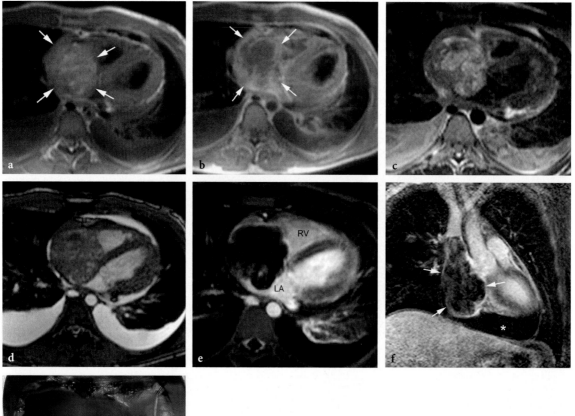

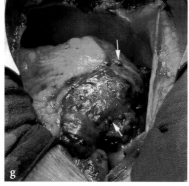

Fig. 12.15a-g. Right atrial angiosarcoma (*arrows*) in a 20-year-old man. The patient experienced a syncope during a football-game. Axial T1-weighted TSE before (**a**) and after (**b**) administration of gadopentetate dimeglumine. Axial T2-weighted STIR TSE-MRI (**c**). Axial cine-MRI using the b-SSFP technique (**d**). Axial (**e**) and coronal (**f**) CE-IR MRI. Macroscopic view on the opened pericardial sac during surgery (**g**). The angiosarcoma is a large mass, almost completely obstructing the RA cavity extending in the RA appendage. The tumor is attached to the lateral wall and extends into the pericardium. Note the presence of an important pericardial effusion (*star*). The angiosarcoma is diffusely metastasized into the pericardium as shown during surgery (*arrows*). (Surgical view, courtesy of P. Herijgers, Leuven, Belgium)

a much rarer primary cardiac sarcoma, may have a similar appearance on MR images and their distinction relies on pathological examination (SATO et al. 1995).

Rhabdomyosarcoma. Rhabdomyosarcoma is the second most frequent primary malignant tumor of the heart. These tumors are composed of malignant cells from striated muscle and occur singly or in multiples anywhere in the heart (SZUCS et al. 1991). The right and left side of the heart are involved with equal frequency, and in a third to a half of the cases the pericardium is involved by direct extension from the myocardium. The prognosis is generally poor. MRI is helpful not only in quantifying the initial extent of the tumor, but also in evaluating its response to chemotherapy (SZUCS et al. 1991). The most common appearance of rhabdomyosarcomas is that of a homogeneous mass, isointense or minimally hyperintense to muscle on T1-weighted images and hyperintense to muscle on T2-weighted images. After Gd-DTPA administration, these tumors enhance markedly (YOUSEM et al. 1990).

Malignant Fibrous Histiocytoma. Malignant fibrous histiocytoma is the most common soft tissue sarcoma in adults, but is distinctly rare as a primary tumor of the heart (MURPHEY et al. 1994; FANG et al. 1996). Malignant fibrous histiocytomas are not infrequently anchored onto the posterior wall in the left atrium, while right-sided tumors are extremely rare (NORITA et al. 1992; TERAMOTO et al. 1995). This tumor may demonstrate clinical similarities with myxoma, and careful anatomopathological examination of multiple sections of the tumor is

necessary to distinguish it from benign tumors, especially myxomas (OUZAN et al. 1990; KASUGAI et al. 1990). However, this tumor is far more aggressive than a myxoma and exhibits a greater tendency for local recurrence and infiltration. The tumors exhibit an intermediate, slightly heterogeneous signal intensity on T1-weighted images and a high signal intensity on T2-weighted images (MAHAJAN et al. 1989; KIM et al. 1989).

Other Cardiac Sarcomas. The heart is occasionally the primary site of other rare sarcomas, including undifferentiated sarcomas, liposarcomas, osteosarcomas, fibrosarcomas, synovial sarcomas, neurofibrosarcomas, leiomyosarcomas, chrondrosarcomas, and Kaposi's sarcomas (Fig. 12.16–18). In a study by Burke et al., in a total of 75 primary cardiac sarcomas, 18 were undifferentiated sarcomas and 9 were osteosarcomas; all of the latter tumors arose in the left atrium (BURKE and VIRMANI 1991; BURKE et al. 1992). Liposarcomas of the heart and pericardium are very rare, while cardiac metastasis of liposarcoma seems to occur more frequently (Fig. 12.16). Most liposarcomas of the heart are tumors with diffuse cardiac involvement. The right ventricle is most frequently involved (PAPA et al. 1994). In contrast to lipomas, liposarcomas display a signal intensity less than that of fat on T1-weighted images, or evidence of inhomogeneity if of high intensity (CONCES et al. 1985; DOOMS et al. 1985). Metastases are common by the time of diagnosis. Leiomyosarcomas predominate in the muscular arteries and great veins, while primary cardiac involvement is extremely rare (LUPETIN et al. 1986; RAAF and RAAF 1994;

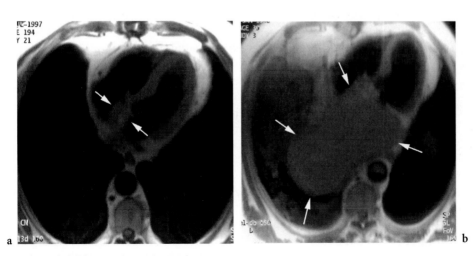

Fig. 12.16a,b. Recurrence of myxoid liposarcoma in the left atrium. **a** Follow-up MRI study 1 year after surgery for left atrial myxoid liposarcoma; axial T1-weighted SE image. **b** Similar image 5 months later. In the first follow-up study, there is an inhomogeneously thickened atrial septum and posterior left atrial wall, highly suggestive of tumor recurrence (*arrows*) (**a**). Five months later (**b**), a huge growth of the tumor recurrence has occurred (*arrows*)

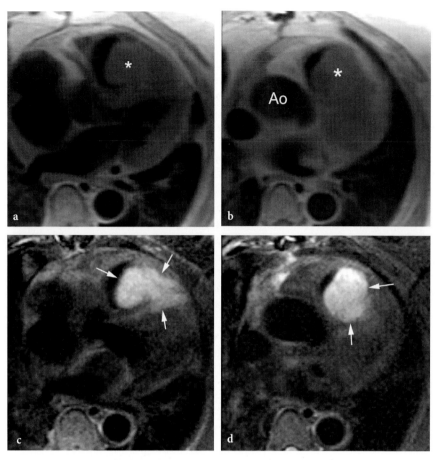

Fig. 12.17a-d.
Leiomyosarcoma of the right ventricular outflow tract in a 64-year-old woman. Axial T1-weighted TSE-MRI (**a, b**), axial T2-weighted STIR-TSE-MRI (**c, d**). The leiomyosarcoma presents a soft-tissue mass subtotally obstructing the RVOT. While isointense to the surrounding myocardium on T1-weighted TSE (*star*), the high signal on strong T2-weighted TSE sequences allows a better determination of the tumor borders (*arrows*)

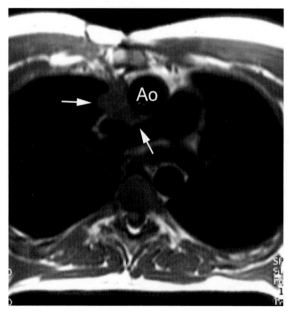

Fig. 12.18. Recurrent synoviosarcoma of the pericardium. Axial turbo SE image. The recurrent synoviosarcoma (*arrows*) is a nodular mass arising anterior to the superior vena cava and lateral to the ascending aorta (*Ao*)

Fig. 12.17). Leiomyosarcomas of the inferior and superior vena cava may directly involve the right atrium. Primary cardiac leiomyosarcomas are usually located in the atria and may invade the pericardium (BORNER et al. 1990; TAKAMIZAWA et al. 1992; KUO et al. 1997). Cardiac Kaposi's sarcoma has been found in patients with acquired immunodeficiency syndrome (AIDS) and in immunosuppressed organ transplant recipients (LANZA et al. 1983; RAAF and RAAF 1994). Kaposi's sarcoma of the heart may present as cardiac masses or as widely disseminated with infiltration of the heart and great vessels (CORALLO et al. 1988; LANGER et al. 1988).

12.4.1.2.2
Lymphoma

Primary cardiac lymphomas are extremely rare, while metastatic involvement of the heart in patients with malignant lymphoma is far more common and results from retrograde lymphatic spread, hematogenous spread, and direction extension from other primary tumor masses (CHILES et al. 2001).

However, since primary cardiac lymphoma is associated with AIDS, an increase in primary cardiac lymphomas may be expected (BALASUBRAMANYAM et al. 1986; GILL et al. 1987). Primary lymphoma of the heart is defined as lymphoma involving only the heart and pericardium (CURTINSINGER et al. 1989; CASTELLI et al. 1989). The clinical course in most patients with primary lymphoma of the heart is remarkably acute in onset and short in duration, and the diagnosis is often not made antemortem. Patients with primary cardiac lymphoma present with pericardial effusion, intracardiac masses, arrhythmias, and other nonspecific cardiac manifestations (Figs. 12.19, 12.20; GILL et al. 1987; CHAO et al. 1995; BOGAERT et al. 1995a). The intracardiac masses frequently arise in the ventricles (GILL et al. 1987). Imaging techniques are helpful for diagnosis but lack specificity (CHOU et al. 1983; COGHLAN et al. 1989; ROBERTS et al. 1990; BOGAERT et al. 1995a). Cytological examination of the pericardial fluid or pericardial biopsy seems to be most suitable for diagnosis because of the frequent involvement of the pericardium. MRI provides accurate information on the cardiac masses and the extent of pericardial fluid, and can be repeated at follow-up.

12.4.1.2.3
Malignant Pericardial Mesothelioma

The incidence of malignant pericardial mesothelioma is approximately 15% of all malignant cardiac tumors (SALCEDO et al. 1992). Mesotheliomas usually cover the visceral and parietal pericardium diffusely, encasing the heart, but generally do not invade the heart. Unlike malignant pleural mesotheliomas, the cardiac variety has no association with prior exposure to asbestos. Although they may be very extensive, they can sometimes be resected. MRI is helpful in depicting tumor localization and expansion, and in delineating the anatomical extent of malignant pericardial mesothelioma. On T1-weighted images, the signal intensity is equal to or a little higher than that of the myocardium, and on T2-weighted images it is the same as or higher than that of fat tissue (GOSSINGER et al. 1988; LUND et al. 1989; VOGEL et al. 1989; KAMINAGA et al. 1993). A heterogeneous signal on T2-weighted images is related to the presence of intratumoral necrosis. Gd-DTPA administration is useful in clarifying the border between the tumor and myocardium (KAMINAGA et al. 1993). The location and MRI sig-

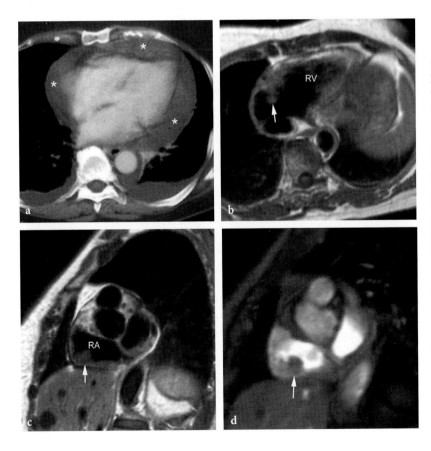

Fig. 12.19a-d. Primary cardiac lymphoma in a 73-year-old woman. a Axial computed tomography. Axial (b) and short-axis (c) T1-weighted SE image. d Short-axis cine MR image, using the spoiled GE-technique. The patient presented initially with an important pericardial effusion (star) (a), which was treated with a pericardiocenthesis. On a subsequent MRI examination of the heart, a small mass was detected laterally in the right atrium (RA; arrow). Because pericardial fluid analysis did not reveal any abnormalities, the RA mass was considered benign, and the patient was dismissed. The patient died 4 months later from massive tumor emboli in the pulmonary arteries. At autopsy, a diffuse involvement by the lymphoma of the entire heart was found. (From BOGAERT et al. 1995a; reprinted with permission from Fortschritte Röentgenstr, Georg Thieme)

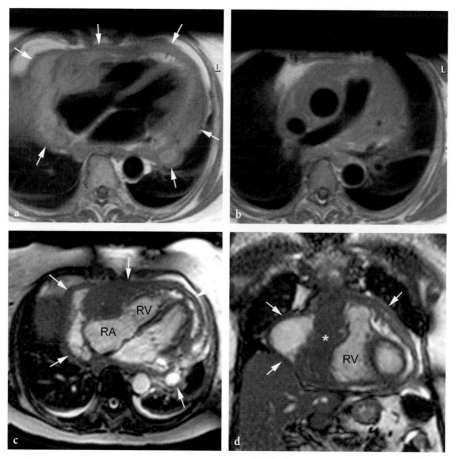

Fig. 12.20a-d. High-grade non-Hodgkin lymphoma invading the heart in a 68-year-old woman. **a, b** Axial T1-weighted TSE-MRI. Axial (**c**) and coronal (**d**) cine MRI, using the b-SSFP technique. Although this patient was diagnosed with a pericardial effusion on cardiac ultrasound, cardiac MRI shows a soft tissue mass diffusely involving the right atrioventricular groove (*star*). The pericardium is diffusely thickened (*arrows*) with a right-sided localized effusion

nal intensity of pericardial mesothelioma resembles those of fibrosarcomas and some metastatic tumors in the pericardial space. However, the latter are more invasive than malignant mesothelioma and tend to invade the intracardiac structures (SALCEDO et al. 1992; KAMINAGA et al. 1993).

12.4.2
Secondary Cardiac Tumors

Secondary tumors of the heart are 20–40 times more frequent than primary tumors of the heart. They may result from direct extension, hematogenous or venous extension, or retrograde flow by lymphatic vessels (CHILES et al. 2001).

12.4.2.1
Direct Extension

Direct extension of a malignant tumor in the pericardium or in the heart occurs from tumors originating in the lung, mediastinum, or breast. Bronchial carcinoma may directly invade the mediastinum, the pericardium, or the heart. Pericardial involvement alone is characterized by a pericardial disruption associated with focal pericardial thickening and pericardial effusion. Irregular thickening of the atrial or ventricular myocardium is the hallmark of myocardial involvement (BARAKOS et al. 1989b). As many as 20% of all patients who die of lymphoma are found to have cardiac involvement at autopsy. The vast majority of these patients, however, do not have symptoms referable to cardiac involvement. The most frequent site of involvement is the pericardium, including the subepicardial fat (TESORO TESS et al. 1993; CHILES et al. 2001). The atrioventricular groove is the most common site of epicardial invasion and often very large deposits occur in it (Fig. 12.21). The cardiac chambers are less frequently involved. Not infrequently tumor may extend through the entire wall of a cardiac chamber or through the atrial septum (ROBERTS et al. 1968). Determination of lymphomatous involvement of the paracardiac spaces, the pericardium, and the heart is important for patients who are treated with radia-

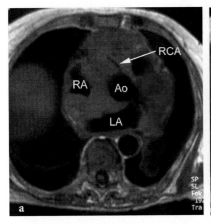 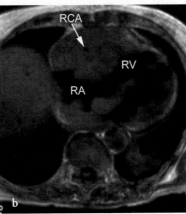

Fig. 12.21 a, b. High-grade mediastinal non-Hodgkin lymphoma diffusely infiltrating the heart. T1-weighted axial SE images. The anterior subepicardial fat and the anterior atrioventricular groove are entirely invaded by lymphomatous tissue, surrounding the right coronary artery (*rca*). There is narrowing of the right atrium due to a tumoral thickening of the lateroposterior wall and the atrial septum. The pericardial sac is displaced anteriorly. Note that the differentiation between retrograde flow by the lymphatic vessels and direct extension is not possible in this case

tion therapy. Generally, lung and cardiac blocks are placed to protect normal heart and lung, but these blocks are modified in the presence of pericardial involvement (JOCHELSON et al. 1983). Also, if the paracardiac disease encompasses a too great area, chemotherapy may be used in addition to radiation therapy.

12.4.2.2
Hematogenous Extension

The incidence of cardiac metastases ranges from 1.5% to 20.6% (average 6%) in autopsies on patients with malignant diseases (ROSENTHAL and BRAUNWALD 1992). There has been a gradual increase in the frequency of cardiac metastases, perhaps as a consequence of the rising frequency of cancer plus the existence of reliable noninvasive diagnostic tests. Cardiac metastases are usually found in patients with disseminated tumors. In particular, pulmonary metastases are usually present. Despite their frequent occurrence in patients with malignant disease, cardiac metastases are usually clinically silent (HEATH 1968). Isolated metastases occurring only in the heart are very unusual. Surgical resection of isolated cardiac metastases can be attempted to improve survival in patients whose primary tumor is well controlled (LEE and FISHER 1989). The most common tumors that metastasize to the heart are of bronchial and breast origin, followed by melanomas, lymphoma, and leukemia (LAGRANGE et al. 1986; HALLALI and HAIAT 1987). Malignant melanoma has a peculiar predilection for metastatic cardiac involvement (accounting for 60% of cases of cardiac metastasis). The pericardium is most frequently affected, while isolated involvement of the myocardium is seldom seen (Fig. 12.22).

Intracardiac metastases from neuroendocrine tumors of the carcinoid type may mimic benign cardiac tumors (e.g., myxoma), and this entity has to be differentiated from valvular abnormalities seen in some patients with carcinoid syndrome.

MRI may be of benefit in defining the size, shape, and extent of metastatic cardiac neoplasms (LEE and FISHER 1989; PAPA et al. 1994). Metastatic deposits appear as focal nodular lesions of the pericardium or myocardium. Myocardial metastases of malignant melanoma tend to be bright on T1- and T2-weighted SE sequences, which is attributable to melanin (CHILES et al. 2001). Adjacent pleural effusion or blood flow provides marked signal contrast, so that myocardial and pericardial lesions are visualized easily, as is the extension of the tumor in the cardiac chamber (BARAKOS et al. 1989b).

12.4.2.3
Venous Extension

The caval and pulmonary veins can serve as conduits for tumor extension toward the heart (Fig. 12.23, 12.24). Intracaval extension is a well-known but rare complication of benign tumors, such as leiomyomatosis arising from a uterine myoma or from the wall of the vessel itself (BASSISH 1974; ROSENBERG et al. 1988; DUNLAP and UDJUS 1990; STEINMETZ et al. 1996), and malignant tumors, e.g., adrenocortical carcinoma (RITCHEY et al. 1987; GODINE et al. 1990), hepatocellular carcinoma (KANEMATSU et al. 1994), Wilms' tumor (GIBSON et al. 1990), renal cell carcinoma (PAUL et al. 1975), recurrent pheochromocytoma (ROTE et al. 1977), endometrial stromal carcinoma (PHILLIPS et al. 1995), and thyroid carcinoma (THOMPSON et al. 1978). Its presence is potentially hazardous, because it can cause caval

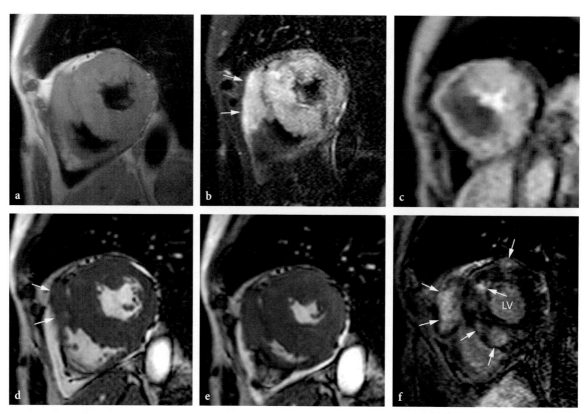

Fig. 12.22a-f. Pericardial and myocardial metastases in 64-year-old man with malignant melanoma. All images are obtained in the cardiac short-axis at midventricular level, T1-weighted TSE-MRI (**a**), T2-weighted STIR-TSE-MRI (**b**), perfusion MRI (**c**), cine MRI, using the b-SSFP technique, at end diastole (**d**) and end systole (**e**) and CE-IR MRI (**f**). The metastastic cardiac involvement presents as a concentric hypertrophy mainly involving the ventricular septum and right ventricular outflow tract (**a, d, e**). On T2-weighted STIR TSE imaging, the left ventricular wall as well as the right ventricular outflow tract wall (*arrows*) appear inhomogeneously hyperintense. Perfusion MRI shows several myocardial perfusion defects, the largest in the center of the ventricular septum (**c**). Although on SPECT imaging the patient presented a normal left ventricular ejection fraction, a diffuse hypokinesia is found most pronounced in the ventricular septum. On the CE-IR MR image, multiple regions of late enhancement are found in the thickened myocardium (*arrows*)

obstruction, extension of the tumor thrombus into the right atrium, causing atrial occlusion, and tumor embolization. Intracardiac leiomyomatosis is a rare complication of right-sided obstruction and should be considered in the differential diagnosis if the patient is of reproductive age and is found to have a mass lesion in the right side of the heart.

Complete excision of tumors showing intracaval extension is necessary to avoid recurrence. Preoperative diagnosis of caval involvement is essential for planning the extent of surgery. For instance, intravascular extension of adrenocortical carcinoma is not a contraindication to radical surgery. Accurate identification is essential to plan treatment and to avoid complications. MRI is perfectly suited to detect the presence and extension of an intracaval tumor thrombus. Although differentiation between the tumor component and the accompanying

bland thrombus is still difficult with MRI, NGUYEN et al. (1996) have recently reported the presence of a patchy flow signal within the cavoatrial thrombus as a pattern of tumoral neovascularity in a patient with a renal granular cell carcinoma.

12.4.2.4
Retrograde Flow by Lymphatic Vessels

This fourth pathway of cardiac involvement occurs from spread from noncontiguous mediastinal lymph nodes via the lymphatic vessels to the heart with predominant epicardial involvement and variable myocardial invasion (Fig. 12.21). Retrograde spread has been shown to be the most common mechanism in lymphomas and may also be seen in cases of lung and breast carcinoma (DELOACH and HAYNES 1953). Disease spreads from the anterior mediastinum to

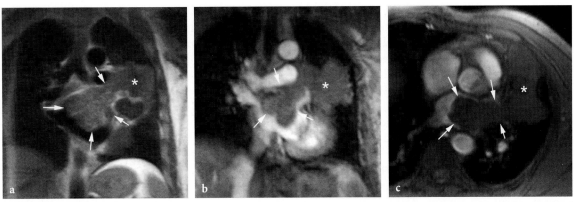

Fig. 12.23a–c. Venous extension of metastatic fibrosarcoma in the left atrium in a 46-year-old man. Coronal T1-weighted TSE-MRI (**a**). Coronal (**b**) and axial (**c**) cine MRI, using the spoiled GE-technique. Large metastatic mass in the left lung (*star*) invades the left atrium (*arrows*) through the left upper lobe pulmonary vein. The left atrial mass is free-floating in the atrial cavity

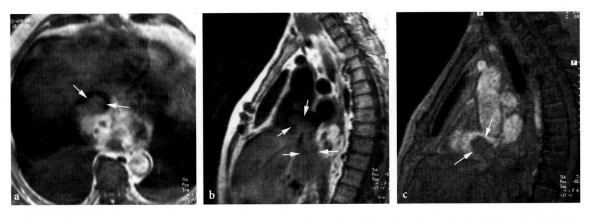

Fig. 12.24 a–c. Intracaval extension of hypernephroma protruding in the right atrium (*arrows*). **a, b** Axial and sagittal T1-weighted SE images. **c** Sagittal cine MR image, using the spoiled GE-technique, through the right atrium and inferior vena cava. An intracaval mass almost completely obliterates the lumen and extends in the right atrium. Note a bilateral pleural effusion

the paracardiac area and pericardium; the hilus may be bypassed and may remain uninvolved, since it is not necessarily part of the drainage (JOCHELSON et al. 1983).

The lymphatics of the visceral pericardium and the heart drain into larger lymphatic vessels which run within the subepicardial fat and drain either to the nodes situated at the base of the heart, between the transverse part of the aorta and the left pulmonary artery, or directly into the anterosuperior mediastinal nodes. The lymphatics of the parietal pericaridium are scanty and run upward along the phrenic nerve over the lateral aspect of the cardiac silhouette and into the anterior mediastinal nodes. A chain of nodes may also be seen posteriorly, running along the pulmonary ligament to the hilus. Lymph nodes that are sometimes present on the parietal pericardial surface, usually in the right hemithorax,

are associated with the lymph drainage from the central part of the diaphragm. Therefore, the nodal areas referred to as pericardiac and paracardiac include the inferior internal mammary, diaphragmatic, paraphrenic, posterior pulmonary ligament, and paraesophageal nodes.

12.4.3
Paracardiac and Extracardiac Tumors

Though an extensive description of the para- and extracardiac tumors is beyond the scope of this chapter, a brief summary will be given. Not only are these tumors more frequent than primary cardiac tumors but, due to their close relation with the pericardium and heart, knowledge of their presentation is required. Paracardial tumors typically arise within the mediastinum, coming into close contact with the heart by direct growth. Pericardial and myocardial involvement occurs by external compression or tumor invasion. Mediastinal masses (e.g., enlarged lymph nodes) often abut the pericardium without penetration of the pericardium (Fig. 12.25). The presence of a normal pericardium and pericardial sinuses provides a natural cleavage plane between the heart and the mediastinal mass. In these cases, usually no pericardial effusion is seen (BARAKOS et al. 1989b). Tumors located in the anterior mediastinum include thymomas, thymolipomas, lymphomas, germ cell tumors, and tumor or masses originating from the thyroid gland. Tumors located in the middle and posterior mediastinum are mostly neurogenic, arise from the esophagus (e.g., esophageal cancer, enteric cyst/duplication), or are related to the trachea or bronchi (e.g., bronchogenic cyst or bronchial cancer).

Magnetic resonance imaging is perfectly suited to describe the relation of the tumor to the heart, and to evaluate cardiac or vascular compression or invasion by the tumor. Furthermore, the signal characteristics on MRI can be used for tissue characterization. For instance, a bronchogenic cyst has a relatively high signal intensity on T1-weighted imaging and a very high signal intensity on T2-weighted imaging (NAKATA et al. 1993). A fluid-fluid level in the cyst may be caused by an intracystic hemorrhage or precipitation of calcium in the dependent part of the cyst (BARGALLO et al. 1993; AYDINGOZ et al. 1997). Thymolipomas are anterior mediastinal masses that may conform to the shape of the adjacent structures, and thus may simulate cardiomegaly or diaphragmatic elevation on chest radiographs. MRI typically demonstrates a mixture of fat and soft tissue signal-intensity characteristics (ROSADO DE CHRISTENSON

et al. 1994). MRI can be helpful in determining the malignancy of thymomas (SAKAI et al. 1992; ENDO et al. 1993; KUSHIHASHI et al. 1996). Benign thymomas are well-defined round or oval masses in the anterior mediastinum with a homogeneous or slightly inhomogeneous signal on T2-weighted images. On the other hand, invasive thymomas usually have an inhomogeneous signal intensity, a multinodular appearance, and a lobulated internal architecture or fibrous septa, and often display irregular borders. Thymic carcinomas demonstrate low signal intensities on both T1- and T2-weighted images and irregular margins, but lack fibrous septa or lobulated internal architecture. Although MRI appears promising, histology is still essential to distinguish benign from malignant mediastinal lesions (MASSIE et al. 1997).

12.4.4
Nontumoral Cardiac Masses and Mimics

12.4.4.1
Thrombus

Cardiac thrombi are much more frequent than cardiac tumors. Recognition and appropriate treatment remains important because of risk of systemic or pulmonary embolization. The formation of thrombi usually occurs in patients with regional or global wall motion abnormalities, such as those that develop after myocardial infarction and in association with dilated cardiomyopathy or atrial fibrillation, especially if mitral valve disease and enlarged atrium and appendage are present (DEPACE et al. 1981). In patients with a myocardial infarction, risk

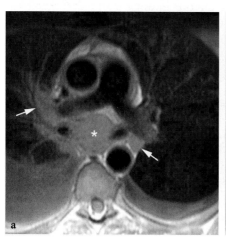
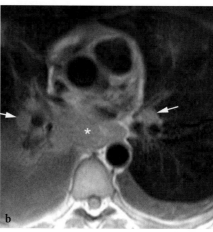

Fig. 12.25a,b. Renal cell carcinoma with enlarged (*star*) and hilar (*arrows*) lymph nodes in a 36-year-old man. Axial T1-weighted TSE-MRI. Bilateral pleural effusion

factors for developing left ventricular thrombus are infarct location, i.e., anterior myocardial infarction, infarct size and extent, and impairment in global and regional left ventricular function. Left ventricular thrombi are often attached to the apex or within a discrete aneurysm or dyskinetic ventricular wall (KEELEY and HILLIS 1996; Fig. 12.26; see also Figs. 12.30–33). Although ventricular thrombi are exceedingly rare in patients with normal ventricular function, they should be considered in patients with coagulation disorders (DEGROAT et al. 1985; CHIN et al. 1988; Fig. 12.27). Left atrial thrombi are generally attached to the posterior left atrial wall by a broad base, so that they are immobile (Fig. 12.28). If they are pedunculated and mobile, distinguishing them from a myxoma may be difficult. Right atrial thrombi are usually found in patients with central venous lines (Fig. 12.29) or patients having enlarged cavities, e.g., restrictive cardiomyopathy.

The primary screening modality for patients with suspected cardiac thrombus is two-dimensional echocardiography. However, false-negative, false-positive, or equivocal findings are not uncommon and are related to inadequate echocardiograms caused by anatomical abnormalities of the patients or to certain characteristics or location of the thrombus (STRATTON et al. 1982; JUNGEHULSING et al. 1992). For instance, large, echogenic, irregular, mobile mural thrombi are easy to detect on echocardiography, while laminated mural thrombi may be difficult to distinguish from myocardium, and slow blood flow in aneurysm may be confused with thrombus. Thrombi located in the ventricular apex are often difficult to assess with TTE (near-field probe).

MRI has a great potential in the diagnosis of suspected cardiac thrombi (JOHNSON et al. 1988). It has already been found, in the 1980s, that cardiac thrombi usually have higher signal intensity than the normal myocardium on SE-MRI, especially on the second echo (DOOMS and HIGGINS 1986). Differentiation between thrombus and slow-flowing blood on SE-MRI, however, may be difficult because of the increased MR signal produced by slow-flow-

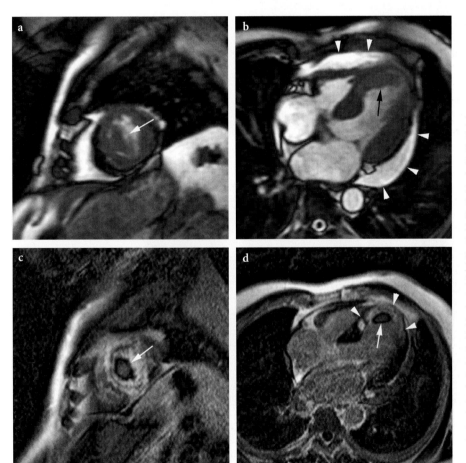

Fig. 12.26a-d. Mural thrombus in a left ventricular apical aneurysm in a 56-year-old man with an old anteroseptal myocardial infarction. Short-axis (**a**) and horizontal long-axis (**b**) cine MR image, using the b-SSFP technique. Short-axis (**c**) and horizontal long-axis (**d**) CE-IR MRI. The thrombus (*arrows*) in the left ventricular apex is nearly isointense to the surrounding myocardium on cine MRI. On CE-IR MRI, the scarred myocardial tissue is hyperintense (*arrowheads*), and easily discernible from the adjacent hypointense thrombus (*arrow*). Note the pericardial effusion on cine MRI (*arrowheads*)

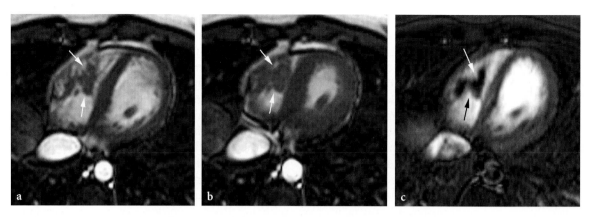

Fig. 12.27a-c. Right ventricular thrombi (*arrows*) in a 19-year-old man with coagulation disorders. Axial cine MRI at end diastole (**a**), and end systole (**b**), using the b-SSFP technique. **c** Axial CE-IR MRI. The thrombus appears as an irregular mass attached to the endocavitary muscular network in the right ventricle. The thrombus is hypointense on CE-IR MRI

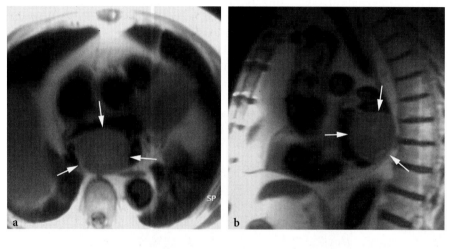

Fig. 12.28 a,b. Left atrial thrombus in a 45-year-old cardiac transplant patient. Axial (**a**) and coronal (**b**) T1-weighted TSE. A well-defined homogeneous mass is broadly attached to the dorsal wall (*arrows*). No enhancement of the thrombus was found after administration of gadopentetate dimeglumine (not shown)

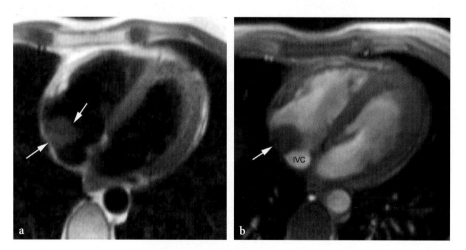

Fig. 12.29a,b. Right atrial thrombus in a patient receiving chemotherapy for testis carcinoma. **a** Axial T1-weighted TSE image; **b** axial cine MRI, using the spoiled-GE-MRI. Thrombi arising in the right atrium are rare but are not infrequently found in patients with intravenous catheters. In this patient a massive thrombus was shown at the tip of the catheter. After anticoagulation therapy the thrombus completely disappeared

ing blood (Fig. 12.30; GOMES et al. 1987; SECHTEM et al. 1989). GE-MRI, in contrast, permits improved differentiation of thrombi from the surrounding blood pool and myocardium (JUNGEHULSING et al. 1992). On GE-MRI, thrombus always shows a lower signal intensity than does blood. The differentiation between thrombus and myocardium on GE-MRI is more difficult because the thrombus is iso- to hyperintense compared with the adjacent surrounding myocardium. Since the thrombotic material differs according to its age and degree of organization, the signal intensity of the thrombus will change due to loss of water, condensation of paramagnetic iron complexes, and sometimes calcification (BAUMGARTNER 1973). A major advantage of GE images is the capability for cine display of cardiac motion and blood flow, i.e., cine MRI. Signal intensity from blood changes slightly during the cardiac cycle, whereas normal anatomical structures or

thrombus maintain a nearly constant signal intensity. Alternative methods that have been reported to distinguish slowly moving blood from thrombus are MRI phase-imaging and MRI tagging (Fig. 12.30; RUMANCIK et al. 1988; AXEL and DOUGHERTY 1989). With the new b-SSFP cine MRI sequences, yielding a significantly higher contrast between blood and surrounding structures than with the spoiled-GE sequences, detection of mural thrombi should be improved (SPUENTRUP et al. 2003). Especially in cardiac views with pronounced in-plane saturation on the spoiled-GE sequences such as the horizontal or vertical long-axis plane, the ventricular apex and the blood-myocardial interface are much more easily accessible on the b-SSFP sequences (Fig. 12.30).

CE-MRI, using an inversion-recovery pulse (CE-IR MRI) to suppress signal of normal myocardial tissue, not only was a major step forward in the detection of myocardial inflammation, infarction,

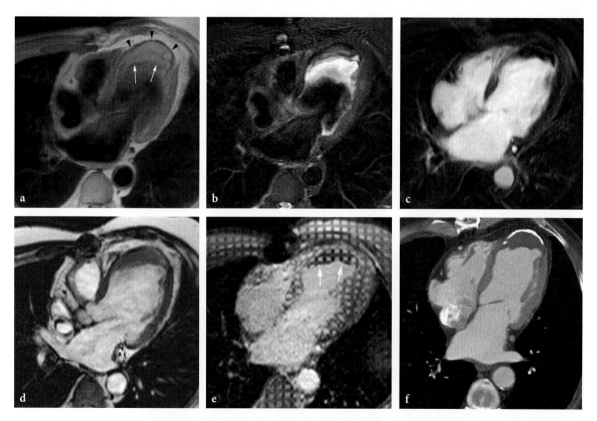

Fig. 12.30a-f. Comparison of imaging techniques to detect large mural thrombus (*arrows*) in a calcified LV apical aneurysm in a 61-year-old man. All images are obtained in the horizontal long-axis plane. **a** T1-weighted TSE-MRI; **b** T2-weighted STIR TSE-MRI; **c** CE-IR MRI TSE; **d** b-SSFP cine MRI; **e** MRI myocardial tagging using the SPAMM technique (after contrast administration); **f** contrast-enhanced computed tomography. The calcified aneurysm is visible as a curvilinear hypointense line (*arrowheads*) on T1-weighted TSE-MRI (**a**). The appearance and signal intensity of the thrombus is different according the used imaging modality. Note the presence of slow-flow adjacent to the thrombus shown as high signal on the T2-weighted STIR TSE image. The MR tagging image shows nicely the nondeformation of the tag lines in the thrombus. Moreover, due to contrast administration, the signal intensity of the tag lines in the thrombus differs from those in the adjacent myocardium

and scarring, but also has been shown to be highly beneficial in detection of intracavitary thrombi. In a recent study by MOLLET et al. (2002), CE-IR MRI yielded a significantly higher number of ventricular thrombi in patients with a recent or a chronic myocardial infarction compared with TTE and b-SSFP cine MRI (Fig. 12.31). Due to a homogeneous, strong enhancement of the left ventricular cavity after gadolinium administration, abnormal in-traventricular structures have a dark appearance. CE-IR MRI allows visualization of small thrombi (less than 1 cm^3; Fig. 12.32), invisible on TTE and cine MRI, e.g., when trapped within endocardial trabeculations (Fig. 12.33). Presence of slow and tur-bulent flow patterns in dysfunctional wall segments and lack of contrast between mural thrombus and adjacent myocardium, even using the new b-SSFP cine MRI techniques, is the most likely explanation

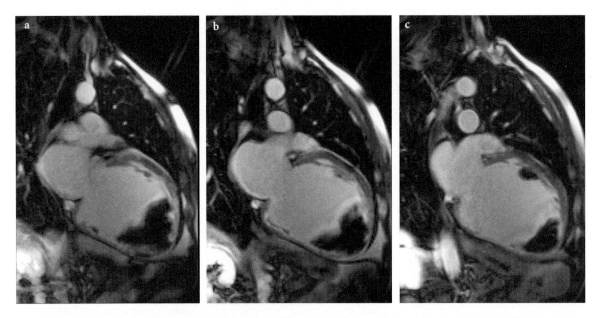

Fig. 12.31a-c. Large LV thrombi in 55-year-old patient with severe ischemic cardiomyopathy. All CE-IR MRI images are obtained along the vertical long-axis. Note the presence of a large apical thrombus (±100 g), and a smaller mural thrombus adjacent to the anterior LV wall. The LV cavity is severely enlarged (i.e., end-diastolic volume: 552 ml) and its function severely impaired (i.e., ejection fraction 7%)

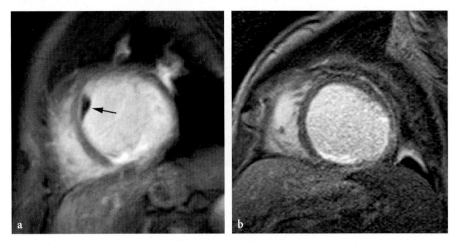

Fig. 12.32a,b. Small septal thrombus before (**a**) and after (**b**) oral anticoagulation in a 43-year-old man with ischemic cardio-myopathy. Short-axis CE-IR-MR images. **a** The mural thrombus is well-visible as hypointense structure (*arrow*) adjacent to the septal wall. **b** On the control MRI study 2 weeks after the start of oral anticoagulation, no residual thrombus is present. (From MOLLET et al. 2002; reprinted with permission from Circulation)

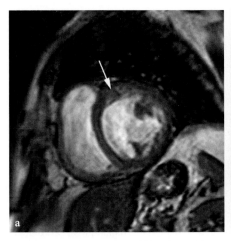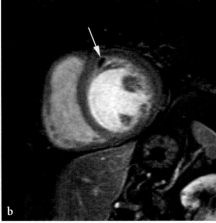

Fig. 12.33a,b. Small thrombus trapped in anterior muscular trabeculations in a 58-year-old man with ischemic cardiomyopathy. **a** Short-axis cine-MRI, using b-SSFP technique; **b** short-axis CE-IR MRI. On the CE-IR MR image, a small, dark thrombus is clearly visible (*arrow*). This thrombus was not detected initially on cine MRI because of its small size and the lack of signal differences with the surrounding myocardium (*arrow*). (From MOLLET et al. 2002; reprinted with permission from Circulation.)

of why small thrombi can be invisible on cine MRI. Similar results have been found in another study (BARKHAUSEN et al. 2002). However, it should be stressed that the CE-IR MRI technique does not allow evaluation of thrombus enhancement and differentiation between subacute and chronic thrombi. This can be achieved using T1-weighted SE- or GE-MRI before and after administration of contrast medium. PAYDARFAR et al. (2001) have reported that subacute clots have a homogeneously low signal, do not enhance with gadolinium, and exhibit magnetic susceptibility effects, while organized clots have an intermediate, heterogeneous signal and show multiple areas of gadolinium enhancement. Especially the enhancement pattern in organized thrombi might impede differentiation with cardiac tumors, e.g., myxoma.

In clinical practice, a combination of the above-discussed MRI techniques with careful analysis of the regions at risk, e.g., infarct area, aneurysmatic ventricular apex and dysfunctional wall segments for the ventricles; and the appendages for the atria, yield the best guarantee not to miss thrombi. The left atrial appendage is usually nicely shown on the vertical long-axis view using b-SSFP and CE-IR MRI sequences (Fig. 12.34).

12.4.4.2
Valvular Vegetations

Valvular vegetations can also be confused with mass lesions by echocardiography. However, in these instances, the echoes generally appear small and movement is limited. Furthermore, the vegetations follow the motion of the valvular cusp to which they are attached. MRI may be useful in clarifying echocardiographic findings and establishing the diagnosis in previously undiagnosed patients (Fig. 12.35). Vegetations may be barely or not visible on SE-MRI but are clearly visible on cine MRI, appearing as areas of low signal at valve leaflets in contrast to the bright blood flow (Fig. 12.36; CADUFF et al. 1996).

Libman-Sacks endocarditis, or the endocardial involvement in patients with systemic lupus erythematosus, is found in up to 50% of hearts at autopsy. It presents as small verrucous vegetations (3–4 mm in size) appearing on the valvular or mural endocardial surface. The posterior leaflet of the mitral valve is most frequently involved. Infrequently, such vegetations may become massive thrombotic lesions, up to 10 mm or even larger (DOHERTY and SIEGEL 1985). Libman–Sacks endocarditis may predispose to infective endocarditis. As in other causes of valvular vegetations, MRI can be helpful in visualization of the valve or mural lesions.

12.4.4.3
Perivalvular Extension of Infection

Perivalvular extension of infection (i.e., cardiac abscess and pseudoaneurysm) is a not infrequent and potentially fatal complication of bacterial endocarditis (CARPENTER 1991). Cardiac abscesses are observed in 20–30% of cases of infective endocarditis and in at least 60% of cases of prosthetic valve endocarditis (THOMAS et al. 1993). The aortic valve

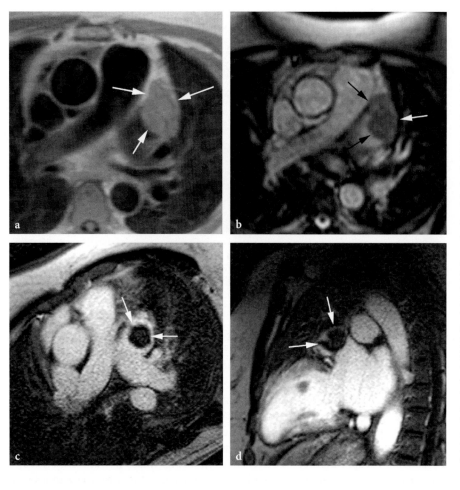

Fig. 12.34a-d. Thrombus in the left atrial appendage in a 70-year-old woman with chronic atrial fibrillation and history of transient ischemic attacks. TTE (not shown) did not reveal abnormalities. Axial, T1-weighted SE-MRI (**a**) shows absence of dark signal (or signal void; *arrows*) in the moderately dilated left atrial appendage. Is it slow flow or thrombus? Axial cine MRI, using the b-SSFP technique, shows gray zone in the left atrial appendage (*arrows*). CE-IR MRI in the axial (**c**) and vertical long-axis plane (**d**) nicely shows the thrombus as a dark, non-enhancing structure in the appendage (*arrows*). (Reprinted in part from BOGAERT et al. 2004; with permission.)

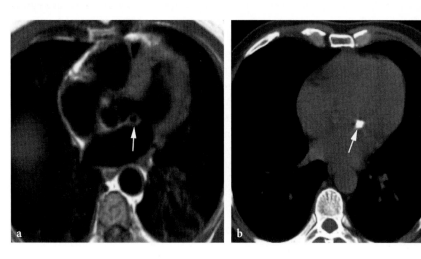

Fig. 12.35a,b. Chronic, calcified vegetation of the mitral valve. **a** Axial T1-weighted SE image; **b** noncontrast-enhanced CT. Small, nodular, centrally hypointense mass at the anterior mitral valve leaflet (*arrows*). The calcified nature as suggested by the absence of signal on SE images is proven on CT

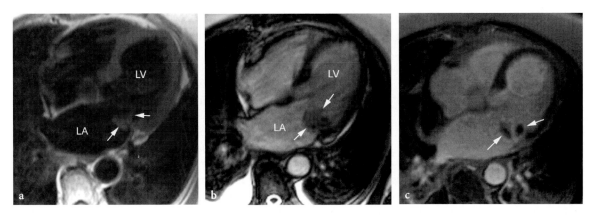

Fig. 12.36a-c. Marantic (nonbacterial, thrombotic) endocarditis (*arrows*) in a 77-year-old woman with bilateral breast cancer. **a** Axial T1-weighted TSE-MRI. **b** Axial cine MRI, using the b-SSFP technique. **c** Axial CE-IR MRI. Presence of irregular mass in the left atrium, and a second smaller mass in the left ventricle, both attached to the lateral part of the mitral valve annulus

ring is more frequently affected than the mitral valve ring. The perivalvular extension of infection (usually involving the mitral-aortic intervalvular fibrosa) may present as a closed purulent collection (i.e., cardiac abscess) or as a cavity contiguous with a cardiac chamber (i.e., pseudoaneurysm; Fig. 12.37). Subsequent rupture of the infected zone of mitral-aortic intervalvular fibrosa or subaortic aneurysm into the left atrium may occur, a condition which should be differentiated from ruptured aneurysm of the sinus of Valsalva (BANSAL et al. 1990).

Although transesophageal echocardiography is the imaging method of choice for the diagnosis of valvular vegetations in infectious endocarditis, the diagnosis of an associated ring abscess is sometimes difficult, especially in patients with valvular prostheses or calcifications, which are an important source of artifacts. MRI may be useful to detect the paravalvular abscess and infectious pseudoaneurysms (JEANG et al. 1986; WINKLER and HIGGINS 1986; FURBER et al. 1997). A cardiac abscess is visible as a heterogeneous low signal-intensity zone on T1-weighted MRI and as high intensity signal on T2-weighted MRI. The inflammatory origin is responsible for the increase in signal after injection of paramagnetic contrast agents. Cine MRI is helpful

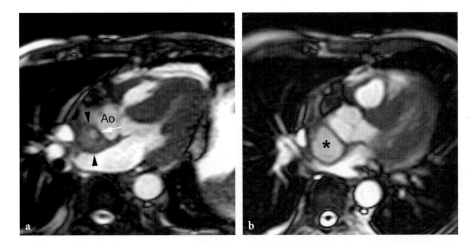

Fig. 12.37a,b. Perivalvular extension of infection in a 52-year-old man with a renal transplant. The patient was admitted with a staphylococcus aureus sepsis. Axial cine MRI at admission (**a**) and 1 week later (**b**). **a** A well-defined, soft tissue structure is visible dorsally of the aorta root (*arrowheads*). Although highly suggestive of a periaortic abscess, because of the presence of a central high-signal spot (*arrow*), a pseudoaneurysm should be also be considered. **b** the control study, 1 week later, clearly shows a presence of a retroaortic pseudoaneurysm (*star*) that fills and empties during the cardiac cycle (information obtained on dynamic cine MRI viewing)

to detect the presence or absence of communication between the abscess cavity and the cardiac chambers. MRI is also recommended in the follow-up of patients with perivalvular extension of infection (Fig. 12.37).

12.4.4.4
Lipomatous Hypertrophy of the Interatrial Septum

Lipomatous hypertrophy of the interatrial septum is, pathogenetically, a hypertrophy of preexisting fat, and not a true neoplasm, and it is not infrequently associated with increased epicardial fat (MEANY et al. 1997). This poorly recognized, but not rare benign condition represents a fat accumulation within the interatrial septum in continuity with the epicardial fat. It is usually anterior to the fossa ovalis. There may be a component posterior to the fossa. Since there is no fat accumulation in the fossa ovalis, lipomatous hypertrophy of the interatrial septum often has a typical bilobed "camel-humped" or "dumbbell-shaped" appearance (Fig. 12.38). The typical appearance and the lipomatous nature, appearing as fat attenuation on CT and high signal intensity on T1-weighted MR images, should suggest lipomatous hypertrophy of the atrial septum and obviate biopsy or excision (LEVINE et al. 1986; APPLEGATE et al. 1987; FISHER and EDMONDS 1988; GAERTE et al. 2002). The differential diagnosis includes nonacute hematoma, lipoma, liposarcoma, hemangioma, and hemorrhage into a preexisting mass. Liposarcoma has a lower signal intensity than that of fat, or evidence of inhomogeneity if of high intensity (DOOMS et al. 1985). In addition, selective fat-suppression techniques can be used to demonstrate the fatty nature and to differentiate lipomatous hypertrophy of the atrial septum from other nonlipomatous conditions (Fig. 12.38).

12.4.4.5
Atrial Septal Aneurysm

An aneurysm of the atrial septum is defined as a diffuse or a localized protrusion of the interatrial septum into the right or left atrium, or both, caused by a bulging of the whole interatrial septum or a bulging of the primary component of the septum through the fossa ovalis. It is an uncommon anomaly and may be associated with other congenital cardiac malformations or with acquired diseases that result in elevated pressures in one atrial chamber with bulging of the septum to the opposite side (HANLEY et al. 1985). Atrial septal aneurysms have been associated with septal defects, atrial arrhythmias, systolic clicks, atrioventricular valve prolapse, systemic and pulmonary embolism, and atrial tumors, and they usually occur at the fossa ovalis (HANLEY et al. 1985; GALLET et al. 1985, BOGAERT et al. 1995b). HANLEY et al. (1985) have observed three types of fossa ovalis aneurysm and one type of aneurysm involving the entire atrial septum. Systemic and pulmonary thromboembolic events in the presence of an atrial septal aneurysm are probably due to thrombus formation within the concave aspect of the aneurysm. The frequently associated atrial septal defect may result in paradoxical emboli (SCHNEIDER et al. 1990).

Diagnosis is usually made by echocardiography, though stagnant blood flow within the cavity of the aneurysm may mimic a cystic mass (SMITH et al. 1990). MRI is helpful in detecting atrial septal aneurysms, though it should be mentioned that low flow or stagnant flow may appear on SE MRI as signal-rich rather than signal-void, thus mimicking a cardiac mass (SMITH et al. 1990). Cine MRI may overcome this shortcoming and may allow a better description of the type and movement of aneurysm (Fig. 12.39; BOGAERT et al. 1995b).

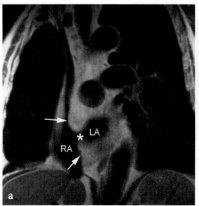
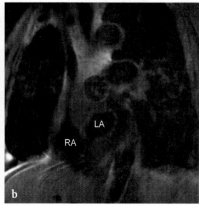

Fig. 12.38a,b. Lipomatous hypertrophy (*arrows*) of the atrial septum (LHAS). **a** Short-axis T1-weighted TSE-MRI; **b** Short-axis T1-weighted TSE-MRI with fat suppression. LHAS is visible on T1-weighted images as a hyperintense bilobated appearance of the atrial septum sparing the fossa ovalis (*star*). The fatty nature can be depicted by means of fat-suppression techniques which will selectively reduce the signal of fat

12.4.4.6
Aneurysm of the Sinus of Valsalva

Aneurysms of the sinus of Valsalva are uncommon entities and, although they are not truly cardiac masses, it is worth mentioning this condition in the differential diagnostic list of cardiac masses. They usually originate from the right coronary sinus, and much less frequently from the noncoronary and the left coronary sinus (DEV et al. 1993). The aneurysms are usually congenital but infrequently they can be acquired (usually endocarditis associated). This condition is usually detected in adults as an incidental finding or by virtue of a complication due to the aneurysm (Fig. 12.40). The most frequent complication is rupture of the aneurysm, usually into the right ventricular outflow tract, right ventricular cavity, or right atrium, and less frequently into the other cardiac chambers or dissecting into the interventricular septum (DEV et al. 1993; ABAD 1995). Other less frequent complications are embolization, compression of the coronary arteries by the aneurysm with subsequent myocardial infarction, and thrombosis of the aneurysm (REID et al. 1990; WIEMER et al. 1996).

The diagnosis is usually made by TTE and TEE, though MRI may be very helpful to demonstrate the aneurysm and to depict the communication between the aorta and the cardiac chambers (OGAWA et al. 1991; RAFFA et al. 1991; HO et al. 1995; KULAN et al. 1996). The latter will be visible on cine MRI as a hypointense jet directed from the aorta into one of the cardiac chambers.

12.4.4.7
Hydatid Cyst

Echinococcosis is endemic in several countries around the Mediterranean Sea. Cardiac involvement in hydatid disease is rare, representing 0.5–2% of all clinical forms of this condition (CACOUB et al. 1991). Because of the risk of potentially lethal complications (due to cyst rupture and massive embolism), early diagnosis and adequate treatment are very important (PASAOGLU et al. 1994). The diagnosis of cardiac echinococcosis is difficult and is based on a series of findings, amongst which hydatid serology and cardiac imaging are particularly important. Hydatid cysts most frequently involve the left ventricular myocardial wall and interventricular septum (KARDARAS et al. 1996). MRI, together with echocardiography and CT, is of considerable importance in the detection of intramyocardial hydatid cysts (ELKOUBY et al. 1990; KULAN et al. 1995; KARDARAS et al. 1996; MACEDO et al. 1997). MRI also allows diagnosis of noncardiac lesions, e.g., pulmonary, hepatic, splenic, and renal involvement, and is helpful in planning surgical intervention.

The detection of intramyocardial cystic lesions is virtually pathognomonic for hydatid disease. These hydatid cysts have a fluid content with a homogeneously hypointense signal intensity on T1-weighted and a homogeneously hyperintense signal on T2-weighted images (KOTOULAS et al. 1996). The pericyst, a thick fibrotic membrane surrounding the hydatid cyst, has a low-signal intensity on T1- and T2-weighted images and this allows differentiation from nonparasitic epithelial cysts (VANJAK et al. 1990; CACOUB et al. 1991; CANTONI et al. 1993; ÜNAL et al. 1995).

12.4.4.8
Pericardial Cyst

Very probably (pleuro)pericardial cysts can be considered as nontumoral masses. They are usually asymptomatic and most frequently arise in the

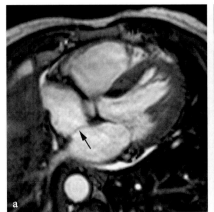
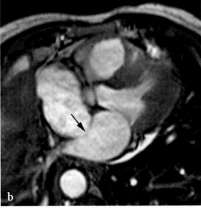

Fig. 12.39a,b. Hypermobile atrial septum in a 62-year-old man. Axial cine MRI, using the b-SSFP technique at 60 ms (**a**) and 170 ms (**b**) after the onset of the QRS wave. At 60 ms, there is a right-sided bulging of the atrial septum (*arrow*), while during systole the atrial septum inverses into a left-sided bulging. This motion is best depicted on dynamic cine MRI views

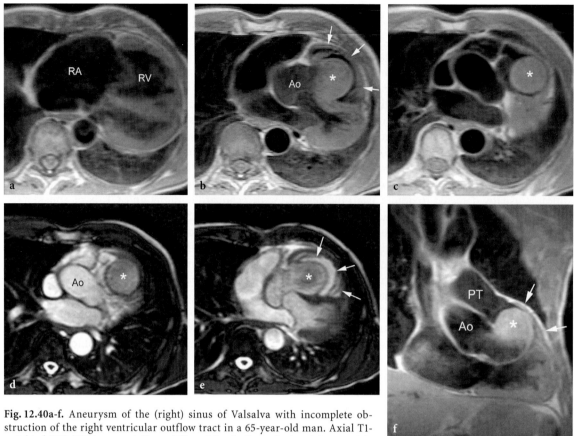

Fig. 12.40a-f. Aneurysm of the (right) sinus of Valsalva with incomplete obstruction of the right ventricular outflow tract in a 65-year-old man. Axial T1-weighted TSE MR images at three different levels through the right ventricle and RVOT (**a-c**). Axial cine MRI at two levels through the RVOT (**d, e**). Oblique T1-weighted TSE MR image through the RVOT (**f**). Left-sided lateral rotation of the cardiac axis due to an important dilatation of the right atrium and ventricle (**a**). Presence of a well-defined, rounded soft-tissue structure (*star*) nearly completely obstructing the right ventricular outflow, causing a gradient of 55 mmHg (*arrows*) (**b-f**). Especially on the cine MRI images, the true nature of this "mass" becomes evident: aneurysmal bulging of the right coronary sinus into the right ventricular outflow tract with subtotal obstruction of the cavity. There was no evidence of any rupture of the aneurysmal wall, leading to the left-to-right shunt

right cardiophrenic angle, followed by the left cardiophrenic angle and, rarely, the anterior or posterior mediastinum. They are usually unilocular and present with a variable diameter. Pericardial cysts are usually discovered during routine radiography. MRI may be very helpful in detecting the water content (VINEE et al. 1992). Pericardial cysts have a low signal intensity on T1-weighted images and a very high signal intensity on T2-weighted images (Fig. 12.41). No enhancement effect of Gd-DTPA is observed. MRI is also helpful in differentiation from other cystic mediastinal structures such as bronchogenic cyst, cystic teratoma, cystic neurogenic tumor, and thymus cyst. Differences in signal intensities on T1-weighted imaging can help in the differentiation, since pericardial cysts have a pure water content with low signal intensities, while the others may have a higher signal intensity due to intracys-

tic hemorrhage or the presence of sebaceous fluid (MURAYAMA et al. 1995) Furthermore, cystic teratomas typically contain fat and calcifications.

12.4.4.9
Gossypiboma or Textiloma

Gossypibomas or textilomas are an iatrogenic cause of cardiac, pericardial, or extracardiac masses. They represent a foreign body reaction surrounding a retained surgical sponge composed of a cotton matrix. Gossypibomas are rare occurrences which are infrequently reported in the literature because of legal implications (BHAT et al. 1997). Their manifestations and complications are so variable that diagnosis is difficult and patient morbidity is significant. A high index of suspicion in a patient who has previously been operated upon will greatly aid

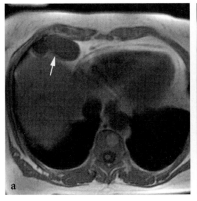 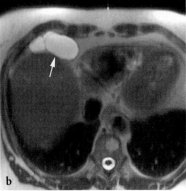 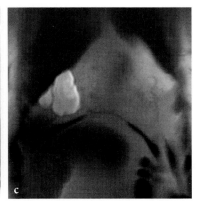

Fig. 12.41a-c. Pleuropericardial cyst (*arrow*) in an asymptomatic 50-year-old man. **a** Axial T1-weighted TSE-MRI. T2-weighted TSE axial (**b**) and coronal (**c**). Bilocular, well-defined soft-tissue structure in the right cardiophrenic angle. The very high signal intensity on T2-weighted MRI sequences is typical for a pleuropericardial cyst

in the diagnosis of this unfortunate complication. Most surgical sponges have radiopaque markers that have a characteristic appearance on plain radiographs (Fig. 12.42). However, the marker may disintegrate over long periods, or sponges used in some countries may not have markers (LERNER and DANG 1997).

Computed tomography, echocardiography, and MRI are particularly important in localizing gossypibomas. Gossypibomas have a typical spongiform pattern on CT images; gas bubbles are the most specific sign for the detection of textilomas but do not indicate abscess formation (KOPKA et al. 1996). The MRI appearances of gossypibomas include masses with low signal intensity on T1- and T2-weighted images, high signal intensity on T1- and T2-weighted images, and heterogeneous signal intensity on T2-weighted images on which the internal architecture suggests retained surgical sponge (MOCHIZUKI et al. 1992; KUWASHIMA et al. 1993; LERNER and DANG 1997). As a result of a pericardial gossypiboma, one or several heart chambers may be compressed. Gossypibomas should be differentiated from postoperative scar formation and tumors (VAN GOETHEM et al. 1991).

12.4.5
Normal Cardiac Anatomy and Variants

Several normal intracardiac structures can mimic pathological masses. Knowledge of these normal variants will reduce the number of false-positively diagnosed cardiac masses. This is particularly important since, with the currently available cardiac imaging modalities, even the smallest cardiac structures are almost perfectly visible. Therefore, the most common normal variants will be described for each cardiac chamber separately and for the pericardium (see also Chapter 4).

12.4.5.1
Right Atrium

Nodular thickening of the posterior right atrial wall is a common finding on cardiac MR images and may resemble a mass lesion (Fig. 12.43; MIROWITZ and GUTIERREZ 1992). Anatomically this nodular thickening corresponds to the *crista terminalis*, which marks the embryological division between the portion of the right atrium that is derived from the sinus venosus, i.e., smooth-walled sinus venarum, and that which is derived from the embryonic atrium, i.e., trabeculated atrium proper and auriculum. The crista terminalis is a prominent muscular ridge that extends along the posterolateral aspect of the right atrium between the orifices of the superior and inferior venae cavae. Inferiorly, it merges with the valve of the inferior vena cava (*eustachian valve*) and the valve of the coronary sinus (*thebesian valve*). In addition, strand-like fibrous structures, known as the *Chiari network*, may arise from the region of the inferior crista terminalis and/or eustachian valve and extend into the right atrial chamber. These structures, which are of variable prominence and have a similar signal intensity to myocardial tissue, are routinely observed on cardiac MRI and should not be mistaken for neoplasms, thrombosis, or inflammation (MEIER and HARTNELL 1994).

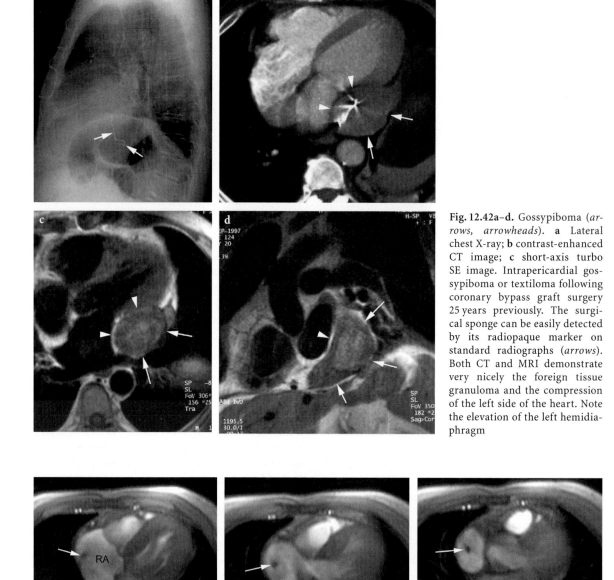

Fig. 12.42a–d. Gossypiboma (*arrows, arrowheads*). **a** Lateral chest X-ray; **b** contrast-enhanced CT image; **c** short-axis turbo SE image. Intrapericardial gossypiboma or textiloma following coronary bypass graft surgery 25 years previously. The surgical sponge can be easily detected by its radiopaque marker on standard radiographs (*arrows*). Both CT and MRI demonstrate very nicely the foreign tissue granuloma and the compression of the left side of the heart. Note the elevation of the left hemidiaphragm

Fig. 12.43a-c. Crista terminalis (*arrows*), presenting as intracavity nodule in right atrium. Axial cine MR images, using the spoiled-GE technique. This muscular structure can be recognized easily by its typical location, i.e., posterolateral wall of the right atrium, connecting the entrances of both caval veins

12.4.5.2
Right Ventricle

The *moderator band*, a thin muscular band, is unique for the right ventricle, which can be very helpful in differentiating the right from the left ventricle in congenital heart malformations. This muscular structure extends from the midinterventricular septum through the cavity of the right ventricle and attaches near the base of the anterior papillary muscle on the free wall of the right ventricle. It may become very prominent in patients with right ventricular enlargement or hypertrophy or both, and may be mistaken for a right ventricular thrombus or tumor (Fig. 12.44). MRI allows detection of the muscular nature of the moderator band, with signal intensities similar to the surrounding myocardium.

12.4.5.3
Left Atrium

While the left atrium has a smooth wall delineation, the left atrial appendage is lined with small, equally spaced muscular pectinate ridges. These pectinate ridges must be distinguished from thrombi. Intracavitary protrusion of the lateral wall at the entrance of the left pulmonary vein in the left atrium is not infrequently mistaken for a cardiac mass on echocardiography. This anatomical variant can be easily recognized on MR images (KING et al. 1998). Furthermore, a variety of extracardiac abnormalities such as hiatal hernia, esophageal carcinoma, bronchogenic cyst, or tortuous descending aorta can simulate masses in the left atrium on echocardiography (MENEGUS et al. 1992). The exact location of these "masses" can be determined by means of MRI.

12.4.5.4
Left Ventricle

Besides the normal papillary muscles and chordae tendinae, in a minority of the population, false tendons or false chordae occur as normal variants in the left ventricle. Rather than connecting the papillary muscles with the valve leaflets, the false chordae are linear structures attached at both ends to the endomyocardium (KEREN et al. 1984). They are asymptomatic and usually accidental findings on echocardiograms.

12.4.5.5
Pericardium

Knowledge of the normal appearance of the pericardium on MR images is necessary to adequately interpret cardiovascular MRI studies (see also Chapter 11). The superior pericardial sinus should not be mistaken for an aortic dissection, anomalous vascular structure, or a nodular mass on MR images (BLACK et al. 1993).

12.4.6
Prosthetic Valves and Other Foreign Devices

Metallic objects such as metallic heart valves, stents, cardiac occluders, vascular clips, and catheters may induce artifacts on the MR images (Figs. 12.45, 12.46). The artifacts are variable and depend on the type and the amount of metal used in the implant and on the type of MRI sequence (SHELLOCK and MORISOLI 1994a, 1994b). Metallic implants induce an alteration of the local magnetic field which leads to loss of signal from the surrounding tissue. For metallic heart valves studied with SE-MRI, artifacts

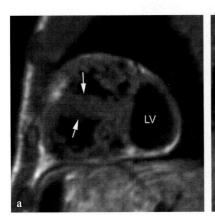 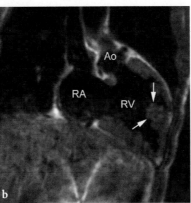

Fig. 12.44 a, b. Hypertrophic moderator band (*arrowheads*) in a patient with transposition of the great arteries. T1-weighted SE images in the cardiac short-axis (**a**) and vertical long-axis (**b**). This MRI study was performed because the patient was suspected on echocardiography to have a thrombus or mass in the right ventricle. The typical location and the signal intensity similar to that of the myocardium allow a correct diagnosis

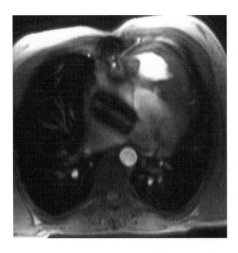

Fig. 12.45. Stent in a venous baffle in a patient with transposition of the great arteries. Axial cine MR image, using the spoiled-GE technique. A venous baffle conducts the systemic venous blood to the left side of the heart and pulmonary arteries. The metallic stent in the "leg" coming from the superior vena cava is visible as a tubular hypointense structure. The lumen of the stent is patent though the intraluminal diameter cannot be exactly assessed as a consequence of metallic susceptibility artifacts

CESARE et al. 1995; WALKER et al. 1995). Physiologic valvular regurgitation can be differentiated from pathological or valvular regurgitation. Artifacts caused by other foreign cardiac devices such as intravascular or coronary stents are similar to those caused by prosthetic valves (MOHIADDIN et al. 1995).

12.5
Conclusions

With the advent of several noninvasive or minimally invasive cardiac imaging modalities such as echocardiography, CT, and MRI, detailed morphological description of the heart, pericardium, great vessels, and mediastinum has become a reality. Even small normal anatomical structures can be very easily recognized and differentiated from pathological structures. The location and extent of cardiac tumors can be precisely evaluated, and the response to treatment can be accurately followed. Though differentiation between benign and malignant tumors, or between tumoral and non-tumoral conditions, is often not feasible without histological proof, cardiac masses can be very accurately depicted or ruled out. Rather than being a primary imaging modality in patients suspected of having a cardiac tumor, MRI can be considered as an excellent "second-line" imaging modality which can be applied to confirm the findings obtained from echocardiography, to determine precisely the tumor location and extent, for tissue characterization, for follow-up of patients under treatment, and to detect early tumor recurrence.

are minimal, since the prosthetic valves cannot be differentiated from the surrounding dark blood. SE-MRI is advantageous in the depiction of anatomical structures such as paravalvular abscesses (BACHMANN et al. 1991). Artifacts, however, are accentuated on GE-MRI (cine MRI). Metallic heart valves are therefore visible as dark areas surrounded by bright blood. Nevertheless, in a majority of cases, qualitative analysis of the valve function and accurate measurement of the blood velocity downstream of the prosthetic heart valve can be performed (DI

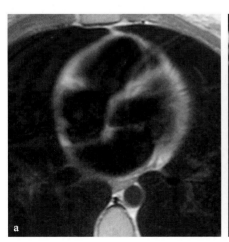

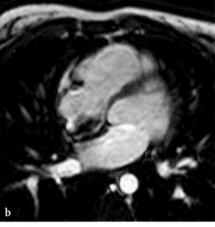

Fig. 12.46a,b. Amplatz occluder in an atrial septal defect. **a** Axial T1-weighted TSE MR image; **b** axial cine MR image, using the b-SSFP technique

12.6
Key Points

- Use a systematic approach to assess cardiac masses:
  - First, determine whether or not the patient has a true cardiac mass
  - Second, determine whether the mass has tumoral or nontumoral characteristics
  - Third, if the mass has features of being a tumor, determine whether the tumor may be benign or malignant
  - Fourth, determine the location, extent, complications, and associated features of the cardiac mass
  - Fifth, use clinical information (e.g., patients' symptoms; history of extracardiac malignancy; heart transplant; restrictive or dilated cardiomyopathy; previous myocardial infarction; etc.) and knowledge about typical location and appearance of cardiac masses for this analysis
- For this systematic approach, use a combination of MRI sequences, often in different imaging planes.
- Nontumoral conditions are much more frequent than cardiac tumors
- Large infiltrative tumors may be clinically silent, while smaller tumors can produce dramatic symptomatology if strategically located with transient obstruction of flow across a valve, or when causing systemic emboli
- A cardiac mass, even small in size, in combination with a pericardial effusion should suggest a cardiac malignancy
- A myxoma has a predilection to arise in the atria near the oval fossa; atrial masses in other locations should be suggestive of nontumoral masses or other cardiac tumors (benign/malignant)
- Angiosarcoma, the most common primary cardiac malignancy, typically arises from the right atrial wall and extends into the pericardium
- Carefully analyze all cardiac MRI studies, for hidden cardiac thrombi, especially in patients with a predilection for thrombus formation
- A combination of cine MRI (using the new b-SSFP techniques) with CE-IR MRI is currently the best approach for thrombus detection

References

Abad C (1995) Congenital aneurysm of the sinus of Valsalva dissecting into the interventricular septum. Cardiovasc Surg 3:563–564

Aggoun Y, Hunkeler N, Destephen M et al (1992) Cardiac rhabdomyomatosis and Bourneville's tuberous sclerosis in the fetus. A propos of 2 cases (in French). Arch Mal Coeur Vaiss 85:609–613

Amparo EG, Higgins CB, Farmer D, Gamsu G, McNamara M (1984) Gated MRI of cardiac and paracardiac masses: initial experience. Am J Roentgenol 143:1151–1156

Aouate P, Artigou JY, Rovany X et al (1988) Contribution of nuclear magnetic resonance in right atrial angiosarcoma. Apropos of a case (in French). Arch Mal Coeur Vaiss 81:1543–1546

Applegate PM, Tajik AJ, Ehman RL, Julsrud PR, Miller FAJ (1987) Two-dimensional echocardiographic and magnetic resonance imaging observations in massive lipomatous hypertrophy of the atrial septum. Am J Cardiol 59:489–491

Araoz PA, Eklund HE, Welch TJ, Breen JF (1999) CT and MR imaging of primary cardiac malignancies. Radiographics 19:1421–1434

Araoz PA, Mulvagh SL, Tazelaar HD, Julsrud PR, Breen JF (2000) CT and MR imaging of benign primary cardiac neoplasms with echocardiographic correlation. Radiographics 20:1303–1319

Arciniegas E, Hakimi M, Farooki ZQ, Green EW (1980) Intrapericardial teratoma in infancy. J Thorac Cardiovasc Surg 79:306–311

Axel L, Dougherty L (1989) Heart wall motion: improved method for spatial modulation of magnetization for me imaging. Radiology 172:349–350

Aydingoz U, Ariyurek M, Selcuk ZT, Demirkazik FB, Baris YI (1997) Calcium within a bronchogenic cyst with a fluid level. Br J Radiol 70:761–763

Bachmann R, Deutsch HJ, Jungehulsing M, et al (1991) Magnetic resonance imaging in patients with heart valve prostheses. Rofo Fortschr Rontgenstr 155:499–505

Bader RS, Chitayat D, Kelly E et al (2003) Fetal rhabdomyoma: prenatal diagnosis, clinical outcome, and incidence of associated tuberous sclerosis complex. J Pediatr 143:620–624

Balasubramanyam A, Waxman M, Kazal HL, Lee MH (1986) Malignant lymphoma of the heart in acquired immune deficiency syndrome. Chest 90:243–246

Bansal RC, Graham BM, Jutzy KR, Shakudo M, Shah PM (1990) Left ventricular outflow tract to left atrial communication secondary to rupture of mitral-aortic intervalvular fibrosa in infective endocarditis: diagnosis by transesophageal echocardiography and color flow imaging. J Am Coll Cardiol 15:499–504

Barakos JA, Brown JJ, Brescia RJ, Higgins CB (1989a) High signal intensity lesions of the chest in MR imaging. J Comput Assist Tomogr 13:797–802

Barakos JA, Brown JJ, Higgins CB (1989b) MR imaging of secondary cardiac and paracardiac lesions. Am J Roentgenol 153:47–50

Bargallo J, Luburich P, Garcia Barrionuevo J, Sanchez Gonzalez M (1993) Fluid-fluid level in bronchogenic cysts. Radiology 186:427–428

Barkhausen J, Hunold P, Eggebrecht H et al (2002) Detection and characterization of intracardiac thrombi on MR imaging. Am J Roentgenol 179:1539–1544

Bassish MS (1974) Mesenchymal tumors of the uterus. Clin Obstet Gynecol 17:51–88

Baumgartner HR (1973) The role of blood flow in platelet adhesion, fibrin deposition, and formation of mural thrombi. Microvasc Rev 5:167–179

Beghetti M, Prieditis M, Rebeyka IM, Mawson J (1998) Images in cardiovascular medicine. Intrapericardial teratoma. Circulation 97:1523–1524

Benetar A, Vaughan J, Nicolini U, Trotter S, Corrin B, Lincoln C (1992) Prenatal pericardiocentesis: its role in the management of intrapericardial teratoma. Obstet Gynecol 79:856–859

Best AK, Dobson RL, Ahmad AR (2003) Best cases from the AFIP. Cardiac angiosarcoma. Radiographics 23:S141-S145

Bhat HS, Mahesh G, Ramgopal KS (1997) "Gossypiboma": an unusual cause of perinephric abscess. J R Coll Surg Edinb 42:277–278

Black CM, Hedges LK, Javitt MC (1993) The superior pericardial sinus: normal appearance on gradient-echo MR images. Am J Roentgenol 160:749–751

Bleiweis MS, Georgiou D, Brundage BH (1994) Detection and characterization of intracardiac masses by ultrafast computed tomography. Am J Card Imag 8:63–68

Bogaert J, Rademakers F, Cappelle L, et al (1995a) High-grade immunoblastic sarcoma: an unusual type of a primary cardiac non-Hodgkin lymphoma. Rofo Fortschr Rontgenstr 162:186–188

Bogaert J, Man F de, Rademakers F et al (1995b) Right atrial tumor arising on an atrial septal aneurysm. Assessment by MR imaging. Clin Imaging 19:172–175

Bogaert J, Taylor AM, Kerckhove F van, Dymarkowski S (2004) Use of the inversion-recovery contrast-enhanced MRI technique for cardiac imaging: spectrum of diseases. Am J Roentgenol AJR 182:609–615

Borner C, Haberbosch W, Hagl S, et al (1990) Primary leiomyosarcoma of the right atrium in an adult patient. Z Kardiol 79:865–869

Bouton S, Yang A, McCrindle BW, et al (1991) Differentiation of tumor from viable myocardium using cardiac tagging with MR imaging. J Comput Assist Tomogr 15:676–678

Brasch RC, Weinmann HJ, Wesbey GE (1984) Contrast-enhanced NMR imaging: animal studies using gadolinium-DTPA complex. Am J Roentgenol 142:625–630

Brizard C, Latremouille C, Jebara VA et al (1993) Cardiac hemangiomas (see comments). Ann Thorac Surg 56:390–394

Brown JJ, Barakos JA, Higgins CB (1989) Magnetic resonance imaging of cardiac and paracardiac masses. J Thorac Imaging 4:58–64

Burke AP, Virmani R (1991) Osteosarcomas of the heart. Am J Surg Pathol 51:289–295

Burke AP, Cowan D, Virmani R (1992) Primary sarcomas of the heart. Cancer 69:387–395

Burke AP, Rosado de Christenson M, Templeton PA, Virmani R (1994) Cardiac fibroma: clinicopathologic correlates and surgical treatment. J Thorac Cardiovasc Surg 108:862–870

Cacoub P, Chapoutot L, Boutin LT duet al (1991) Hydatid cyst of the interventricular septum. Contribution of magnetic resonance imaging (in French). Arch Mal Coeur Vaiss 84:1857–1860

Caduff JH, Hernandez RJ, Ludomirsky A (1996) MR visualization of aortic valve vegetations. J Comput Assist Tomogr 20:613–615

Cantoni S, Frola C, Gatto R, et al (1993) Hydatid cyst of the interventricular septum of the heart: MR findings. Am J Roentgenol 161:753–754

Carpenter JL (1991) Perivalvular extension of infection in patients with infectious endocarditis. Rev Infect Dis 13:127–138

Castelli MJ, Mihalov ML, Posniak HV, Gattuso P (1989) Primary cardiac lymphoma initially diagnosed by routine cytology: case report and literature review. Acta Cytol 30:662–664

Chao TY, Han SC, Nieh S, Lan GY, Lee SH (1995) Diagnosis of primary cardiac lymphoma. Report of a case with cytologic examination of pericardial fluid and imprints of transvenously biopsied intracardiac tissue. Acta Cytol 39:955–959

Chiles C, Woodard PK, Gutierrez FR, Link KM (2001) Metastatic involvement of heart and pericardium: CT and MR imaging. Radiographics 21:439–449

Chin WW, van Tosh A van, Hecht SR, Berger M (1988) Left ventricular thrombus with normal left ventricular function in ulcerative colitis. Am Heart J 116:562–563

Chou ST, Arkles LB, Gill GD, et al (1983) Primary lymphoma of the heart: a case report. Cancer 52:744–747

Coghlan JG, Paul VE, Mitchell AG (1989) Cardiac involvement by lymphoma: diagnostic difficulties. Eur Heart J 10:765–768

Colucci V, Alberti A, Bonacina E, Gordini V (1995) Papillary fibroelastoma of the mitral valve. A rare cause of embolic events. Tex Heart Inst J 22:327–331

Conces DJ, Vix VA, Klatte EC (1985) Gated MR imaging of left atrial myxomas. Radiology 156:445–447

Corallo S, Mutinelli MR, Moroni M et al (1988) Echocardiographic detects myocardial damage in AIDS: prospective study in 102 patients. Eur Heart J 9:887–892

Curtinsinger CR, Wilson MJ, Yoneda K (1989) Primary cardiac lymphoma. Cancer 64:521–525

DeGroat TS, Parameswaran R, Popper PM, Kotler MN (1985) Left ventricular thrombi in association with normal left ventricular wall motion in patients with malignancy. Am J Cardiol 56:827–828

DeLoach JF, Haynes JW (1953) Secondary tumors of the heart and pericardium. Review of subject and report of 137 cases. Arch Intern Med 91:224–249

DePace NL, Soulen RL, Kotler MN, Mintz GS (1981) Two dimensional echocardiographic detection of intraatrial masses. Am J Cardiol 48:954–960

De Roos A, Weijers E, Duinen S van, Wall EE van der (1989) Calcified right atrial myxoma demonstrated by magnetic resonance imaging. Chest 95:478–479

Dev V, Goswami KC, Shrivastava S, Bahl VK, Saxena A (1993) Echocardiographic diagnosis of aneurysm of the sinus of Valsalva. Am Heart J 126:930–936

Di Cesare E, Enrici RM, Paparoni S et al (1995) Low-field magnetic resonance imaging in the evaluation of mechanical and biological heart valve function. Eur J Radiol 20:224–228

Doherty NE, Siegel RJ (1985) Cardiovascular manifestations of systemic lupus erythematosus. Am Heart J 110:1257–1265

Dooms GC, Higgins CB (1986) MR imaging of cardiac thrombi. J Comput Assist Tomogr 10:415–420

Dooms GC, Hricak H, Sollitto RA, Higgins CB (1985) Lipomatous tumors and tumors with fatty components: MR imaging potential and comparison of MR and CT results. Radiology 157:479–483

Dunlap HJ, Udjus K (1990) Atypical leiomyoma arising in an hepatic vein with extension into the inferior vena cava and right atrium. Report of a case in a child. Pediatr Radiol 20:202–203

Edwards FH, Hale D, Cohen A, Thompson L, Pezzella AT, Virmani R (1991) Primary cardiac valve tumors. Ann Thorac Surg 52:1127–1131

Elkouby A, Vaillant A, Comet B, Malmejac C, Houel J (1990) Cardiac hydatidosis. Review of recent literature and report of 15 cases (in French). Ann Chir 44:603–610

Endo M, Adachi S, Kusumoto M et al (1993) A study of the utility of the MR image for the diagnosis of thymic tumors - imaging and pathologic correlation. Nippon Igaku Hoshasen Gakkai Zasshi 53:1–10

Engberding R, Daniel WG, Erbel R et al (1993) Diagnosis of heart tumours by transoesophageal echocardiography: a multicentre study in 154 patients. European Cooperative Study Group. Eur Heart J 14:1223–1228

Fang CY, Fu M, Chang JP, Eng HL, Hung JS (1996) Malignant fibrous histiocytoma of the left ventricle: a case report. Chang Keng I Hsueh 19:187–190

Fisher MS, Edmonds PR (1988) Lipomatous hypertrophy of the interatrial septum. Diagnosis by magnetic resonance imaging. J Comput Tomogr 12:267–269

Fisher MR, Higgins CB, Andereck W (1985) MR imaging of an intrapericardial pheochromocytoma. J Comput Assist Tomogr 9:1103–1105

Fueredi GA, Knechtges TE, Czarnecki DJ (1989) Coronary angiography in atrial myxoma: findings in nine cases. Am J Roentgenol 152:737–738

Funari M, Fujita N, Peck WW, Higgins CB (1991) Cardiac tumors: assessment with Gd-DTPA enhanced MR imaging. J Comput Assist Tomogr 15:953–958

Furber A, Geslin P, Le Jeune JJ et al (1997) Value of MRI with injection of gadolinium in the diagnosis of mitral ring abscess. Apropos of a case (in French). Arch Mal Coeur Vaiss 90:399–404

Gaerte SC, Meyer CA, Winer-Muram HT, Tarver RD, Conce DJ Jr (2002) Fat-containing lesions of the chest. Radiographics 22:S61–S78

Gallet B, Malergue MC, Adams C et al (1985) Atrial septal aneurysm – a potential cause of systemic embolism. Br Heart J 53:292–297

Gamsu G, Starck D, Webb WR, Moore EH, Sheldon PE (1984) Magnetic resonance of benign mediastinal masses. Radiology 151:709–713

Gibson JM, Hall CM, Dicks MC, Finn JP (1990) Intracardiac extension of Wilms' tumour: demonstration by magnetic resonance. Br J Radiol 63:568–569

Gill PS, Chandraratna AN, Meyer PR, Levine AM (1987) Malignant lymphoma: cardiac involvement at initial presentation. J Clin Oncol 5:216–224

Glazer HS, Gutierrez FR, Levitt RG, Lee JK, Murphy WA (1985) The thoracic aorta studied by MR imaging. Radiology 157:149–155

Godine LB, Berdon WE, Brasch RC, Leonidas JC (1990) Adrenocortical carcinoma with extension into inferior vena cava and right atrium: report of 3 cases in children. Pediatr Radiol 20:166–168

Gomes AS, Lois JF, Child JS, Brown K, Batra P (1987) Cardiac tumors and thrombus: evaluation with MR imaging. AJR Am J Roentgenol 49:895–899

Gomi T, Ikeda T, Sakurai J, Toya Y, Tani M (1994) Cardiac pheochromocytoma. A case report and review of the literature. Jpn Heart J 35:117–124

Gossinger HD, Siostrzonek P, Zangeneh M et al (1988) Magnetic resonance imaging findings in a patient with pericardial mesothelioma. Am Heart J 115:1321–1322

Grebenc ML, Rosado-de-Christenson, Burke AP, Green CE, Galvin JR (2000) Primary cardiac and pericardial neoplasms: radiologic-pathologic correlation. Radiographics 20:1073–1103

Grebenc ML, Rosado de Christenson, Green CE, Burke AP, Galvin JR (2002) From the archives of the AFIP. Cardiac myxoma: imaging features in 83 patients. Radiographics 22:673–689

Grote J, Mugge A, Schfers HJ, Daniel WG, Lichtlen PR (1995) Multiplane transoesophageal echocardiography detection of a papillary fibroelastoma of the aortic valve causing myocardial infarction. Eur Heart J 16:426–429

Hamilton BH, Francis IR, Gross BH et al (1997) Intrapericardial paragangliomas (pheochromocytomas): imaging features. Am J Roentgenol 168:109–113

Hananouchi GI, Goff WB (1990) Cardiac lipoma: six-year follow-up with MRI characteristics, and a review of the literature. Magn Reson Imaging 8:825–828

Hanley PC, Tajik AJ, Hynes JK et al (1985) Diagnosis and classification of atrial septal aneurysm by two-dimensional echocardiography: report of 80 consecutive cases. J Am Coll Cardiol 6:1370–1382

Hanson EC (1992) Cardiac tumors: a current perspective. NY State J Med 92:41–42

Haouzi A, Danchin N, Renoult E et al (1989) Cardiac pheochromocytoma. Failure of classic non-invasive diagnostic methods (in French). Arch Mal Coeur Vaiss 82:97–100

Hatabu H, Gefter WB, Axel L et al (1994) MR imaging with spatial modulation of magnetization in the evaluation of chronic central pulmonary thromboemboli. Radiology 190:791–796

Heath D (1968) Pathology of cardiac tumors. Am J Cardiol 21:315–327

Herrera CJ, Mehlman DJ, Hartz RS, Talano JV, McPherson DD (1992) Comparison of transesophageal and transthoracic echocardiography for diagnosis of right sided cardiac lesions. Am J Cardiol 70:964–966

Herrmann MA, Shankerman RA, Edwards WD, Shub C, Schaff HV (1992) Primary cardiac angiosarcoma: a clinico-pathologic study of six cases. J Thorac Cardiovasc Surg 103:655–664

Ho VB, Kinney JB, Sahn DJ (1995) Ruptured sinus of Valsalva aneurysm: cine phase-contrast MR characterization. J Comput Assist Tomogr 19:652–656

Hoffmann U, Globits S, Schima W et al (2003) Usefulness of magnetic resonance imaging of cardiac and paracardiac masses. Am J Cardiol 92: 890–895

Ichikawa T, Ohtomo K, Uchiyama G, Fujimoto H, Nasu K (1995) Contrast-enhanced dynamic MRI of adrenal masses: classification of characteristic enhancement patterns. Clin Radiol 50:295–300

Janigan DT, Husain A, Robinson NA (1986) Cardiac angiosarcomas. A review and a case report. Cancer 57:852–859

Jeang MK, Fuentes F, Gately A, Byrnes J, Lewis M (1986)

Aortic root abscess. Initial experience using magnetic resonance imaging. Chest 89:613–615

Jochelson MS, Balikian JP, Mauch P, Liebman H (1983) Peri- and paracardial involvement in lymphoma: a radiographic study of 11 cases. Am J Roentgenol 140:483–488

Johnson DE, Vacek J, Gollub SB, Wilson DB, Dunn M (1988) Comparison of gated cardiac magnetic resonance imaging and two-dimensional echocardiography for the evaluation of right ventricular thrombi: a case report with autopsy correlation. Cathet Cardiovasc Diagn 14:266–268

Jungehulsing M, Sechtem U, Theissen P, Hilger HH, Schicha H (1992) Left ventricular thrombi: evaluation with spin-echo and gradient-echo MR imaging. Radiology 182:225–229

Kaminaga T, Yamada N, Imakita S, Takamiya M, Nishimura T (1993) Magnetic resonance imaging of pericardial malignant mesothelioma. Magn Reson Imaging 11:1057–1061

Kanematsu M, Imaeda T, Minowa H et al (1994) Hepatocellular carcinoma with tumor thrombus in the inferior vena cava and right atrium. Abdom Imaging 19:313–316

Kaplan PA, Williams SM (1987) Mucocutaneous and peripheral soft tissue hemangiomas. MR findings. Radiology 163:163–168

Kardaras F, Kardara D, Tselikos D et al (1996) Fifteen year surveillance of echinococcal heart disease from a referral hospital in Greece. Eur Heart J 17:1265–1270

Kasarskis EJ, O'Connor W, Earle G (1988) Embolic stroke from cardiac papillary fibroelastomas. Stroke 19:1171–1173

Kasugai T, Sakurai M, Yutani C et al (1990) Sequential malignant transformation of cardiac myxoma. Acta Pathol Jpn 40:687–692

Kawasuji M, Matsunaga Y, Iwa T (1989) Cardiac phaeochromocytoma of the interatrial septum. Eur J Cardiothorac Surg 3:175–177

Keeley EC, Hillis LD (1996) Left ventricular mural thrombus after acute myocardial infarction. Clin Cardiol 19:83–86

Kemp JL, Kessler RM, Raizada V, Williamson MR (1996) Case report. MR and CT appearance of cardiac hemangioma. J Comput Assist Tomogr 20:482–483

Keren A, Billingham ME, Popp RL (1984) Echocardiographic recognition and implications of ventricular hypertrophic trabeculations and aberrant bands. Circulation 70:836–842

Kiaffis MG, Powell AJ, Geva T (2002) Magnetic resonance imaging evaluation of cardiac tumor characteristics in infants and children. Am J Cardiol 89:1229–1233

Kim EE, Wallace S, Abello R et al (1989) Malignant cardiac fibrous histiocytomas and angiosarcomas: MR features. J Comput Assist Tomogr 13:627–632

King MA, Vrachliotis TG, Bergin CJ (1998) A left atrial pseudomass: potential pitfall at thoracic MR imaging. JMRI 8:991–993

Klarich KW, Enriquez-Sarano M, Gura GM, Edwards WD, Tajik AJ, Seward JB (1997) Papillary fibroelastoma: echocardiographic characteristics for diagnosis and pathologic correlation. J Am Coll Cardiol 30:784–790

Klima T, Milam JD, Bossart MI, Cooley DA (1986) Rare primary sarcomas of the heart. Arch Pathol Lab Med 110:1155–1159

Konermann M, Sorge HB, Grotz J, Josephs W, Hotzinger H (1989) Hemangioma of the left coronary artery with a fistula into the pulmonary artery (in German). Dtsch Med Wochenschr 114:1363–1366

Kopka L, Fischer U, Gross AJ, Funke M, Oestmann JW, Grabbe E (1996) CT of retained surgical sponges (textilomas): pitfalls in detection and evaluation. J Comput Assist Tomogr 20:919–923

Kotoulas GK, Magoufis GL, Gouliamos AD et al (1996) Evaluation of hydatid disease of the heart with magnetic resonance imaging. Cardiovasc Intervent Radiol 19:187–189

Kulan K, Tuncer C, Kulan C et al (1995) Hydatid cyst of the interventricular septum and contribution of magnetic resonance imaging. Acta Cardiol 50:477–481

Kulan K, Kulan C, Tuncer C, Komsuoglu B, Zengin M (1996) Echocardiography and magnetic resonance imaging of sinus of Valsalva aneurysm with rupture into the ventricle. J Cardiovasc Surg Torino 37:639–641

Kuo CS, Hsu HC, Huang CH, Liu SM, Ho CH (1997) Leiomyosarcoma of the left atrium: a case report. Chung Hua I Hsueh Tsa Chih 59:136–140

Kupferwasser I, Mohr-Kahaly S, Erbel R et al (1994) Three-dimensional imaging of cardiac mass lesions by transesophageal echocardiographic computed tomography. J Am Soc Echocardiogr 7:561–570

Kushihashi T, Fujisawa H, Munechika H (1996) Magnetic resonance imaging of thymic epithelial tumors. Crit Rev Diagn Imaging 37:191–259

Kuwashima S, Yamato M, Fujioka M, et al (1993) MR findings of surgically retained sponges and towels: report of two cases. Radiat Med 11:98–101

Lagrange JL, Despins P, Spielman M et al (1986) Cardiac metastases. Case report on an isolated cardiac metastasis of a myxoid liposarcoma. Cancer 58:2333–2337

Langer E, Mischke U, Stommer P, Harrer T, Stoll R (1988) Kaposi's sarcoma with pericardial tamponade in AIDS. Dtsch Med Wochenschr 29:1187–1190

Lanza RP, Cooper DK, Cassidy MJ, Barnard CN (1983) Malignant neoplasms occurring after cardiac transplantation. JAMA 249:1746–1748

Lee R, Fisher MR (1989) MR imaging of cardiac metastases from malignant fibrous histiocytoma. J Comput Assist Tomogr 13:126–168

Lerner CA, Dang HP (1997) MR imaging of a pericardial gossypiboma (letter). Am J Roentgenol 169:314

Levine RA, Weyman AE, Dinsmore RE et al (1986) Noninvasive tissue characterization: diagnosis of lipo-matous hypertrophy of the atrial septum by nuclear magnetic resonance imaging. J Am Coll Cardiol 7:688–692

Lie JT (1989) Petrified cardiac myxoma masquerading as organized atrial mural thrombus. Arch Pathol Lab Med 113:742–745

Lund JT, Ehman RL, Julsrud PR, Sinak LJ, Tajik AJ (1989) Cardiac masses: assessment by MR imaging. Am J Roentgenol 152:469–473

Lupetin AR, Dash N, Beckman I (1986) Leiomyosarcoma of the superior vena cava: diagnosis by cardiac gated MR. Cardiovasc Intervent Radiol 9:103–105

Macedo AJ, Magalhaes MP, Tavares NJ, et al (1997) Cardiac hydatid cyst in a child. Pediatr Cardiol 18:226–228

Mahajan H, Kim EE, Wallace S, et al (1989) Magnetic resonance imaging of malignant fibrous histiocytoma. Magn Reson Imaging 7:283–288

Manger WM, Gifford RWJ (1990) Pheochromocytoma. In:

Laragh JH, Brenner BM (eds) Hypertension. Raven, New York, pp 1639–1650

Massie RJ, Van Asperen PP, Mellis CM (1997) A review of open biopsy for mediastinal masses. J Paediatr Child Health 33:230–233

Matsuoka H, Hamada M, Honda T et al (1996) Morphologic and histologic characterization of cardiac myxomas by magnetic resonance imaging. Angiology 47:693–698

Matteucci C, Busi G, Biferali F, Paventi S (1997) Tardive pseudo-ischemic presentation of cardiac rhabdomyoma (in Italian). G Ital Cardiol 27:583–587

McAllister HGJ (1979) Primary tumors and cysts of the heart and pericardium. Curr Probl Cardiol 4:1–11

McAllister HA, Fenoglio JJ (1978) Tumors of the cardiovascular system. Armed Forces Institute of Pathology, Washington, DC, pp 1–39

McFadden PM, Lacy JR (1987) Intracardiac papillary fibroelastoma: an occult cause of embolic neurologic deficit. Ann Thorac Surg 43:667–669

Meany JFM, Kazerooni EA, Jamadar DA, Korobkin M (1997) CT appearance of lipomatous hypertrophy of the interatrial septum. Am J Roentgenol 168:1081–1084

Meier RA, Hartnell GG (1994) MRI of right atrial pseudomass: is it really a diagnostic problem? J Comput Assist Tomogr 18:398–401

Menegus MA, Greenberg MA, Spindola-Franco H, Fayemi A (1992) Magnetic resonance imaging of suspected atrial tumors. Am Heart J 123:1260–1268

Mirowitz SA, Gutierrez FR (1992) Fibromuscular elements of the right atrium: pseudomass at MR imaging. Radiology 182:231–233

Mitchell DG, Burk DL, Vinitski S, Rifkin MD (1987) The biophysical basis of tissue contrast in extracranial MR imaging. Am J Roentgenol 149:831–837

Mochizuki T, Takehara Y, Ichijo K, et al (1992) Case report: MR appearance of a retained surgical sponge. Clin Radiol 46:66–67

Mohiaddin RH, Roberts RH, Underwood R, Rothman M (1995) Localization of a misplaced coronary artery stent by magnetic resonance imaging. Clin Cardiol 18:175–177

Mollet NR, Dymarkowski S, Volders W et al (2002) Visualization of ventricular thrombi with contrast-enhanced magnetic resonance imaging in patients with ischemic heart disease. Circulation 106: 2873–2876

Mosthaf FA, Gieseler U, Mehmel HC, Fischer JT, Gams E (1991) Left bundle-branch block and primary benign heart tumor (in German). Dtsch Med Wochenschr 116:134–136

Mugge A, Daniel WG, Haverich A, Lichtlen PR (1991) Diagnosis of noninfective cardiac mass lesions by two-dimensional echocardiography. Comparison of the transthoracic and transesophageal approaches. Circulation 83:70–78

Murayama S, Murakami J, Watanabe H et al (1995) Signal intensity characteristics of mediastinal cystic masses on T1-weighted MRI. J Comput Assist Tomogr 19:188–191

Murphey MD, Gross TM, Rosenthal HG (1994) From the archives of the AFIP. Musculoskeletal malignant fibrous histiocytoma: radiologic-pathologic correlation. Radiographics 14:807–826

Naka N, Ohsawa M, Tomita Y,et al (1995) Angiosarcoma in Japan. Cancer 75:989–996

Nakata H, Egashira K, Watanabe H et al (1993) MRI of bronchogenic cysts. J Comput Assist Tomogr 17:267–270

Neuerburg JM, Bohndorf K, Sohn M, et al (1989) Urinary bladder neoplasms: evaluation with contrast-enhancement MR imaging. Radiology 172:739–743

Nguyen BD, Westra WH, Zerhouni EA (1996) Renal cell carcinoma and tumor thrombus neovascularity: MR demonstration with pathologic correlation. Abdom Imaging 21:269–271

Norita H, Ohteki H, Todaka K, et al (1992) Malignant fibrous histiocytoma of the heart. Nippon Kyobu Geka Gakkai Zasshi 40:1933–1937

Ogawa T, Iwama Y, Hashimoto H, Ito T, Satake T (1991) Noninvasive methods in the diagnosis of ruptured aneurysm of Valsalva. Usefulness of magnetic resonance imaging and Doppler echocardiography. Chest 100:579–581

Oshima H, Hara M, Kono T, et al (2003) Cardiac hemangioma of the left atrial appendage: CT and MR findings. J Thorac Imaging 18:204–206

Ouzan J, Joundi A, Chapoutot L et al (1990) Malignant histiocytofibroma of the heart simulating myxoma of the left atrium (in French). Arch Mal Coeur Vaiss 83:1011–1013

Oyama N, Oyama N, Komatsu H (2003) Left ventricular asynchrony caused by an intramuscular lipoma. Computed tomography and magnetic resonance dectection. Circulation 107:e200–e201

Papa MZ, Shinfeld A, Klein E, Greif F, Ben AG (1994) Cardiac metastasis of liposarcoma. J Surg Oncol 55:132–134

Parmley LF, Salley RK, Williams JP, Head G3 (1988) The clinical spectrum of cardiac fibroma with diagnostic and surgical considerations: noninvasive imaging enhances management. Ann Thorac Surg 45:455–465

Pasaoglu I, Dogan R, Pasaoglu E, Tokgozoglu L (1994) Surgical treatment of giant hydatid cyst of the left ventricle and diagnostic value of magnetic resonance imaging. Cardiovasc Surg 2:114–116

Paul JG, Rhodes DB, Skow JR (1975) Renal cell carcinoma presenting as right atrial tumor with successful removal using cardiopulmonary bypass. Ann Surg 181:471–473

Paydarfar D, Krieger D, Dib N et al (2001) In vivo magnetic resonance imaging and surgical histopathology of intracardiac masses: distinct features of subacute thrombi. Cardiology 95:40–47

Phillips MR, Bower TC, Orszulak TA, Hartmann LC (1995) Intracardiac extension of an intracaval sarcoma of endometrial origin. Ann Thorac Surg 59:742–744

Pinelli G, Carteaux JP, Mertes PM, et al (1995) Mitral valve tumor revealed by stroke. J Heart Valve Dis 4:199–201

Raaf HN, Raaf JH (1994) Sarcomas related to the heart and vasculature. Semin Surg Oncol 10:374–382

Raffa H, Mosieri J, Sorefan AA, Kayali MT (1991) Sinus of Valsalva aneurysm eroding into the interventricular septum. Ann Thorac Surg 51:996–998

Reid PG, Goudevenos JA, Hilton CJ (1990) Thrombosed saccular aneurysm of a sinus of Valsalva: unusual cause of a mediastinal mass. Br Heart J 63:183–185

Ritchey ML, Kinard R, Novicki DE (1987) Adrenal tumors: involvement of the inferior vena cava. J Urol 38:1134–1136

Roberts CS, Gottdiener JS, Roberts WC (1990) Clinically undetected cardiac lymphoma causing fatal congestive heart failure. Am Heart J 120:1239–1242

Roberts WC, Glancy DL, Vita VT de (1968) Heart in malignant lymphoma (Hodgkin's disease, lymphosarcoma, reticulum cell sarcoma and mycosis fungoides). A study of 196 autopsy cases. Am Heart J 22:85–108

Rosado de Christenson ML, Pugatch RD, Moran CA, Galobardes J (1994) Thymolipoma: analysis of 27 cases. Radiology 193:121–126

Rosenberg JM, Marvasti MA, Obeid A, Johnson LW, Bonaventura M (1988) Intravenous leiomyomatosis: a rare cause of right sided cardiac obstruction. Eur J Cardiothorac Surg 2:58–60

Rosenthal DS, Braunwald E (1992) Cardiac manifestations of neoplastic disease. Saunders, Philadelphia, pp 1752–1760

Rote AR, Flint LD, Ellis FH (1977) Intracaval extension of pheochromocytoma extending into the right atrium: surgical management using intracorporeal circulation. N Engl J Med 296:1269–1271

Rumancik WM, Naidich DP, Chandra R et al (1988) Cardiovascular disease: evaluation with MR phase imaging. Radiology 166:63–68

Sakai F, Sone S, Kiyono K et al (1992) MR imaging of thymoma: radiologic-pathologic correlation. Am J Roentgenol 158:751–756

Salcedo EE, Cohen GI, White RD, Davison MB (1992) Cardiac tumors: diagnosis and management. Curr Probl Cardiol 17:73–137

Sato Y, Togawa K, Ogawa K, et al (1995) Magnetic resonance imaging of cardiac hemangiopericytoma. Heart Vessels 10:328–330

Schneider B, Hanrath P, Vogel P, Meinertz T (1990) Improved morphologic characterization of atrial septal aneurysm by transesophageal echocardiography: relation to cerebro-vascular events. J Am Coll Cardiol 16:1000–1009

Sechtem U, Tscholakoff D, Higgins CB (1986) MRI of the abnormal pericardium. Am J Roentgenol 147:245–252

Sechtem U, Theissen P, Heindel W et al (1989) Diagnosis of left ventricular thrombi by magnetic resonance imaging and comparison with angiocardiography, computed tomography and echocardiography. Am J Cardiol 64:1195–1199

Semelka RC, Shoenut JP, Wilson ME, Pellech AE, Patton JN (1992) Cardiac masses: signal intensity features on spin-echo, gradient-echo, gadolinium-enhanced spin-echo, and TurboFLASH images. J Magn Reson Imaging 2:415–420

Shahian DM, Labib SB, Chang G (1995) Cardiac papillary fibroelastoma (see comments). Ann Thorac Surg 59:538–541

Shellock FG, Morisoli SM (1994a) Ex vivo evaluation of ferromagnetism, heating, and artifacts produced by heart valve prostheses exposed to a 1.5-T MR system. J Magn Reson Imaging 4:756–758

Shellock FG, Morisoli SM (1994b) Ex vivo evaluation of ferromagnetism and artifacts of cardiac occluders exposed to a 1.5-T MR system. J Magn Reson Imaging 4:213–215

Singh RN, Burkholder JA, Magovern GJ (1984) Coronary arteriography as an aid in the diagnosis of angiosarcoma of the heart. Cardiovasc Intervent Radiol 7:40–43

Smith AJ, Panidis IP, Berger S, Gonzales R (1990) Large atrial septal aneurysm mimicking a cystic right atrial mass. Am Heart J 120:714–716

Spuentrup E, Mahnken AH, Kühl HP et al (2003) Fast interactive real-time magnetic resonance imaging of cardiac masses using spiral gradient echo and radial steady-state free precession sequences. Invest Radiol 38:288–292

Stanford W, Galvin JR, Weiss RM, Hajduczok ZD, Skorton DJ (1991) Ultrafast computed tomography in cardiac imaging: a review. Semin Ultrasound CT MR 12:45–60

Steinmetz OK, Bedard P, Prefontaine ME, Bourke M, Barber GG (1996) Uterine tumor in the heart: intravenous leiomyomatosis. Surgery 119:226–229

Stratton JR, Ligthy GW, Pearlman AS (1982) Detection of left ventricular thrombus by two-dimensional echocardiography: sensitivity, specificity, and causes of uncertainty. Circulation 66:156–164

Szucs RA, Rehr RB, Yanovich S, Tatum JL (1991) Magnetic resonance imaging of cardiac rhabdomyosarcoma. Quantifying the response to chemotherapy. Cancer 67:2066–2070

Takamizawa S, Sugimoto K, Tanaka H, et al (1992) A case of primary leiomyosarcoma of the heart. Intern Med 31:265–268

Teramoto N, Hayashi K, Miyatani K et al (1995) Malignant fibrous histiocytoma of the right ventricle of the heart. Pathol Int 45:315–319

Tesoro Tess JD, Biasi S, Balzarini L et al (1993) Heart involvement in lymphomas. The value of magnetic resonance imaging and two-dimensional echocardiography at disease presentation. Cancer 72:2484–2490

Thomas D, Desruennes M, Jault F, Isnard R, Gandjbakhch I (1993) Cardiac and extracardiac abscesses in bacterial endocarditis (in French). Arch Mal Coeur Vaiss 86:1825–1835

Thompson NW, Brown J, Orringer M, Sisson J, Nishiyama R (1978) Follicular carcinoma of the thyroid with massive angioinvasion: extension of tumor thrombus to the heart. Surgery 83:451–457

Uchida S, Obayashi N, Yamanari H, et al (1992) Papillary fibroelastoma in the left ventricular outflow tract. Heart Vessels 7:164–167

Ünal M, Tuncer C, Serce K, et al (1995) A cardiac giant hydatid cyst of the interventricular septum masquerading as ischemic heart disease: role of MR imaging. Acta Cardiol 50:323–326

Urba WJ, Longo DL (1986) Primary solid tumors of the heart. In: Kapoor AS (ed) Cancer and the heart. Springer, New York Berlin Heidelberg, pp 62–75

Van Goethem JW, Parizel PM, Perdieus D, Hermans P, Moor J de (1991) MR and CT imaging of paraspinal textiloma (gossypiboma). J Comput Assist Tomogr 15:1000–1003

Vanjak D, Moutaoufik M, Leroy O et al (1990) Cardiac hydatidosis: contribution of magnetic resonance imaging. Report of a case (in French). Arch Mal Coeur Vaiss 83:1739–1742

Varghese JC, Hahn PF, Papanicolaou N, et al (1997) MR differentiation of phae-chromocytoma from other adrenal lesions based on qualitative analysis of T2 relaxation times. Clin Radiol 52:603–606

Vinee P, Stover B, Sigmund G et al (1992) MR imaging of the pericardial cyst. J Magn Reson Imaging 2:593–596

Vogel HJ, Wondergem JH, Falke TH (1989) Mesothelioma of the pericardium: CT and MR findings. J Comput Assist Tomogr 13:543–544

Walker PG, Pedersen EM, Oyre S et al (1995) Magnetic resonance velocity imaging: a new method for prosthetic heart valve study. J Heart Valve Dis 4:296–307

Watanabe M, Takazawa K, Wada A et al (1994) Cardiac myxoma with Gamna-Gandy bodies: case report with MR imaging. J Thorac Imaging 9:185–187

Wiemer J, Winkelmann BR, Beyersdorf F et al (1996) Multiplicity of clinical symptoms and manifestations of unruptured aneurysms of the sinus of Valsalva. Three case reports. Z Kardiol 85:221–225

Williams ES, Kaplan JI, Thatcher F, Zimmerman G, Knoebel SB (1980) Prolongation of proton spin lattice relaxation times in regionally ischemic tissue from dog hearts. J Nucl Med 21:449–453

Winkler ML, Higgins CB (1986) MRI of perivalvular infectious pseudoaneurysms. Am J Roentgenol 147:253–256

Wolf JE, Lambert B, Pilichowski P et al (1987) Value of magnetic resonance imaging in a lipoma of the left ventricle (in French). Arch Mal Coeur Vaiss 80:1801–1805

Yanagisawa H (1991) Left ventricular intramyocardial rhabdomyoma suggested by coronary angiography. Cardiology 79:146–150

Yousem DM, Lexa FJ, Bilaniuk LT, Zimmerman RI (1990) Rhabdomyosarcomas in the head and neck: MR imaging evaluation. Radiology 177:683–686

Zerhouni EA, Parish DM, Rogers WJ, Yang A, Shapiro EP (1988) Human heart: tagging with MR imaging - a new method for noninvasive assessment of myocardial motion. Radiology 169:59–63

13 Valvular Heart Disease

Andrew M. Taylor and Jan Bogaert

CONTENTS

A. M. Taylor MD, MRCP, FRCR
Cardiothoracic Unit, Institute of Child Health and Great Ormond Street Hospital for Children, London WC1N 3JH, UK
J. Bogaert MD, PhD
Department of Radiology, Gasthuisberg University Hospital, Catholic University of Leuven, Herestraat 49, 3000 Leuven, Belgium

13.1
Introduction

Over the last 5 years, the principles of valvular heart disease assessment with magnetic resonance imaging (MRI) have not changed significantly. By measuring both flow in the great vessels and right and left ventricular volumes by cardiovascular MRI, valvular function can be accurately and reproducibly quantified. However, what has changed is the speed with which a complete assessment of valvular function and associated pathology can be performed, with improved MR hardware and software that enables rapid acquisition of MR data. With these improvements, assessment of valvular function on a routine basis has become a reality.

When investigating cardiac valves, the information required can be divided into four categories:
- Clarification of the affected valve after auscultation of the heart
- Definition of the valvular anatomy (valve leaflet number, leaflet thickness, presence of infective endocarditis)
- Assessment of valvular function (degree of valvular stenosis or regurgitation)
- Definition of the effect of the valvular dysfunction on other cardiac structures and function (ventricular size, function and mass, pulmonary artery pressure, great vessel anatomy)

These questions can be addressed by combining echocardiography with X-ray angiography. However, cardiovascular MRI can now provide much of the required information in a single investigation that is safe, noninvasive, without exposure to X-rays.

In this chapter, we will present an overview of the MRI techniques that are currently used in the assessment of valvular heart disease, provide protocols for the cardiovascular MRI assessment of valvular heart disease, and identify new areas of development in this field. We will also discuss the advantages and limitations of cardiovascular MRI with reference to more conventional imaging modalities for investigating valvular heart disease.

13.2
Conventional Imaging Modalities

13.2.1
Transthoracic Echocardiography

Transthoracic echocardiography remains the most important and easily accessible investigation for the assessment of valvular heart disease (CARABELLO and CRAWFORD 1997). The technique is noninvasive, safe, portable and accurate at localizing the diseased valve. Quantification of valvular stenosis and valve area can be easily performed (CURRIE et al. 1985); however, echocardiography is less good at quantifying valvular regurgitation (HATLE and ANGELSON 1992; SMITH and XIE 1998). A semiquantitative assessment can be achieved by measuring the regurgitant jet length and width, but there is poor correlation to X-ray angiographic measurements (ABBASI et al. 1980; QUINONES et al. 1980; BOLGER et al. 1988). Several echocardiography methods have been developed in an attempt to quantify valvular regurgitation, but all have their limitations. The regurgitant fraction can be calculated, but this is time-consuming; only patients with isolated valvular regurgitation can be readily assessed (ROCKEY et al. 1987); and echocardiography only provides an estimate of ventricular function (BOEHRER et al. 1992). Imaging of the proximal isovelocity surface area has been proposed. However, this technique relies on the assumption that the regurgitant jet orifice is both flat and circular, which is not the case for most patients (UTSUNOMIYA et al. 1991). A final limitation of transthoracic echocardiography is that the imaging plane may be restricted by the lack of good acoustic windows.

13.2.2
Transesophageal Echocardiography

Transesophageal echocardiography is valuable in the assessment of left atrial thrombus (MANNING

et al. 1993), atrial septal wall defects (HAUSMANN et al. 1992), and aortic dissection (TICE and KISSLO 1993; LAISSY et al. 1995). In the assessment of valvular heart disease, the technique may clarify valvular anatomy in patients with infective endocarditis (PEDERSEN et al. 1991) or in patients with poor acoustic windows. With regard to functional assessment, it is less accurate than transthoracic echocardiography because of difficulties with Doppler alignment and has all the limitations of transthoracic echocardiography in the assessment of valvular regurgitation, in addition to being an invasive procedure. A unique use for transesophageal echocardiography is in the intraoperative assessment of valvular function for monitoring and evaluating surgical and percutaneous interventions (FIX et al. 1993; BRYAN et al. 1995).

13.2.3
X-ray Angiography

X-ray angiography has been regarded as the gold standard investigation of valvular heart disease, against which other imaging modalities should be compared (SANDLER et al. 1963; SELLERS et al. 1964; CARROLL 1993). Valvular stenosis can be quantified by calculating the transvalvular gradients and valve areas using the Gorlin formula (GORLIN and GORLIN 1951). However, the grading system used for the assessment of valvular regurgitation is both imprecise and inaccurate. Although generally regarded as safe, the technique is associated with a mortality of approximately 0.1%, and other complications occur such as myocardial infarction, arterial embolization, thrombosis, and dissection (DAVIS et al. 1979). Also the use of ionizing radiation during the procedure is not ideal (COHEN 1991). In general, X-ray angiography should only be regarded as necessary if the pulmonary artery pressure needs accurate measurement, if the coronary artery anatomy needs defining, or if there is a discrepancy between the clinical symptoms and the noninvasive investigations.

13.2.4
Radionuclide Angiography

The main use of radionuclide angiography is in the monitoring of ventricular function in order to assess when interventions should take place (RIGO et al. 1979; SORENSON et al. 1980). The technique can also be used to calculate the regurgitant fraction, but again only when regurgitation in a single valve is present. As with X-ray angiography, the use of ionizing radiation is not ideal, especially as serial measurements of ventricular function are necessary.

13.3
MRI of Cardiac Valves

MRI can provide good functional information about both valvular stenosis and regurgitation, and allows accurate assessment of ventricular function and relevant cardiac and vascular anatomy.

13.3.1
Morphology

13.3.1.1
Valve Leaflets

Normal valves are fast-moving, low proton-density, fine structures that are difficult to visualize with con-

ventional spin-echo (SE) "black-blood" imaging, due to respiratory motion and averaging. However, newer fast SE sequences allow for the acquisition of data at defined points in the cardiac cycle during a single breath-hold (Fig. 13.1). When thickened and immobile valve leaflet identification is more common.

Using spoiled gradient-echo (GE) or balanced steady-state free precession (b-SSFP) cine imaging, the moving leaflets are easily seen, because blood flowing over the valve tips leads to signal loss, secondary to eddies and mild turbulence (KIVELITZ et al. 2003) (Fig. 13.2).

Despite these improvements in defining valve leaflet morphology, echocardiography remains the investigation of choice for imaging valve leaflet anatomy.

13.3.1.2
Thrombus

It is important to identify the presence of thrombus in the atria, particularly in the presence of mitral stenosis or valvular disease with atrial fibrillation.

SE imaging can identify atrial thrombus, but care must be taken to distinguish between slow-moving

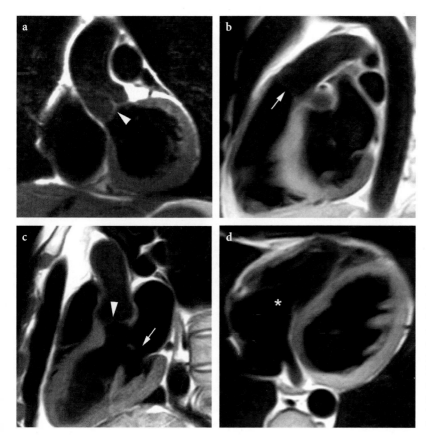

Fig. 13.1a-d. T1-weighted fast spin-echo (FSE) images of the cardiac valves. a Oblique coronal view of the aortic valve (*arrowhead*). b Oblique sagittal view of the pulmonary valve (*white arrow*). c Left ventricle inflow/outflow view of the mitral valve (*arrow*) and aortic valve (*arrowhead*). d Axial view (systole) of the tricuspid valve (*star*)

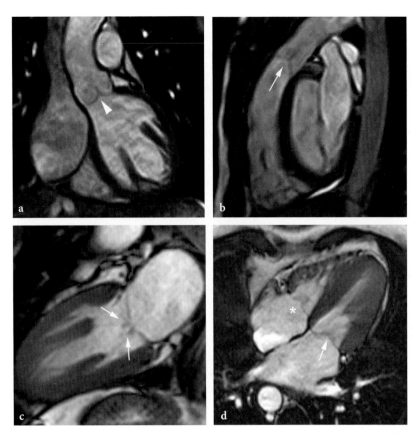

Fig. 13.2a-d. Balanced steady-state free precession (b-SSFP) images of the valves. **a** Oblique coronal view of the aortic valve (*arrowhead*). **b** Oblique sagittal view of the pulmonary valve (*arrow*). **c** Vertical long-axis view of the mitral valve. The *arrows* indicate the insertion points of the chordae tendinae into the tips of the valve leaflets. **d** Four-chamber view (systole) of the tricuspid (*star*) and mitral valves (*arrow*)

blood that may appear as increased signal on these images (Dooms and Higgins 1986). Cine MRI and velocity mapping should thus be used to confirm the presence and size of any apparent mass (Fig. 13.3).

Thrombus can also be distinguished from other atrial masses using gadolinium (Gd)-based contrast agents (Weinmann et al. 1984). Recently, we have shown that late-enhancement MRI that has been developed for myocardial infarct imaging (see Chap. 8) can be utilized to image thrombus (Bogaert et al. 2004). Images are acquired using inversion-recovery contrast-enhanced MRI (3D T1-weighted turbo-field-echo technique) performed 10-20 min after intravenous injection of Gd-diethylene triamine penta-acetic acid (DTPA) (0.2 mmol/kg body weight). The inversion time is adjusted for optimal suppression of normal myocardial signal (inversion time approx. 200–300 ms). Enhancement of the blood-pool is excellent to depict abnormal intraluminal structures, such as thrombi (Fig. 13.3b).

13.3.1.3
Endocarditis

Only very large vegetations can be demonstrated by SE MRI. Fast GE imaging has been shown to be helpful in clarifying echocardiographic findings in aortic valve vegetations (Caduff et al. 1996). MRI can be invaluable in the identification of abscesses (Jeang et al. 1986) or if infection has spread outside the heart (Fig. 13.4). Furthermore, sinus of Valsalva rupture, secondary to endocarditis, can be seen on MR images

13.3.2
Valvular Regurgitation

Currently none of the conventional imaging techniques can accurately define valvular regurgitation and it is here that MRI has particular value. Cardiovascular MR can image the regurgitant jet in any plane, and thus a 3D appreciation of the jet can be acquired. Furthermore, MRI can quantify the regurgitant volume, either as an absolute value or as the regurgitant fraction. Such a noninvasive quantification of the degree of valvular regurgitation, in combination with information about ventricular function, is of particular clinical relevance for the timing of valve replacement.

MR assessment of valvular regurgitation severity can be evaluated by using the following techniques:

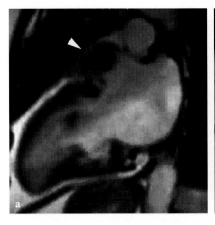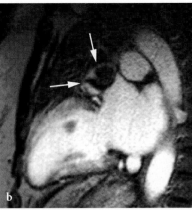

Fig. 13.3. a Vertical long-axis b-SSFP image showing thrombus in the left atrial appendage (*arrowhead*). **b** Vertical long-axis contrast-enhanced MR image, using T1-weighted 3D fast-field-echo technique (TR 4.3 ms, TE 1.3 ms, inversion time 240 ms), obtained 8 min after injection of 0.2 mmol/kg of Gd-DTPA, showing thrombus in left atrial appendage (*arrows*)

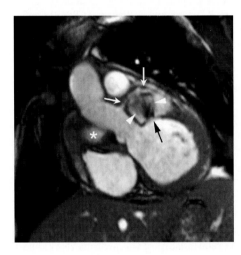

Fig. 13.4. Aortic root pseudoaneurysm following aortic valve replacement for endocarditis. The pseudoaneurysm surrounds the aorta (*star* and *white arrowheads*), and displaces the left main stem coronary artery (*white arrows*). *Black arrow* shows communication between LV and pseudoaneurysm, which fills during each cardiac contraction

- Qualitative assessment of signal loss on cine MR images
- Quantitative assessment by measurement of ventricular volumes
- Quantitative assessment by phase-contrast velocity mapping

13.3.2.1
Qualitative Assessment with Cine Gradient-Echo Imaging

In cine MRI using the spoiled-GE technique, dephasing of the proton spins, secondary to turbulent flow, leads to signal loss (EVANS et al. 1988).

Imaging over multiple frames (20–40) enables accurate assessment of the turbulent flow, throughout the cardiac cycle. For regurgitant lesions the signal loss can be graded in a similar way to X-ray angiography: grade 1 = signal loss close to the valve; grade 2 = signal loss extending into the proximal chamber; grade 3 = signal loss filling the whole of the proximal chamber; grade 4 = signal loss in the receiving chamber throughout the relevant half of the cardiac cycle (Fig. 13.5) (UNDERWOOD et al. 1987a; SECHTEM et al. 1987). This qualitative method has been validated, but is unable to separate turbulent volumes when dual valve disease exists (e.g., aortic regurgitation and mitral stenosis), and there remains poor reproducibility of the technique between centers (SECHTEM et al. 1988; WAGNER et al. 1989; GLOBITS et al. 1991). In addition, signal loss is very dependent on MR parameters such as echo time (TE), and jet size is easily underestimated when it impinges on the myocardial wall, as has been known from echocardiography for some years.

With the increasing use of b-SSFP cine imaging in cardiovascular MRI (ZUR et al. 1990), qualitative assessment of signal loss has become less useful. Though b-SSFP white-blood images are much quicker to acquire with better endocardial/blood pool definition than conventional GE imaging (PERELES et al. 2001; BARKHAUSEN et al. 2001), the sequence is designed to be relatively flow-insensitive. This results in reduced visualization of flow disturbance secondary to valvular regurgitation, in particular when regurgitation is mild. Thus, in subjects who are being imaged for other reasons, incidental detection of mild valvular regurgitation may not be apparent on b-SSFP cine imaging.

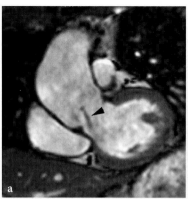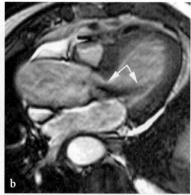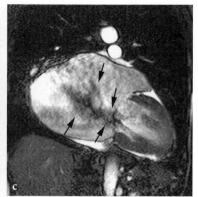

Fig. 13.5a-c. Balanced-SSFP images. **a** Oblique coronal left ventricular outflow tract view. Grade 1–2 aortic regurgitation (*black arrowhead*) in a patient with aortic root dilatation due to Marfan syndrome. **b** Oblique axial left ventricle inflow/outflow view. Grade 3 aortic regurgitation (*white arrows*). **c** Vertical long-axis view. Grade 4 mitral regurgitation (*black arrows*); note the massively dilated left atrium. (Image **c**: Courtesy of F. Melonas, R. Truter, and G. Wagner, SCP MRI Center, Cape Town, South Africa)

13.3.2.2
Quantitative Evaluation of Ventricular Volume Measurement

MRI can now be regarded as the best available in vivo technique for the measurement of ventricular volumes (see Chap. 6) (SAKUMA et al. 1993; BOGAERT et al. 1995; GROTHUES et al. 2002). In particular, b-SSFP imaging enables good blood-pool/endocardial contrast images to be acquired in a single breath-hold (MOON et al. 2002; ALFAKIH et al. 2003). Using a set of short-axis cuts covering the length of the ventricles, in combination with Simpson's rule, the stroke volumes of both the right and the left ventricle can be measured (DULCE et al. 1993) (see Chap. 6).

In normal individuals there is a 1:1 relationship between these stroke volumes. Any discrepancy between the ventricular volumes in a patient with regurgitation will identify the regurgitant volume. The main limitation of this technique, when used alone, is that only patients with a single regurgitant valve can be assessed. Overall imaging times are now significantly shorter than 5 years ago. In general, one or two short-axis images can be acquired in a single breath-hold, and newer sequence implementations enable the acquisition of a complete short-axis stack in a single breath-hold (LEE et al. 2002; HORI et al. 2003; TAYLOR et al. 2004). Thus, a complete MRI assessment of ventricular volumes can be performed in approximately 40 min (20 min acquisition time, 20 min analysis time (BELLENGER et al. 2000).

13.3.2.3
Quantitative Evaluation with Velocity Mapping

For velocity mapping, phase information and not magnitude information is displayed. The application of short-lived magnetic gradients allows each point in the imaging plane to be encoded with a phase shift that is directly proportional to the velocity at that point. Because phase shifts can arise from other factors, a second velocity-compensated phase image is acquired, and subtraction yields the actual phase relationship of the protons (NAYLER et al. 1986; UNDERWOOD et al. 1987b). Velocity encoding can be applied in any direction (through-plane, left to right, up and down), though for flow quantification through-plane imaging is used, and the size of the velocity window defined for increased sensitivity. Stationary material is represented as mid-gray, while increasing velocities in either direction are shown in increasing grades of black or white (Fig. 13.6). It is important to define the velocity encode window as close to the peak velocity as possible, to reduce aliasing of peak velocities, while maintaining sensitivity for flow measurements.

Measurement of the spatial mean velocity for all pixels in a region of interest of known area enables the calculation of the instantaneous flow volume at any point in the cardiac cycle. Calculation of the flow volume per heart beat can be made by integrating the instantaneous flow volumes for all frames throughout the cardiac cycle. This technique has been validated in vitro and in vivo, and is extremely accurate and reproducible (FIRMIN et al. 1987; MEIER et al. 1988; BOGREN et al. 1989a). It now represents the

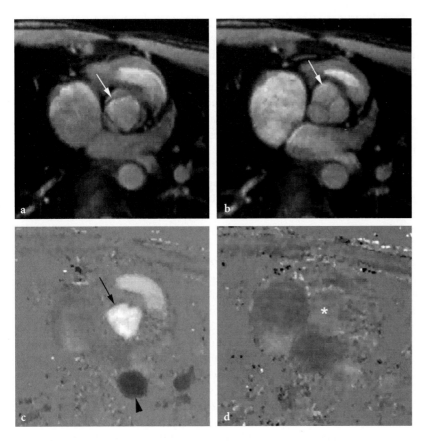

Fig. 13.6a-d. Phase-contrast velocity map, TE 5 ms, velocity-encoding window ±1.5 m/s. **a, b** Magnitude image at level of aortic root (*white arrow*) during **a** systole and **b** diastole. The opening and closing of the three valve leaflets can be clearly seen. **c, d** Velocity image in the same imaging plane during **c** systole and **d** diastole. Stationary material is represented as midgray, while flow toward the head in the aortic root is represented by white pixels (*black arrow* in **c**, and flow toward the feet in the descending aorta (*arrowhead in* **c**) is represented by black pixels. There is little or no flow in the aortic root during diastole (*star*) during valve closure

best available in vivo technique for flow measurements. Quantification of the right ventricular (RV) and left ventricular (LV) outputs can be compared using through-plane flow measurements from the proximal ascending aorta and pulmonary trunk (1:1 ratio in normal individuals) (KONDO et al. 1991), thus allowing quantification of pulmonary to systemic shunting (and vice versa) (see Chap. 15.3).

The severity of regurgitation can be defined as follows (SECHTEM et al. 1988):
- Mild: regurgitant fraction 15–20%
- Moderate: regurgitant fraction 20–40%
- Severe: regurgitant fraction >40%

Conventionally, phase-contrast GE images are acquired during shallow respiration over several minutes. Faster imaging can be performed, and it is now possible to acquire real-time phase-contrast data (KORPERICH et al. 2004).

13.3.2.4
Issues Related to MRI Functional Measurements

There are several technical issues that must be addressed when performing phase-contrast velocity mapping. Firstly, phase-contrast imaging should be performed as close to the center of the main magnet field (B_0) as possible. This ensures phase errors introduced by eddy currents and Maxwell terms are kept to a minimum.

Secondly, the imaging plane should be perpendicular to the vessel. This ensures that the velocity vectors of the majority of the voxels are perpendicular to the imaging plane. This can be achieved by planning the through-plane imaging position from two perpendicular views (e.g., LV outflow tract plane and LV inflow/outflow plane for the aortic valve) (see Figs. 5.5–5.8).

Thirdly, the imaging plane should not be at the level of the valve, but just proximal or distal to the valve annulus. This ensures that artifacts secondary to eddy currents and the complex motion of the valve annulus are kept to a minimum. One possible method to compensate for motion of the valve annulus through the imaging plane is to use a moving slice velocity-mapping (or slice tracking) technique (KOZERKE et al. 1999). This experimental method enables the imaging slice to follow the valve annulus during the cardiac cycle, reducing velocity offsets and demonstrating discrepancies in conventional measurements of aortic and mitral regurgitation measurements by cardiovascular MR (Kozerke et al. 2001a).

And finally, it is important to have a degree of quality control with regard to ventricular volumes and flow measurements, and it is worthwhile performing two validation experiments on one's own scanner. The first validation is to use a flow phantom and compare MR measured flows with those acquired using a bucket and stopwatch method (Fig. 13.7). Such an experiment will only be possible in centers with access to a flow phantom, but will help confirm the accuracy of your own scanner. The second validation can be performed in any center and involves assessing ventricular volumes and flow measurements in normal healthy volunteers. In this group of subjects, the stroke volume of the ventricles calculated from the ventricular volume assessment should equal the net forward flow measured by phase-contrast velocity mapping. Thus, the normal subjects act as their own control for all the measurements acquired.

13.3.3
Valvular Stenosis

The presence of valvular stenosis can be identified by signal loss seen in cine MR images. Velocity map-

ping may then be used to establish an accurate peak velocity across the valve to quantify the severity of the stenosis. The use of the mean velocity across the caval veins and mitral valve can be used to describe the inflow curves for the atrioventricular valves (Mohiaddin et al. 1990). Concomitant changes in myocardial mass, due to increase in afterload, can be precisely assessed with cine MRI.

13.3.3.1
Qualitative Assessment with Cine Gradient-Echo Imaging

For stenotic lesions, the degree of signal loss is dependent on the degree of stenosis and the echo time used. Thus, for shorter echo times less proton spin dephasing can take place and more signal is recovered (DeRoos et al. 1989; Kilner et al. 1991). Figure 13.8 demonstrates the relationship between the echo time and the peak velocity across a stenosis. Thus, in more severe stenosis, a lower echo time must be used to prevent signal loss in the images.

As with the qualitative assessment of valvular regurgitating, signal loss is less marked on the increasingly used b-SSFP cine imaging, due to the design and short TE of this sequence. It is thus much more difficult to get a feel for the peak velocity with

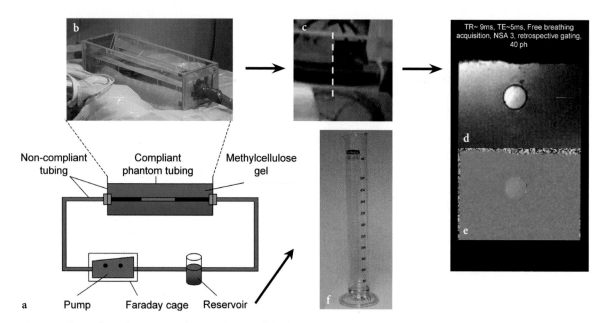

Fig. 13.7a-f. MR flow phantom. **a** Schematic layout of the flow phantom. A programmable pump is used to create pulsatile flow for the range of flows seen in the aorta and pulmonary trunk. **b, c** Compliant tubing set in methylcellulose gel is used to mimic the compliant vessel. **d, e** MR phase-contrast imaging is performed to measure flow, through-plane, in the compliant tubing (*dotted line*) – **d** magnitude image, **e** velocity map. **f** The flowing fluid (water with dilute gadolinium to give the same T1 as blood) is collected over 1 min to give a flow in milliliters per minute, which is then correlated to the MR flow calculations

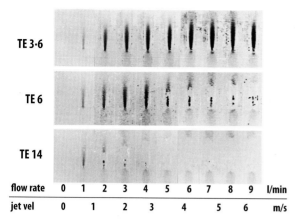

| flow rate | 0 | 1 | 2 | 3 | 4 | 5 | 6 | 7 | 8 | 9 | l/min |
| jet vel | 0 | | 1 | | 2 | | 3 | | 4 | | 5 | | 6 | | m/s |

Fig. 13.8. In vitro jet velocity mapping. Velocity maps obtained with MRI of flow – increased from left to right – through the test stenosis, showing the significance of shortening the TE from 14 ms (*bottom*) to 6 ms (*center*) and 3.6 ms (*top*). Only the 3.6-ms TE sequence allows mapping of high-velocity jets, up to a maximum tested velocity of 6.0 m/s. (Reprinted with permission from KILNER et al. 1991)

b-SSFP sequences than with conventional spoiled-GE cine imaging.

Valve area can also be measured on cine MR images, and this measurement has been shown to correlate well with Doppler echocardiography and catheterization (SONDERGAARD et al. 1993a; FRIEDRICH et al. 2002).

13.3.3.2
Quantitative Evaluation with Velocity Mapping

Direct measurement from the phase-contrast velocity map enables measurement of the peak velocity across the valve, and application of the modified Bernoulli equation enables an estimate of the gradient across the valve:

$$\Delta P = 4V^2 \qquad (1)$$

where *P is* the pressure drop across the stenosis (in millimeters of mercury) and *V is* velocity (in meters per second). The technique is comparable with Doppler echocardiography valvular stenosis measurements and has an in vitro accuracy of 4% (SIMPSON et al. 1993). The main advantage of the technique over echocardiography is that the velocity jet can be aligned easily in any direction without the limitation of acoustic windows.

Imaging can be performed through-plane (velocity jet perpendicular to the imaging plane) or in-plane (velocity jet parallel to the imaging plane). Both strategies have their advantages and disadvan-

tages. For the in-plane method, the entire jet can be visualized, and the point within the jet of peak velocity easily identified. However, not all jets are easily aligned in a single 2D plane, and, for tight narrow jets, there may be partial volume averaging and motion within the imaging slice, and the peak velocity may not be accurately depicted. For through-plane imaging, the jet will always pass through the imaging plane, but, as only part of the stenotic jet is sampled, the peak velocity may not be measured. It is thus best to use a combination of the two strategies with initial definition of the jet in-plane and quantification with through-plane imaging at the site of maximum velocity on the in-plane image.

Selection of the correct velocity-encode gradient is essential to maintain sensitivity and accuracy of measurements, while avoiding aliasing. Most scanners now have a fast phase-contrast velocity-mapping sequence that can be acquired in approximately 15–20 s. This enables an estimate of the peak velocity to be made before progressing to the more time-consuming conventional phase-contrast velocity-mapping sequence.

Using data acquired from phase-contrast flow curves, the continuity question can be used to calculate valve area. For the aortic valve, velocity is measured below the valve in the left ventricular outflow tract (LVOT) and above the valve in the aorta (Ao). The velocity time integral (VTI) is measured for systolic forward flow in both planes (CARUTHERS et al. 2003) (Fig. 13.9). The aortic valve area A_{Ao} (centimeters squared) is given by:

$$A_{Ao} = A_{LVOT}(VTI_{LVOT}/VTI_{Ao}) \qquad (2)$$

where A_{LVOT} is LVOT area (centimeters squared), VTI_{LVOT} is LVOT VTI, and VTI_{Ao} is Ao VTI].

13.3.4
Aortic Valve

13.3.4.1
Aortic Regurgitation

A protocol for imaging patients with aortic regurgitation is shown in Fig. 13.10. Regurgitant aortic jets are best visualized in the coronal or oblique coronal plane. Estimation of the signal void volume is possible (AURIGEMMA et al. 1991; NISHIMURA 1992; OHNISHI et al. 1992), but care must be taken to ensure that all the jet has been visualized. The most accurate method for quantifying the regurgitant fraction is

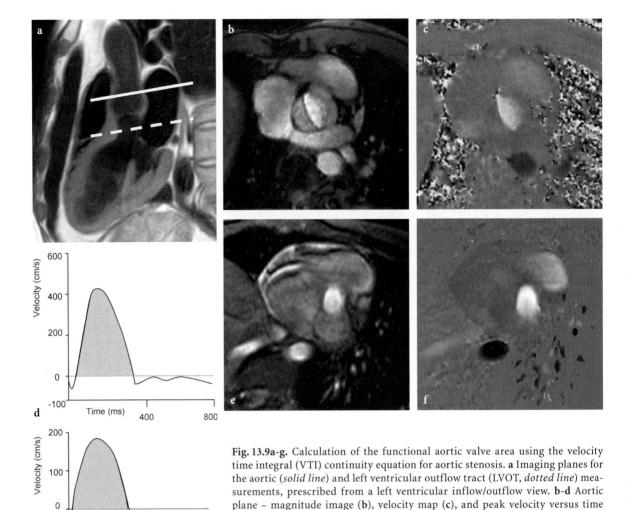

Fig. 13.9a-g. Calculation of the functional aortic valve area using the velocity time integral (VTI) continuity equation for aortic stenosis. **a** Imaging planes for the aortic (*solid line*) and left ventricular outflow tract (LVOT, *dotted line*) measurements, prescribed from a left ventricular inflow/outflow view. **b-d** Aortic plane – magnitude image (**b**), velocity map (**c**), and peak velocity versus time curve (**d**). **e-g** LVOT plane – magnitude image (**e**), velocity map (**f**), and peak velocity vs. time curve (**g**). The summation of the area under the curve (*black shading*) during systole is the VTI. See Eq. 2

with phase-contrast velocity-encoding in the slice direction, in an oblique axial plane above the aortic valve. In order to ensure that the velocity vectors for the majority flow are through-plane in this image, it is best to use two perpendicular images through the ascending aorta and prescribe the oblique axial plane perpendicular to both (see also Fig. 5.5).

A through-plane velocity window of ±1.5 m/s should be set if there is isolated aortic regurgitation. If significant aortic stenosis is present, a dual velocity window, with a high systolic setting of ±5 m/s, changing to ±1.5 m/s for the diastolic frames, may be necessary. Aortic regurgitation volume is the amount of retrograde diastolic flow and is measured in milliliters per beat or liters per minute (milliliters per beat × heart rate) (Fig. 13.11). The aortic regurgitant fraction is given by:

Regurgitant fraction (%) =

$$\frac{\text{Aortic retrograde flow (mL/beat)} \times 100}{\text{Aortic forward flow (mL/beat)}} \quad (3)$$

A good correlation has been demonstrated between ventricular volume measurements and velocity mapping in the ascending aorta, for the calculation of aortic reguritant fractions (SONDERGAARD et al. 1993b). Interstudy reproducibility has been demonstrated to be high and thus the technique is ideal for long-term patient follow-up (DULCE et al. 1992).

Some debate still remains as to the positioning of the plane across the aorta. Current in vivo experience suggests that a position between the coronary ostia and the aortic valve may be most accurate (CHATZIMAVROUDIS et al. 1997). Positions above the coronary ostia lead to inaccuracies secondary

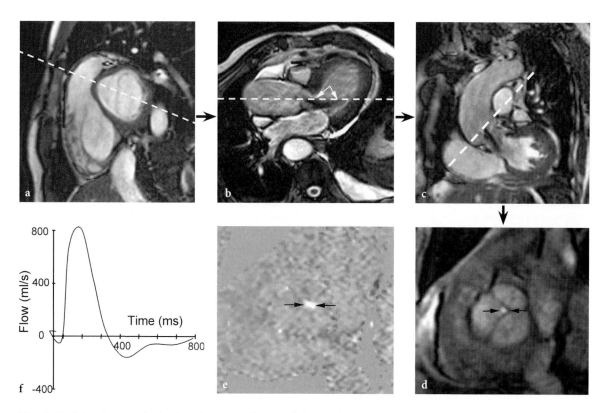

Fig. 13.10a-f. Aortic regurgitation imaging protocol. **a** Basal short-axis b-SSFP cine frame. **b** A plane prescribed through the mitral valve and aortic valve on the basal short-axis view yields the left ventricular inflow/outflow view, which shows grade 2 aortic regurgitation. **c** A perpendicular plane through the jet of regurgitation yields an oblique coronal plane through the aortic valve and LV outflow tract. **d, e** An oblique axial plane in the aortic root, just above the aortic valve at the level of the coronary artery openings, is then defined from both **b** and **c** for phase-contrast velocity mapping. **d** Magnitude image. **e** Velocity map in early diastole shows a narrow jet of aortic regurgitation due to lack of coalition of the valve leaflets centrally (*black arrows*). **f** Flow versus time plot for the ascending aorta. Antegrade flow calculated at 120 ml/beat, retrograde flow 30 ml/beat, and aortic regurgitant fraction 25%

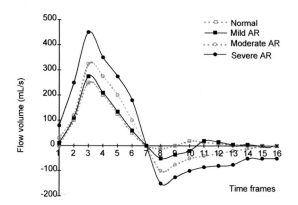

Fig. 13.11. Plots of flow volume versus time frames per cardiac cycle. Measurements were made in the ascending aorta for a normal subject and patients with increasing severity of aortic regurgitation (*AR*). Each point on the graphs represents the blood flow in the aorta for each image in the cardiac cycle. Negative values represent retrograde flow during diastole. Integration of the area under the curve for antegrade and retrograde flow enables calculation of the regurgitant volume per cardiac cycle (milliliters per beat)

to coronary flow and aortic compliance. Further in vivo studies need to be performed to confirm these findings. The commercial application of moving-slice velocity mapping would be a potential aid for slice positioning (KOZERKE et al. 2001a).

Aortic regurgitation can be caused by abnormalities of the aortic leaflets or annulus or be secondary to dilatation of the aortic root. The etiologies of aortic regurgitation are given in Table 13.1.

In acute aortic regurgitation (bacterial endocarditis, aortic dissection, and trauma), ventricular adaptation does not occur and there is a rapid increase in LV filling pressures, reduced cardiac output, increased left atrial pressure, pulmonary edema, and ultimately shock. In chronic aortic regurgitation, the initial response is LV hypertrophy, as compensation for increased wall stress secondary to volume overload. However, over time, the main hemodynamic response to aortic regurgitation is dilatation of the left ventricle and reduction in ventricular function.

Table 13.1 Causes of aortic regurgitation

Valvular causes
  Congenital bicuspid aortic valve
  Rheumatic heart disease
  Bacterial endocarditis
  Myxomatous valve associated with cystic medial necrosis
  Aortic valve prolapse

Secondary to dilatation of the aortic annulus
  Marfan syndrome
  Syphilitic aortitis
  Ankylosing spondylitis
  Reiter disease
  Rheumatoid arthritis
  Ehlers–Danlos syndrome

Secondary to aortic dissection
  Deceleration trauma
  Hypertension

Though medical treatments can be used to deal with the symptomatic effects of aortic regurgitation, surgical valvular replacement remains the treatment option for moderate/severe aortic regurgitation. The timing of surgery is important and is a balance between operating too soon (operative risks, insertion of a valve that will not last for ever, lifelong anticoagulation) and operating too late (irreversible left ventricular failure). Currently, operative timing depends on symptoms, chest X-ray appearance, echocardiographic findings, and the longitudinal changes in these parameters (Bonow et al. 1998). With improving surgical techniques, noninvasive methods of investigation and enhanced knowledge of the natural history and prognosis, there has been progressively earlier application of surgery for both severe aortic and mitral regurgitation (Borer and Bonow 2003) (Table 13.2).

MRI protocols, as outlined above, by providing accurate, quantifiable, and reproducible measurements of regurgitant volume may contribute to the development of more specific criteria for the timing of surgery. As yet, no large-scale cardiovascular MRI studies addressing these issue have been published, though velocity mapping in the ascending aorta has now been performed to analyze the therapeutic effects of ACE inhibition in patients with aortic regurgitation (Globits et al. 1996). MRI has demonstrated the beneficial effects of the therapy and is able to identify those patients with aortic regurgitation who respond favorably to angiotensin-converting enzyme (ACE) inhibition.

13.3.4.2
Aortic Stenosis

Aortic stenosis can be divided into sub-valvular stenosis, valvular stenosis, and supra-valvular stenosis. The hemodynamic consequence of all forms of aortic stenosis is concentric LV hypertrophy. The causes of aortic stenosis are outlined in Table 13.3. Supravalvular aortic stenosis is discussed in the chapter about congenital heart disease (see Chap. 15.4.3). Sub-valvular aortic stenosis can be congenital or, more commonly in adults, occurs secondary to hypertrophic cardiomyopathy (see Chap. 9.4.1). The remainder of this section will concentrate on valvular aortic stenosis.

MRI of aortic stenosis is outlined in Fig. 13.12. The alignment of the jet and definition of the veloc-

Table 13.3 Causes of aortic stenosis

Acquired
  Degenerative (fibrocalcific senile aortic stenosis)
  Rheumatic heart disease
Congenital
  Subvalvular
  Valvular – bicuspid aortic valve
  Supravalvular

Table 13.2 Schema for selecting asymptomatic patients with aortic regurgitation for aortic valve replacement (*AVR*). (*CHF*, congestive heart failure; *LVEF_rest*, left ventricular ejection fraction at rest; *FS_rest*, fractional shortening at rest; *LVID_s*, left ventricular systolic dimension; Δ, change from rest to exercise; *ESS*, end-systolic stress; *LVID_d*, left ventricular diastolic dimension. All dimensions from echocardiography). (Adapted from Borer and Bonow 2003)

Group	AVR replacement	Criteria	Progression to CHF or death (%/year)
I	Definite	Subnormal $LVEF_{rest}$ and/or FS_{rest}	25
II	Strongly considered; definite if ≥2 criteria met	$LVID_s$ ≥55 mm, ≥25 mm/m^2 $\Delta LVEF > -5\%$ $\Delta LVEF - \Delta ESS$ Index $\geq -17\%$	10-20
III	Consider; definite if ≥1 group II criteria also met	$LVID_d$ ≥80 mm "Rapid" $\downarrow LVEF_{rest}$, FS_{rest} "Rapid" $\uparrow LVID_s$, $LVID_d$	7-10

ity-encode window are important variables. The jet core appears as high signal sandwiched between two jets of low signal. For most scanners, the shortest TE sequence will now be used and manual selection of the TE is less common. However, if TE selection is still necessary, the TE and velocity window should be set to aim for greatest signal-to-noise and velocity sensitivity, though, if the shortest TE and largest velocity window are defined, most clinically significant jets will be accounted for.

Good in vivo agreement has been demonstrated for a wide range of pressure gradients across the aortic valve (3–148 mmHg) between MR velocity mapping and Doppler echocardiography and X-ray angiography (EICHENBERGER et al. 1993). In our own practice, we have found it easiest to interpret velocity maps parallel to the jet, as this reveals the jet length in relationship to pre- and poststenotic flows (KILNER et al. 1993a).

Valve area can also be assessed, using either direct visualization of the valve area on cine images (FRIEDRICH et al. 2002; JOHN et al. 2003) (Fig. 13.13) or the application of the continuity equation to MR data (CARUTHERS et al. 2003) (Fig. 13.9). For direct measurement of valve area, the area of flow through-plane at the level of the origin of the flow jet is performed. The results of this technique to date have been conflicting. FRIEDRICH et al. (2002) have demonstrated that direct MR measurement of aortic valve area agree well with aortic area calculated at cardiac catheterization ($r=0.78$), and less well with that calculated at echocardiography ($r=0.52$); while JOHN et al. (2003) have demonstrated good agreement between MR measurements and echocardiography ($r=0.96$), but poor agreement between MR and cardiac catheterization ($r=0.44$). When MR assessment of velocity profiles in the LVOT and aorta was performed and the continuity equation applied (see

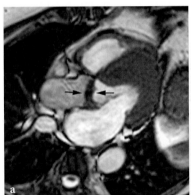
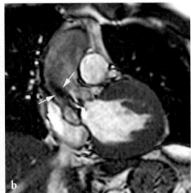
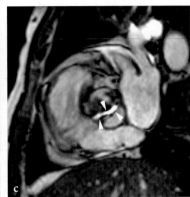

Fig. 13.12a-c. Balanced-SSFP images of severe aortic stenosis. **a** Oblique coronal plane through the aortic valve and LVOT in systole shows a tight jet of signal loss (turbulence) in the ascending aorta (*white arrows*). **b** Left ventricular inflow/outflow view through the aortic valve and LVOT in diastole shows marked thickening of the aortic valve (*black arrows*). **c** Through-plane image in the aortic root above the aortic valve in systole. The narrow jet of turbulent flow can be clearly seen (*white arrowheads*)

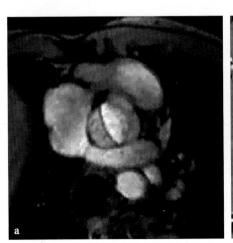
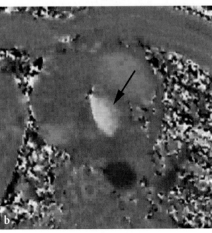

Fig. 13.13a,b. Bicuspid aortic valve (*arrow*). **a** Magnitude image in systole – note the "fish mouth" appearance of the aortic valve aperture, when compared with normal valve opening as shown in Fig. 13.6. **b** Velocity map in systole – forward flow is shown as *white*

Eq. 2 above), there was good agreement between the MR method and similar data acquired with echocardiography (r=0.83) (CARUTHERS et al. 2003).

When imaging aortic stenosis it is also important to assess LV mass and aortic root dimensions. LV mass is increased in aortic stenosis and can be used as a guide to the significance of the aortic stenosis with a reduction in LV hypertrophy seen after aortic valve replacement (RAJAPPAN et al. 2000; SANDSTEDE et al. 2000; LAMB et al. 2002; SENSKY et al. 2003). The aortic root may be dilated secondary to aortic stenosis, and this is well documented in patients with bicuspid aortic valve (ALEGRET et al. 2003; NOVARO et al. 2003; NKOMO et al. 2003). In patients with angina and aortic stenosis, visualization of the coronary arteries is often requested to exclude ischemic heart disease as a contributing factor to the symptoms. At present, this is best performed by direct X-ray cardiac catheterization.

LV contraction can also be assessed using myocardial tagging. In patients with pressure-overloaded hypertrophied ventricles, there is an increase in apical rotation that leads to increased torsion of the left ventricle (NAGEL et al. 2000; SANDSTEDE et al. 2002), and delay and prolongation of diastolic untwisting (NAGEL et al. 2000). Not only do such studies help improve our understanding of cardiac physiology in aortic stenosis, but also they may help clinically to distinguish pathological causes of LV hypertrophy from physiological changes that can occur in the "athlete" heart (see Chap. 9.3). Furthermore, 1 year after aortic valve replacement for aortic stenosis, there is normalization of LV torsion, and monitoring such parameters in patients over time may aide in defining the optimal time for operative intervention in aortic stenosis (SANDSTEDE et al. 2002).

13.3.5
Mitral Valve

13.3.5.1
Mitral Regurgitation

There is good correlation between the signal loss caused by mitral regurgitation on spoiled-GE cine MR images and Doppler and X-ray angiographic grading (AURIGEMMA et al. 1990) (Fig. 13.14). The regurgitant jet is best visualized in either the horizontal or the vertical long-axis plane. MR imaging has the advantage of being able to define lesions in subjects with poor acoustic windows. For alignment of the optimal imaging planes for the mitral valve, see Fig. 5.6.

There are three methods for quantifying mitral regurgitation with cardiovascular MR:

For isolated mitral regurgitation, ventricular volume measurements provide an accurate method for quantifying mitral regurgitation (HUNDLEY et al. 1995):

$$\text{Regurgitant volume (ml/beat)} = \text{LVSV (ml/beat)} - \text{RVSV (ml/beat)} \qquad (4)$$

$$\text{Regurgitant fraction (\%)} = [\text{Regurgitant volume (ml/beat)} \times 100] / [\text{LVSV (ml/beat)}] \qquad (5)$$

where LVSV is LV stroke volume and RVSV is RV stroke volume.

Secondly, when other valvular disease is present, the mitral regurgitant volume can be calculated from the LV stroke volume and phase-contrast velocity-mapping flow measurements in the aorta:

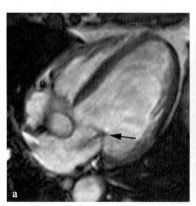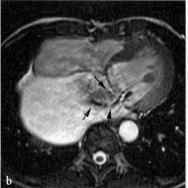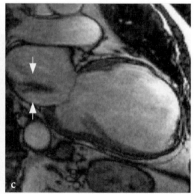

Fig. 13.14a-c. Balanced-SSFP images of mitral incompetence **a, b** Horizontal long-axis views. Grade 2 mitral incompetence (*black arrows*). **c** Vertical long-axis view of grade 3 mitral incompetence (*white arrows*) in a patient with mitral annulus dilatation secondary to ischemic heart disease. (Image **b**: Courtesy of F. Melonas, R. Truter and G. Wagner, SCP MRI Center, Cape Town, South Africa)

Regurgitant volume (ml/beat) = LVSV
(ml/beat) – aortic forward flow (ml/beat)   (6)

A third proposed method for quantifying mitral regurgitation involves calculation of the difference between ventricular outflow and ventricular inflow (FUJITA et al. 1994). Velocity mapping in the ascending aorta can be used to assess ventricular outflow, while velocity mapping at the mitral valve annulus during diastole can be used to assess inflow (Fig. 13.15). Thus:

Regurgitant volume (ml/beat) = LV inflow
(ml/beat) – aortic forward flow (ml/beat)   (7)

Using this method, MRI is able to demonstrate different mitral regurgitant volumes for groups with mild, moderate, and severe mitral regurgitation, defined at echocardiography. There is also good correlation between the calculated regurgitant fraction and the grading of mitral regurgitation severity at Doppler echocardiography (FUJITA et al. 1994).

When assessing mitral regurgitation with MRI, it is important to image the left atrium to assess the left atrial size and exclude the presence of thrombi.

As with aortic regurgitation, mitral regurgitation may be acute or chronic (see Table 13.4). The main

hemodynamic consequence of chronic mitral regurgitation is gradual LV dilatation and ultimately LV failure. Importantly, long-term survival is less good if surgical repair is performed when the LV ejection fraction is less than 60% (ENRIQUEZ-SARANO et al. 1994). Thus, cardiovascular MRI is well placed as an imaging tool that can accurately quantify and reproducibly monitor the severity of mitral regurgitation and the hemodynamic consequences on LV function. Again, no large-scale clinical studies have assessed the use of MRI for defining the timing of surgical repair of mitral regurgitation.

Table 13.4 Causes of mitral regurgitation

Acute
　Bacterial endocarditis
　Myocardial infarction with involvement of the papillary
　　muscle
Chronic
　Rheumatic heart disease
　Mitral valve prolapse syndrome
　Marfan syndrome
　Congenital
　Idiopathic hypertrophic subaortic stenosis
　Persistent ostium primum ASD with cleft mitral valve
　Functional – secondary to dilatation of the mitral
　　annulus in LV dilatation

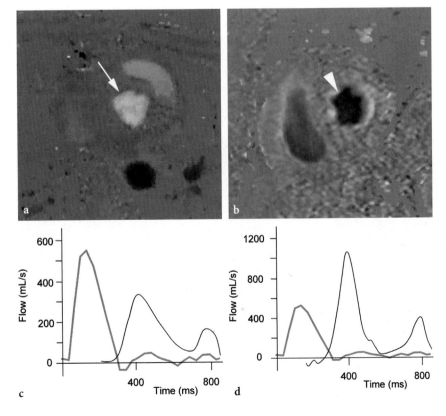

Fig. 13.15a-d. Measurement of mitral regurgitation by using velocity-encoded MR to measure the difference between outflow across the proximal ascending aorta (a) and inflow across the mitral annulus (b). Phase images acquired at the level of the proximal part of ascending aorta (arrow in a) and the mitral annulus (arrowhead in b). The graphs show the flow volume versus time frame for mitral in-flow (black curve) and aortic outflow (red curve) in a normal subject (c) and in a patient with mitral regurgitation (d). The difference in the areas under the two curves is the volume of mitral regurgitation

13.3.5.2
Mitral Stenosis

Restrictive opening of the mitral valve in mitral stenosis is most commonly secondary to rheumatic heart disease (Table 13.5). Elevation of left atrial outflow resistance occurs when the mitral valve area is below 2.5 cm^2. This leads to an increase in the diastolic transmitral gradient, which can be assessed by measuring the peak velocity across the mitral valve.

Table 13.5 Causes of mitral stenosis

Congenital
Rheumatic heart disease
Obstruction
Thrombus
Myxoma
Tumor

Peak velocity measurements at MR across the mitral valve (short-axis view below the mitral valve) correlate well with Doppler measurements at echocardiography (HEIDENREICH et al. 1995). Because of the complicated shape of the stenotic jet in most patients, through-plane measurements of velocity are more accurate than in-plane measurements (Fig. 13.16). Valve area can also be measured.

Velocity-mapping flow curves show loss of the normal dual peaks, with high velocities throughout diastole. The flow curves can be used to determine the mitral pressure half-time (the time taken for the pressure gradient to fall to half its peak value), a useful echocardiographic indicator of mitral stenosis severity:

$$\text{Valve area (cm}^2) = 220 \text{ Pressure half-time (ms)} \quad (8)$$

The severity of mitral stenosis can also be estimated by measuring pulmonary vein flow. In severe mitral stenosis this flow is reversed (MOHIADDIN et al. 1991a).

The consequences of mitral stenosis, left atrial enlargement, pulmonary edema and RV dysfunction and pulmonary regurgitation, secondary to pulmonary hypertension, can all be assessed. In particular, the presence of atrial thrombus should be evaluated in all patients in both atria (secondary to atrial fibrillation).

13.3.6
Pulmonary Valve

Difficulties with the alignment of the acoustic window for Doppler echocardiographic investigation has made MR velocity mapping a useful tool in the investigation of the pulmonary valve and pulmonary arteries (BOGREN et al. 1989b; MOHIADDIN et al. 1991b; REBERGEN et al. 1993). The imaging protocols for aortic stenosis and regurgitation apply for investigation of the pulmonary stenosis (Fig. 13.17) and pulmonary regurgitation (Fig. 13.18).

For pulmonary stenosis, measurement and visualization of the pulmonary valve is best performed in a sagittal or oblique sagittal plane. For the quantification of pulmonary regurgitation and RV out-

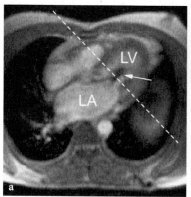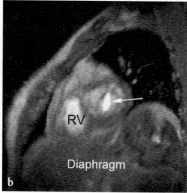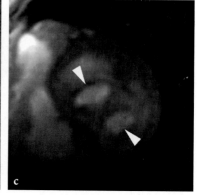

Fig. 13.16a-c. Mitral stenosis. **a** Axial GE image in mid-diastole. Turbulent flow is seen through the mitral valve (*arrow*). *Dotted white lines* represent the image plane for the short-axis image. **b** Short-axis GE image in mid-diastole. Flow through the mitral valve is shown as bright pixels (*arrow*). The valve orifice area can be easily measured. *LA*, Left atrium; *LV*, left ventricle; *RV*, right ventricle. **c** b-SSFP basal short-axis view of a rare example of a double mitral valve orifice (*arrowheads*)

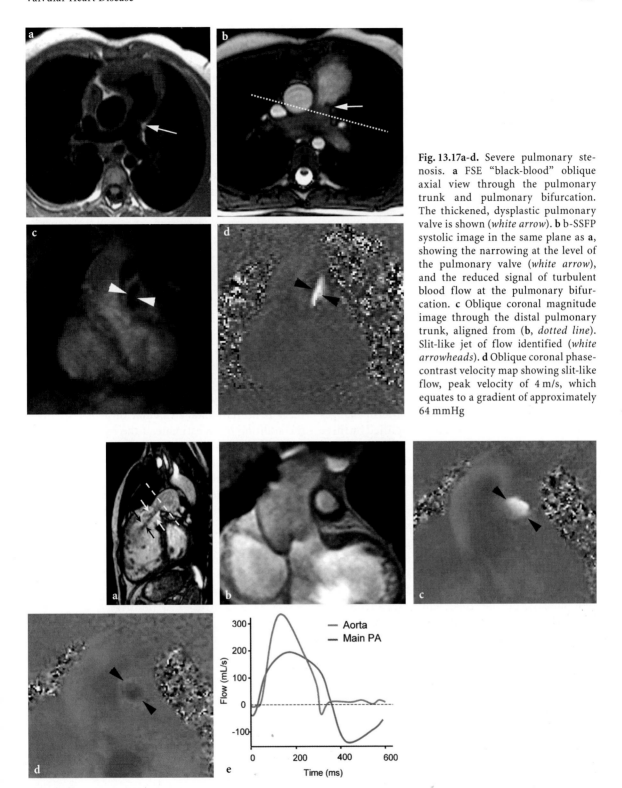

Fig. 13.17a-d. Severe pulmonary stenosis. **a** FSE "black-blood" oblique axial view through the pulmonary trunk and pulmonary bifurcation. The thickened, dysplastic pulmonary valve is shown (*white arrow*). **b** b-SSFP systolic image in the same plane as **a**, showing the narrowing at the level of the pulmonary valve (*white arrow*), and the reduced signal of turbulent blood flow at the pulmonary bifurcation. **c** Oblique coronal magnitude image through the distal pulmonary trunk, aligned from (**b**, *dotted line*). Slit-like jet of flow identified (*white arrowheads*). **d** Oblique coronal phase-contrast velocity map showing slit-like flow, peak velocity of 4 m/s, which equates to a gradient of approximately 64 mmHg

Fig. 13.18a-e. Moderate/severe pulmonary regurgitation, in a patient, 25 years after total repair of tetralogy of Fallot with a transannular patch. **a** Oblique sagittal right ventricular outflow tract view, diastolic frame, showing signal loss in the right ventricle secondary to pulmonary regurgitation (*arrows*). **b** Magnitude image through the proximal pulmonary trunk, aligned along the *dotted line* shown in **a**. Phase-contrast velocity mapping in systole (**c**) and in diastole (**d**) – *white* signal signifies forward flow during systole and *black* signifies reverse flow during diastole (*black arrowheads*). **e** Flow curve for pulmonary regurgitation; regurgitant fraction is 30%

flow curves, imaging the main pulmonary trunk in cross-section in a coronal or oblique axial plane is most accurate. These images should be prescribed from two perpendicular RVOT views to ensure that the majority of blood flow is perpendicular to the imaging plane (see Fig. 5.8) (KIVELITZ et al. 2003).

13.3.6.1
Clinical Importance of Pulmonary Regurgitation

Pulmonary regurgitation is an important sequelae of surgical repair of the RV outflow tract in many congenital heart disease conditions, in particular after complete repair for tetralogy of Fallot. Cardiovascular MR imaging has been used to quantify these changes, demonstrating elevated RV end-diastolic and end-systolic volumes and reduced RV ejection fraction in patients with severe pulmonary regurgitation (HELBING et al. 1996; SINGH et al. 1998; DAVLOUROS et al. 2002; TULEVSKI et al. 2003). Chronic RV volume overload has long been regarded as a rather benign consequence of pulmonary regurgitation in this clinical setting. However, there is increasing evidence that RV function may be irreversibly compromised by such long-term changes (THERRIEN et al. 2000). This is exemplified by three findings that have been demonstrated by cardiovascular MRI. First, RV ejection fraction has been shown to be significantly lower in patients with both RV pressure and volume overload as compared to RV pressure-overload alone (TULEVSKI et al. 2003). Second, an abnormal RV response to stress [either physiological (ROEST et al. 2002) or pharmacological (TULEVSKI et al. 2003)] has been demonstrated in patients with pulmonary regurgitation and tetralogy of Fallot. In normal subjects, RV ejection fraction increases during stress, while, in patients with tetralogy of Fallot, RV function remains remains unchanged or reduced during stress. And thirdly, there appears to be no improvement in RV function following pulmonary valve replacement (THERRIEN et al. 2000; VLIEGEN et al. 2002; RAZAVI et al. 2004) (see Sect. 13.3.9.1).

The accurate quantification of pulmonary incompetence and its effects on the right ventricle with cardiovascular MRI should help define the natural history of this condition and the response to treatment. Ultimately this may enable the definition of parameters that can be used to optimize treatment interventions.

13.3.7
Tricuspid Valve

Examination of the tricuspid valve is as for the mitral valve. The regurgitant jet of tricuspid regurgitation is best visualized in the transverse plane (Fig. 13.19). Velocity mapping in the superior vena cava can demonstrate tricuspid regurgitation, the causes of which are similar to mitral regurgitation. Tricuspid regurgitation of varying degrees is most commonly seen secondary to dilatation of the right ventricle, often due to mitral valve pathology and/or pulmonary hypertension. An important cause of tricuspid regurgitation that should be considered when there is thickening of the valve leaflet is carcinoid syndrome (Fig. 13.20). Tricuspid regurgitation can also occur after blunt trauma. It should be noted that trivial tricuspid regurgitation is a common finding in normal subjects (WAGGONER et al. 1981). For alignment of the optimal imaging planes for the tricuspid valve, see Fig. 5.7.

As with echocardiography, quantification of the tricuspid regurgitation is possible by measuring the peak velocity within the regurgitant flow jet. If there is no pulmonary valvular or artery stenosis, the addition of an estimate of the right atrial pressure (RA_{Pa}) to the calculated pressure difference between the right atrium and right ventricle (ΔP across the tricuspid valve, calculated using the modified Bernoulli equation), can give an estimate of the RV systolic pressure (RVS_{Pa}) and pulmonary artery pressure (PA_{Pa}).

Thus, tricuspid $\Delta P = 4(V_{max})^2$ $\qquad$ (9)

and,

$$RVS_{Pa} \; (mmHg) = PA_{Pa} \; (mmHg) =$$
$$RA_{Pa} \; (mmHg) + \Delta P \; (mmHg) \qquad (10)$$

where RA_{Pa}, the right atrial pressure, is estimated at 10 mmHg.

The tricuspid valve orifice is larger than the mitral orifice. Tricuspid stenosis is uncommon but can be easily diagnosed on GE cine images. Tricuspid atresia is easily identified on SE images.

13.3.7.1
Ebstein's Anomaly

Ebstein's anomaly is a congenital abnormality of the tricuspid valve. The septal and mural leaflets are more apically placed than normal, resulting in a malfunctioning, regurgitant tricuspid valve and atrialization of the right ventricle (ANDERSON et al.

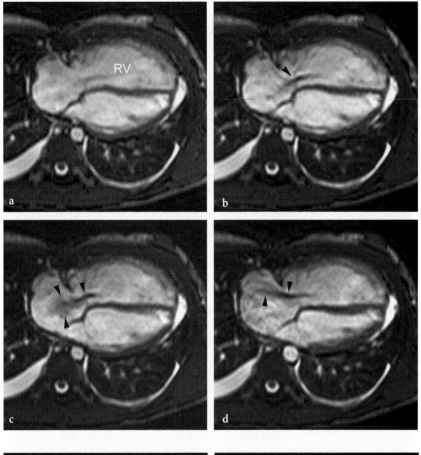

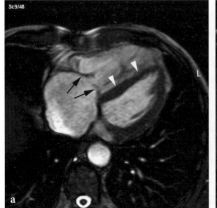

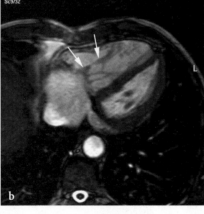

Fig. 13.19a-d. Balanced-SSFP 4-chamber images of tricuspid regurgitation (*arrowheads*) throughout systole. Time from the R wave: **a** 0 ms, **b** 50 ms, **c** 100 ms, **d** 200 ms

Fig. 13.20a,b. Carcinoid syndrome of the heart. **a, b** b-SSFP 4-chamber images at two different levels, showing thickened, stiff tricuspid valve (*black arrows* in **a**), and subvalvular apparatus (*white arrows* in **b**). The right ventricle is enlarged with flattening of the septum (*arrowheads* in **a**). This leads to nonclosure of tricuspid valve at end-systole, with important tricuspid regurgitation

1979). The consequence is gross right atrial enlargement and raised right atrial pressure. The anomaly is usually associated with an atrial septal defect (ASD) and there is thus right-to-left shunting at the atrial level and subsequent cyanosis. Ultimately, Ebstein's anomaly results in gross enlargement of the cardiac contour on the plain chest radiograph. Treatment is problematic, though expert surgical repair of the tricuspid valve is possible in some centers.

MRI can be used to assess valve morphology, quantify ventricular function, and size right atrial enlargement (Fig. 13.21).

13.3.8
Mixed Valvular Disease

The measurement of both RV and LV stroke volumes with cine MRI, in combination with velocity-map-

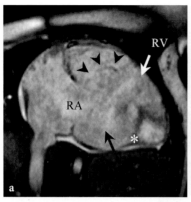
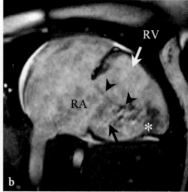
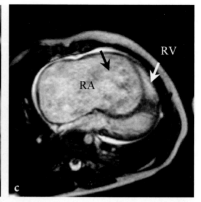

Fig. 13.21a-c. Ebstein's anomaly. Coronal long-axis view through the right atrium (*RA*) and right ventricle (*RV*), showing the apical displacement of the mural tricuspid valve leaflet (*asterisk*), and the normal sited antero-superior leaflet (*arrowheads*) in diastole (**a**) and systole (**b**). **c** Axial plane. In all three images the *black arrow* identifies "atrialization" of the right ventricle

ping measurement of pulmonary and aortic flow, permits the quantification of valvular regurgitation in all four valves, even if aortic, mitral, pulmonary, and tricuspid regurgitation are all present. Aortic and pulmonary regurgitation are calculated from the velocity maps and diastolic reverse flow, and subtraction of the systolic forward flow from the LVSV and RVSV yields the amount of mitral and tricuspid regurgitation, respectively.

13.3.9
Prosthetic Valves

For nonbiological prosthetic valves and stented biological valves, the applied magnetic field is distorted by differences in the local magnetic fields between the prosthesis and the biological tissue, and by eddy currents induced in the valve. These phenomena lead to signal loss around the prosthesis (Fig. 13.22). These artifacts can be very severe on GE images and

may degrade the image significantly. This makes imaging turbulent jets in the vicinity of the prosthesis difficult; however, velocity mapping distal to the image artifact can still be accurately performed. Homografts, autografts, and stentless porcine valve replacements do not cause signal artifact and can be imaged normally.

All valvular prostheses can be safely imaged, at current field strengths, except for Starr-Edwards mitral pre-6000 series valves used from 1960 to 1964, at field strengths of greater than 0.35 T (RANDALL et al. 1988; SHELLOCK 1988; SHELLOCK et al. 1993). Very few of the aforementioned prosthetic valves still remain in situ.

MRI offers an ideal method for the noninvasive follow-up of patients after valvular surgery (DEUTSCH et al. 1992). In vitro, the accuracy of MR velocity measurements distal to a wide variety of valvular prostheses has been confirmed by laser Doppler anemometry (FONTAINE et al. 1996). The assessment of prosthetic valve function at low

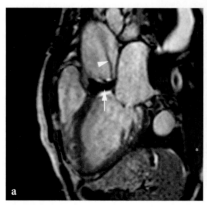
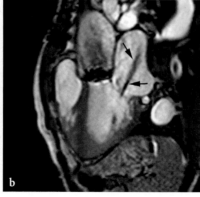

Fig. 13.22a,b. Aortic prosthetic valve with associated mitral incompetence. **a** b-SSFP left ventricular inflow/outflow view showing artifact related to prosthetic valve (*white arrow*), and mild jet of turbulent flow in the aortic root (*white arrowhead*). **b** b-SSFP image in a parallel imaging plane to (**a**), but in plane with the mitral valve, reveals grade 2/3 mitral regurgitation (*black arrows*)

field strength (0.2 T) has also been demonstrated (DiCesare et al. 1995). Useful clinical follow-up has been reported in patients following aortic root reconstruction, where not only was prosthetic valve function assessed, but the aortic graft, LV outflow tract, and proximal coronary arteries were all evaluated (Lepore et al. 1996).

13.3.9.1
Ventricular Response to Valve Replacement

Several small studies have now demonstrated a short-term (6 months to 1 year) reduction in MR-measured LV mass following aortic valve replacement (Rajappan et al. 2000; Sandstede et al. 2000; Lamb et al. 2002; Sensky et al. 2003). This reduction in LV mass is independent of the prosthesis type (porcine or mechanical) and is of the order of a 19–26% reduction in LV mass at 6 months (Sensky et al. 2003), though the LV mass reduction does not reach that of the normal population by 1 year (Sandstede et al. 2000).

LV end-diastolic volumes decrease after aortic valve replacement for both aortic stenosis (Sandstede et al. 2000; Lamb et al. 2002; Sensky et al. 2003) and aortic regurgitation (Lamb et al. 2002); and though LV function improves after aortic valve replacement for aortic stenosis (Sandstede et al. 2000; Lamb et al. 2002), ejection fraction remains the same in patients treated for regurgitation of the aortic valve (Lamb et al. 2002).

For pulmonary regurgitation, cardiovascular MRI has demonstrated abolition/reduction in pulmonary regurgitation in patients with tetralogy of Fallot treated with conventional surgical pulmonary valve replacement (Vliegen et al. 2002) and, more recently, in young patients treated with percutaneous pulmonary valve stent insertion (Bonhoeffer et al. 2002; Razavi et al. 2004) (Fig. 13.23).

Despite the reduction in pulmonary regurgitation, there is no change in the RV ejection fraction for both treatment methods; though it should be noted that to date (2004) postprocedural MRI studies have been performed at rest, and improvements in RV function during stress may be identified. The lack of significant improvement in resting RV function after treatment may reflect irreversible changes in RV function/contractility and raises the possibility that pulmonary valve competence should be restored in this patient group before RV function deteriorates (Therrien et al. 2000). The optimal timing for pulmonary valve replacement is not yet known, and several imaging modalities (echocardiography, quantifiable exercise testing, cardiovascular MRI) in combination will probably be used to help elucidate this information.

13.3.9.2
Velocity Mapping in the
Aorta After Aortic Valve Replacement

Two-dimensional velocity mapping profiles in the aorta, just downstream of aortic valve prosthesis, have been shown to be abnormal, when compared with normal aortic valve flow (Botnar et al. 2000; Kozerke et al. 2001b). These studies demonstrate an increased peak velocity during systolic forward flow (1.9±0.4m/s versus 1.2±0.03m/s, respectively) (Botnar et al. 2000), with a distinct pattern of two lateral jets and one central jet of antegrade flow (Botnar et al. 2000; Kozerke et al. 2001b). There was also diastolic reverse flow, with a RF of approximately 15% (Botnar et al. 2000; Kozerke et al. 2001b).

Velocity vector mapping is possible when 3D phase-contrast cine imaging is performed. The technique has been used to define helical and retro-

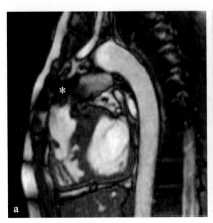
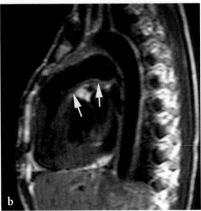

Fig. 13.23a-b. MR imaging after percutaneous pulmonary valve-stent (PPVS) insertion. **a** b-SSFP oblique sagittal RVOT view, showing artifact secondary to the metallic component of the PPVS (*asterisk*). **B** TSE "black-blood" image in the same plane as **a** shows that the PPVS is widely patent. The stent position on the inferior wall of the pulmonary homograft is seen between the two *arrows*

grade flow patterns in the aortic arch of healthy subjects (KILNER et al. 1993b) and flow patterns in the left ventricles of both healthy subjects and patients with dilated ischemic cardiomyopathy (MOHIADDIN 1995). In valvular disease, a potential use for this technique may be in defining the position of prosthetic valves to improve postvalvular flow characteristics. In vitro studies are ongoing, and preliminary results with tilting disc prostheses suggest that, for aortic valve replacement, better flow characteristics can be achieved if the larger of the two valve orifices is positioned toward the inner aortic wall and not the outer wall. Such simple changes in prosthesis position may result in less aortic dilatation postvalve replacement and longer valve lifetimes.

Preliminary 3D velocity mapping has also now been performed in patients with bileaflet aortic valve prosthesis (KOZERKE et al. 2001c), revealing complex flow patterns that vary considerably between patients (Fig. 13.24).

13.3.10
Magnetic Resonance Spectroscopy

There is limited experience with MR spectroscopy and valvular heart disease in the clinical setting. It is known that a reduction in the phosphocreatine to ATP (PCr/ATP) ratio occurs in patients with heart failure (CONWAY et al. 1991) and can be a useful predictor of cardiovascular morbidity in patients with dilated cardiomyopathy (NEUBAUER et al. 1997a). Such changes in the PCr/ATP ratio have been confirmed in patients with aortic valve disease and New York Heart Association class III symptoms of heart failure (NEUBAUER et al. 1997b). Furthermore, patients with aortic stenosis have been shown to have a reduced PCr/ATP ratio (NEUBAUER et al. 1997b; BEYERBACHT et al. 2001), which normalizes following aortic valve replacement (BEYERBACHT et al. 2001).

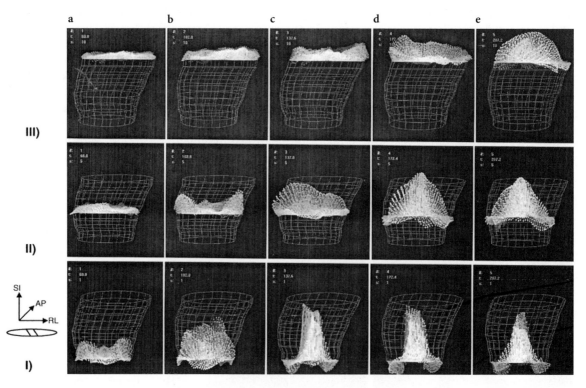

Fig. 13.24a-e. Velocity vectors of consecutive heart phases separated by 35 ms starting 68 ms after R-wave for three different distances downstream from the bileaflet valve. Flow is initially accelerated by the opening leaflets toward the vessel walls (*Ia*). Later, flow emerges through the fully opened valve as seen in (*Ic-e*). Reverse velocities are found adjacent to the vessel wall in areas corresponding to the lateral orifices of the valve (*Ic-e*). As flow travels downstream, high-velocity jets decay (*II-III*). Nonaxial velocity components are accentuated in regions following the outer curvature of the aorta (*IIc-e and IIId-e*). (Reprinted with permission from KOZERKE et al. 2001c)

A large-scale prospective study, with measurement of both pre- and post-valve-replacement PCr/ATP ratios, needs to be performed to assess the use of MR spectroscopy for optimizing treatment of aortic valve disease.

As cardiovascular MRI becomes more cost-effective and easily accessible, its use for the accurate assessment of valvular heart disease in clinical cardiology will increase and enable physicians to better predict the optimal treatment for their patients with valvular heart disease.

13.4
Future Directions

Future improvements in MR scanner hardware and sequences will improve the speed of MR assessment of valvular heart disease, with the acquisition of ventricular volume and great-vessel flow data in a single breath-hold. Improvements in analysis software, in particular the development of robust, automated ventricular volume contour tracking, will reduce laborious postprocessing.

The techniques for MR valvular heart disease assessment are well validated and well established. However, what are lacking are large-scale, long-term studies of the physiological natural history of valvular heart disease and the consequences of treatment, either medically or surgically with valve replacement. Such studies with the described accurate MRI techniques should enable improved timing for optimal valve replacement to balance the risks of surgery and prosthetic valve insertion and irreversible ventricular dysfunction.

13.5
Conclusion

MRI can provide important information about valvular function. Both stenotic and regurgitant lesions can be quantified for all four valves. Quantification can also be performed even when multiple valves are affected. Anatomical information with regard to leaflet number, valve thickness, and the presence of endocarditis is still best provided by echocardiography.

MRI offers the only noninvasive, accurate, and reproducible method for quantifying valvular regurgitation, with no X-ray exposure. In combination with accurate ventricular function assessment, cardiovascular MRI is ideal for the long-term follow-up and evaluation of patients awaiting valvular surgery. However, long-term studies using MRI in such a role need to be performed to define the optimal timings for these interventions.

13.6
Key Points

- Accurate flow and ventricular measurements are the cornerstone of assessment of valvular heart disease
- Confirmation of the accuracy of these technique should be confirmed for each individual scanner using flow phantoms and/or normal healthy subjects
- MRI is the best available noninvasive method for quantification of valvular regurgitation
- Accurate quantification of all valves can be performed, even when mixed valvular disease is present
- MRI is the best available noninvasive method for the quantification of the consequences of valvular dysfunction, in particular for the assessment of ventricular function and LV mass
- Larger-scale studies are required to establish whether MRI assessment of valvular regurgitation will be able to optimize treatment timings (surgical or interventional cardiology)
- MRI assessment of valve leaflets remains limited

Acknowledgements
We would like to acknowledge the following for their help and support with cardiovascular MR: From Great Ormond Street Hospital for Children, London, UK: Professor John Deanfield and Professor Philipp Bonhoeffer of the Cardiothoracic Unit; Dr. Cathy Owens, Rod Jones, Wendy Norman, and Clare Thompson of the Department of Radiology; and Dr. Angus McEwan of the Anesthetic Department. From the MR Unit, Guy's Hospital, London, UK: Dr. Reza Razavi, Dr. Vivek Muthurangu, and Dr. Sanjeet Hegde. We would also like to thank Dr. Philip Kilner and Professor Dudley Pennell from the Cardiothoracic Unit, Royal Brompton Hospital, London, UK, for their contribution to the version of this chapter that was published in the first edition of this handbook.

References

Abbasi AS, Allen MW, Decristofaro D, Ungar I (1980) Detection and estimation of the degree of mitral regurgitation by range-gated pulsed Doppler echocardiography. Circulation 61:143–149

Alegret JM, Duran I, Palazon O et al (2003) Prevalence of and predictors of bicuspid aortic valves in patients with dilated aortic roots. Am J Cardiol 91:619–622

Alfakih K, Plein S, Thiele H, et al (2003) Normal human left and right ventricular dimensions for MRI assessed by turbo gradient echo and steady-stae free precession imaging sequences. J Magn Reson Imaging 17:323–329

Anderson KR, Zuberbuhler JR, Anderson RH, Becker AE, Lie JT (1979) Morphologic spectrum of Ebstein's anomaly of the heart: a review. Mayo Clin Proc 54:174–180

Aurigemma G, Reichek N, Schiebler M, Axel L (1990) Evaluation of mitral regurgitation by cine MRI. Am J Cardiol 66:621–625

Aurigemma G, Reichek N, Schiebler M, Axel L (1991) Evaluation of aortic regurgitation by cardiac cine MRI: planar analysis and comparison to Doppler echocardiography. Cardiology 78:340–347

Barkhausen J, Ruehm SG, Goyen M, et al (2001) MR evaluation of ventricular function: true fast imaging with steady-state precession versus fast low-angle shot cine MR imaging: feasibility study. Radiology 219:264–269

Bellenger NG, Francis JM, Davies CL, Coats AJ, Pennell DJ (2000) Establishment and performance of a magnetic resonance cardiac function clinic. J Cardiovasc Magn Reson 2:15–22

Beyerbacht HP, Lamb HJ, Laarse A van der et al (2001) Aortic valve replacement in patients with aortic stenosis improves myocardial metabolism and diastolic function. Radiology 219:637–643

Boehrer JD, Lange RA, Willard JE, Grayburn PA, Hillis LD (1992) Advantages and limitations of methods to detect, localise and quantitate intracardiac left-to-right shunting. Am Heart J 124:448–455

Bogaert JG, Bosmans HT, Rademakers FE et al (1995) Left ventricular quantification with breath-hold MR imaging: comparison with echocardiography. MAGMA 3:5–12

Bogaert J, Taylor AM, Kerkhove F van, Dymarkowski S (2004) Use of inversion recovery contrast-enhanced MRI for cardiac imaging: spectrum of applications. AJR Am J Roentgenol 182:609–615

Bogren HG, Klipstein RH, Firmin DN, et al (1989a) Quantification of antegrade and retrograde blood flow in the human aorta by magnetic resonance velocity mapping. Am Heart J 117:1214–1222

Bogren HG, Klipstein RH, Mohiaddin RH et al (1989b) Pulmonary artery distensibility and blood flow patterns: a magnetic resonance study of normal subjects and patients with pulmonary arterial hypertension. Am Heart J 118:990–999

Bonhoeffer P, Boudjemline Y, Qureshi SA et al (2002) Percutaneous insertion of the pulmonary valve. J Am Coll Cardiol 39:1664–1669

Bolger AF, Eigler NL, Maurer G (1988) Quantifying valvular regurgitation: limitations and inherent assumptions of Doppler technique. Circulation 78:1316–1318

Bonow RO, Carbello B, DeLeon AC et al (1998) ACC/AHA guideline for the management of patients with valvular heart disease. J Am Coll Carddiol 32:1486–1588

Borer JS, Bonow RO (2003) Contemporary approach to aortic and mitral regurgitation. Circulation 108:2432–2438

Botnar R, Nagel E, Scheidegger MB, et al (2000) Assessment of prosthetic aortic valve performance by magnetic resonance velocity imaging. MAGMA 10:18–26

Bryan AJ, Barzilai B, Kouchoukos NT (1995) Transesophageal echocardiography and adult cardiac operations. Ann Thorac Surg 59:773–779

Caduff JH, Hernandez RJ, Ludomirsky A (1996) MR visualization of aortic valve vegetations. J Comput Assist Tomogr 20:613–615

Carabello BA, Crawford FA (1997) Valvular heart disease. N Engl J Med 337:32–41

Carroll JD (1993) Cardiac catheterisation and other imaging modalities in the evaluation of valvular heart disease. Curr Opin Cardiol 8:211–215

Caruthers SD, Jiuan Lin S, Brown P et al (2003) Practical value of cardiac magnetic resonance imaging for clinical quantification of aortc valve stenosis. Comparison with echocardiography. Circulation 108:2236–2243

Chatzimavroudis GP, Walker PG, Oshinski JN, et al (1997) Slice location dependence of aortic regurgitation measurements with MR phase velocity mapping. Magn Reson Med 37:545–551

Cohen BL (1991) Catalogue of risks extended and updated. Health Phys 61:317–335

Conway MA, Allis J, Ouwerkerk R, et al (1991) Detection of low phosphocreatinine to ATP ratio in failing hypertrophied human myocardium by P magnetic resonance spectroscopy. Lancet 338:973–976

Currie PJ, Seward JB, Reeder GS et al (1985) Continuous wave Doppler echocardiographic assessment of the severity of calcific aortic stenosis: a simultaneous Doppler-catheter correlative study in 100 adult patients. Circulation 71:1162–1169

Davis K, Kennedy J, Kemp H, et al (1979) Complications of coronary arteriography from the collaborative study of coronary artery surgery (CASS). Circulation 59:1105–1112

Davlouros PA, Kilner PJ, Hornung TS et al (2002) Right ventricular function in adults with repaired tetralogy of Fallot assessed with cardiovascular magnetic resonance imaging: detrimental role of right ventricular outflow aneurysm or akinesia and adverse right-to-left ventricular interaction. J Am Coll Cardiol 40:2044–2052

DeRoos A, Reichek N, Axel L, Kressel HY (1989) Cine MR imaging in aortic stenosis. J Comput Assist Tomogr 13:421–425

Deutsch HJ, Bachmann R, Sechtem U et al (1992) Regurgitant flow in cardiac valve prosthesis: diagnostic value of gradient echo nuclear magnetic resonance imaging in reference to transesophageal two-dimensional color Doppler echocardiography. J Am Coll Cardiol 19:1500–1507

DiCesare E, Enrici RM, Paparoni S et al (1995) Low-field magnetic resonance imaging in the evaluation of mechanical and biological heart valve function. Eur J Radiol 20:224–228

Dooms G, Higgins CB (1986) MR imaging of cardiac thrombi. J Comput Assist Tomogr 10:415–420

Dulce MC, Mostbeck GH, O'Sullivan M, et al (1992) Severity of aortic regurgitation: interstudy reproducibility of measurements with velocity-encoded cine MRI. Radiology 185:235–240

Dulce MC, Mostbeck GH, Friese KK, Caputo GR, Higgins CB (1993) Quantification of the left ventricular volumes and function with cine MR imaging: comparison of geometric models with three-dimensional data. Radiology 188:371–376

Eichenberger AC, Jenni R, Schulthess GK von (1993) Aortic valve pressure gradients in patients with aortic valve stenosis: quantification with velocity-encoded cine MR imaging. AJR Am J Roentgenol160:971–977

Enriquez-Sarano M, Tajik A, Schaff H et al (1994) Echocardiographic prediction of survival after surgical correction of organic mitral regurgitation. Circulation 90:830–837

Evans AJ, Blinder RA, Herfkens RJ et al (1988) Effects of turbulence on signal intensity in gradient echo images. Invest Radiol 23:512–518

Firmin DN, Nayler GL, Klipstein RH, Underwood SR, Longmore DB (1987) In vivo validation of MR velocity imaging. J Comput Assist Tomogr 11:751–756

Fix J, Isada L, Cosgrove D, et al (1993) Do patients with less than "echo-perfect" results from mitral valve repair by intraoperative echocardiography have a different outcome? Circulation 88:39–48

Fontaine AA, Heinrich RS, Walker PG et al (1996) Comparison of magnetic resonance imaging and laser Doppler anemometry velocity measurements downstream of replacement heart valves: implications for in vivo assessment of prosthetic valve function. J Heart Valve Dis 5:66–73

Friedrich MG, Schulz-Menger J, Poetsch T, et al (2002) Quantification of valvular aortic stenosis by magnetic resonance imaging. Am Heart J 144:329–334

Fujita N, Chazouilleres AF, Hartiala JJ et al (1994) Quantification of mitral regurgitation by velocity encoded cine nuclear magnetic resonance imaging. J Am Coll Cardiol 23:951–958

Globits S, Mayr H, Frank H et al (1991) Quantification of regurgitant lesions by MRI. Int J Card Imaging 6:109–116

Globits S, Blake L, Bourne M et al (1996) Assessment of haemodynamic effects of ACE inhibition therapy in chronic aortic regurgitation by using velocity-encoded cine magnetic resonance imaging. Am Heart J 131:289–293

Gorlin R, Gorlin SG (1951) Hydraulic formula for calculation of the area of the stenotic mitral valve, other valves and central circulatory shunts. Am Heart J 41:1–29

Grothues F, Smith GC, Moon JC et al (2002) Comparison of interstudy reproducibility of cardiovascular magnetic resonance with two-dimensional echocardiography in normal subjects and in patients with heart failure or left ventricular hypertrophy. Am J Cardiol 90:29–34

Hatle L, Angelson B (1992) Doppler ultrasound in cardiology: physical principles and clinical applications. Lea and Febiger, Philadelphia

Hausmann D, Daniel WG, Mugge A, Ziemer G, Pearlman AS (1992) Value of transesophageal color Doppler echocardiography for detection of different types of atrial septal defect in adults. J Am Soc Echocardiogr 5:481–488

Heidenreich PA, Steffens JC, Fujita N, et al (1995) The evaluation of mitral stenosis with velocity-encoded cine MRI. Am J Cardiol 75:365–369

Helbing WA, Niezen RA, Le Cessie S, et al (1996) Right ventricular diastolic function in children with pulmonary regurgitation after repair of tetralogy of Fallot: volumetric evaluation by magnetic resonance velocity mapping. J Am Coll Cardiol 28:1827–1835

Hori Y, Yamada N, Higashi M, Hirai N, Nakatani S (2003) Rapid evaluation of right and left ventricular function and mass using real-time True-FISP cine MR imaging without breath-hold: comparison with segmented True-FISP cine MR imaging with breath-hold. J Cardiovasc Magn Reson 5:439–450

Hundley WG, Li HF, Willard JE et al (1995) Magnetic resonance imaging assessment of the severity of mitral regurgitation. Circulation 92:1151–1158

Jeang MK, Fuentes F, Gately A, Byrnes J, Lewis M (1986) Aortic root abscess – initial experience using magnetic resonance imaging. Chest 89:613–615

John AS, Dill T, Brandt RR et al (2003) Magnetic resonance to assess the aortic valve area in aortic stenosis. How does it compare to current diagnostic standards? J Am Coll Cardiol 42:519–526

Kilner PJ, Firmin DN, Rees RSO et al (1991) Valve and great vessel stenosis: assessment with MR jet velocity mapping. Radiology 178:229–235

Kilner PJ, Manzara CC, Mohiaddin RH et al (1993a) Magnetic resonance jet velocity mapping in mitral and aortic valve stenosis. Circulation 87:1239–1248

Kilner PJ, Yang GZ, Mohiaddin RH, Firmin DN, Longmore DB (1993b) Helical and retrograde secondary flow patterns in the aortic arch studied by three-dimensional mag-netic resonance velocity mapping. Circulation 88:2235–2247

Kivelitz DE, Dohmen PM, Lembcke A et al (2003) Visualization of the pulmonary valve using cine MR imaging. Acta Radiology 44:172–176

Kondo C, Caputo GR, Semelka R, Shimakawa M, Higgins CB (1991) Right and left ventricular stroke volume measurements with velocity encoded cine NMR imaging: in vivo and in vitro evaluation. AJR Am J Roentgenol 157:9–16

Korperich H, Gieseke J, Barth P et al (2004) Flow volume and shunt quantification in pediatric congenital heart disease by real-time magnetic resonance velocity mapping. A validation study. Circulation (in press)

Kozerke S, Scheidegger MB, Pedersen EM, Boesiger P (1999) Heart motion adapted cine pahse-contrast flow measurements through the aortic valve. Magn Reson Med 42:970–978

Kozerke S, Schwitter J, Pedersen EM, Boesiger P (2001a) Aortic and mitral regurgitation: quantification using moving slice velocity mapping. J Magn Reson Imaging14:106–112

Kozerke S, Hasenkam JM, Nygaard H, et al (2001b) Heart motion-adapted MR velocity mapping of blood velocity distribution downstream of aortic valve prostheses: initial experience. Radiology 218:548–555

Kozerke S, Hasenkam JM, Pedersen EM, Boesiger P (2001c) Visualization of flow patterns distal to aortic valve prostheses in humans using a fast approach for cine 3D velocity mapping. J Magn Reson Imaging 13:690–698

Laissy JP, Blanc F, Soyer P et al (1995) Thoracic aortic dissection: diagnosis with transesophageal echocardiography versus MR imaging. Radiology 194:331–336

Lamb HJ, Beyerbacht HP, Roos A de et al (2002) Left ventricular remodelling early after aortic valve replacement:

differential effects on diastolic function in aortic valve stenosis and aortic regurgitation. J Am Coll Cardiol 40:2182–2188.

Lee VS, Resnick D, Bundy JM, et al (2002) Cardiac function: MR evaluation in one breath hold with real-time true fast imaging with steady state precession. Radiology 222:835–842

Lepore V, Lamm C, Bugge M, Larsson S (1996) Magnetic resonance imaging in the follow-up of patients after aortic root reconstruction. Thorac Cardiovasc Surg 44:188–192

Manning WJ, Silverman DI, Gordon SP, Krumholz HM, Douglas PS (1993) Cardioversion from atrial fibrillation without prolonged anticoagulation with use of transesophageal echocardiography to exclude the presence of atrial thrombi. N Engl J Med 328:750–755

Meier D, Maier S, Boesiger P (1988) Quantitative flow measurements on phantoms and on blood vessels with MR. Magn Reson Med 8:25–34

Mohiaddin RH (1995) Flow patterns in the dilated ischaemic left ventricle studied by MR imaging with velocity vector mapping. J Magn Reson Imaging 5:493–498

Mohiaddin RH, Wann SL, Underwood R, et al (1990) Vena caval flow: assessment with cine MR velocity mapping. Radiology 177:537–541

Mohiaddin RH, Amanuma M, Kilner PJ, et al (1991a) MR phase-shift velocity mapping of mitral and pulmonary venous flow. J Comput Assist Tomogr 15:237–243

Mohiaddin RH, Paz R, Theodoropolus S et al (1991b) Magnetic resonance characterization of pulmonary arterial blood flow following single lung transplantation. J Thorac Cardiovasc Surg 101:1016–1023

Moon JCC, Lorenz CH, Francis JM, Smith GC, Pennell DJ (2002) Breath-hold FLASH and FISP cardiovascular MR imaging: left ventricular volume differences and reproducibility. Radiology 223:789–797

Nagel E, Stuber M, Burkhard B et al (2000) Cardiac rotation and relaxation in patients with aortic valvular stenosis. Eur Heart J 21:582–589

Nayler GL, Firmin DN, Longmore DB (1986) Blood flow imaging by cine magnetic resonance. J Comput Assist Tomogr 10:715–722

Neubauer S, Horn M, Cramer M et al (1997a) Myocardial phosphocreatine-to-ATP ratio is a predictor of mortality in patients with dilated cardiomyopathy. Circulation 96:2190–2196

Neubauer S, Horn M, Pabst T et al (1997b) Cardiac high-energy phosphate metabolism in patients with aortic valve disease assessed by ^{31}P-magnetic resonance spectroscopy. J Invest Med 45:453–462

Nishimura F (1992) Oblique cine MRI for the evaluation of aortic regurgitation: comparison with cineangiography. Clin Cardiol 66:621–625

Nkomo VT, Enriquez-Sarano M, Ammash NM et al (2003) Bicuspid aortic valve associated with aortic dilatation: a community-based study. Arterioscler Thromb Vasc Biol 23:351–356

Novaro GM, Tiong IY, Pearce GL, et al (2003) Features and predictors of ascending aortic dilatation in association with a congenital bicuspid aortic valve. Am J Cardiol 92:99–101

Ohnishi S, Fukui S, Kusuoka H, et al (1992) Assessment of valvular regurgitation using cine MRI coupled with phase

compensating technique: comparison with Doppler color flow mapping. Angiology 43:913–924

Pedersen WR, Walker M, Olson JD et al (1991) Value of transesophageal echocardiography as an adjunct to transthoracic echocardiography in evaluation of native and prosthetic valve endocarditis. Chest 100:351–356

Pereles FS, Kapoor V, Carr JC et al (2001) Usefulness of segmented trueFISP cardiac pulse sequence in evaluation of congenital and acquired adult cardiac abnormalities. AJR Am J Roentgenol 177:1155–1160

Quinones MA, Young JB, Waggoner AD, et al (1980) Assessment of pulsed Doppler echocardiography in detection and quantification of aortic and mitral regurgitation. Br Heart J 44:612–620

Randall PA, Kohman LJ, Scalzetti EM, Szeverenyi NM, Panicek DM (1988) Magnetic resonance imaging of prosthetic cardiac valves in vitro and in vivo. Am J Cardiol 62:973–976

Rajappan K, Melina G, Bellenger NG et al (2000) Evaluation of left ventricular function and mass after Medtronic Freestyle versus homograft aortic root replacement using cardiovascular magnetic resonance. J Heart Valve Dis 11:60–65

Razavi R, Muthurangu V, Taylor AM, Hegde SR, Bonhoeffer P (2004) Magnetic resonance assessment of percutaneous pulmonary valve-stent implantation (abstract). J Cardiovasc Magn Reson 6:429

Rebergen SA, Chin JGJ, Ottenkamp J, Wall van der, Roos A de (1993) Pulmonary regurgitation in the late post-opera-tive follow-up of tetralogy of Fallot. Circulation 88:2257–2266

Rigo P, Alderson PO, Robertson RM, Becker LC, Wagner HN (1979) Measurement of aortic and mitral regurgitation by gated cardiac blood pool scans. Circulation 60:306–312

Rockey R, Sterling LL, Zoghbi WA, et al (1987) Determination of the regurgitant fraction in isolated mitral regurgitation by pulsed Doppler two-dimensional echocardiography. J Am Coll Cardiol 7:1273–1278

Roest AAW, Helbing WA, Kunz P et al (2002) Exercise MR imaging in the assessment of pulmonary regurgitation and biventricular function in patients after Tetralogy of Fallot repair. Radiology 223:204–211

Sakuma H, Fujita N, Foo TK et al (1993) Evaluation of left ventricular volume and mass with breath-hold cine MR imaging. Radiology 188:377–380

Sandler H, Dodge HT, Hay RE, Rackley CE (1963) Quantification of valvular insufficiency in man by angiocardiography. Am Heart J 65:501–513

Sandstede JJW, Beer M, Hofmann S et al (2000) Changes in left and right ventricular cardiac function after valve replacement for aortic stenosis determined by cine MR imaging. J Magn Reson Imaging 12:240–246

Sandstede JJW, Johnson T, Harre K et al (2002) Cardiac systolic rotation and contraction before and after valve replacement for aortic stenosis. AJR Am J Roentgenol 178:953–958

Sechtem U, Pflugfelder PW, White RD, et al (1987) Cine MR imaging: potential for the evaluation of cardiovascular function. AJR Am J Roentgenol 148:239–246

Sechtem U, Pflugfelder PW, Cassidy MM, et al (1988) Mitral and aortic regurgitation: quantification of regurgitant volumes with cine MR imaging. Radiology 167:425–430

Sellers RD, Levy MJ, Amplatz K, Lillehei CW (1964) Left retrograde cardioangiography in acquired cardiac disease: technique, indication and interpretation. Am J Cardiol 14:437–445

Sensky PR, Loubani M, Keal RP, et al (2003) Does the type of prosthesis influence early left ventricular mass regression after aortic valve replacement? Assessment with magnetic resonance imaging. Am Heart J 146:e13

Shellock FG (1988) MR imaging of metallic implants and materials: a compilation of the literature. AJR Am J Roentgenol 151:811–814

Shellock FG, Morisoli S, Kanal E (1993) MR procedures and biomedical implants, materials and devices: 1993 update. Radiology 189:587–599

Simpson IA, Maciel BC, Moises V et al (1993) Cine magnetic resonance imaging and color Doppler flow mapping displays of flow velocity, spatial acceleration and jet formation: a comparative in vitro study. Am Heart J 126:1165–1174

Singh GK, Greenberg SB, Yap YS, et al (1998) Right ventricular function and exercise performance late after primary repair of tetralogy of Fallot with transannular patch in infancy. Am J Cardiol 81:1378–1382

Smith MD, Xie GY (1998) Current echocardiography-Doppler approaches to the quantification of valvular regurgitation. Cardiol Rev 6:168–181

Sondergaard L, Lindvig K, Hildebrandt P et al (1993a) Valve area and cardiac output in aortic stenosis. Am Heart J 127:1156–1164

Sondergaard L, Lindvig K, Hildebrandt P, et al (1993b) Quantification of aortic regurgitation by magnetic resonance velocity mapping. Am Heart J 125;1081–1090

Sorenson SG, O'Rourke RA, Chaudhuri TK (1980) Non-invasive quantification of valvular regurgitation by gated equilibrium radionuclide angiography. Circulation 62:1089–1098

Taylor AM, Dymarkowski S, Meerleer K de et al (2004) Validation and application of single breath-hold cine Cardiac MR for ventricular function assessment in children with congenital heart disease (abstract). J Cardiovasc Magn Reson 6:409

Therrien J, Siu SC, McLaughlin PR, et al (2000) Pulmonary valve replacement in adult late after repair of Tetralogy of Fallot: are we operating too late? J Am Coll Cardiol 36:1670–1675

Tice FD, Kisslo J (1993) Echocardiography in the diagnosis of thoracic aortic pathology. Int J Card Imaging [Suppl 2] 9:27–38

Tulevski II, Hirsch A, Dodge-Khatami A, et al (2003) Effect of pulmonary valve regurgitation on right ventricular function in patients with chronic right ventricular pressure overload. Am J Cardiol 92:113–116

Underwood SR, Firmin DN, Mohiaddin RH et al (1987a) Cine magnetic resonance imaging of valvular heart disease (abstract). Proc Soc Magn Reson Imaging 2:723

Underwood SR, Firmin DN, Klipstein RH, Rees RSO, Longmore DB (1987b) Magnetic resonance velocity mapping: clinical application of a new technique. Br Heart J 57:404–412

Utsunomiya T, Ogawa T, Doshi R, et al (1991) Doppler color flow "proximal isovelocity surface area" method for estimating volume flow rates: effects of orifice shape and machine factors. J Am Coll Cardiol 17:1103–1111

Vliegen HW, Straten A van, Roos A de et al (2002) Magnetic resonance imaging to assess the hemodynamic effects of pulmonary valve replacement in adults late after repair of tetralogy of Fallot. Circulation 106:1703–1707

Waggoner AD, Quinones MA, Young JB et al (1981) Pulsed Doppler echocardiography detection of right-sided valve regurgitation. Experimental results and clinical significance. Am J Cardiol 47:279–283

Wagner S, Auffermann W, Buser P, et al (1989) Diagnostic accuracy and estimation of the severity of valvular regurgitation from the signal void on cine magnetic resonance imaging. Am Heart J 118:760–767

Weinmann HJ, Lanaido M, Mutzel W (1984) Pharmacokinetics of Gd-DTPA/dimeglumine after iv injection. Physiol Chem Phys Med NMR 16:167–172

Zur Y, Wood ML, Neuringer LJ (1990) Motion-insensitive, steady-state free precession Imaging. Magn Reson Med 16:444–459

14 Coronary Artery Disease

Jan Bogaert, Steven Dymarkowski and Andrew M. Taylor

CONTENTS

J. Bogaert MD, PhD; S. Dymarkowski MD, PhD
Department of Radiology, Gasthuisberg University Hospital,
Catholic University of Leuven, Herestraat 49, 3000 Leuven,
Belgium
A. M. Taylor, MD, MRCP, FRCR
Cardiothoracic Unit, Institute of Child Health and Great
Ormond Street Hospital for Children, London, WC1N 3JH,
UK

14.1
Introduction

Coronary heart disease is the leading cause of morbidity and mortality in the developed countries, and the World Health Organization estimate that it will be the leading cause of morbidity and mortality worldwide by 2020 (Reddy and Yusuf 1998). Catheter-based X-ray coronary angiography is considered the technique of choice for detecting, quantifying and treating atherosclerotic coronary lesions. This technique, however, has many limitations and, because of its invasive nature, it is not suited as a screening modality. The substantial technical progress in magnetic resonance (MR) imaging, electron beam computed tomography (EBCT) and multi-slice computed tomography (MSCT) in the last decade has opened new horizons to study the coronary arteries non-invasively, and therefore to compete with catheter-based coronary angiography. Although non-invasive coronary artery imaging with MR imaging is highly challenging and, to date (2004), should still be considered as emerging, it has the potential to provide unique information about the presence, extent and severity of coronary artery disease (CAD). Three-dimensional angiographic or "luminographic" MR imaging techniques can detect or exclude the presence of stenotic atherosclerotic lesions, while MR flow techniques can be applied to assess the severity of a stenotic lesion on the distal coronary flow. In addition, MR imaging techniques are under development to visualize the coronary artery wall, enabling assessment of wall remodelling and plaque characterization. The above-mentioned techniques can also be applied to study the patient with recurrent anginal symptoms after percutaneous coronary intervention (PCI) or coronary artery bypass graft (CABG) surgery. Unlike EBCT or MSCT, coronary MR angiography does not require iodinated contrast agents or X-ray radiation and therefore has the potential to become a more widespread and easy-to-use screening tool to investigate subjects at high risk for developing atherosclerosis and acute coronary syndromes. Coronary MR imaging techniques can also be part of a broader cardiac investigation where, within a single MR imaging study, valuable and often unique information can be obtained with regard to ventricular function, myocardial perfusion and myocardial viability in patients with ischemic heart disease. Since most coronary MR imaging techniques are still premature for clinical use, the different approaches and strategies currently used are extensively discussed. In addition, the current and potential clinical indications, as well as the role of MR imaging compared with MSCT and EBCT, are highlighted in this chapter.

14.2
Pathogenesis and Pathophysiology of Coronary Artery Disease

Atherosclerosis, the disease process underlying CAD, is a systemic disease of the arterial vessel wall that causes distinct clinical manifestations, depending on the affected circulatory bed and the characteristics of the individual lesions (Fuster et al. 1999; Fuster and Gotto 2000). Atherosclerosis develops silently over several decades and begins as early as young adulthood (Strong et al. 1997). Since clinical complications such as myocardial infarction and stroke usually occur in asymptomatic, apparently healthy middle-aged or older people, identification of high-risk subjects, assessment of the atherosclerotic burden, and application of appropriate preventive strategies (e.g. improvement of plaque stability with lipid-lowering medication) during the presymptomatic detection of the disease, is considered a major challenge for the 21st century (Celermajer 1998; Grundy et al. 1999).

According to the criteria of the American Heart Association Committee on Vascular Lesions, coronary artery plaques and plaque progression can be subdivided into five phases of progression and six different lesion types (classified according to Stary; Stary et al. 1992). The pathogenesis of atherosclerosis is complex and a detailed description is beyond the scope of this chapter. In brief, the influx of lipids and/or accumulation into the vessel wall leads to remodelling of the arterial wall, which consists of fatty accumulation, and an increased number of macrophages (Fuster 1994). Type I–III lesions are mainly differentiated by their proportions of lipids, macrophages and smooth muscle cells and whether the lipid is intra- or extracellular. The potential for clinical problems, however, begins when the process of lipid influx and accumulation continues (Fig. 14.1). A type IV lesion, i.e. atheroma, has a predominance of extracellular lipid, mainly diffuse; and a type Va lesion, i.e. fibroatheroma, has a high lipid content, mainly localized, and a very thin capsule (Stary et al. 1995). Both lesions can evolve into the more fibrotic and stenotic types Vb (mainly calcified) and Vc (mainly fibrotic) lesions. However, both type IV and Va lesions also have a tendency for acute rupture with a change in their geometry, and subsequent thrombus formation may lead to the type VI, i.e. complicated, lesions (Fig. 14.1). Disruption-prone plaques in the coronary arteries, the so-called "vulnerable plaques" tend to have a thin fibrous cap (cap thickness 65–150 μm), a large lipid core (plaque type IV–Va), a high number of macrophages, and a low number of smooth muscle cells. These vulnerable plaques are often only modestly stenotic, and therefore angiographically silent.

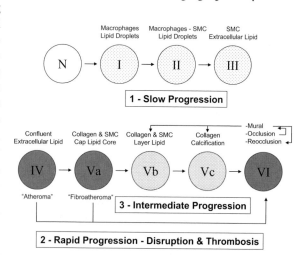

Fig. 14.1. Evolution of coronary artery disease. (Adapted from Zaman et al. 2000). SMC, smooth muscle cells

The absence or near absence of luminal narrowing can be explained by the phenomenon of positive remodelling; as the arterial wall is not a static, immutable structure. Remodelling of the arterial wall can occur by increasing its external diameter to accommodate the plaque without narrowing the lumen – positive remodelling. Negative remodelling is the opposite phenomenon, with a reduction of the internal diameter and luminal narrowing, and is usually found in plaque type Vb and Vc. Disruption of a coronary artery plaque in general leads to an acute or unstable coronary syndrome (unstable angina, acute myocardial infarct, sudden coronary death). The degree of lesion disruption determines the nature of the ensuing clinical state (STARY et al. 1995). The deeper the disruption or ulceration, the more the lipid core, collagen, tissue factor and other elements are exposed, with a thrombotic occlusion that is relatively persistent (2–4 h or longer) and that may result in acute myocardial infarction. In some cases, however, a deep plaque injury cannot be identified. The thrombus appears to be superimposed on a de-endothelialized but otherwise intact plaque. This type of superficial plaque injury is called plaque erosion (DAVIES 1996).

In contrast to small lipid-rich lesions that are prone to disruption, severely stenotic lesions tend to be fibrotic and stable (KRAGEL et al. 1991). These fibrotic and/or calcified lesions typically narrow the coronary artery lumen, causing symptoms of myocardial ischemia (angina). Severe stenoses tend to progress to total thrombotic occlusion approximately three times more often than less severe lesion, but less frequently lead to infarction, probably because of well-developed collateral vessels.

The concept of plaque vulnerability and assessment of a vulnerability index for future acute ischemia events (determined by the absolute number of vulnerable plaques present) has recently led a consensus report defining "the vulnerable patient" (NAGHAVI et al. 2003a, 2003b). First, all types of atherosclerotic plaques with a high likelihood of thrombotic complications and rapid progression should be considered as vulnerable plaques (Table 14.1). However, they are not the only culprit factors for the development of acute coronary syndromes. "Vulnerable blood" (prone to thrombosis) and "vulnerable myocardium" (prone to fatal arrhythmia) play an important role in the outcome. Therefore, the term "vulnerable patient" may be more appropriate and should be used for identification of subjects with a high likelihood of developing cardiac events in the near future. The non-invasive coronary imag-

Table 14.1. Markers of vulnerability. Adapted from NAGHAVI et al. (2003b)

Plaque morphology – Plaque structure
– Plaque cap thickness
– Plaque lipid core size
– Plaque stenosis (luminal narrowing)
– Remodelling (positive versus negative remodelling)
– Colour (yellow, red)
– Collagen content versus lipid content
– Mechanical stability
– Calcification burden and pattern
– Shear stress
Plaque activity – Plaque function
– Plaque inflammation
– Endothelial denudation or dysfunction
– Plaque oxidative stress
– Superficial platelet aggregation and fibrin deposition
– Rate of apoptosis
– Angiogenesis, and intraplaque haemorrhage
– Matrix-digesting enzyme activity in the cap
– Certain microbial antigens
Other factors
– Transcoronary gradient of serum markers of vulnerability
– Total burden of coronary artery disease (coronary calcium score)
– Systemic indexes of inflammation
– Endothelial dysfunction
– Blood coagulability (vulnerable blood)
– Myocardial susceptibility to develop arrhythmia (vulnerable myocardium)

ing techniques such as MR imaging and computed tomography (CT) might have an important role in identifying these vulnerable patients.

14.3
Challenges for Non-invasive Coronary Artery Imaging

Catheter-based or X-ray coronary angiography is the indisputable reference standard for the detection of coronary artery stenosis (Table 14.2). It uses a photographic approach with selective injection of iodinated contrast material in to the left (LCA) and right coronary artery (RCA). Images are obtained with a high temporal resolution (60 images/s) and a high spatial resolution (0.1×0.1 mm^2). Projectional images of the coronary arteries are obtained without interference of the cardiac chambers in different standardized image planes. Computed techniques are available for quantitative analysis of coronary artery stenoses (QCA) techniques. The fluoroscopic approach allows cine viewing and provides informa-

Table 14.2. Strengths and limitations of catheter-based coronary angiography

Strengths
- Reference technique for CA anatomy and stenosis detection
- Photographic approach
- High temporal resolution (60 images/s)
- High spatial resolution (0.1x0.1 mm²)
- Selective injection of LCA – RCA
- Projectional images without interference of cardiac chambers
- Detailed and large coverage of CAs
- Fluoroscopic approach with cine viewing provides information on CA flow patterns
- Therapeutic procedures (e.g. balloon dilatation – stenting – stem cell procedures)

Limitations
- Narrowing of lesion expressed to calibre of adjacent "normal" segments
- Risk of underestimation of CA stenoses
- "Luminography"": no information about CA wall, arterial remodelling or plaque morphology
- Vulnerable (often non-stenotic) plaque not detected
- Irradiation – expensive
- Significant morbidity (e.g. CA – aortic dissection) and mortality
- Significant number of negative studies (up to 25%)
- Not useful as screening technique

tion on coronary flow patterns (e.g. thrombolysis in myocardial infarction (TIMI) flow patterns after revascularization of coronary artery stenoses). X-ray coronary angiography is not only a diagnostic technique, but is also often used for therapeutic procedures such as balloon angioplasty, coronary artery stenting and, more recently, the injection of autologous stem cells in patients with an acute myocardial infarction. As shown in Table 14.2, X-ray coronary angiography has several shortcomings. For example, since coronary atheromatosis is a diffuse disease, expression of the degree of coronary artery narrowing to the calibre of adjacent "normal" segments, is prone to underestimation of the severity of coronary artery stenosis. The angiographic or luminographic type of imaging obtained by X-ray angiography provides no information about the presence of wall remodelling or about the coronary plaque morphology. Thus, vulnerable plaques, with often a mild or moderate narrowing of the coronary artery lumen, are not detected on coronary angiography. The catheter-based approach has a significant morbidity (e.g. coronary or aortic dissection) and mortality and, because of its invasive nature, is not applicable as a screening technique. Also, there are a significant number of negative studies (up to 25%) in patients with a clinical suspicion of

coronary artery disease. Other important issues to consider are the X-ray dose, the injection of a considerable amount of iodinated contrast material and the expense of the procedure.

A good, non-invasive alternative to conventional coronary angiography has to meet several challenges, as shown in Table 14.3. Coronary arteries are small, tortuous vessels (size 2–5 mm) embedded in the epicardial fat and located on a curved cardiac surface. Coronary artery anatomy and its branching pattern are highly variable. Coronary artery flow and velocity patterns are complex, with differences between LCA and RCA. Furthermore, when significant coronary artery stenosis is present, the contribution of collateral flow should be assessed. Coronary artery motion, due to respiration and cardiac pump function, is a major problem for non-invasive imaging techniques and has a strong impact on image quality. As a consequence, non-invasive coronary artery imaging is a compromise between various parameters: spatial resolution, acquisition window, volume coverage, signal-to-noise ratio (SNR) and contrast-to-noise ratio (CNR; Fig. 14.2). Other issues such as metal artefacts due to coronary stents or bypass clips, or coronary atherosclerotic calcifications should be considered.

Table 14.3. Challenges for non-invasive coronary artery imaging

- Small vessel size (2–5 mm)
- Long, tortuous and curved CA course along the cardiac surface
- Physiology of CA blood flow
  - Flow patterns
  - Velocities
  - Collateral flow
- Cardiac and CA motion (different for the 3 main CAs)
- Respiratory motion
- Epicardial fat
- Spatial resolution
- Volume coverage
- Metal artefacts from CA stents and CABG clips

14.4
History of Coronary MR Imaging

The quest to non-invasively demonstrate the coronary arteries with MR imaging started in the early 1990s. Since then, huge progress has been made, starting from hardly detectable coronary arteries and moving towards a reliable and reproducible assessment of large portions of the coronary artery tree in a reasonable imaging time in the current

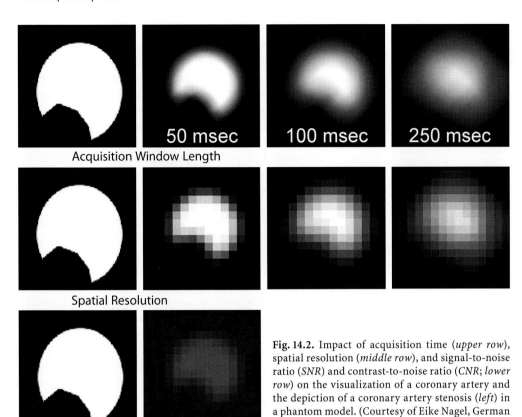

Acquisition Window Length

Spatial Resolution

SNR – CNR

Fig. 14.2. Impact of acquisition time (*upper row*), spatial resolution (*middle row*), and signal-to-noise ratio (*SNR*) and contrast-to-noise ratio (*CNR; lower row*) on the visualization of a coronary artery and the depiction of a coronary artery stenosis (*left*) in a phantom model. (Courtesy of Eike Nagel, German Heart Institute, Berlin, Germany)

era. A brief review of the history of coronary MR angiography gives the reader a good idea of the technical evolution, and the approaches and strategies that have been used to study the coronary arteries. Although most review papers use "generations" to define the major steps in coronary MR angiography, this subdivision in different generations is somewhat artificial and prone to confusion and discussion (BUNCE and PENNELL 1999; WIELOPOLSKI et al. 2000; FAYAD et al. 2002). For example, the navigator-echo ("second" generation) and breath-hold ("third" generation) techniques are two different approaches that are still used for coronary MR angiography; but, based on their subdivision, third-generation techniques might be falsely considered as superior to second-generation techniques. For an extensive review of coronary MR angiography techniques and its history, let us refer the reader to the excellent book edited by André Duerinckx on this interesting topic (DUERINCKX 2002).

Although imaging of the coronary arteries by MR was initially noted in 1987 (PAULIN et al. 1987; GOMES et al. 1987), with visualization of small segments of native coronary vessels and bypass grafts, the real start of coronary artery imaging by MR, coronary

MR angiography (or magnetic resonance coronary angiography, MRCA), coincided with the introduction of ultrafast imaging techniques in 1991. These techniques relied upon a combination of segmental acquisition of data in κ-space to minimize cardiac motion, and the use of a single breath-hold to minimize respiratory motion artefacts (ATKINSON and EDELMAN 1991). Edelman and colleagues used a two-dimensional (2D), ECG-triggered, κ-space segmented MR sequence to study coronary arteries (Fig. 14.3; EDELMAN et al. 1991). Its subsequent value for visualizing the course of the coronary arteries and detecting coronary artery disease has been evaluated by several groups (MANNING et al. 1993a; DUERINCKX and URMAN 1994; MOHIADDIN et al. 1996; NITATORI et al. 1995; POST et al. 1997; YOSHINO et al. 1997). For several reasons, this so-called first generation of techniques has been totally abandoned. Two-dimensional imaging techniques are not well suited to the study of the tortuous course of coronary arteries. Only portions of the coronary arteries can be visualized within each breath-hold and the inconsistency of breath-hold position makes coronary artery imaging, even for experienced investigators in the field, a difficult task. The absence

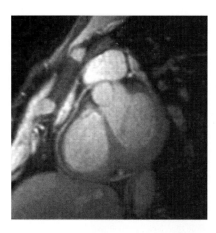

Fig. 14.3. 2D coronary MR angiography of the right coronary artery (RCA) using the breath-hold segmented κ-space spoiled gradient-echo (GE) technique

of dedicated cardiac receiver coils necessitates the examination of patients in a prone position, which most find uncomfortable and difficult to sustain. Furthermore, the high number of repeated breath-holds is usually too exhausting to study cardiac patients in a comfortable way.

Because of the severe limitations of the 2D breath-hold approach, investigators have explored several alternatives to overcome these problems and improve image quality. They can be summarized as: (a) three-dimensional (3D) imaging approaches, (b) techniques to suppress respiratory motion either by using navigators or acquisition during breath-hold, and (c) use of intravascular contrast agents. Three-dimensional imaging offers the advantages of higher SNR, shorter echo times, more isotropic voxel resolution, and the ability to examine the data set with a multi-planar reformatting technique. Moreover, the complex course of the coronary arteries necessitates a 3D approach. Although the initial attempts at using signal averaging (without breath-holding) for 3D coronary imaging did not produce very good results (PASCHAL et al. 1993; HOFMAN et al. 1995a; LI et al. 1996), SCHEIDEGGER and colleagues were the first to use sophisticated 3D imaging display technology (SCHEIDEGGER et al. 1994, 1996). This and other pioneering work on 3D coronary MR imaging has formed the basis for the development of currently used 3D coronary MR angiography techniques. More recent improvements in MR imaging technology with stronger gradient systems, shorter rise times and more sophisticated ECG triggering devices have further contributed to current high-quality sub-millimetre 3D visualization of the coronary arteries.

Navigator echoes (NE) rely upon an MR pulse to determine the motion of the diaphragm (a surrogate of respiratory motion). This enables MR images to be acquired during continuous regular breathing and open the way for higher spatial-resolution coronary MR angiography with increased patient comfort. Navigator techniques were first described in 1993–1994 (WANG et al. 1996), but, because the initial proposed implementations had severe shortcomings, they have undergone several improvements (DANIAS et al. 1997; McCONNELL et al. 1997a). Though this technique has been implemented on existing 2D coronary MR angiography techniques, to improve image quality either by providing feedback to the patient for repeated breath-holds (as to when to hold his/her breath) or by feeding information back to the MR computer, NEs have been generally used in combination with 3D coronary MR angiography techniques. The NE pulse most often determines the motion of the diaphragm, but in some implementations it directly monitors the motion of portions of the left ventricular wall. For the repeated breath-holding versions, inconsistent breath-holding is no longer a problem, as the patient receives feedback as to when to stop breathing. For the non-breath-hold versions, the regularity of the breathing pattern during the long scan acquisition (sometimes up to 15 min) is important. It has been recommended that: the NE window be placed around end-expiratory position; subjects should not sleep; and scan efficiency should be monitored and, if necessary, the NE window repositioned (TAYLOR et al. 1997). Because of these and similar recommendations, many adaptations and improvements to NE schemes have been made to improve their efficacy, including adaptive windowing (to correct for upward creep of the diaphragm in the supine position after 15–20 min) and the use of three orthogonal NE (to minimize motion in all three directions; DANIAS et al. 1997; McCONNELL et al. 1997b; TAYLOR et al. 1997). Once implemented, this technique requires less expertise and training, because a 3D transaxial slab covering the top of the heart and aortic root can be acquired and images can be analysed later. Potential problems with the NE coronary MR angiography technique are: (a) the length of each acquisition, up to 12–15 min in some cases, compare with a single 15- to 20-s breath-hold; and (b) difficulty obtaining a good NE position (up to 50% failure in normal volunteers in initial studies).

Breath-hold 3D techniques (so-called third-generation) are an alternative to NE techniques and were first described in 1995 by Piotr Wielopolski

(WIELOPOLSKI et al. 1995). These techniques may provide the ultimate compromise between user-friendliness and acquisition speeds. The entire coronary anatomy can be acquired in a single breath-hold with isotropic resolution. Using a segmented echoplanar imaging (EPI) technique, with thin slabs oriented along the course of the coronaries, high spatial-resolution images of the coronaries can be obtained in a single breath-hold. This approach, using small-volume scan acquisitions oriented along the coronaries, is called VCATS (volume coronary arteriography using targeted scans; WIELOPOLSKI et al. 1998). Other groups have used a fat-suppressed, 3D-segmented, ECG-triggered TurboFLASH, with acquisition of small volumes during breath-hold.

Dynamic contrast-enhanced MR angiography (CE-MRA), first described by Martin Prince, has totally changed the way thoracic and body MR angiography are performed today (PRINCE 1994). Although CE-MRA started out with relatively long acquisition times (greater than 1 min), it can now be used within very short breath-hold periods (7- to 23-s breath-holds to study the aorta or the pulmonary arteries). The same non-ECG-triggered technique was applied for native coronary artery and CABG imaging (VAN ROSSUM et al. 1997; VRACHLIOTIS et al. 1997). In order to acquire ECG-triggered MRA of native coronary vessels, pulse sequences with faster acquisition rates, κ-space data segmentation, data interpolation and other technical tricks are required.

Initial experience with extravascular MR contrast agents indicated that very high doses of gadolinium would be needed for 2D-breath-hold coronary MR angiography. With bolus arrival timing to catch the first pass of the gadolinium contrast agent, image quality improvements have been obtained (improved SNR and CNR) for the 3D coronary MR angiography techniques.

14.5
Coronary MR Angiography: Strategies

14.5.1
Respiratory Motion

14.5.1.1
Free-Breathing Coronary MR Angiography

Free-breathing coronary MR angiography is at present a commonly used and robust technique for studying the coronary arteries (Table 14.4). By using

Table 14.4. Current strategies used for anatomical assessment of coronary arteries

Breathing motion compensation
 – navigators
 – breath-hold

Contrast enhancement techniques
 – magnetization transfer contrast (MTC)
 – T2-preparation pulse
 – steady-state imaging
 – (intravascular) contrast agents
 – fat-suppression techniques
 – arterial spin-labelling

Fast imaging techniques
 – echoplanar imaging (EPI)
 – parallel imaging

High spatial-resolution techniques
 – 3D spoiled-GE techniques (TFE/FLASH)
 – 3D balanced-SSFP (b-TFE/true-FISP/FIESTA)
 – 3D turbo spin-echo (TSE)

κ-space filling techniques
 – 3D Cartesian
 – 3D radial
 – 3D spiral

Volume coverage techniques
 – CA targeted approach (VCATS)
 – whole-heart coronary MR angiography

Black-blood imaging
 – 3D TSE
 – 3D balanced SSFP

NE algorithms that correct for respiratory-induced coronary artery motion, 3D coronary MR angiography sequences can be performed during free-breathing with the effects of respiratory motion on image quality largely eliminated (FIRMAN and KEEGAN 2001). Since its introduction in the mid-1990s, the NE technique has been refined into a reliable and easy-to handle tool that is often used in routine cardiac MR imaging for a variety of clinical applications (SPUENTRUP et al. 2002a). Not only is the patient's comfort improved, as repeated, often exhausting, breath-holds are avoided, but the risk of misregistration by breath-hold inconsistency is limited (CHUANG et al. 1997). The success of coronary MR imaging in uncooperative or minimally cooperative patients (e.g. paediatric and elderly populations) depends on the use of NE-based MR imaging sequences. Free-breathing coronary MR angiography, however, takes significantly longer than breath-hold coronary MR angiography, since only a small part of each respiratory cycle is used for data acquisition. As already mentioned, the optimization of cardiac MR sequences is a compromise between different, often conflicting parameters (e.g. spatial resolution, temporal resolution, SNR, CNR, total imaging time and volume coverage). Breath-hold techniques opt to gather all data during a single breath-hold, but have to make sacrifices between these various parameters, with trade-off in optimal spatial and temporal resolution, and volume coverage. By removing the time constraints of breath holding, the NE-based coronary MR angiography techniques can choose for an improved spatial resolution (e.g. to improve coronary artery stenosis quantification), for a shorter acquisition duration per cardiac cycle (e.g. to limit image blurring due to coronary artery motion), or for a more extensive volume coverage (e.g. whole-heart coronary MR angiography), at the expense of a longer total imaging time (WEBER et al. 2003).

NE are an accurate method for measuring motion in MR imaging (EHMAN and FELMLEE 1989). The earlier-used, retrospective NE-gating techniques have been abandoned because of the need to over-sample the acquisition (typically by a factor of 5), considerably prolonging the total imaging time with the risk of respiratory drifting and sub-optimal results (LENZ et al. 1989; HOFMAN et al. 1995a; POST et al. 1996; LI et al. 1996). The currently implemented NE techniques use prospective algorithms, applying either a selective 2D radiofrequency pulse to excite the signal in a column of approximately circular cross-section (a "pencil beam"; HARDY and CLINE 1989), or a spin-echo sequence, with the planes selected by the 90° and 180° radiofrequency pulses being either orthogonal or at an angle such that the spin echo signal is formed from a column of rectangular or parallelogram cross-section (FIRMIN and KEEGAN 2001). These NEs are usually positioned perpendicular on the dome of the right hemidiaphragm (Fig. 14.4). During image acquisition, the cranio-caudal or superior–inferior motion of the diaphragm at the liver/ lung interface is measured (CHUANG et al. 1997). The spatial resolution of the NE in the long-axis direction is 1 mm. This real-time, prospective NE-gating technique uses a tolerance range (or gating window), usually at end-expiration. The width of this gating window usually is 5 mm. If the respiratory position is within this gating window, data are accepted. Otherwise, data are rejected and re-acquired during the next heartbeat (WANG and EHMAN 2000). The efficiency of this real-time navigator approach (often called "scan efficiency") is expressed as the numbers of acquisitions accepted divided by the total number of heartbeats used for completing a scan (STUBER et al. 1999b). A scan efficiency of 50%, for example, refers to a scan in which, on average, data acquired from every other heartbeat are accepted for reconstruction. Using a similar approach, Stuber et al. have reported a scan efficiency of 60% in healthy volunteers and 43% in patients (STUBER et al. 1999b). Patient instruction before coronary MR angiography can be helpful to improve scan efficiency. It is recommended that patients are instructed to perform regular, shallow breathing and to avoid changes in depth of breathing during the acquisition. It is important to consider that, during respiration, the diaphragmatic motion or shift is not the same as the coronary shift (WANG et al. 1995; DANIAS et al. 1997). To effectively suppress coronary artery motion, a scaling (or correction) factor between both needs to be known. A correction factor of 0.6 in the superior–inferior direction has been recommended by Wang and co-workers for the base of the heart (WANG et al. 1995; DANIAS et al. 1997). In ten healthy volunteers, a relative displacement of 0.57±0.26 (measured at the origin of the RCA) has been demonstrated. Optionally, an additional scaling of 0.12 can be used to correct for motion in the

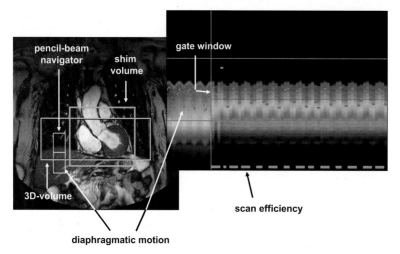

Fig. 14.4. Real-time prospective navigator-echo (NE) technique. Coronal scout MR image (*left*). The pencil-beam navigator is positioned on the dome of the right hemidiaphragm. The up- and downward motion of the diaphragm is shown as a *red curve* (*right*). The gating window, indicated by the *blue lines*, determines whether or not the shots are accepted for data reconstruction. The scan efficiency is indicated by the *green line*

anterior–posterior direction (BÖRNERT et al. 1999; STUBER et al. 1999b). This superior–inferior scaling factor is, however, not the same between individuals, as shown by the relative large standard deviation (WANG et al. 1995; KEEGAN et al. 2002; MANKE et al. 2002). Therefore, the use of a fixed scaling factor might lead to non-optimal motion suppression, stressing the need to use subject-specific correction factors (TAYLOR et al. 1997). In a recent study by Keegan and co-workers using a free-breathing acquisition, significantly smaller motion correction factors for slice-following applications were found than fixed value of 0.6 (derived from breath-hold acquisitions; KEEGAN et al. 2002). Another important issue for effective motion correction is that the motion (and motion direction) in the acquired image needs to be the same as the motion measured by the NE. Therefore, the time between the NE and the image echo needs to be as short as possible (TAYLOR et al. 1997; SPUENTRUP et al. 2001). Taylor et al. have shown that, to maintain a measurement error of less than 0.5 mm (peak respiratory velocity is about 10 mm/s), the time lapse should be less than 50 ms. To improve sharpness of coronary artery visualization, Stuber et al. have proposed, in addition to navigator gating, an adaptive prospective real-time motion correction of the image volume position ("gate and track approach"; STUBER et al. 1999c). Adaptation or correction of the measured volume is related to the distance from the end-expiratory level to the detected interface position. Real-time motion correction is performed prospectively only if the position of the measured interface is within the gating window. The position of the imaged 3D volume can be adapted prospectively for all three spatial coordinates, which allows optimal correction for the different spatial courses of the LCA and RCA tree (STUBER et al. 1999c). If the gate and track approach is used, the shortest time delay (less than 40 ms) between NE and image echo is necessary for high-resolution coronary MR angiography (SPUENTRUP et al. 2002b, 2002c).

Particularly in long coronary MR angiography scans, the respiratory motion statistics may change because of diaphragm drift effects or macroscopic patient motion (TAYLOR et al. 1997). Wang and Ehman have proposed the use of an additional NE immediately following the image sequence as an effective means of retrospectively correcting for motion and moreover to overcome the problem of a fixed scaling factor (WANG and EHMAN 2000). Respiratory drift might also be corrected by the motion-adapted gating (MAG) algorithm that uses three navigators distributed over one cardiac cycle, enabling an instant and automatic analysis of the motion statistics of the diaphragm in real time (SINKUS and BÖRNERT 1999). If necessary, the algorithm changes gating parameters without user interaction being required. Motion-adapted gating, based on the concept of κ-space weighting, has been proposed by Weiger and co-workers to reduce respiratory motion artefacts, to increase coronary vessel sharpness and to improve scan efficiency (WEIGER et al. 1997; JHOOTI et al. 1999; WEBER et al. 2002). κ-space reordering techniques take advantage of the inhomogeneous signal distribution in κ-space, with highest signal amplitudes in the centre of κ-space and gradually decreasing information content in the periphery of κ-space. With motion-adaptive gating, the "important" profiles are acquired during a small diaphragmatic displacement, while profiles of "lesser importance" are subject to broader or larger displacement conditions (HUBER et al. 2001). The use of a method of ordering the data acquisition in real-time according to the navigator position enables the use of a larger navigator acceptance window (and hence improved scan efficiency) while maintaining image quality. The Brompton group in London has proposed several 2D reordering schemes (e.g. hybrid-ordered phase encoding, HOPE), while the Beth Israel group in Boston has described a "true" 3D κ-space reordering technique in conjunction with a 3D imaging approach (BUNCE et al. 2001b; HUBER et al. 2001). Recently, Plein et al. have proposed a novel technique to synchronize cardiac and respiratory motion with the aid of an external respirator (cuirass-type respirator; PLEIN et al. 2003a). Their preliminary results show a significant gain in imaging time with preserved SNR, CNR and image quality.

The position of the NE in most studies has been on the dome of the right hemidiaphragm. Although the dome is somewhat less mobile than the posterior or lateral portions of the diaphragm, the dome is generally selected for NE monitoring because it is perpendicular to the direction of motion over a wide range of motion and consequently results in a sharp edge, easily suited to edge detection techniques. Alternative locations for the NE include the heart–lung interface (at the level of the left anterior descending coronary artery (LAD); McCONNELL et al. 1997b). Although a NE position close to the coronary arteries is strategically appealing (no correction for scaling necessary), Stuber and co-workers have found only minor quantitative differences in vessel diameter, CNR, and SNR, compared with a diaphragmatic NE positioning (STUBER et al. 1999c). Nguyen et al. have recently reported direct monitoring of coronary artery motion with a cardiac fat NE (NGUYEN et al. 2003). Recently a study by the same group, reporting their preliminary experience on in vivo coronary MR angiography at 3 T in humans, has recommended a NE position at the heart–liver interface instead of the lung–liver interface (STUBER et al. 2002a).

14.5.1.2
Breath-Hold Coronary MR Angiography

Breath-hold imaging has become the current standard approach for MR imaging of the heart. Cardiac morphology, function, perfusion, flow measurements and viability studies are routinely performed in breath-hold, and these fast techniques have largely abandoned the conventional, time-consuming MR sequences over the last decade. The breath-hold approach is also appealing for coronary artery MR imaging. The 2D breath-hold coronary MR angiography technique, described by Edelman and colleagues in 1991 (EDELMAN et al. 1991), was a major step forward in coronary MR angiography. However, as mentioned above, coronary artery imaging is probably one of the most demanding areas in imaging of the human body, and definitely at the edge of what is currently achievable on a technical MR imaging level. Thus, to obtain images with a high spatial resolution and sufficiently high temporal resolution in a single breath-hold, only small 3D volumes can be covered. This approach was introduced by Piotr Wielopolski and colleagues (WIELOPOLSKI et al. 1995, 1998). VCATS uses small volumes (24 mm thick) targeted along the course of the coronaries. On a single, end-expiratory breath-hold 3D localizer, covering the entire heart, multiplanar reformation (MPR) images are generated

that are used for planning of the double-obliquely oriented, 3D slabs containing the coronary segment of interest. The entire coronary artery tree is consistently covered in fewer than 13 breath holds, taking 16–22 heartbeats at end-expiration. The VCATS technique can acquire a true section thickness of 2 mm and an in-plane resolution of 1.5×0.75 mm in 21 heartbeats, but, at this spatial resolution, noise prevails (WIELOPOLSKI et al. 1998). To improve SNR, a low-readout bandwidth (necessitating longer acquisition times and thus a free-breathing approach) and use of contrast agents might be helpful. In a clinical study from the same Rotterdam group using the VCATS technique, the assessability of the different coronary arterial segments ranged from an excellent 91% assessability for the left main stem coronary artery (LM) and proximal LAD to a poor 38% assessability for the mid left circumflex coronary artery (LCx; VAN GEUNS et al. 2000). The Northwestern Group from Chicago have applied a combination of real-time NE with 3D breath-hold coronary MR angiography to the above-mentioned problems (SHEA et al. 2001; Figs. 14.5 and 14.6). A multiple breath-hold imaging method in which a segment of κ-space is acquired in each breath-hold increases the spatial resolution, SNR and coronary artery coverage of the VCATS technique. A real-time slab following a technique using NEs for motion detection is used to correct for slab position differences between breath-holds. A similar approach has been proposed by the Beth Israel group, combining 3D breath-hold coronary artery imaging with real-time NE technology (STUBER et al. 1999d).

The question arises as to whether or not it is best to acquire image data during end-expiration or end-inspiration. On the one hand, long breath-holds such as necessary for coronary MR angiography (e.g. 16–22 heartbeats) are often difficult to sustain at end-expiration for patients. On the other hand,

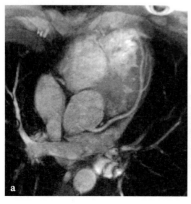 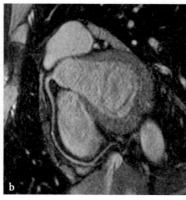

Fig. 14.5a,b. Breath-hold 3D coronary MR angiography using the balanced steady-state free precession (b-SSFP; true-fast imaging in steady-state precession, FISP, technique; Courtesy of Debiao Li, Northwestern University, Chicago, USA). Left main stem coronary artery and left anterior descending coronary artery (**a**), and RCA (**b**). The length per breath-hold was 24–30 s

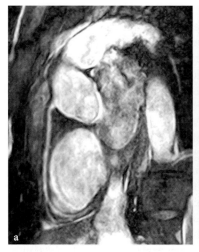 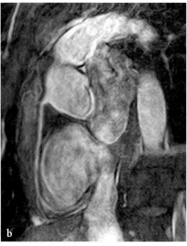

Fig. 14.6a,b. Comparison between 3D coronary MR angiography (b-SSFP technique) using the breath-hold approach (**a**) and NE approach (**b**). In both approaches the number of shots acquired per cardiac cycle was 32 (acquisition window length: 160 ms)

Holland and colleagues report that breath-holding does not eliminate motion of the diaphragm. Based on a study of normal volunteers, they have calculated that the average total diaphragm displacement during a 20-s breath-hold at end-inspiration is 11 mm (HOLLAND et al. 1998). At end-expiration the average total diaphragm displacement was only 3 mm, with an average diaphragm velocity of 0.15 mm/s. During both end-inspiration and end-expiration there was a gradual upward creep of the diaphragm during the short, 20-s period of breath-holding. It was a linear and gradual motion at end-expiration for all volunteers; but at end-inspiration it was more irregular, with time-varying velocities in some of the volunteers. Thus, if possible, end-expiration should be used for image data acquisition. If the patient has trouble holding his/her breath for the required duration (12–16 s), one can lower the matrix size or increase the data acquisition length by taking a larger number of views per κ-space segment. Another interesting approach to improve breath-hold lengths is pre-oxygenation of patients (MCCARTHY et al. 2003). In a study in healthy volunteers, oxygen was administered at a rate of 4 l/min for 2 min before the start of imaging (subjects were instructed not to hyperventilate because of the risk of coronary artery spasm). Breath-hold length increased from 56 s (range, 21–173 s) before to 92 s (range, 33–241 s) after oxygen administration. As a result voxel size decreased from 0.8×1.1×4 mm^3 on the room-air images to 0.8×0.9×2.6 mm^3 on the post-oxygen images. Not only is the subject's comfort increased, but this approach produces images with an increased spatial resolution and improved vessel wall delineation. Although these long breath-holds are not achievable in patients with coronary artery disease, Marks et al. have shown that oxygen administration allows patients with chronic pulmonary disease to more than double their average maximum breath-hold duration (MARKS et al. 1997).

14.5.2
Coronary Artery Motion and Acquisition Window

Another major source of coronary artery motion, besides bulk motion of the heart due to respiration, is motion induced by cardiac pump activity and pulsatile arterial flow patterns. With an ultra-short acquisition time per image (approximately 15–30 ms for digital images), coronary artery motion is perfectly "frozen" in X-ray coronary angiography. Real-time, high-frequency imaging of the coronary arteries during injection of contrast media allows not only the acquisition of sharp coronary artery images, but also the visualization of coronary artery motion during the cardiac cycle and respiration (WANG et al. 1999). The acquisition length for coronary MR angiography images is unfortunately too long to freeze coronary artery motion. The total measurement time necessary to fill κ-space takes about 2.6 s for a breath-hold 3D coronary MR angiography sequence (using an acquisition length of 120 ms per heartbeat and a total of 22 heartbeats) and, for the free-breathing approach, approximately 13 s (using a data acquisition length or "shot duration" of 80 ms per heartbeat, and a total of 164 shots). Different strategies have been developed that cope with these motion problems and attempt to reduce vessel blurring.

Cardiac motion and thus also coronary artery motion can be suppressed by synchronizing the image acquisition to the repetitive pattern of cardiac contraction and relaxation. This is usually achieved by ECG triggering (the different currently used ECG techniques are discussed in Chaps. 1 and 3). Next, the length of data acquisition per heartbeat needs to be adjusted to reduce cardiac motion artefacts. This can be done by varying the number of refocusing echoes (for fast spin-echo sequences) or the number of shots (for gradient-echo sequences). Several other methods to reduce the acquisition length are discussed below. Whereas this adjustment is important for achieving the best image quality for assessment of gross cardiac anatomy or cardiac function, it becomes crucial when studying small structures such as the coronary arteries, since the faintest residual motion will lead to image blurring and unsharpness.

Assessment of the coronary artery motion pattern and velocities with biplane conventional angiography, EBCT and MR imaging have shown a highly variable pattern throughout the cardiac cycle, with important differences between the left and right coronary artery systems, and with a large variation between individuals (WANG et al. 1999; ACHENBACH et al. 2000; KIM et al. 2001a). Coronary artery displacement and velocities are much higher for the RCA than for the LAD. This can be explained by the anatomical location of the RCA within the anterior atrioventricular groove, which is prone to larger displacement and higher velocities due to the base to apex contraction of the heart during systole, which is not seen for the LAD in the anterior interventricular groove. Achenbach and colleagues have shown that coronary artery motion is most pronounced during early systole, early diastole and atrial contraction; and minimal during isovolumic relaxation and diastasis (ACHENBACH et al. 2000). Diastasis, or the mid-diastolic period between early ventricular filling and atrial contraction, is a relative rest period with minimal cardiac motion (Figs. 14.7 and 14.8). Diastasis is typically preceded by a gradual slowing of motion, as a result of the normalization of pressures between the atria and ventricles, but is always followed by abrupt motion, owing to the onset of atrial contraction. Wang et al. have found a huge variation in the length of this rest period, ranging from 66 to 333 ms, with a mean of 161 ms for the LCA and from 66 to 200 ms with a mean of 120 ms for the RCA (WANG et al. 1999). The length of this rest period is closely related to the cardiac frequency. The duration of the rest period decreases as the heart rate increases. For a heart rate less than 45 beats per minute, the rest period is approximately 200 and 300 ms for the RCA and LCA, respectively. As the heart rate increases from 45 to 65 beats/min, the rest period decreases to about 70 ms for both coronary arteries. For a heart rate greater than 65 beats/min, the rest period stays at 70 ms. The findings of Wang and colleagues have important implications for coronary MR angiography. First, in patients with a normal heart rate, the rest period is short and the data acquisition should be limited and synchronized as well as possible to this brief rest period. Second, in patients with heart rates below 55–60 beats/min, longer acquisition times can be used, thus enabling reduction in the total acquisition time without deterioration in image quality.

Precise determination of the timing of the rest period within the cardiac cycle is essential, especially in patients with heart rates above 55–60 min. Different approaches have been used to estimate this period of diastasis. Most of the earlier studies on coronary MR angiography used a fixed delay of 500 ms, with an adjustment of ±100 ms according to heart rate. Empirical estimations for diastasis can be calculated with the Weissler or Stuber formulae (WEISSLER et al. 1968; STUBER et al. 1999b). The trigger delay in the Stuber empirical formula is obtained as: trigger delay (milliseconds) = [(RR interval (milliseconds)−350)×0.3]+350. This definition takes advantage of the relatively constant duration of the systolic part of the cardiac cycle (±350 ms). This trigger delay was adjusted to sample the low κ-space profiles in diastasis. Empirical formulae have the advantage that they are easy to implement into the coronary MR angiography sequence. However, because these estimations are based on data from heart sounds or electrocardiography, they do or might not represent the actual cardiac motion that is occurring during data acquisition. Direct assessment of the optimal delay for coronary MR angiographic data acquisition window in the cardiac cycle is therefore probably the most correct approach. Direct assessment can be obtained by a breath-hold cine pre-scan at a fixed location (e.g. long-axis scan through the proximal or mid-portion of the RCA and LCx) with a high temporal resolution (FOO et al. 2000; KIM et al. 2001a; Fig. 14.7) or by an ECG-triggered navigator cardiac motion scan (WANG et al. 2001). The Beth Israel group have found a significant improvement in RCA imaging using a subject-specific determination of the diastasis period (compared with the heart-rate-dependent delay; KIM et al. 2001a). Imaging of the RCA vessel wall is only feasible with the subject-specific method, while the coronary wall can not be identified with the heart rate-dependent formula.

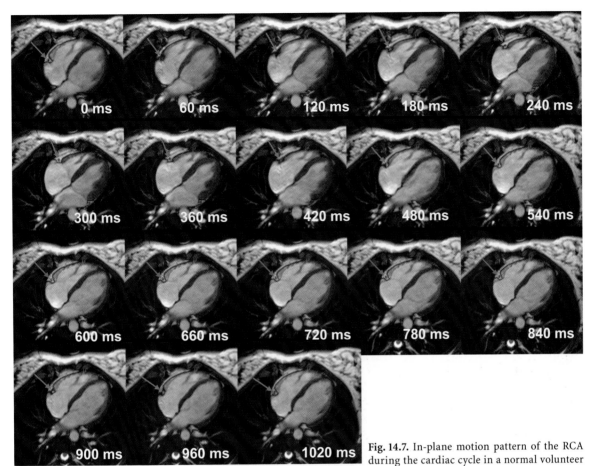

Fig. 14.7. In-plane motion pattern of the RCA during the cardiac cycle in a normal volunteer with a heart rate of 56 beats/min. Axial cine MRI using the b-SSFP technique (time frame 60 ms). The *arrow* indicates the RCA in the anterior atrioventricular groove. The data acquisition should be adjusted to the period of minimal cardiac motion, i.e. diastasis. In this volunteer the ideal period for imaging is between 600 and 840 ms after the R-wave (*green arrow*). The other cardiac phases are characterized by substantial motion and are consequently suboptimal for coronary artery imaging (*red arrow*)

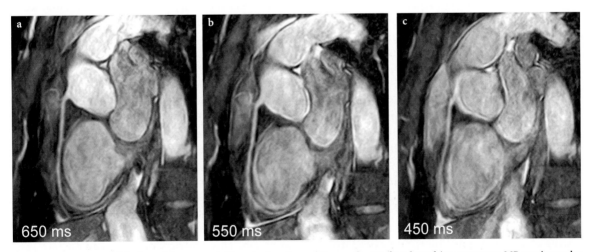

Fig. 14.8a-c. Impact of timing of data acquisition during the cardiac cycle. 3D free-breathing coronary MR angiography of RCA using the b-SSFP technique. Image acquisition at 650 ms after the R-wave (**a**) perfectly fits with cardiac diastasis as shown by the sharp delineation of the RCA and its branches. Images at 550 ms (**b**), and 450 ms (**c**) after the R-wave are obtained too early, i.e. during early ventricular filling. They are characterized by image blurring, vessel unsharpness, and loss in visualization of CA branches

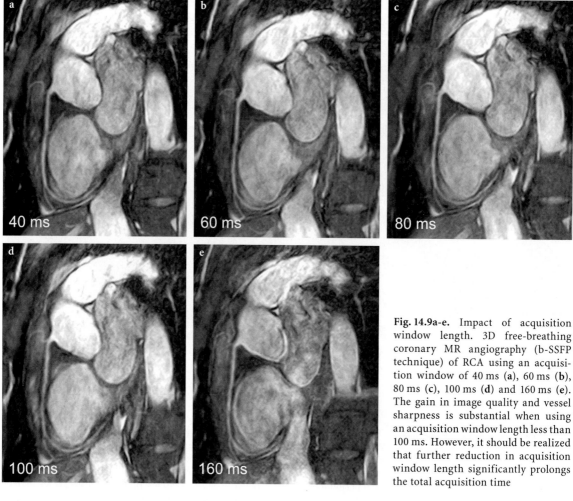

Fig. 14.9a-e. Impact of acquisition window length. 3D free-breathing coronary MR angiography (b-SSFP technique) of RCA using an acquisition window of 40 ms (**a**), 60 ms (**b**), 80 ms (**c**), 100 ms (**d**) and 160 ms (**e**). The gain in image quality and vessel sharpness is substantial when using an acquisition window length less than 100 ms. However, it should be realized that further reduction in acquisition window length significantly prolongs the total acquisition time

Determination of the length of the rest period might be interesting since, in patients with long coronary rest periods, extended acquisitions windows can be used with consequently shortened scanning times (Fig. 14.9). In a study by Plein and colleagues, from Leeds, UK, a subject-specific cardiac acquisition window in combination with motion-adapted respiratory gating (see 14.5.1.1) was used (PLEIN et al. 2003b). On a long-axis cine MR pre-scan through the atrioventricular grooves the timing and duration of the rest-period in each subject were determined and the acquisition length was subsequently adjusted. The motion-adapted gating used a 2-mm acceptance window for the central 35% of κ-space and a 6-mm window for the outer 65% of κ-space. Compared with the conventional technique (consisting of a fixed acquisition window of 73 ms, and a timing of the rest period estimated by the Stuber empirical formula, in combination with a fixed 5-mm gating window at end-expiration, with real-time correction for the accepted data within the gating window), scanning times with the adaptive technique were reduced by a factor of 2.3 for the RCA, and by a factor of 2.2 for the LCA without loss in image quality. This was mainly the result of longer rest periods up to 200 ms, usually found in patients with heartbeats less than 60 beats/min.

Another interesting approach to reduce cardiac motion effects is to adjust the κ-space sampling with the motion amplitude (WANG et al. 2000). The idea is that the centre of κ-space, where the majority of MR signal resides, is sampled during the quiescent diastasis period, and the edge of κ-space is sampled before and after diastasis. The traditionally used, centric κ-space sampling, in contrast, maximizes signal at the centre of κ-space by acquiring it at the beginning of the acquisition window when the spins are fresh. This centric view order can contain substantial cardiac motion effects, because of residual motion of the early, fast filling. Faster data acquisition not only shortens the scan time, but might be beneficial for the image quality, since the acquisi-

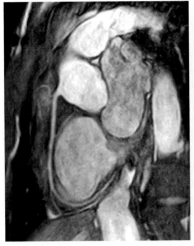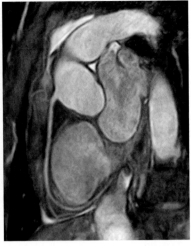

Fig. 14.10a,b. Impact of parallel imaging. 3D free-breathing coronary MR angiography (b-SSFP technique) of RCA without (**a**) and with parallel imaging (SENSE technique). Parallel imaging can be used to shorten acquisition window length and thus to reduce motion-related artefacts. Note also the improvement in overall image quality (constant level appearance effect)

tion window length can be reduced. The recent introduction of a new generation of MR scanners with stronger gradients (30 mT/m) and faster gradient switching systems has led to a significant shortening of sequence parameters (such as TR and TE).

Hybrid gradient-echo/EPI sequences are an effective method to reduce scan times. However, in the heart the EPI technique is prone to artefacts. Partial Fourier encoding can be used to halve the acquisition time and obtain reasonable coverage and in-plane spatial resolution (WIELOPOLSKI et al. 1998). However, partial Fourier acquisitions can produce signal intensity changes and distortions in the image, especially in gradient-echo acquisitions. A new and interesting approach to shorten the acquisition time per heartbeat, and therefore to increase image sharpness, is by using parallel imaging (e.g. SENSE, GRAPPA; Fig. 14.10). Sensitivity encoding (SENSE) uses multiple MR receive-coil elements to encode spatial information in addition to traditional gradient encoding (PRUESSMANN et al. 2001; VAN DEN BRINK et al. 2003). Requiring less gradient encodings translates into shorter scan times, which is beneficial for coronary MR angiography. Acceleration of the coronary MR angiography acquisition might be obtained by simultaneous acquisition of multiple rather than one 3D stack (MANKE et al. 2001). This approach uses not only diastasis, but also the period of isovolumic relaxation for image acquisition. One 3D stack is positioned through the LCA and measured during isovolumic relaxation, the second stack covering the RCA measured in diastasis. This two-stack approach yields a total scan time reduction of 50%, with an image quality equivalent to standard, single-stack coronary MR angiography.

14.5.3
Contrast Generation

One of the most difficult technical issues for coronary MR angiography is the differentiation of the coronary artery lumen from the surrounding tissues, in particular epicardial fat. Different methods to increase the visibility of the coronary arteries have been explored. Nowadays, a combination of techniques is used. In summary, generation of signal in coronary arteries is usually based on differences in physical properties between the coronary artery blood and surrounding structures. This can be related to differences in flow patterns, or to differences in T1- or T2-relaxation behaviour between blood and surrounding tissues. Differences in relaxation behaviour between tissues can be enhanced by using paramagnetic contrast agents. The visualization of coronary arteries can be indirectly enhanced by suppressing the signal of the surrounding tissues (e.g. fat saturation techniques, magnetization-transfer contrast techniques, T2-preparation pulse). Other techniques such as spin labelling use another approach to generate contrast in the coronary artery lumen and might be a valuable alternative. The visualization of coronary arteries will also benefit from the use of other dedicated cardiac surface coils and techniques such as CLEAR (i.e. constant level appearance).

14.5.3.1
Sequence Design

The generation of "bright blood" in the coronary arteries can be based on different mechanisms. In 1991, Edelman and colleagues described a segmented κ-space 2D FLASH (fast low-angle shot technique) gradient-echo sequence to study the coronaries arteries in a single breath-hold (EDELMAN et al. 1991). Characteristics of this sequence are the small flip angle of the excitation pulse and the use of a gradient spoiler at the end of each repetition time (TR) to destroy the remaining transverse magnetization and thus create T1-weighted contrast ("spoiled-GE" technique). For 2D imaging, the creation of contrast between flowing blood and surrounding stationary tissues is based on the inflow of fully relaxed spins and the progressive saturation of the stationary spins in the image slice – described as "inflow enhancement". The highest contrast is obtained with through-plane flow, while in-plane vessel segments suffer from decreased signal within the vessel. Before the introduction of CE-MRA, 2D-FLASH was a commonly used technique for studying human vessels by MR imaging. As discussed above, the applicability of 2D techniques for coronary artery imaging, however, is limited (see Sect. 14.4). The 3D-FLASH technique, as presented by Li and co-workers in 1993, overcomes many of the limitations of the 2D approach for coronary artery imaging, but suffers from inherent problems related to sequence design, especially if acquisition of data is performed during breath-holding (LI et al. 1993). Similar to 2D imaging, for 3D imaging the magnetization of blood has a large signal at the beginning of the 3D acquisition but is progressively saturated for each subsequent excitation experienced by the blood in the imaging volume. By using a central ordering encoding of the 3D section optimal signal can be achieved (HOLSINGER and RIEDERER 1990). To speed up data acquisition for breath-hold coronary MR angiography, the repetition time needs to be shortened at the expense of a larger bandwidth, and as a consequence lower SNR, which may be a limiting factor. Moreover, due to the magnetization recovery during the trigger delay time, the images have limited blood inflow-related signal enhancement. Therefore, the contrast between blood and myocardium is often not adequate for clear visualization of certain coronary segments. T2 preparation or magnetization transfer contrast (MTC) are necessary to improve contrast but at the expense of reduced SNR. Injection of contrast media is necessary to shorten the blood T1, and thus to improve SNR and CNR (DESHPANDE et al. 2001b). Free-breathing 3D-FLASH or TFE (turbo-field-echo) coronary MR angiography is much less restricted by the need to speed up data acquisition, allowing the use of smaller bandwidths and the creation of higher intravoxel signal without injection of contrast (STUBER et al. 1999b).

Truly balanced steady-state free precession (b-SSFP) acquisition of the heart has become feasible with the recent improvements in gradient (shorter repetition times) and field shimming capabilities (CARR et al. 2001). The commercial name of the b-SSFP sequence differs between vendors: True-FISP (fast imaging in steady-state precession – Siemens), balanced-TFE (balanced-turbo-field-echo – Philips), and FIESTA (fast imaging employing steady-state acquisition – General Electric). Because of significant improvement in blood SNR and blood-myocardium CNR as compared to FLASH, these sequences have been evaluated recently for both breath-hold (DESHPANDE et al. 2001b) and free-breathing (GIORGI et al. 2002a; SPUENTRUP et al. 2002b) coronary MR angiography. In b-SSFP imaging, the transverse magnetization is maintained between successive RF pulses, because the net gradient moments are zero in all three directions and no RF spoiling is implemented. The signal intensity in the b-SSFP sequence is T2/T1 weighted, and the contrast between blood and myocardium is therefore enhanced because blood has a much higher T2/T1 than myocardium. A higher SNR are obtained than in magnetization-spoiled techniques (FLASH and TFE technique), because the coherent transverse magnetization contributes to the signal in successive TRs. Giorgi and colleagues compared a 3D-balanced TFE sequence with a 3D-TFE sequence in volunteers. The image quality of both the RCA and LCA was significantly better for the balanced sequence, and significantly longer segments of the coronary arteries and more side branches were visualized compared with the TFE sequence (GIORGI et al. 2002a; Fig. 14.11; Table 14.5). These findings are supported by a study of Spuentrup and colleagues, who also reported an improvement in coronary artery border delineation (SPUENTRUP et al. 2002b). Compared with the TFE-technique, the balanced-TFE technique with "T2-like" contrast characteristics enables an improvement in differentiation between small epicardial coronary arteries (medium high signal intensity) and adjacent pericardial sac (high signal intensity; BOGAERT and DUERINCKX 1995; GIORGI et al. 2002a).

As an alternative to the "bright-blood" techniques, Stuber and colleagues recently proposed a free-breathing, 3D high-resolution, "black-blood" fast spin-echo coronary MR angiography sequence (STUBER et al. 2001a, 2001b). A modified type of this sequence is also used for coronary wall imaging (see Sect. 14.6). Three-dimensional spin-echo coronary sequences have intrinsically higher SNR than bright-

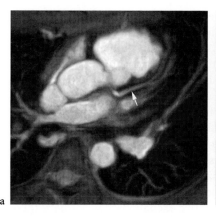
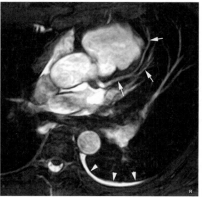

a   b

Fig. 14.11a,b. Coronary MR angiography sequence design, spoiled GE-technique (**a**) versus b-SSFP technique (**b**). Imaging of the LM and LAD in a normal subject. Improved vessel sharpness and substantially improved visualization of longer portions of LAD and the first diagonal branch (*arrows*) with the b-SSFP technique. Note also the improved depiction of other thoracic vessels such as the pulmonary and mammary arteries. Since the b-SSFP technique is mainly T2-weighted, fluid-containing structures such as pleural effusions (*arrowheads*) show much higher signal intensities and are therefore better depicted than on the spoiled GE technique. (Partially adapted from GIORGI et al. 2002b.)

Table 14.5. Effects of coronary MR angiography sequence on length of continuous depiction of coronary arteries

	No.	RCA	LM	LAD	LCx
Breath-hold Approach					
3D spoiled-GE technique (contrast-enhanced)					
LI et al. (2001a)	16-V	109±25		78±14[a]	
Free-breathing with retrospective respiratory gating					
3D spoiled-GE technique					
LI et al. (1996)	12-V	126±19	11±1	116±20	97±13
Free-breathing with real-time prospective navigator					
3D spoiled-GE technique (volume targeted)					
BOTNAR et al. (1999a)	12-V	84±14		53±11[a]	
BUNCE et al. (2001a)	46-P	56±21	12±5	30±11	16±9
KIM et al. (2001b)	109-P	91±19		74±10[a]	40±11
GIORGI et al. (2002a)	15-V	95±27	8±3	79±24	61±18
SOMMER et al. (2002)	107-P	69±26	19±5	55±22	44±17
WEBER et al. (2002)	15-V/P	129±19	12±1	117±21	47±5
BOGAERT et al. (2003)	19-P	90±31	7±2	72±15	31±15
3D b-SSFP Technique (volume targeted)					
GIORGI et al. (2002a)	15-V	112±27	8±3	92±21	71±18
SPUENTRUP et al. (2002c)	10-V	81±24		61±7[a]	39±11
3D-b-SSFP technique (whole-heart)					
WEBER et al. (2003)	12-V	107±32		117±34[a]	69±36
3D-black-blood technique (volume targeted)					
STUBER et al. (2001b)	8-V	112±22		64±6[a]	26±9
3 Tesla					
3D-spoiled-GE technique (volume targeted)					
STUBER et al. (2002a)	9-V	122±35		83±9[a]	52±6

Results are expressed in millimetres, and as shown as mean±standard deviation
Abbreviations: LAD, left anterior descending artery; LCx, left circumflex artery; LM, left main stem artery; No., Number of subjects; P, patient; RCA, right coronary artery; V, volunteer
[a]Combined LM–LAD length

blood sequences, which may be traded for improved spatial resolution. Currently, in plane-resolutions up to 400 µm are achievable. Other advantages of the spin-echo technique are the reduced susceptibility to turbulent flow in regions of focal stenosis, a reduced sensitivity to artefacts induced by metallic implants, and a high CNR. To create black-blood, a dual inversion-recovery pre-pulse is applied, with an inversion properly chosen to null the signal of inflowing blood at the level of interest (FLECKENSTEIN et al. 1991; SIMONETTI et al. 1996). The coronary artery lumen appears as a region of low signal intensity with surrounding high signal intensity from epicardial fat and myocardium. The length of the coronary arteries visualized with black-blood techniques is comparable with currently available bright-blood techniques (see Table 14.5). The precise role of the black-blood technique in patients with coronary artery disease needs further research. For instance, it is not known yet whether it is suited to studying coronary artery lesions that have low or no signal on spin-echo sequences such as heavily fibrotic and/or calcified stenotic plaques.

14.5.3.2
Magnetization Preparation Techniques

The epicardial coronary arteries are embedded in the (sub)epicardial fat. By suppressing the fat signal,

contrast between coronary blood pool and the surrounding tissue can be enhanced (MANNING et al. 1993a; Fig. 14.12). Fat suppression can be achieved by pre-saturation of the longitudinal magnetization of fat prior to imaging (HAASE et al. 1985) or by using a spectral selective RF-excitation pulse (MEYER et al. 1990). The latter excites only the water signal within the selected slice. Both have advantages and disadvantages. The pre-saturation method is experimentally simple, but the T1-relaxation process of the fat signal may hamper its relaxation characteristics, particularly for longer sequences. The use of spectral-selective excitation does not have these disadvantages. However, the use of an RF excitation pulse between each readout limits the shortest available echo time. This in turn leads to a prolonged acquisition window and may be disadvantageous with respect to T2* effects, secondary to flow and motion problems that can occur during the long RF pulse. In a study by Börnert and colleagues, comparing both fat suppression techniques, no significant differences were found in objective and subjective image parameters (BÖRNERT et al. 2002). It is, however, important to realize that fat has a steady-state signal close to that of blood in b-SSFP imaging because of their similar T2/T1 ratios. A spectral selective fat saturation pre-pulse, however, disturbs the steady-state magnetization and leads to magnetization oscillations, and to off-resonance effects during data

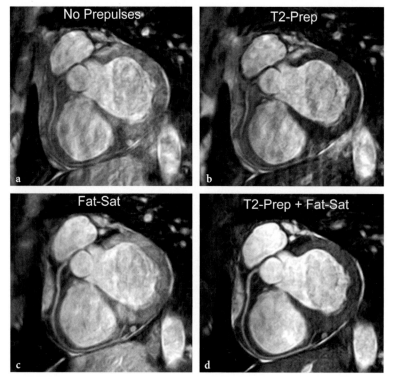

Fig. 14.12a-d. Beneficial effects of magnetization preparation pulses for coronary artery imaging. 3D free-breathing coronary MR angiography (b-SSFP technique) of the RCA in a normal subject. Compared with the coronary MR angiography sequence without preparation pulses (a), use of T2-prep(aration) technique (b) suppresses the signal of myocardial tissue, while the fat-suppression technique (*Fat Sat*) (c) eliminates the signal of epicardial and mediastinal fat. A combination of both techniques (d) substantially improves overall image quality, which favours visualization of the coronary arteries

acquisition. The subsequent signal fluctuations in κ-space lead to image artefacts such as ghosting and blurring (DESHPANDE et al. 2001b). A substantial reduction in image artefacts, higher SNR and better overall image quality is found when using a linearly increasing flip angle series of dummy pre-pulses during the magnetization preparation (DESHPANDE et al. 2003). Another benefit of the application of a fat saturation pulse is the suppression of the subcutaneous and mediastinal fat, reducing the breathing artefacts in the coronary MR angiography images.

Magnetization transfer contrast (MTC) pulses and T2 preparation pulses are magnetization prepulses that are useful for improving coronary artery visualization by suppressing the signal of the myocardium. This is especially useful for coronary arteries in close contact with the myocardium (e.g. mid and distal portions of the LAD and the side branches).

The MTC technique, described by Wolff and Balaban, consists of the off-resonance application of low-power RF pulses to selectively saturate hydrogen protons with short T2 (WOLFF and BALABAN 1989; WOLFF et al. 1991). A 30–60% drop in myocardial signal was found with the use of MTC prepulses (BALABAN et al. 1991; LI et al. 1993). As a result, the contrast difference between tissues with a short (myocardium) and long T2 (arterial blood) can be enhanced, at the expense of SNR.

The T2-magnetization preparation scheme, as originally proposed by Brittain and co-workers, is based on the fact that the T2 of myocardium (±50 ms) is considerably less than that of arterial blood (±250 ms; BRITTAIN et al. 1995). The T2 prep uses a 90° RF pulse to flip the M_z magnetization vector into the M_{xy} plane and is most beneficial in sequences with low inflow contrast (for further sequence details, see BRITTAIN et al. 1995; BOTNAR et al. 1999a). Shea et al. have found that a T2-prep length of approximately 40 ms yields the best CNR between blood and myocardium without compromising the SNR (SHEA et al. 2002). Not only the myocardium but also other tissues with a short T2 relaxation time are suppressed, for example cardiac veins with deoxygenated blood (20% O_2 saturation, T2: 35 ms) and epicardial fat (BOTNAR et al. 1999a; Fig. 14.12). Moreover, both MTC and T2-preparation pulses decrease the signal from the coronary artery wall, providing a more realistic measure of the coronary vessel diameter (BOTNAR et al. 1999a). Since the addition of a T2-prep pulse has a negative influence on SNR, it is mainly the b-SSFP sequence with a higher SNR than the spoiled gradient-echo sequence that benefits from this T2-prep pulse, because adequate SNR is still available for coronary artery visualization.

14.5.3.3
Contrast Agents

Although improved sequence design in combination with magnetization preparation techniques has led to a significant improvement in coronary artery visualization with coronary MR angiography, some issues such as low SNR, especially in breath-hold coronary MR angiography, are more difficult to solve. Use of T1-shortening contrast agents in combination with ultrafast 3D MR angiography techniques, described by Marty Prince in 1994, has become the current standard for MR angiography of the entire body, ranging from the intracerebral vessels to the peripheral arteries (PRINCE 1994). Also for coronary artery imaging, this technique should be appealing. It provides a flow-independent mechanism for blood/background contrast, which is important for visualizing coronary arteries with slow flow and for accurate delineation coronary vessel lumen (JOHANSSON et al. 1999; LORENZ and JOHANSSON 1999; ZHENG et al. 2001). Improved blood SNR with efficient T1-shortening contrast agent may allow for increased spatial resolution and reduced imaging time, which in turn may reduce potential image artefacts caused by cardiac and respiratory motion during a long scan.

In 1998, Goldfarb and Edelman reported an ECG-triggered, breath-hold, gadolinium-enhanced 3D-FLASH technique for imaging the coronaries. In a single breath-hold of 24 heartbeats, a 6-cm-thick 3D volume positioned transversally at the base of the heart was scanned during the first pass of 40 ml of gadopentate dimeglumine (GOLDFARB and EDELMAN 1998). A pre-scan with a small bolus of contrast is necessary to determine the bolus arrival time. Since only a single slab was obtained in this study, the coverage of the coronary artery tree was limited to its proximal portion. Therefore, Li and colleagues proposed a VCATS technique for better coverage (LI et al. 2001a; DESHPANDE et al. 2001a). Two injections of 20 ml of contrast agent cover the left and right coronary artery system in two breath-holds. The contrast between blood and non-blood tissues (mainly myocardium) can be further improved by the addition of an inversion pulse prior to data acquisition (HOFMAN et al. 1999). For maximal blood–myocardium contrast, the appropriate length of the inversion time needs to be determined (Li et al. 2001a,b). Zheng and co-workers have found a T1 of blood less than 80 ms optimal for contrast-enhanced coronary MR angiography (Zheng et al. 2001). With an inversion time between 200 and 300 ms, the blood magnetization is almost fully recovered (T1s less than 100 ms for blood during the first pass of 20- to 40-ml injections of contrast agent). Conversely, the magnetization of myocardium with T1s of 400–600 ms is nullified with these inversion times.

Extracellular contrast agents have a short intravascular half-life because of rapid diffusion through the extracellular space and fast renal excretion. Therefore, data acquisition should be synchronized to the passage of contrast through the coronaries arteries, and because of the rapid extravasation contrast need to be (re-)injected for each coronary MR angiography acquisition (Ho et al. 2001). Because of dose-related safety reasons and the cost of the contrast agent, the number of (breath-hold) acquisitions is limited and thus also an extended coverage of the coronary arteries. Moreover, breath-hold, contrast-enhanced coronary MR angiography, when compared with retrospective, free-breathing coronary MR angiography, does not significantly improve coronary artery visualization or stenosis detection (Kessler et al. 1999). Therefore, contrast-enhanced coronary MR angiography would benefit from the use of "intravascular" or "blood-pool" contrast agents that have a long intravascular half-life. The effectiveness of different, new intravascular contrast agents (e.g. iron particles and albumin-bound gadolinium) has been tested in animals [MS-325, Li et al. 1998); BSA-(Gd-DTPA), Hofman et al. 1999; Gadomer-17, Li et al. 2001b; P792, Taupitz et al. 2001; VSOP-C91, Taupitz et al. 2002] as well as in normal subjects and patients [MS-325, Stuber et al. 1999a; NC100150, Taylor et al. 1999; Klein et al. 2000; AMI-25 (Endorem), van Geuns et al. 2000; Feruglose, Bedaux et al. 2002a; SH L 643A, Herborn et al. 2003]. These studies consistently report an improved blood-to-myocardium CNR compared with non-enhanced images, and a prolonged and persistent blood-to-myocardium CNR improvement compared with extracellular contrast agents. Their use in assessing patients with coronary artery stenoses needs further evaluation. Despande and Li recently investigated the potential benefits of T1-shortening agents in improving the blood–myocardium contrast using the new 3D b-SSFP coronary MR angiography sequence. Their preliminary results show a net increase of 78% in blood–myocardium CNR for post-contrast imaging over pre-contrast imaging (Deshpande and Li 2003).

14.5.3.4
Arterial Spin-Labelling or -Tagging

Conventional coronary MR angiography techniques display the coronary artery blood-pool and the surrounding structures, including the myocardium, the blood in the cardiac cavities, and the great vessels. This representation of the coronary artery lumen is not analogous to the "luminography" obtained with conventional X-ray coronary angiography. Such "luminographic" images may be obtained with bolus tagging (Nishimura et al. 1988), also called spin-lock flow tagging (Azhari et al. 2001), and MR arterial spin-tagging or -labelling (projection MR angiography) techniques (Stuber et al. 2002a). Bolus tagging has the potential to provide information on flow rates and directions as well as on the anatomy of the studied vessels. Nishimura and co-workers have used a selective inversion-recovery method to tag the upstream blood and then follow the flow into the imaged region (Nishimura et al. 1988). The signal from the selectively tagged blood is obtained by subtraction of this first image from a second image, acquired without tagging. Since the original report in 1988, several variations and improvements of this bolus tagging technique have been presented (Foo et al. 1989; Burstein 1991; Azhari et al. 2001). Recently, Stuber and colleagues have further refined this bolus tagging technique. They have combined a 2D-selective "pencil" excitation for aortic spin-tagging with a 3D-interleaved spiral sequence with free-breathing and real-time NE technology. The pencil beam is positioned along the long axis of the ascending aorta. Two sets are required, one without (unlabelled) and one with aortic spin-tagging (labelled). During the time delay between spin tagging and imaging (delay time 200–300 ms), the inverted spins wash into the targeted volume by the aortic blood flow into the coronary arteries. After subtraction of both data sets (one with and one without preceding spin labelling), the inverted spins in the coronary arteries are selectively visualized while the surrounding static tissue is completely suppressed. In this fashion, arterial spin-labelling allows for selective visualization of the coronary artery lumen. In arterial spin-labelling with projection coronary MR angiography, sufficient motion artefact suppression is especially important, because any motion, with resultant blurring and ghosting, would lead to severe subtraction errors between the subsequent scans, reduced background suppression and reduced vessel border definition (Stuber et al. 2002a; Spuentrup et al. 2003).

14.5.3.5
Catheter-Directed, Contrast-Enhanced Coronary MR Angiography

With the recent improvements in the field of cardiovascular interventional MR imaging, some X-ray-guided interventional procedures such as balloon angioplasty, stent placement, inferior vena cava filter placement, and embolization can be performed under MR imaging guidance (HWANG et al. 2002). Catheter-directed intra-arterial CE-MRA has emerged as a potentially important tool in these interventions because of its ability to produce rapid vascular roadmaps, similar to those obtained with X-ray angiography (OMARY et al. 2002a, 2002b). Advantages over conventional intravenous CE-MRA include the ability to inject contrast agent selectively into the artery of interest, simple synchronization of contrast injection and image acquisition, and reduced background tissue enhancement. Intra-arterial injections also have the advantage of reduced contrast agent dosage when compared with intravenous injections, thereby enabling multiple injections during a single imaging session. In a recent paper, Green and colleagues have reported their preliminary results on coronary artery imaging with intra-arterial injections of diluted contrast agent (GREEN et al. 2003). The clinical value of these new, emerging techniques for studying the coronary arteries is at present unknown.

14.5.4
Spatial Resolution

The issue of spatial resolution becomes increasingly important with decreasing size of the object of interest. For coronary artery imaging, the main challenge is to accurately detect and quantify atherosclerotic stenotic lesions in vessels with a calibre ranging from 5 mm proximally, to 1 or 2 mm in the distal parts and side branches. X-ray coronary angiography, with a pixel size ~0.1×0.1 mm, allows full coverage of the epicardial coronary arteries and branch vessels. The pixel size in MR imaging is obtained by the ratio of the field-to-view (FOV) to the acquisition matrix. The voxel size is the pixel size multiplied by the slice thickness. Thus, spatial resolution will increase if the FOV decreases, the acquisition matrix increases or the slice thickness is reduced. However, the increase in spatial resolution is inversely related to the SNR. A higher spatial resolution is desired, but can only be acquired if the

SNR and CNR are sufficient (Fig. 14.2). In fact, the gain in spatial resolution can be inefficient if the image becomes too noisy as a result of using too small a voxel size. So, for each image, there is an optimal compromise between SNR, CNR and spatial resolution.

The issue of spatial resolution in coronary MR angiography is definitely more complicated than in any other part of the human body, as not only the SNR, but other parameters such as coronary artery motion, acquisition window and total scan time have a major influence on the achievable spatial resolution. Thus, even though spatial resolution similar to X-ray angiography may theoretically be obtained, several parameters pose major technical challenges to a successful high-resolution visualization of the coronary vessels. The large size of the chest has both a negative impact on pixel size and SNR. Use of a rectangular FOV, and fold-over suppression techniques are helpful for increasing the pixel size. Moreover, SNR can be increased by using cardiac-dedicated, phased array surface coils positioned as closely as possible to the coronary arteries. 3D sequences not only allow for better depiction of curved and tortuous vessels than 2D sequences, but also provide a higher SNR and therefore enable the acquisition of smaller pixel and voxel sizes. Zero-filling techniques enable the reconstructed slice thickness to be halved (e.g. from 3-mm obtained to 1.5-mm reconstructed slice thickness) and thus reduce partial volume artefacts (DU et al. 1994). Isotropic scanning is particularly important for coronary artery imaging (BOTNAR et al. 2000a). Since the spatial resolution is equal in all directions in isotropic voxels, the accuracy of imaging coronary arteries becomes independent of the scan positioning, and the coronary artery delineation in the through-plane direction is improved. The risk of creating partial volume artefacts in tortuous vessels is minimized, and there is a clear benefit for the reconstruction algorithms (MPR, MIP, volume rendering techniques). However, total imaging times are significantly longer than in anisotropic scanning and the smaller voxels yield a lower SNR. Since the available time for coronary artery imaging per heartbeat is limited to a small period during the cardiac cycle, increase in spatial resolution will inevitably lead to longer total scan times, which may become too long for breath-holding, unless a larger bandwidth is used. The latter, however, significantly reduces the SNR and necessitates the administration of contrast agents. As discussed in Sect. 14.5.6, imaging at a high field-strength might at least partially overcome the above limitations. In Table 14.6

Table 14.6. Characteristics of breath-hold and free-breathing coronary MR angiography versus coronary CT angiography

| | MR | | CT |
	Free-Breathing	Breath-Hold	
Spatial resolution (mm)	0.7×1.0×3.0	1.1×1.1×3.0	0.6×0.6×0.75 (16-slice)
	0.5×0.5×1.5(reconstructed)		0.4×0.4×0.6 (64-slice)
Acquisition window (ms)	70–100	120–150	83–165
Total scan time	Several minutes	Multiple breath-holds	±16 sec
Approach	Targeted–whole-heart	Targeted	Whole-heart
ECG trigger/gating	Prospective triggering	Prospective triggering	Retrospective gating
Contrast agent needed	No	Advisable	Yes
Impact CA calcifications	Minimal	Minimal	Large
Influence heart rate	Moderate	Minimal	Large
Irradiation	No	No	Yes
Operator (training)	Experience needed	Experience needed	Less experience needed
CA stenosis detection	Possible	Possible	Possible
CA stenosis quantification	Not possible	Not possible	Possible (?)
CA wall visualization	Difficult	Difficult	Possible
Comprehensive study, including:			
- cardiac function	Yes	Yes	Yes
- myocardial perfusion	Yes	Yes	Research
- late enhancement	Yes	Yes	Research

voxel sizes that are currently used for breath-hold and free-breathing coronary MR angiography are shown.

14.5.5
κ-space Strategies

Different acquisition schemes can be used for filling κ-space. Traditionally, the Cartesian scheme is applied with a centric-ordered (low–high) κ-space acquisition scheme (see Chap. 1). The limitations of the acquisition window length per heartbeat have stimulated the search for alternative, more efficient and faster sampling schemes such as EPI, spiral imaging and radial imaging (Fig. 14.13). Rectilinear EPI has been used to image coronary arteries in normal volunteers with some success (BÖRNERT and JENSEN 1995; YANG et al. 1998; SLAVIN et al. 1998). However, artefacts induced by flow may potentially degrade images, causing ghosting, misregistration and loss of spatial resolution (BUTTS and RIEDERER 1992). A second alternative strategy is spiral coronary MR angiography (TAYLOR et al. 2000a; DIRKSEN et al. 2003). Thedens and co-workers have utilized a "stack of spirals" to traverse 3D κ-space rapidly and thus to reduce imaging time (THEDENS et al. 1999). Spiral κ-space data acquisition of the coronary arteries with a single-interleaf spiral yields a higher SNR, and CNR and image quality than the Cartesian data-

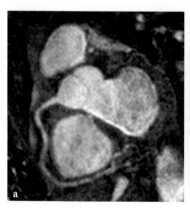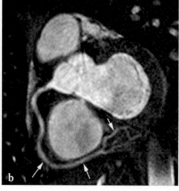

Fig. 14.13a,b. κ-space strategies, Cartesian versus spiral imaging. (Courtesy of Tim Leiner MD, University of Maastricht, Maastricht, The Netherlands). 3D free-breathing coronary MR angiography of the RCA in a normal subject, using a 70-ms acquisition window length with a Cartesian (**a**) and a spiral κ-space fill-in strategy (**b**). Compared with the Cartesian acquisition scheme, use of the spiral acquisition scheme substantially improves vessel sharpness, with depiction of longer portions of the RCA (*arrows*)

acquisition for the same scanning time (BÖRNERT et al. 2001a, 2001b). Using a double-interleaf spiral, a 50% reduction in scanning time is found with a still-higher SNR and a similar image quality when compared with the standard Cartesian approach. Technically, spiral-based trajectories have improved flow and motion characteristics compared with the Cartesian approach. However, an important limitation of the spiral technique is its sensitivity to off-resonance chemical-shift effects or main-field inhomogeneities, leading to blurring of images (KEEGAN et al. 1999). These artefacts can be reduced by using effective fat suppression techniques and conjugate phase reconstruction to correct for the off-resonance effects induced by the variation in the main field. The radial κ-space acquisition schemes use a priority for the central κ_y and κ_z profiles, while the most peripheral κ_y and κ_z profiles are not sampled. In radial imaging, a "stack of stars" approach is used for sampling along two directions, while, in the remaining direction, Fourier encoding is used. This enables substantial reduction in the scanning time (±20–25%) without reducing the in-plane or through-plane spatial resolution compared with Cartesian acquisition schemes (STUBER et al. 2002b; GIORGI et al. 2002a). In a recent study by Spuentrup and colleagues, radial b-SSFP scanning yielded reduced motion artefacts and superior vessel sharpness when compared with Cartesian b-SSFP, at the expense of a somewhat lower CNR (SPUENTRUP et al. 2004).

14.5.6
High Field Strength Coronary MR Angiography

The recent approval of 3.0-T systems for clinical use has opened new perspectives for overcoming some of the limitations encountered on 1.5-T systems, in particular, suboptimal SNR, which limits spatial resolution and the ability to visualize the distal and branch vessel coronary segments (STUBER et al. 2002b). Since SNR is directly related to the strength (β_0) of the static magnetic field, improved SNR and spatial resolution can be expected from 3.0-T systems. However, a number of potential adverse affects have been reported at higher field strengths, such as susceptibility artefacts, reduced T2* and increased T1 RF field distortions. At high field strength, reliable ECG triggering becomes more challenging owing to the amplified magneto-hydrodynamic effects. Furthermore, the flexibility of sequence design is less because of increased RF deposition. Stuber and colleagues have used a free-breathing, real-time NE 3D-TFE sequence, adjusted for 3.0 T, to study the coronary arteries in volunteers in a 3.0-T system (STUBER et al. 2002b; Fig. 14.14). The pencil beam of the respiratory NE was positioned at the heart–liver interface. Using vector ECG, QRS triggering remained accurate despite the enhanced T-wave at 3.0 T (FISCHER et al. 1999). Compared with 1.5-T coronary MR angiography, using a similar sequence and voxel size, 3.0 T yielded visualization of longer segments of the coronary arteries with similar diameters and vessel sharpness, but with an increased SNR and CNR (Fig. 14.15). The increase in SNR and CNR enabled reduction in the voxel size of ±50% (from 1.0×0.7×3 mm to 0.6×0.6×3 mm), maintaining high image quality and improving visualization of the small-diameter branching vessels (see Table 14.5). These preliminary studies demonstrate that 3.0-T coronary MR angiography is feasible, and, with further fine-tuning of the sequence, 3.0 T might become the preferred field-strength to study the coronary artery lumen and wall.

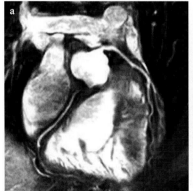
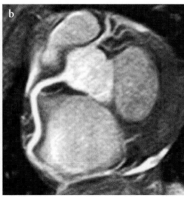

Fig. 14.14a,b. 3.0-T coronary MR angiography using the 3D free-breathing b-SSFP technique. Examples of imaging of the right and left coronary artery system in two normal subjects (**a**, **b**). (Courtesy of Matthias Stuber, Johns Hopkins University Medical School, Baltimore, USA)

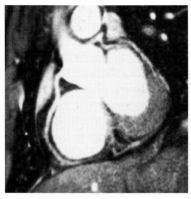

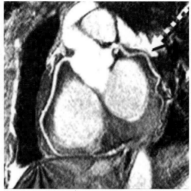

a   b

Fig. 14.15a,b. Comparison between 1.5-T and 3.0-T coronary MR angiography using the free-breathing b-SSFP technique in the same subject. At higher field strength, the CA vessel delineation and anatomical detail is improved (*dashed arrow*). (Courtesy of Matthias Stuber, Johns Hopkins University Medical School, Baltimore, USA)

14.6
Coronary Artery Wall and Plaque Imaging: Strategies

The issue of non-invasive assessment of arterial wall remodelling and plaque morphology is at present considered a "hot" topic in cardiology. Atherothrombosis is often the first presentation of atheromatosis in otherwise asymptomatic patients, and if vital organs (e.g. heart, brain) are involved the consequences can be dramatic (acute myocardial infarction, sudden death, stroke) and the related medical cost for treatment enormous. Screening for vulnerable plaques with non-invasive imaging modalities in patients at risk, in combination with appropriate medical treatment could significantly reduce the atherothrombosis-related morbidity and mortality. The superior contrast resolution of MR imaging, improved MR hardware, new sequence designs and development of tissue-specific MR contrast agents have stimulated several groups to explore the role of MR imaging in the assessment of the atheromatosis-prone arterial wall (aorta, carotid arteries, coronary arteries and peripheral arteries).

Because the constraints for MR vessel wall imaging are by and large similar to those of coronary MR angiography, the different strategies discussed in Sect. 14.5 can be applied for imaging of the vessel wall: breath-hold and free-breathing strategies, timing of image data acquisition, κ-space sampling strategies, etc. At present three types of sequences have been proposed for wall imaging; 3D fast spin-echo (FAYAD et al. 2000), 3D-spiral (BOTNAR et al. 2000b; KIM et al. 2002) and 3D-radial b-SSFP (SPUENTRUP et al. 2003; Fig. 14.16). Black-blood properties are obtained using an inversion (pre-)pulse with an inversion time properly chosen to null the signal of blood (FLECKENSTEIN et al. 1991). A fat-suppression pulse (spectral inversion recovery pre-pulse) is applied for improved contrast to the surrounding tissue. For signal enhancement of the targeted coronary artery vessel wall a 2D pencil beam local re-inversion pulse is applied along the main coronary artery axis immediately after the non-selective inversion pulse (BOTNAR et al. 2001). Both breath-hold (FAYAD et al. 2000; WORTHLEY et al. 2001) and free-breathing (BOTNAR et al. 2000b) approaches are available for coronary vessel wall imaging. The preliminary results of coronary vessel wall MR imaging in animal models, healthy volunteers and small patient groups are encouraging. In a porcine model, wall thickness and wall area measurements of experi-

a   b

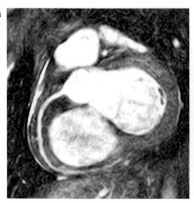

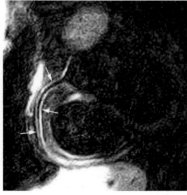

Fig. 14.16a,b. Coronary artery wall imaging using the dark-blood 4th-order local inversion 3D spiral imaging technique. Bright-blood (a) versus dark-blood (b) technique of the RCA in a normal subject. The CA wall is shown as a thin (curvilinear) line (*arrows*) between the dark CA lumen and hypointense epicardial fat. (Courtesy of Matthias Stuber, Johns Hopkins University Medical School, Baltimore, USA)

mentally induced coronary artery lesions obtained with high-resolution MR imaging correspond well the histological measurements (WORTHLEY et al. 2000a). Fayad and colleagues have measured a wall thickness of 0.75±0.17 mm in normal, healthy volunteers (FAYAD et al. 2000). Their results are comparable with the results of the Beth Israel group for normal wall thickness (1.0±0.2 mm; BOTNAR et al. 2000b). In patients with non-significant coronary artery disease (i.e. 10–50%-diameter reduction at X-ray angiography), Kim and colleagues were able to demonstrate positive (outward) arterial remodelling (GLAGOV et al. 1987; KIM et al. 2002).

In an ex vivo animal study, Worthley and colleagues have been able to characterize and differentiate the different components (i.e. calcified, lipid-rich, fibrocellular and hemorrhagic regions) of coronary atherosclerotic plaques with high-resolution MR imaging (in-plane resolution of 156×156 µm; WORTHLEY et al. 2000b). These findings open new avenues for the non-invasive study of the natural history of coronary atheromatosis and to better understand the complex relationship between arterial remodelling, vessel inflammation and plaque rupture. However, it should be noted that spatial resolution as well as coronary and respiratory motion have a strong impact on the accuracy of the wall thickness measurements (SCHÄR et al. 2002, 2003). Low-resolution images tend to overestimate wall area and underestimate lumen area; and deteriorate the shape of an object. With current clinically used in-plane resolutions (500–1,000 µm), an overestimation of 20% for a diseased, 2-mm-thick coronary artery wall and 45% overestimation for a normal, 1-mm-thick coronary artery wall is found. Visual discrimination of the different layers (fibrous cap, lipid core and smooth muscle) in the arterial wall is possible if the spatial resolution is ≥1 pixel per tissue layer. A thin fibrous cap (50 µm) overlying a lipid ring or eccentric lipid core necessitates ≥2 pixels across these two adjacent tissue layers for visual cap detection. The precision of motion correction (gating window width) for respiratory motion should be ≤3 times the thickness of the tissue layer. These boundaries should be considered for in vivo characterization of atherosclerotic plaques. In the near future, improvement in spatial resolution might be expected from high field-strength scanning, use of tissue-specific contrast agents (KOOI et al. 2003) and intravascular coils (WORTHLEY et al. 2003). In a recent paper, Botnar and colleagues have reported their preliminary results on RCA vessel wall imaging on a 3.0-T system (BOTNAR et al.

2003), using a similar sequence design to the 1.5-T system adjusted to the 3.0 T requirements (BOTNAR et al. 2000b). A favourable SNR (50% gain in SNR compared with 1.5 T) and CNR have been reported. Quantitative measurements such as lumen diameter (3.2±0.6 mm) and wall thickness (0.9±0.3 mm) compare well with the abovementioned values obtained on a 1.5-T system.

14.7
Coronary Blood Flow Assessment: Strategies

X-ray angiography does not provide accurate information about the physiological significance of a stenosis, in particular stenoses of intermediate severity (40–70%), on the coronary artery flow. In lesions of intermediate severity, assessment of the functional significance is important, since this information has a significant influence on patient management (WHITE et al. 1984; MARCUS et al. 1988). Coronary artery flow has a typical biphasic pattern, with the highest flow and velocity in mid-diastole. The functional significance of a coronary artery stenosis can be evaluated by measuring the ratio of maximal hyperaemic coronary flow to the baseline coronary flow (GOULD et al. 1974). Normal coronary arteries are characterized by a threefold augmentation of their blood flow after administration of a coronary vasodilator such as adenosine or dipyridamole. In the presence of a flow-limiting stenosis in an epicardial coronary artery, the downstream vascular bed in the myocardium demonstrates a compensatory dilatation to maintain blood flow, and the ability to achieve augmentation in coronary blood flow is limited. As a consequence, the flow reserve is markedly reduced in a coronary artery with a significant stenosis. Intra-coronary Doppler measurement is an established technique to determine coronary flow and flow reserve, but this technique is available only during cardiac catheterization (WHITE 1993; JOYCE et al. 1994). MR imaging has a unique potential for non-invasive measurement of flow in vessels and across valves (see Chaps. 1, 13). Although highly challenging, MR flow measurements can be performed in the small cardiac vessels (coronary arteries, coronary sinus) and in CABG vessels, during rest and during hyperaemia using fast velocity-encoded cine MR imaging techniques (EDELMAN et al. 1993; SAKUMA et al. 1999; HUNDLEY et al. 2000; SCHWITTER et al. 2000).

Another approach to assess coronary perfusion and myocardial blood flow is assessment of blood flow in the coronary sinus, which represents approximately 96% of total myocardial blood flow (LUND et al. 2000). By measuring myocardial mass with cine MR imaging, the average coronary blood flow per gram of myocardial mass can be quantified by using non-invasive MR imaging. A close correlation is found between the estimated myocardial blood flow obtained by coronary sinus flow MR measurement and PET flow data (SCHWITTER et al. 2000; KOSKENVUO et al. 2001). Bedaux and colleagues have applied this technique to quantify the flow velocity and volume flow in the great cardiac vein, which has a close anatomic relationship to the LAD. The flow in the great cardiac vein is found to be mainly systolic and pointing in the inverse direction to the predominantly diastolic flow in the LAD (BEDAUX et al. 2001).

To assure accurate coronary flow measurements with MR imaging, at least four important sources of error should be taken into consideration – partial volume effects, misalignment of flow axis and flow-encoding gradients, intravoxel dispersion, and through- and in-plane motion (TANG et al. 1993; MARCUS et al. 1999; NAGEL et al. 1999). With the currently achievable in-plane resolution of approximately 1×1 mm, only a few pixels will be effectively located within the coronary artery lumen, while many pixels will be located at the boundary between the lumen and the vessel wall. This may reduce significantly the accuracy of MR measurements, with differences of up to 60% between MR and intravascular Doppler measurements (TANG et al. 1993). Accuracy can be improved when peak velocities (highest in the centre of the vessel and thus less dependent on partial volume effects) are used instead of volume flow; though Hofman and colleagues have found that, with ~3 pixels per vessel diameter, accurate blood volume flow rates can be determined (HOFMAN et al. 1995b). Intra-voxel phase dispersion can be reduced by an improvement in spatial resolution, leading to more homogeneous flow velocities within one voxel. Misalignment can be reduced by careful planning of the image plane perpendicular to the coronary vessel of interest. Coronary arteries move significantly during data acquisition. Through-plane motion can be corrected for by measuring and subtracting the velocity of the adjacent myocardium from the flow velocity within the vessel. In-plane motion cannot be corrected for. In-plane motion is higher for the RCA (6–12 cm/s; HOFMAN et al. 1996) than for the LAD (2–5 cm/s; SAKUMA et al. 1999), causing blurring of the vessel boundaries and overestimation of the volume flow. This is most problematic during ejection and fast filling. To obtain accurate flow measurements, the acquisition window should be less than 25 ms for the RCA, and less than 120 ms for the LAD (HOFMAN et al. 1998).

Coronary MR flow measurements can be performed in breath-hold as well during free breathing with use of the NE technique (NAGEL et al. 1999; SAKUMA et al. 1999; KEEGAN et al. 2004). Both approaches have advantages and disadvantages. A higher temporal and spatial resolution can be achieved with the free-breathing technique, but this approach might be problematic due to its longer scan time when using pharmacological stress. It should be noted that coronary blood flow measurement with breath-hold imaging may be different from physiological blood flow during regular breathing, since breath-holding can change the intrathoracic pressure, which affects the systemic venous return to the heart and thus decreases the cardiac output (29.0±6.3%) when breath-holding at deep inspiration is employed (FERRIGNO et al. 1986).

14.8
Coronary Artery Bypass Graft Imaging: Strategies

In general, the strategies used for coronary artery imaging are also applicable to CABG imaging, but CABG imaging deals with specific problems (see Sect. 14.11.5). Imaging is focused either on angiographic depiction of the bypass graft, assessment of flow patterns (volume flow and velocities) and flow reserve, or a combination of both techniques (Fig. 14.17). For the angiographic assessment of CABG grafts, black-blood as well as bright-blood techniques have been used in the past (WHITE et al. 1987; RUBINSTEIN et al. 1987; AURIGEMMA et al. 1989; GALJEE et al. 1996). The newer, b-SSFP bright-blood techniques and, for breath-hold, ultrafast contrast-enhanced MR angiography have been used for CABG MR angiography (WINTERSPERGER et al. 1998; KALDEN et al. 1999; BUNCE et al. 2003a). Bypass graft flow and flow reserve assessment uses the same approach and strategies as applied to coronary artery flow measurement, but should take into account differences in the flow profiles and flow reserves that are related to the type of graft, the position along the graft where the flow is quantified, and the flow patterns in the distal run-off vessels.

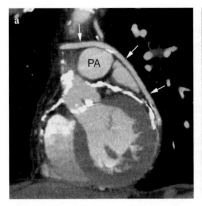 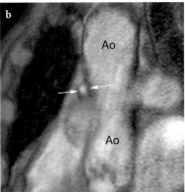 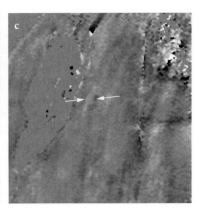

Fig. 14.17a–c. Coronary artery bypass graft (CABG) imaging and flow assessment in a patient with a venous jump graft. Contrast-enhanced ECG-gated CT (**a**), magnitude (**b**) and phase image (**c**) using velocity-encoded cine MRI. The course of the jump vein is well shown on the CT images (**a**). Perpendicular-positioned views through the vein graft allow assessment of flow patterns and quantification of flow volumes (*arrows*) (**b, c**). *Ao*, Aorta

14.9
Practical Approach for Coronary MR Angiography

14.9.1
Patient Setup and Patient Instructions

Patient setup is similar to other cardiovascular MR indications (see Chap. 3). Patients are positioned supine with the ECG-leads on the anterior left hemithorax. Although, in a recent paper, Stuber and colleagues have reported an improved coronary visualization in a prone position, similar to the 2D-approaches used in the early 1990s, this uncomfortable position is not suitable for patient studies (DUERINCKX et al. 1995; STUBER et al. 2001c). Patient instructions are important to improve the success of coronary MR angiography. The non-breath-hold sequences are much simpler, as they require virtually no patient instructions besides a recommendation to breathe regularly and to keep still during the scan. For the breath-hold techniques, the patient should be instructed on how to hold their breath during a non-forced, normal end-expiration for the duration of each scan and these manoeuvres should be practiced for several minutes prior to the start of the scan. It is important to work on this with the patient prior to starting the MR scan to obtain breath-holding that is as consistent as possible. For contrast-enhanced coronary MR angiography, the patient needs an intravenous line, preferentially with a continuous perfusion of small amount of physiologic fluid to assure an open line prior to injection.

14.9.2
Cookbook Approach to Free-Breathing Coronary MR Angiography

The Beth Israel group from Boston was the first to propose a standardized, stepwise approach to free-breathing coronary MR angiography (http://www.bidmc.harvard.edu: Cookbook Coronary MRA). A cookbook offers several advantages:

- It ensures that coronary arteries are always studied in the same way
- Studies can be performed by technicians with experience in cardiac imaging, and total imaging can be shortened
- Improvements in sequence designs can be updated in the cookbook without changing the cookbook strategy

The protocol includes four or five different scans, all of which are performed during free breathing. For coronary artery localization and for NE positioning at the right hemidiaphragm, two localizers are utilized (scan 1 and 2). The first localizer is a vector ECG-triggered, free-breathing, multi-slice 2D segmented gradient-echo scan with nine transverse, nine coronal and nine sagittal interleaved acquisitions of the thorax (acquisition duration 1 min). On these images, the NE is positioned at the dome of the right hemidiaphragm (see Fig. 14.4). Scan 2 is a low-resolution, 3D-segmented, gradient-echo scout scan (TFE-EPI, or balanced TFE with parallel imaging), which is used for the localization of the targeted 3D volumes that constitute the final sub-millimetre MR angiography scans (Bogaert et al. 2003; Giorgi et al. 2002a). This low spatial-resolution scan is oriented transversely through the origin and course of the RCA and LCA. The scan results in a 3D slab consisting of 40 slices with a reconstructed slice thickness of 2.5 mm and an in-plane resolution of 1.39×1.82 mm. T2-preparation and fat-saturation pulses are applied just prior to data acquisition to obtain high contrast between the blood and myocardium and between fat and other structures, respectively. This scan, as well as the following scans, are obtained during diastasis, using an empirical formula (Stuber et al. 1999b) or a direct assessment of the optimal delay time (Foo et al. 2000; Kim et al. 2001a).

To precisely target the scan volumes of the submillimetre scans (scan 3–5), a three-point plan scan is applied to locate the RCA and LCA on the low spatial-resolution scan. For the RCA (scan 3), the RCA is depicted in three locations (proximal, mid and a distal segment of the RCA) on transverse images (Fig. 14.18). These three points define the geometry of the centre plane of the imaged 3D volume, subsequently applied for the sub-millimetre coronary MR angiography sequence (Stuber et al. 1999b). This 3D volume covers not only the anterior atrioventricular groove, but also the posterior atrioventricular groove containing the LCx. For

the left coronary tree, two scans are performed. Scan 4 is positioned tangentially to the surface of the left anterolateral part of the heart ("tangential" view), using the LM, the mid-LAD and mid LCx as landmarks (Fig. 14.19). The landmarks on the LAD and LCx should be positioned carefully to assure the longest coverage of the left coronary tree, including the diagonal branching vessels. Scan 5 is a perpendicular view through the LM and entire length of the LAD ("perpendicular" view), using the LM, mid-LAD and distal LAD as landmarks (Fig. 14.20). On the perpendicular view, the small, septal branches of the LAD are often visible (Fig. 14.21). In this way, the LM, LCx and LAD (but not the RCA) are scanned in two perpendicular planes. As a result, longer segments of the LCA tree, and more of its branching vessels are visualized. Also, the visualization and description of stenotic lesions benefits from this approach, since lesions are scanned in-plane (with a better in-plane resolution) at least in one direction. Not infrequently, the accompanying coronary veins are visible on the MR angiography scans (Fig. 14.22). The American Heart Association classification system to define and number the different CA segments can also be applied to coronary MR angiography (Austen et al. 1975; Fig. 14.23).

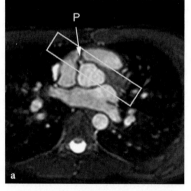

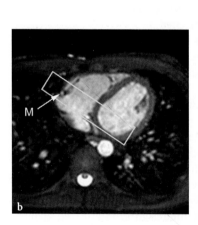

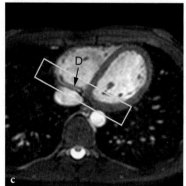

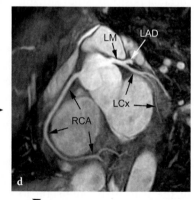

Fig. 14.18a-d. Positioning of RCA. Indication of the position of the proximal (*P*), mid (*M*) and distal (*D*) part of the RCA on the low spatial-resolution images allows determination of a small volume (indicated in *yellow*) covering the entirety of the RCA in the anterior

atrioventricular groove. This small 3D volume usually visualizes also the left main stem coronary artery (*LM*), the proximal left anterior descending coronary artery (*LAD*), and the left circumflex coronary artery (*LCx*) in the posterior atrioventricular groove

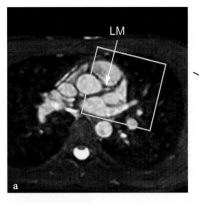

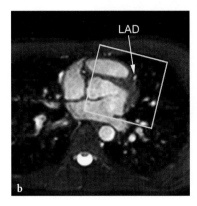

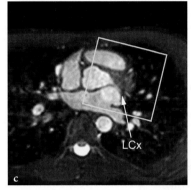

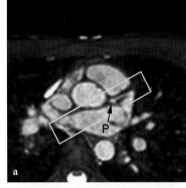

Fig. 14.19a-d. Tangential view to study LM, and the proximal and mid portions of the LAD and LCx. To determine the ideal volume (indicated in *yellow*), the position of the LM, mid portions of the LAD and LCx are indicated on the transverse low spatial resolution images

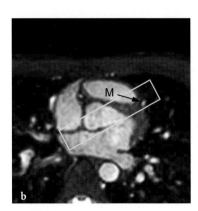

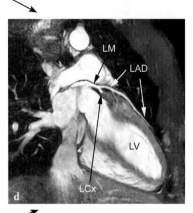

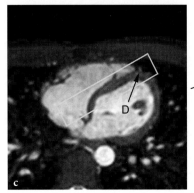

Fig. 14.20a-d. Perpendicular view to study LM, and the LAD in the anterior interventricular groove. The position of the LM (*P*), and the mid (*M*) and distal (*D*) portions of the LAD are indicated on the low spatial resolution images

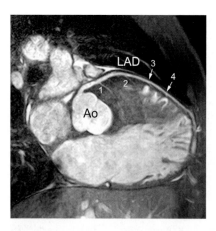

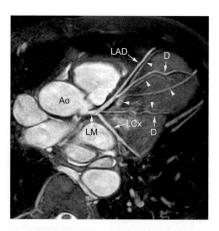

Fig. 14.21. Septal (perforator) branches of LAD. Perpendicular view of LAD, using 3D free-breathing coronary MR angiography (b-SSFP technique). With current available spatial resolution, the branching vessels such as the septal perforator branches (*1, 2, 3, 4*) are frequently visible on coronary MR angiography

Fig. 14.22. Coronary arteries and accompanying veins of left coronary tree. Tangential view of left coronary tree, using 3D free-breathing coronary MR angiography (b-SSFP technique). The LM, LAD and two diagonal branches (*D*), and LCx are visible as high-signal intensity vessels on the anterolateral surface of the left ventricle. The accompanying veins draining in the great cardiac vein (*arrowheads*) have a lower signal intensity due to the suppression of the venous blood by the T2 pre-pulse

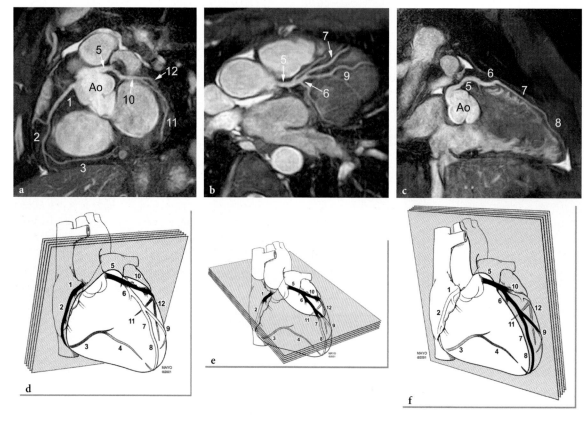

Fig. 14.23a-f. Coronary artery segment definition. Coronary MR angiography, using 3D free-breathing coronary MR angiography (b-SSFP technique) through the anterior and posterior atrioventricular groove (**a**), tangential (**b**) and perpendicular (**c**) view of left coronary artery tree. Corresponding anatomical drawings of segmental coronary artery anatomy (**d–f**) (from Gerber et al. 2003b; by permission of the Mayo Foundation for Medical Education and Research. All rights reserved). (*1*) proximal RCA; (*2*) middle RCA; (*3*) distal RCA; (*4*) posterior descending artery; (*5*) LM; (*6*) proximal LAD; (*7*) middle LAD; (*8*) distal LAD; (*9*) first diagonal branch; (*10*) proximal LCx; (*11*) middle LCx; (*12*) posterolateral branch. Ao, Aorta

The sequence design of the sub-millimetre scan is shown is Fig. 14.24. It starts with a flow-insensitive T2-prepulse for contrast enhancement (60 ms), is followed by a NE (20 ms), a spectrally selective fat-saturation pulse (20 ms) and a localized anterior saturation pre-pulse (REST; 8 ms), and finally the high-resolution MR coronary angiography sequence itself. The REST pulse, positioned on the anterior chest wall, is an effective means of suppressing breathing-related artefacts from the anterior chest wall. Different types of high-resolution MR coronary angiography sequences are currently available: 3D-segmented κ-space TFE (or FLASH sequence), and 3D-segmented SSFP (balanced TFE or true FISP). As discussed above, different κ-space sampling strategies can be used (Cartesian, radial, spiral). Usually a low to high fill-in of the κ-space is applied. With a field of view of 360 mm and a 512×360 matrix, an in-plane acquisition resolution of 0.7×1.0 mm is obtained. The 3D-slab consists of 20 slices of 1.5 mm reconstructed thickness, resulting in a coverage of 30 mm. Scans are reconstructed to a voxel size of 0.54×0.54×1.5 mm by additional zero-filling. Image quality can be further improved by using CLEAR for all scans in order to correct for the non-uniform cardiac coil sensitivity (based on the separate reference scan which determines the coil sensitivity profiles for all cardiac coil elements, the same reference scan that is also used for sensitivity encoding in the scout scan).

A new approach for free-breathing coronary MR angiography, recently described by Oliver Weber and colleagues, is "Whole-Heart" coronary MR angiography (WEBER et al. 2003). It represents a simplified version of the cookbook approach and consists of only two scans. After a localizer (similar to scan 1 in the cookbook), used for positioning of the NE, a transverse-oriented, sub-millimetre, high-resolution coronary MR angiography scan (balanced-TFE) is obtained which covers the entire heart. With 120–140 axial slices (in-plane reconstructed resolution of 0.54×0.54 mm) and a slice thickness of 0.75 mm, the heart is nearly completely, "isotropically" scanned. Advantages of this approach are its simplicity (reduction from 5 to 2 scans, without need to use double-obliquely targeted volumes for optimal coronary artery scanning), and reduction in total scan time. In the study by Weber and colleagues, a scan efficiency of 48% was found. Mean acquisition duration was 5.36 min (range 3.30–11.51 min) for the targeted volumes and 13.48 min (range 7.18 – 20.18 min) for the whole-heart volume. The near isotropic scanning permits multi-planar reconstruction without loss in image quality, with limited problems related to partial-volume effects (Fig. 14.25) (see Table 14.5 for coronary artery lengths obtained with the whole-heart approach).

14.9.3
Practical Approach to Breath-Hold Coronary MR Angiography

Wielopolski and colleagues have proposed an interactive, stepwise approach for 3D breath-hold coronary MR angiography (WIELOPOLSKI et al. 1998). The first step involves the acquisition of a scout volumetric data set during end-expiration, with a 3D multi-shot segmented EPI sequence to cover the entire heart. The heart volume localizer data are subsequently loaded into an MPR platform, to interactively compute the optimal orientation for imaging of the different segments of the coronary arteries. The optimal double-oblique plane and slab position containing the coronary segment of interest are implemented into an end-expiratory breath-hold 3D segmented turbo FLASH (or currently the SSFP) sequence (VCATS). This procedure of localization and imaging is continued and repeated until all necessary orientations covering all major coronary

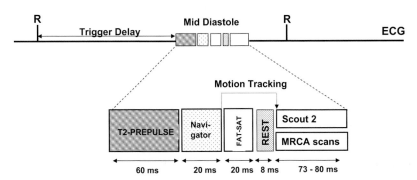

Fig. 14.24. 3D free-breathing coronary MR angiography sequence design

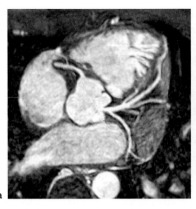
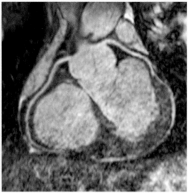

a   b

Fig. 14.25a,b. Whole-heart coronary MR angiography in a normal subject. Reconstruction in an oblique axial image plane of the original data set shows the LM, LAD, LCx, the origin of the RCA and several CA branches (**a**); and reconstruction along the atrio-ventricular grooves shows the RCA, LM and LCx (**b**). (The post-processing program used for reconstruction was the Soap-Bubble tool, Philips Medical Systems, Best, The Netherlands)

segments are examined. In just 7 breath-holds, the major coronary segments can be visualized: (1) plane along LM, proximal LCx, and proximal LAD (transverse); (2) plane of proximal RCA (transverse); (3) plane along distal RCA and PDA (oblique); (4) plane through aortic root and proximal RCA and LM (oblique); (5) plane along LCx (oblique); (6) plane along middle and distal LAD (oblique); (7) plane along middle RCA (oblique; van Geuns et al. 2000). A detailed description of the optimal positioning of the different volumes can be found in Wielopolski et al. (1998). These VCATS scans obtained in end-expiratory breath-holds of 24 heartbeats have a FOV of 240×320 mm^2, a slab thickness of 24–32 mm, a reconstructed slice thickness of 1.5 mm, an in-plane resolution of 1.4 to 2.0×1.0 to 1.2 mm^2 and an acquisition length of 110 ms (van Geuns et al. 2000; Li et al. 2001a). Magnetization preparation techniques include the use of magnetization transfer irradiation or a T2-prepulse for myocardium-blood CNR enhancement and a chemical-shift fat-suppression pulse. As discussed in Sect. 14.5.3.3, use of intravenous, T1-shortening contrast agents is highly beneficial in breath-hold coronary MR angiography to increase the SNR.

14.10
Post-Processing Techniques for Coronary MR Angiography

The coronary arteries have a complex, often tortuous course on the curved surface of the heart. Moreover, especially on the left side, the coronary artery tree has side branches. Using current 3D volumetric acquisition techniques, the majority of the epicardial coronary arteries can be imaged in a single, 3D volume, but only small portions of the coronary arter-

ies will be visible on the individual reconstructed images. Therefore, to facilitate coronary arterial depiction, post-processing of the images is necessary. With the advent and wide clinical use of ultrafast contrast-enhanced MR angiography techniques, post-processing techniques such as maximum intensity projection (MIP), multi-planar reformations (MPR), and surface (SR) and volume rendering (VR) from 3D data sets are currently available on most clinical MR scanners and off-line workstations (van Ooijen et al. 2003). Three-dimensional rendering of coronary arteries is one type of post-processing that requires segmentation of the data (Doyle et al. 1993; Börnert and Jensen 1995). To execute this 3D rendering routine, "seeds" are placed in both the left and right coronary vessels, and thresholds are set to discriminate individual coronary vessels from adjacent structures (Doyle et al. 1993). Segmentation of the left coronary system with its many branches is much more involved than the RCA segmentation. Recently, Etienne and colleagues have introduced an elegant "Soap-Bubble" tool for visualization and quantitative analysis of 3D coronary MR angiograms (Etienne et al. 2002). This quantitative software tool facilitates MPR of 3D volume-targeted coronary MR angiography data sets, while also providing quantitative measures such as SNR, CNR, vessel length and diameter, and local vessel sharpness. The user interactively specifies a curved sub-volume, enclosed in the 3D coronary MR angiography data set, which closely encompasses the coronary arterial segments and branches that are represented in one 2D representation (Fig. 14.26). All the voxels that are not included in this user-prescribed sub-volume are discarded and are not used for subsequent visualization and analysis. Typically 20–60 points are needed for the left coronary system, and 10–20 points for the right coronary system, taking ~3 min and ~8–10 min, respectively. Regenfus and

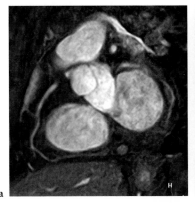 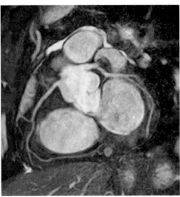

a   b

Fig. 14.26a,b. Thin maximum intensity projection (MIP) (**a**) versus soap-bubble (**b**) post-processing of 3D free-breathing coronary MR angiography of RCA, LM and LCx in a normal subject. The complex 3D course of the coronary arteries can only be partially visualized using a thin MIP (**a**). With more sophisticated 3D post-processing techniques, such as the soap-bubble tool (Philips Medical Systems, Best The Netherlands), the complete course of the CAs and several branches (**b**) can be shown in a single image

colleagues have compared the (conventional) MIP versus original source images in patients with coronary artery stenosis (REGENFUS et al. 2003). They have found no significant differences in overall accuracy for stenosis detection between the processed and unprocessed images. However, the MIP post-processing is compromised by a higher number of images that could not be evaluated owing to overlap of coronary arteries with adjacent structures.

14.11
Clinical Applications for Coronary MR Angiography

14.11.1
Congenital Anomalies of the Coronary Arteries

Congenital anomalies of the coronary arteries tend to be primary and are usually not associated in adults with other types of congenital heart diseases. They are, however, associated with an increased risk of sudden cardiac death, infective endocarditis and ischemic cardiomyopathy (WALKER and WEBB 2001). These anomalies can be classified into three large groups: anomalous origin, anomalous distribution, and anomalous drainage of the coronary artery (ANNÉ et al. 2000). Of clinical relevance are the haemodynamically significant congenital coronary anomalies.

14.11.1.1
Anomalous Origin of the Coronary Arteries

Although anomalous origin and epicardial course of the coronary arteries is an uncommon entity, it can be the cause of chest pain and sudden cardiac death, often in a younger asymptomatic population

(DAVIS et al. 2001). Together with hypertrophic cardiomyopathy and arrhythmogenic right ventricular dysplasia, anomalous origin of the coronary artery is the most frequent cause of sudden cardiac death in competitive young athletes (PELLICIA 2001). The incidence has been reported to be between 0.3 and 1.0% of the normal population, although this is probably an underestimate, as many asymptomatic individuals may be unrecognised (CLICK et al. 1989; DESMET et al. 1992; GARG et al. 2000). From an anatomical point of view, the anomalies are classified according to the coronary artery involved, the origin of the anomalous coronary artery and the anatomic course of the proximal segment. From a clinical point of view, the anomalies are divided into "benign" and "malignant" lesions, the latter have an increased risk for developing myocardial ischemia and sudden cardiac death.

Anomalous origins represent one-third of all coronary artery anomalies. They can present as anomalies in the coronary ostia, e.g. high take-off, multiple ostia, single ostium, and congenital hypoplasia, or as anomalies in the origin and proximal anatomic course of the coronary arteries, or as a combination of both. Most of the anomalies in coronary ostia are benign and have normal myocardial perfusion. The commonest type of multiple ostia is separate origins of the RCA and conus branch; less common are separate origins of the LAD and LCx (Fig. 14.27). Single coronary artery is extremely rare and the clinical relevance in adults is limited (LIPTON et al. 1979; DESMET et al. 1992; WALKER and WEBB 2001). Approximately 60% of all coronary arteries with an anomalous origin and course involve an isolated LCx originating from separate ostium within the right sinus of Valsalva, or as a proximal branch of the RCA This entity has a retro-aortic course and is totally asymptomatic (Fig. 14.28). The remaining 40% of coronary anomalies involve the

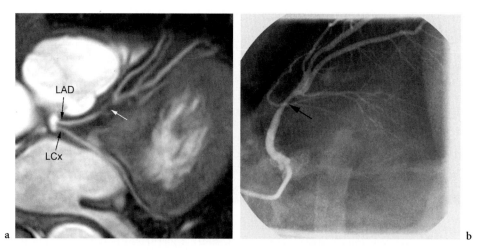

Fig. 14.27a,b. Separate origin of LAD and LCx from the left sinus of Valsalva in a female patient with a 50% stenosis in the proximal LAD. 3D free-breathing coronary MR angiography using a tangential view (b-SSFP technique) (**a**), and X-ray coronary angiography with selective injection in LAD (**b**). The absence of the LM, and the origin of the LAD and LCx directly from the left coronary sinus, as well as the focal narrowing of the LAD (*arrow*), are clearly visible on coronary MR angiography. The LAD stenosis, however, looks more severe on coronary MR angiography than on X-ray coronary angiography. (X-ray coronary angiography, courtesy of Walter Desmet, Dept of Cardiology, UZ Leuven, Leuven, Belgium)

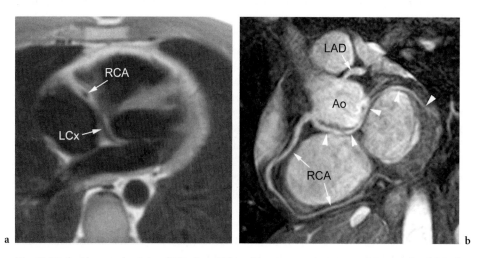

Fig. 14.28a,b. Abnormal origin of LCx from RCA with retro-aortic course of the proximal LCx in a young male patient referred for MRI to exclude arrhythmogenic right ventricular dysplasia. On the axial spin-echo MR images (**a**), a curvilinear hypointense structure is visible behind the left ventricular outflow tract and aortic root. The vascular anomaly, i.e. an abnormal origin of the LCx from the RCA with retro-aortic course of the proximal LCx (*arrowheads*), is confirmed on 3D free-breathing coronary MR angiography (b-SSFP technique) (**b**)

RCA and LCA (BUNCE et al. 2003b). The association of coronary artery anomalies and sudden cardiac deaths ("malignant" forms) appears to be exclusively found in patients with an interarterial vessel, in whom the anomalous vessel passes between the aortic root and RV outflow tract or pulmonary artery (LEBERTHSON et al. 1974). This can be the LCA originating from the right sinus of Valsalva or RCA, the LAD originating from the right sinus of Valsalva or RCA with a LCx originating from the left sinus of Valsalva, or the RCA originating from the LCA of

left sinus of Valsalva (Fig. 14.29). The precise mechanism leading to myocardial ischemia and sudden cardiac death in these patients is still controversial. Very likely, this long interarterial segment is compressed during exercise or other stress conditions, leading to exertional chest pain, syncope, myocardial ischemia and infarction, and potential sudden death. Other mechanisms causing symptoms can be related to a decrease in coronary artery blood flow due to a kinking of the LCA at its origin from the RCA by an increased angulation caused by disten-

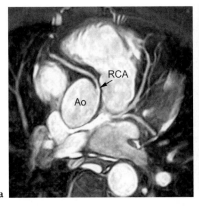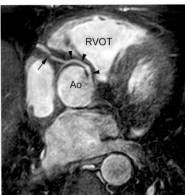

a   b

Fig. 14.29a,b. Abnormal origin of the RCA from the left sinus of Valsalva, in two different patients with symptoms of myocardial ischemia (**a**, **b**). 3D free-breathing coronary MR angiography (b-SSFP technique). The interarterial course of the proximal RCA between the aorta and right ventricular outflow tract (*RVOT*) is clearly visible on the axial images (*arrowheads*). The focal narrowing (*arrow*) of the more distal RCA in patient (**b**) is suggestive of a CA stenosis

sion of the aorta during increased cardiac activity (DAVIS et al. 2001). In young athletes dying from anomalous coronary artery origin and course, the anomalous interarterial segment is most frequently due to a LCA rather than a RCA (23 and 4 deaths, respectively), presumably owing to the more important distribution of LCA blood supply (WALKER and WEBB 2001). In patients with anomalous coronary artery, it is vital to identify the precise anatomic arrangement to enable an appropriate management plan to be followed (i.e. surgical reconstruction or bypass graft surgery, and medical therapy).

Although very uncommon, another group of coronary artery anomalies not mentioned yet are patients with an origin of the coronary artery from the pulmonary trunk. In 90% of these subjects, the LCA arises from the pulmonary artery (ALCAPA). From birth, the myocardium is perfused at low oxygen tension and pressure, stimulating the development of collaterals from the RCA. However, the benefit of collaterals is often offset by a "steal" mechanism, whereby blood passing from the RCA to LCA branches flows retrogradely through the LCA back into the pulmonary artery, thus creating a left-to-right shunt. Without surgical correction this condition is associated with a high mortality in infancy.

One of the earliest and most widely accepted applications for coronary MR angiography has been the detection of congenital anomalies of the origin and the proximal course of the coronary arteries (DOUARD et al. 1988; DUERINCKX et al. 1995; POST et al. 1995; MCCONNELL et al. 1995, 2000; WHITE et al. 1999; TAYLOR et al. 2000b; BUNCE et al. 2003b). Even with multiple projections, the precise location of the proximal course of the vessel in a patient with an abnormal origin of a coronary artery can be difficult to depict with conventional angiography (BUNCE et al. 2003b). Other techniques such as transthoracic echocardiography fail to visualize the ostium of the

RCA in 20% of patients, while the more distal parts are often not interpretable (PELLICCIA 2001). In contrast, 3D coronary MR angiography provides reliable visualization of the root of the arteries and the coronary artery tree. Its tomographic approach enables precise description of the origin and course of the different coronary arteries. Moreover, coronary MR angiography can be combined with functional MR studies, rest–stress coronary artery flow studies, rest–stress myocardial perfusion studies, and late-enhancement MR studies of myocardium. In this way, a single imaging technique enables assessment of the impact of a proximal coronary artery anomaly on the distal coronary flow, the perfusion and function of the myocardial perfusion territory, and depiction of myocardial damage, i.e. infarction and fibrosis, as a result of repeated periods of prolonged myocardial ischemia (BUNCE et al. 2001b; GIORGI et al. 2002b).

14.11.1.2
Myocardial Bridging

Anomalous intramyocardial course of the epicardial coronary artery, also known as "myocardial bridging" is a common finding at autopsy and during cardiac catheterization, but the clinical significance remains controversial (WALKER and WEBB 2001). Myocardial bridges are most commonly localized in the middle segment of the LAD, at a depth of 1–10 mm, with a typical length of approx. 10–30 mm (MÖHLENKAMP et al. 2002). The clinical presentation includes angina, myocardial infarction, left ventricular dysfunction, paroxysmal AV blockade and sudden cardiac death. However, considering the prevalence of myocardial bridging, these complications are rare. Myocardial bridges are diagnosed on coronary angiography by the typical "milking effect" induced by systolic compression of the tunnelled segment. Non-invasive detection of myocardial bridges with CT and MR imaging are appealing, because these techniques visualize not only the coronary artery lumen, but also the surrounding tissues such as the myocardium (Fig. 14.30). However, it should be stressed that the use of magnetization preparation pulses (MTC pulses and T2 preparation pulses) to enhance the blood/ myocardium CNR, in coronary MR angiography, suppresses the myocardial signal and thus will inevitably hamper the visualization of the myocardial bridge. Also, current acquisition times for cardiac CT are too long to accurately assess the severity of compression of the intramyocardial coronary segment during systole.

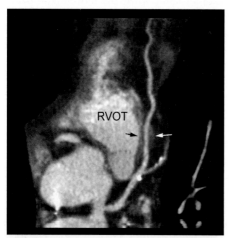

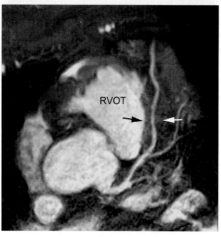

Fig. 14.30a,b. Myocardial bridging of the mid LAD in a patient with symptoms of myocardial ischemia. Contrast-enhanced ECG-gated CT (**a**), 3D free-breathing coronary MR angiography (b-SSFP technique) (**b**). The focal intramyocardial course (*arrows*) of the LAD near the right ventricular outflow tract (*RVOT*) is more easily visible on cardiac CT than on coronary MR angiography. This is related to the use of a T2-preparation pre-pulse which suppresses the signal of myocardium and therefore makes differentiation with epicardial fat more difficult

Other approaches such as MR flow measurements in the LAD might be appealing to assess the severity of myocardial bridging.

14.11.1.3
Coronary Arteriovenous Fistulae

Coronary arteriovenous fistulae are the most common clinically significant congenital coronary anomaly (WALKER and WEBB 2001). They are anomalies of termination and comprise 50% of all coronary anomalies, and can be congenital or acquired. Congenital arteriovenous fistulae are usually isolated and result from an incomplete obliteration of the primitive myocardial sinusoids. Acquired fistulae may be infectious, traumatic or iatrogenic in aetiology. Although they arise from both coronary arteries, the right side is slightly more affected (55–60%). Coronary artery fistulae usually drain directly into the right side of the heart or venous structures (pulmonary trunk, coronary sinus, superior vena cava). A fistula results in a left-to-right shunt, except in the rare cases where it terminates in a left chamber of the heart . If there is a large shunt, the involved coronary artery is grossly enlarged, elongated and tortuous, and commonly contains saccular aneurysms that may progressively dilate. Those with a large shunt may develop heart failure, myocardial ischemia or infarction, infective endocarditis or rupture of an associated aneurysm. Those with smaller shunts tend to be asymptomatic and undergo investigation because a continuous murmur is audible. Although cardiac catheterization with coronary angiography is the standard method for defining the fistula and establishing its functional significance, MR imaging is helpful for 3D visualization of the complex anatomical details of coronary arteriovenous fistulas (coronary MR angiography) (Fig. 14.31) and assessment of the functional impact by quantifying the left-to right shunt volumes (phase-contrast MR imaging) and right and left ventricular volumes (DUERINCKX et al. 1999, 2000; ANNÉ et al. 2000).

14.11.1.4
Coronary Artery Imaging in Congenital Heart Diseases

Embryologically, the coronary arterial bed arises from three components: the sinusoids (which go on to develop into myocardium), the in situ vascular endothelial network and the coronary buds (from which the aortopulmonary trunk arises; WALKER

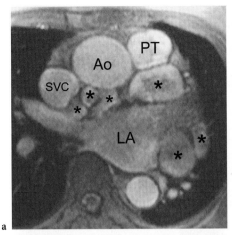

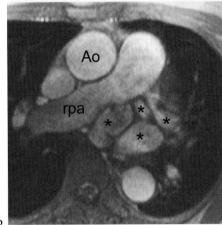

Fig. 14.31a,b. Coronary arteriovenous fistulae in an elderly female patient with symptoms of cardiac failure. Bright-blood cine MRI, using the spoiled-GE technique. Several dilated coronary vessels (*stars*) are visible along the left coronary artery tree. Velocity-encoded cine MRI showed a left to right shunt with a shunt ratio (QP/QS) of 1.45. Ao, Aorta; SVC, superior vena cava; LA, left atrium; PT, pulmonary trunk; rpa, right pulmonary artery

and WEBB 2001). The coronary ostia form early, but the distal coronary pattern develops later, after formation of the ventricular masses. The ostia arise from the two aortic cusps situated next to the aortopulmonary septum. The origin of the LAD is influenced by the development of the pulmonary conus. Hence, in tetralogy of Fallot (characterized by uneven septation and hypoplasia of the pulmonary infundibulum), an abnormal origin of the LAD from the RCA is not uncommon. Ventricular morphology largely determines the coronary pattern; for example, in ventricular inversion, the coronary arteries are also inverted. The distribution and size of the epicardial coronary vessels are strictly related to the extent of their dependent myocardium. A lack of myocardium would induce hypoplasia of the myocardium and, conversely, a reduction in myocardium mass would cause a relative hypoplasia of its coronary branch (ANGELINI 1989) (Fig. 14.32). In patients with congenital heart disease, coronary MR angiography has a complementary role to X-ray coronary angiography (TAYLOR et al. 2000b) (Fig. 14.33). Not only is the incidence of anomalous coronary arteries much higher in patients with congenital heart disease (3–36%), but detailed information regarding the coronary artery is necessary to avoid damage to the arteries in patients undergoing cardiac surgery. Since a high number of these patients have abnormally related great vessels, the identification of the relationship of the coronary arteries with X-ray angiography is much more difficult than it is for normal cardiac anatomy.

Coronary MR angiography may have a role in the postoperative assessment of coronary artery patency in patients who have undergone the arterial switch operation for transposition of the great

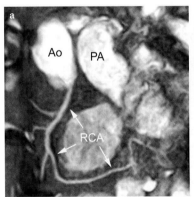

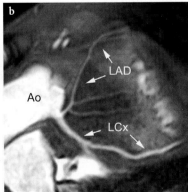

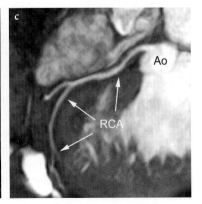

Fig. 14.32a-c. Coronary MR angiography in a patient with transposition of the great arteries, using 3D free-breathing coronary MR angiography (b-SSFP technique). The proximal course of the three CAs is clearly visible. The small calibre of the LAD and its branches is related to the hypoplasia of the morphological left ventricle. Ao, Aorta; PA, pulmonary artery

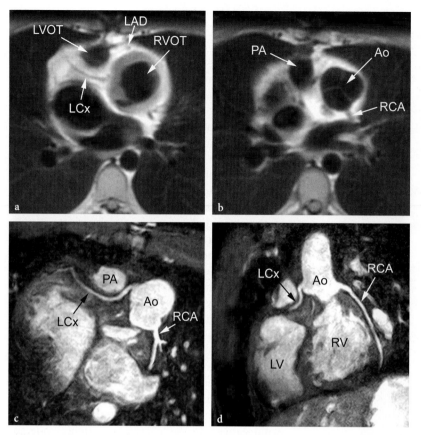

Fig. 14.33a-d. Coronary artery anatomy in a patient with congenitally corrected transposition of the great arteries. Axial T1-weighted fast spin-echo MRI (**a**, **b**), 3D free-breathing coronary MR angiography using the b-SSFP technique in the axial plane (**c**) and short-axis plane through the atrioventricular valves (**d**). In this patient the thick-walled muscular infundibulum of the morphological right ventricle is connected to the aortic valve. The origin and proximal parts of the RCA and LCx are clearly visible on coronary MR angiography

arteries. This surgical procedure has become the treatment of choice for transposition of the great arteries. Good mid-term prognosis for the operation has been reported recently, with most complications and mortality occurring within the 1st year of life (PRÊTRE et al. 2001). The majority of the deaths during this period are secondary to myocardial ischemia/infarction associated with relocation of the coronary arteries at operation. However, little is known about the natural history of the coronary morphology in children as they grow. Due to issues related to repeated X-ray exposure (FAULKNER et al. 1986), morbidity associated with the procedure itself and potential toxicity of iodinated contrast agents, screening of this group of subjects with X-ray coronary angiography is not feasible. In a recent study, Taylor and colleagues obtained diagnostic-quality images of the coronary artery ostium and proximal coronary in 72% of coronary artery images using free-breathing, real-time NE 3D coronary MR angiography. This figure rose to a 100% in subjects older than 11 years (TAYLOR et al. 2004). No ostial stenoses were seen and, in all 16 subjects (mean age, 10.8±1.3 years), the proximal course of the coronary arteries was visualized (see also Fig. 15.29). In their study, coronary MR angiography was combined with cine MR imaging to evaluate ventricular function, and contrast-enhanced MR imaging to assess myocardial damage. Two sub-endocardial viability defects were detected, corresponding to known compromise of the artery supplying that territory. Global left and right ventricular function were preserved, with no regional wall abnormalities.

14.11.2
Coronary Artery Vasculitis

Kawasaki disease is an acute vasculitis of unknown aetiology that predominantly occurs in young children and produces coronary artery aneurysms in 15–25% of untreated cases (KATO et al. 1996). Coronary artery aneurysms may rupture, thrombose or develop stenotic lesions that cause myocardial ischemia. Serial evaluation of the distribution and size of coronary artery aneurysms is necessary for risk stratification and therapeutic management. Although transthoracic echocardiography is often sufficient for this purpose initially, visualization and characterization of the coronary arteries become progressively more difficult as children grow. Serial evaluation with X-ray angiography carries risks associated with its invasive nature and exposure to ionizing radiation (VITIELLO et al. 1998). Although, in a recent paper, Sohn and colleagues reported on the role of MDCT in the detection and follow-up of coronary artery aneurysms due to Kawasaki disease, the considerable X-ray dose of repeated CT investigations seriously limits its role as follow-up technique in the paediatric population (SOHN et al. 2003). Coronary MR angiography on the other hand is totally harmless, and the technique has become sufficiently robust to be used in the paediatric population. In the late 1990s, several groups investigated the use of this technique in a limited number of patients with Kawasaki disease (DUERINCKX et al. 1997; FLACKE et al. 2000; MOLINARI et al. 2000). More recently, two larger patient studies have been published. Greil et al. have compared real-time NE 3D-free-breathing coronary MR angiography with conventional angiography in six patients with Kawasaki disease (GREIL et al. 2002). They have found complete agreement between both techniques in the detection of coronary artery aneurysms (n=11), coronary artery stenoses (n=2), and coronary occlusions (n=2). Moreover, an excellent correlation is found for the maximal diameter

and length of the coronary artery aneurysms. In the second study, 14 young patients with Kawasaki disease (mean age 22±31 months) were studied with MR imaging (VICK et al. 2003). The study protocol included: real-time NE 3D-free-breathing coronary MR angiography, T2-weighted fast spin-echo MR imaging and CE-MRA of the peripheral arteries, with the results compared with echocardiography. Coronary artery diameters are comparable between both techniques, but MR angiography demonstrate distal coronary artery regions that are often not well seen echocardiographically. In patients with acute Kawasaki disease, increased signal intensity surrounding coronary artery aneurysm sites on T2-weighted images is found. Moreover, several large aneurysms have been found in peripheral arteries with CE-MRA. Further evaluation of MR imaging in patients with Kawasaki disease is now necessary following these initial positive results. Furthermore, since patients are prone to development of coronary artery stenosis with subsequent development of myocardial ischemia, coronary flow assessment and other MR imaging techniques to detect myocardial ischemia and infarction might be interesting to investigate patients with Kawasaki disease (Fig. 14.34).

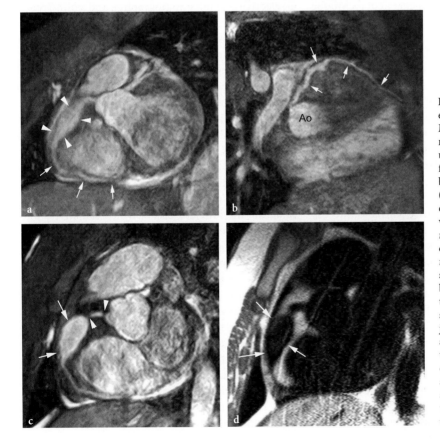

Fig. 14.34a-d. Kawasaki's disease. 3D free-breathing coronary MR angiography (b-SSFP technique) of RCA (a), LM and LAD using a perpendicular view (b); follow-up study 1 year later with bright-blood (c) and black-blood (d) coronary MR angiography of RCA. A fusiform aneurysm is visible in the proximal RCA (*arrowheads*) with normalization of the calibre more distally (*arrows*) (a). The LM and LAD show some mild enlargements in calibre (b). On the follow-up study, the bright-blood images strongly suggest the presence of a stenosis just proximally to the aneurysm, as well as an ostial stenosis of the RCA. (*arrowheads*). The size of the aneurysm on bright-blood and black-blood images is fairly similar, which virtually excludes the presence of the peripheral thrombus in the aneurysm

Takayasu's arteritis is a chronic vasculitis involving the aorta and its main branches, the pulmonary arteries and the coronary tree, and needs to be considered in a young patient with angina, in particular when pulses are absent. It may lead to stenosis with obstruction caused by fibrosis and thrombus formation or aneurysm formation due to weakening of the vessel wall. Although cardiac features are present in up to 40% of cases, angina pectoris is rarely a presenting feature, reported in 6–16% of cases. Angina pectoris is usually caused by premature coronary disease, in particular involving the ostia of the coronary arteries, but may be related to extrinsic compression of the coronary tree or a steal phenomenon (MALIK et al. 2003). At present, the role of coronary MR angiography is not yet defined.

14.11.3
Coronary Artery Disease

14.11.3.1
Coronary Artery Stenosis Detection

As discussed in the previous paragraphs, coronary MR angiography has become an excellent technique for the non-invasive visualization of the origin and course of the coronary arteries. However, the biggest question remains unanswered: What is the current value and clinical role of coronary MR angiography in detecting CAD? And is it an acceptable alternative to X-ray coronary angiography? Moreover, as several recent publications have suggested a promising role for MR imaging of the coronary artery vessel wall and characterization of atherosclerotic plaques, new expectations have been created.

Since the early 1990s, several patient studies using coronary MR angiography for assessing CAD have been published, reporting variable success for imaging coronary artery stenoses with a wide range of sensitivities and specificities (PENNELL et al. 1993; MANNING et al. 1993b; DUERINCKX and URMAN 1994; POST et al. 1996, VAN GEUNS et al. 1999, 2000; SANDSTEDE et al. 1999; HUBER et al. 1999; LETHIMONNIER et al. 1999; SARDANELLI et al. 2000; REGENFUS et al. 2000, 2002; KIM et al. 2001b; SOMMER et al. 2002; WEBER et al. 2002; BOGAERT et al. 2003; Fig. 14.35–38). Comparison of the different studies is difficult for several reasons (Table 14.7). There have constantly been technical improvements in coronary MR angiography techniques over time, and what initially was considered as innovative is nowadays completely outdated. Although this technical progress has led to a much more reliable and robust visualization of longer coronary arterial segments and side branches, improved coronary artery image quality and vessel sharpness, surprisingly this has not been reflected in an improved accuracy of coronary artery stenosis detection. Most studies used X-ray coronary angiography as reference technique to compare the coronary MR angiography results. The criteria for comparison, however, differed between studies. Some studies included only the segments that were visible on coronary MR angiography for comparison, others used only the proximal segments or segments with a minimal coronary artery diameter (e.g. ≥2 mm) as inclusion criteria. There were interstudy differences between the definitions of a significant coronary artery stenosis, e.g. 50% versus 70% stenosis.

Statistical analysis has also differed widely between studies. While most studies used a comparison of individual coronary segments, others used the entire coronary artery for comparison or expressed results on a per-patient basis. The criteria to include a patient are not always clear, and might lead to bias of results. Although most studies mention a consecutive inclusion of patients (e.g. scheduled for an elective coronary angiography), and a blind reading of the coronary MR angiography studies, these issues are difficult to verify when assessing the published data. Multi-centre studies with a central, blind reading of studies are one way to make results more believable, and only a few studies to date have used receiver operating characteristic (ROC) curves as a more efficient way to display the relationship between sensitivity and specificity, for expressing their results (DUERINCKX et al. 1995; BOGAERT et al. 2003). For these ROC analyses, a degree-of-confidence decision task is used, i.e. confidence from 1 (definitely normal) to 5 (definitely abnormal), to define the four cut-offs at which sensitivity and specificity are calculated and the ROC curves are plotted. The closer a ROC is situated to the upper left hand-corner of the graph, the more accurate is the coronary MR angiography (Fig. 14.39). Another way to express the clinical feasibility is the assessment of confidence levels between two independent readers, using the kappa statistic to measure the agreement between readers.

The following points should be considered from the patient studies. The accuracy of stenosis detection is strongly dependent on the image quality (DUERINCKX et al. 1995; WIELOPOLSKI et al. 2000; SOMMER et al. 2002; BOGAERT et al. 2003). As soon as the image qual-

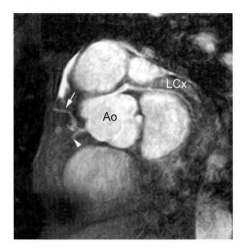

Fig. 14.35. Total occlusion of proximal RCA (*arrowhead*) with collateral circulation by the conal artery (*arrow*). These findings were confirmed on cardiac catheterization (images not shown)

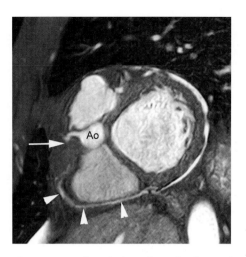

Fig. 14.36. Total occlusion of proximal RCA (*arrow*) with retrograde filling of distal RCA (*arrowheads*) by collaterals from LCA system. These findings were confirmed on cardiac catheterization (images not shown)

Table 14.7. Detection of coronary artery stenoses: comparison of sensitivity and specificity (>50% stenoses) of the different 3D coronary MR angiography techniques with conventional invasive coronary angiography

Technique Study	No. of Patients	No. of Lesions	No. of Patients, Vessels or Segments Excluded (%)	Sensitivity (%)	Specificity (%)
3D-Breath-hold, non-contrast enhanced					
- Van Geuns et al. (2000)	38	41	85 segments (31)	68	97
3D-Breath-hold, contrast enhanced					
- Regenfus et al. (2000)	50	56	82 segments (23)	86	91
- Regenfus et al. (2002)[a]	32	25	53 segments (24)	87	92
3D Retrospective respiratory gating					
- van Geuns et al. (1999)	32	26	52 segments (26)	50	91
- Sandstede et al. (1999)	30		7 patients (23)	81	89
- Huber et al. (1999)	20		45 segments (31)	79	54
- Sardanelli et al. (2000)	42	67	39 segments (14)	82	89
- Regenfus et al. (2002)[a]	32	25	69 segments (31)	60	89
3D Real-time prospective navigator					
- Lethimonnier et al. (1999)	20	53	3 patients (15)	65	93
- Kim et al. (2001b)	109	94	123 segments (16)	93	42
- Sommer et al. (2002)	107	95	all proximal/mid included	74	63
- Weber et al. (2002)	11	16	26 segments (30)	88	94
- Bogaert et al. (2003)	21	29	59-56 segments (31-29)	44 /55[b]	95 / 84[b]

Sensitivity and specificity are expressed on a segmental basis
[a]Same patient group
[b]Values for reader A and B

ity drops, a large number of image artefacts are created, which can be misinterpreted as representing lesions (and vice versa), and which inevitably lead to a drop in the degree of confidence of lesion assessment. Image quality is often not predictable, but usually there is a drop in image quality between healthy volunteers and patients. Potential explanations for the lower image quality in patients are irregularities in heart rhythm or breathing pattern and breath-hold capacity, patient constitution (such as presence of lung emphysema in elderly patients) or technical issues such as suitability of NE technique in patients.

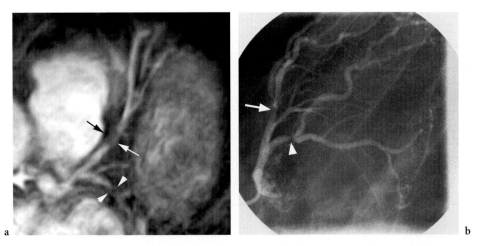

Fig. 14.37a,b. Haemodynamically significant stenosis of proximal LAD (*arrows*) and proximal LCx (*arrowheads*) on coronary MR angiography (**a**), confirmed by X-ray coronary angiography (**b**). (X-ray coronary angiography, courtesy of Walter Desmet, Dept of Cardiology, UZ Leuven, Leuven, Belgium)

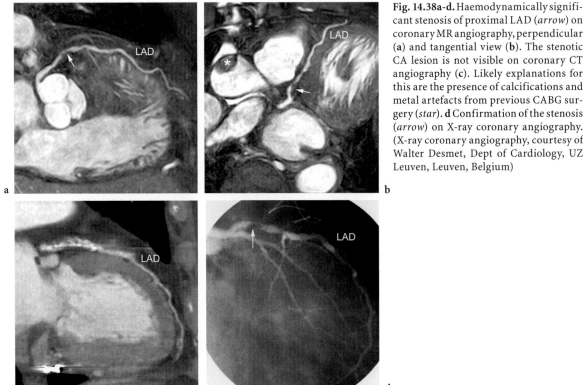

Fig. 14.38a-d. Haemodynamically significant stenosis of proximal LAD (*arrow*) on coronary MR angiography, perpendicular (**a**) and tangential view (**b**). The stenotic CA lesion is not visible on coronary CT angiography (**c**). Likely explanations for this are the presence of calcifications and metal artefacts from previous CABG surgery (*star*). **d** Confirmation of the stenosis (*arrow*) on X-ray coronary angiography. (X-ray coronary angiography, courtesy of Walter Desmet, Dept of Cardiology, UZ Leuven, Leuven, Belgium)

The more distal a lesion from the origin, the more difficult it is to detect. This is related to the smaller vessel size and less-reliable image quality. Assessment of coronary artery stenosis in most studies is limited to the proximal half of the major coronary arteries, excluding the more distal parts and side branches. Although coronary artery stenosis detection is feasible in a considerable number of patients, quantification of the degree of stenosis is not. With the currently available in-plane spatial resolution of 0.7×0.7 mm even in the larger proximal coronary arterial portions, distinction between

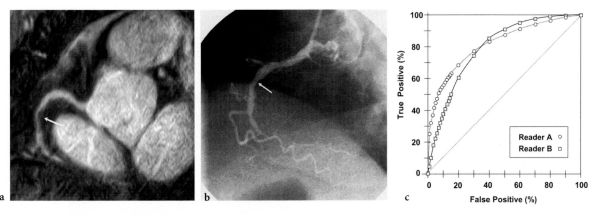

Fig. 14.39a,b. Haemodynamically significant stenosis in mid-RCA in 61-year old male patient on 3D free-breathing coronary MR angiography using spoiled GE technique (**a**), confirmed by X-ray coronary angiography (**b**). Corresponding receiver operating characteristic (ROC) curves (area under the curve: reader A, 0.82; reader B, 0.80) for the detection of haemodynamically significant CA stenoses on coronary MR angiography in 21 patients by two independent readers (**c**). (From BOGAERT et al. (2003). Reprinted with permission of *Radiology*.)

a 40% and 60% stenosis is not possible (Fig. 14.27). Therefore, at present the role of MR imaging as a first-line test that can be used to select patients for cardiac catheterization, seems limited. In diffuse atherosclerotic vessels, stenosis detection is hardly possible. Some other issues such as the influence of plaque composition on stenosis detection are not yet clarified. For example, what is the influence of atherosclerotic plaque calcification on the assessment on the coronary artery stenosis detection? What are the best coronary MR angiography techniques to detect fresh thrombi? New approaches such as combining coronary MR angiography with vessel wall imaging have the advantage that luminographic abnormalities can be directly compared with underlying abnormalities in the arterial wall (SPUENTRUP et al. 2003). From a clinical point of view, it has to be said that coronary artery wall imaging is still a research topic limited to a few centres. In the coming years, this novel technique will certainly become more widely available for evaluation of its clinical value.

Thus, to conclude, assessment of coronary artery stenosis with coronary MR angiography is promising but is still premature for routine clinical use. In some groups of patients, however, MR imaging may be considered for exclusion of coronary artery stenosis. For example, to rule out coronary stenosis in patients with a low likelihood of CAD, scheduled for aortic valve surgery, or, in patients in whom a cardiac catheterization forms a risk (e.g. aortic dissection) or is contraindicated (e.g. renal insufficiency, allergy to contrast media). Moreover, as pointed out

in a recent study by Plein and co-workers, coronary MR angiography might be part of a comprehensive MR imaging protocol (PLEIN et al. 2002). In a 1-h scan, diagnostic information was obtained on cardiac function (short- and long-axis cine imaging), inducible myocardial ischemia (rest and adenosine stress perfusion), coronary artery patency (coronary MR angiography), and myocardial viability (delayed enhancement) in patients with coronary artery disease. From a cost-effective point of view, these kind of comprehensive protocols will become of utmost importance for keeping fast-growing medical expenses under control.

14.11.3.2
Coronary Artery Stent Imaging and Assessment of Coronary Artery Restenosis

To improve the immediate and long-term results of balloon angioplasty, new forms of catheter-based therapies have been developed. Coronary artery stent placement has taken the lead in the treatment of obstructive coronary arterial disease and is applied in more than 50% of patients undergoing non-surgical coronary artery interventional procedures (PEPINE et al. 1996). Coronary arterial stents are typically made of stainless steel or tantalum. After implantation in the artery, they are endothelialized and incorporated into the vessel wall. Initially it was recommended that MR studies should be postponed for 4–8 weeks after stent implantation until the endothelialization had occurred, because it was believed that endothelialization opposed possible dislodgement. Several studies since then have shown that, at a field strength of 1.5 T, MR studies less than 8 weeks after coronary stent placement can be considered to be safe, and the risk of stent heating and stent migration, and subsequent stent thrombosis and myocardial infarction and cardiac death is low (SCOTT and PETTIGREW 1994; STROHM et al. 1999; HUG et al. 2000; SCHROEDER et al. 2000; GERBER et al. 2003a). The artefact size, created by the stent, differs according to the type and size of stent, the MR imaging sequence used and the orientation to the main magnetic field (HUG et al. 2000; MAINTZ et al. 2002). Fast spin-echo images had minimal artefacts, while larger artefacts are seen on the turbo gradient-echo and echo-planar images. Coronary artery stents typically appear as well-defined areas of signal void on coronary MR angiography (SARDANELLI et al. 2002; Fig. 14.40). MR-lucent stents, allowing assessment of the CA lumen, are currently under development.

Although improved medical treatment regimes have significantly reduced the risk of stent occlusion, this risk is still estimated to be in the range of 20–40% (SERRUYS et al. 1994). To date, several MR imaging approaches are under investigation to evaluate patients with suspected stent occlusion or re-stenosis, by either direct assessment of the stent patency (DUERINCKX et al. 1998) or indirect evaluation of the distal coronary artery flow (and flow reserve) (SAITO et al. 2001; SARDANELLI et al. 2002; NAGEL et al. 2003). Radiofrequency penetration into the stents is strongly influenced by the stent material (MAINTZ et al. 2002). For example, tantalum stents demonstrate minimal intraluminal signal attenuation, while steel stents show pronounced intraluminal signal voids. So, future stent design should be focused on the MR imaging characteristics to allow optimal intrastent imaging. Another new, interesting approach for imaging the stent lumen is to use the stent as a receiver coil itself (QUICK et al. 1999, 2002). Low signal in the distal coronary artery on bright-blood coronary artery MR angiography has been reported to occur in stent restenosis, in a small groups of patients (SARDANELLI et al. 2002). Saito and co-workers measured coronary flow reserve repeatedly for 6 months after stent placement and found a significant reduction in coronary flow reserve in patients with an angiographically confirmed re-stenosis at 6 months (2.26±0. 49 at 1 month versus 1.52±0.09 at 6 months). In patients without re-stenosis, coronary flow reserve remained normal (2.31±0.30 at 1 month versus 2.52±0.25 at 6 months; SAITO et al. 2001). Two other studies have found similar results in patients

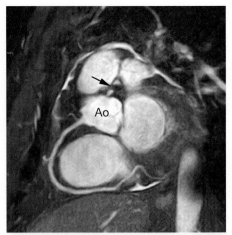

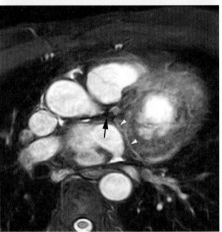

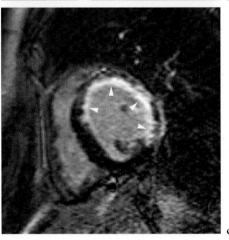

Fig. 14.40a-c. Patient with in-stent restenosis. Stent in LM visible as area of signal void (*arrow*) on MR coronary angiography (**a, b**). In contrast to the normal appearance of the (dominant) RCA, the LCx is very thin and the LAD is not visible. On late-enhancement MR imaging using the contrast-enhanced inversion-recovery technique, a large infarct is visible involving the anterior and lateral LV wall (LAD and LCx perfusion territory)

with stent restenosis (HUNDLEY et al. 2000; NAGEL et al. 2003). However, the optimal coronary flow reserve threshold for detecting stent restenosis differs significantly between the two studies (1.2 versus 2.0, respectively).

14.11.3.3
Coronary Artery Bypass Graft Imaging and Patency Assessment

Surgical placement of a coronary artery bypass graft is an effective and frequently performed intervention for patients with coronary artery stenoses. The procedure results in reduced angina symptoms and cardiovascular mortality (MYERS et al. 1999). However, the 10-year patency rate for saphenous vein grafts is only 40–60% as a result of a combination of early thrombosis, intimal hyperplasia and accelerated atherosclerosis (BOURASSA 1994). For internal mammary artery grafts, survival is better, with up to 90% of grafts patent at 10 years. Conventional angiography is commonly performed to investigate bypass graft and native vessel patency in patients who present with recurrent angina. The altered vascular anatomy and the need to image additional vessels, results in prolonged, more difficult procedures with increased exposure to ionizing radiation and increased renal toxicity to contrast agents. MR imaging has been used to non-invasively assess CABG patency with several techniques; black-blood spin-echo sequences (WHITE et al. 1987; RUBINSTEIN et al. 1987), different bright-blood gradient-echo sequences (AURIGEMMA et al. 1989; GALJEE et al. 1996; LANGERAK et al. 2002) and CE-MRA techniques (BUNCE et al. 2003a). Coronary artery bypass graft MR angiography has yet to reach the level of reliability required for clinical use (Table 14.8). Graft stenosis often occurs at the site of the anastomosis with the native coronary artery, a location where MR imaging encounters spatial resolution problems, and hence reduced consistency in image quality. Bypass graft angiography encounters similar problems induced by respiratory and cardiac motion as for imaging native coronary artery stenosis.

Metallic clip artefacts remain a problem. Arterial grafts are small, tortuous vessels that are difficult to assess with MR techniques. In a recent study by Langerak and colleagues, diagnostic accuracy of approximately 80% was observed after exclusion of patients with stents and another 11% of patients with insufficient image quality (LANGERAK et al. 2002). Although the ROC areas under the curve were acceptable for identifying graft occlusion

Table 14.8. Specific problems related to CABG imaging

- Physiology of flow pattern(s) in CA bypass grafts
- Differences in flow physiology between different CA bypass graft types, i.e. single versus sequential graft, venous versus arterial graft
- Influence by concomitant alterations in microvasculature
- Tortuous appearance of bypass grafts
- Ability to assess concomitant stenoses in distal coronary vessels (run-off vessels)
- Spatial resolution at the suture with the native CA
- Metallic vascular clips
- Postoperative changes in mediastinum
- Associated pulmonary diseases, i.e. chronic obstructive pulmonary disease and pulmonary emphysema

(0.89), significantly lower values were found for assessing ≥50% and ≥70% stenotic lesions. A similar pattern was found for the interobserver agreement. In another recent study, comparing CE-MRA with b-SSFP angiography, 84% of the venous grafts were correctly identified as patent and only 45% correctly identified as occluded with b-SSFP MR angiography versus 85% and 73%, respectively, for cardiac-gated CE-MRA (BUNCE et al. 2003a). Both techniques are unreliable for accurately assessing graft stenosis or stenosis within the distal native vessels.

An alternative to CABG angiography is assessment of flow patterns and flow reserve using the phase-contrast technique (GALJEE et al. 1996; FURBER et al. 1999; MILLER et al. 1999; LANGERAK et al. 2003a). Defining cut-off or threshold values for different degrees of graft stenosis, however, is complicated. The flow pattern in the bypass graft is influenced by the type of graft used (vein versus arterial), the number of bypass anastomoses to the coronary arteries (single versus sequential), the flow pattern in the distal epicardial coronary arteries (i.e. right versus LCA tree, normal run-off versus diseased run-off) and microcirculation, and the location within the graft where the flow is measured (ISHIDA et al. 2001). Moreover, the flow pattern may be influenced by concurrent anterograde flow through native coronary arteries and in collateral vessels. The aorta and mammary arteries have a high systolic forward flow, whereas the coronary arteries (mainly the LAD) have the largest forward flow during diastole. So, proximal measurements in the internal mammary artery preferentially show a systolic pattern, distal measurements a diastolic pattern, while in between a transition pattern will be found. Single and sequential grafts are functionally different grafts as sequential grafts show significantly higher volume flow and velocity values (GALJEE et al. 1996; LANGERAK et al.

2001, 2003a), a phenomenon probably related to the lower resistance in sequential grafts. Langerak and colleagues found a baseline total flow of 25±9 ml/min and a maximal total flow of 65±33 ml/min during adenosine infusion in normal single grafts, versus 41±15 ml/min and 99±36 ml/min, respectively, in sequential grafts. The graft flow reserve was 2.7 for both types of grafts (LANGERAK et al. 2001), a value that corresponds to those measured with intravascular Doppler flow wires. In another study by the Leiden Group, baseline and stress velocities were measured in different types of bypass grafts, and cut-off points were determined to differentiate between grafts with and without stenosis (LANGERAK et al. 2003b). The best results were obtained using velocity reserve to detect bypass stenoses in single vein grafts. MR flow mapping was used by the same group to examine the beneficial effects of percutaneous intervention (PCI) in patients with graft stenosis (LANGERAK et al. 2003a).

Ishida and colleagues have measured the flow volumes, and the diastolic-to-systolic peak velocities ratio in internal mammary artery-to-coronary artery bypass grafts (ISHIDA et al. 2001). Flow measurements in the midpoint of the internal mammary artery show a mean flow rate of 80±38 ml/min in the non-stenotic group versus 17±5 ml/min in the stenotic group ($p<0.01$). Moreover, a reversal in diastolic-to-systolic peak velocity ratios is found in the stenotic group (0.61±0.44) as compared to the non-stenotic group (1.88±0.96; $p<0.01$). The flow reserve ratios, however, are not significantly different between the two groups. In another recent study, Bedaux and colleagues have used an algorithm combining resting flow (<20 ml/min) and graft flow reserve (<2) for detecting a significant stenosis in the graft or distal run-off vessel (BEDAUX et al. 2002b). This study combines the approach of previous studies where either flow volumes, graft flow velocities or velocity reserves were independently used to demonstrate significant stenosis in the graft or distal run-off vessels. This algorithm had a sensitivity and specificity of 78% and 80%, respectively, for detecting grafts with significant stenosis or diseased run-off. However, it should be stressed that, because of significant overlap in values of basal flow and flow reserve ratio between patients with and without a graft or distal run-off vessel stenosis, application of these values in the individual patient should be interpreted with care.

14.12
Coronary MR Angiography compared with Coronary CT Angiography

Another emerging coronary imaging technique, and at present definitely the closest competitor for coronary MR angiography, is coronary CT angiography (see Table 14.6) (Fig. 14.41). Considerable progress has been achieved in the field of non-invasive or minimally invasive coronary imaging with multi-slice spiral computed tomography (MSCT; BUDOFF et al. 2003). With the use of 4-slice MSCT scanners, promising results have been published; however, cardiac motion and calcium deposits in the coronary artery wall render a substantial number of scans incompletely interpretable (NIEMAN et al. 2002a; GERBER et al. 2003b; KUETTNER et al. 2004). Motion artefacts limit proper assessment, particularly at higher heart rates (GIESLER et al. 2002). With the advent of newer-generation MSCT scanners, equipped with more (8, 16, 40, 64) and thinner detector rows (0.6 mm), improved in-plane resolution (0.4 mm × 0.4 mm) and increased rotation speed (330 ms), several of the previous problems can be solved (NIEMAN et al. 2002b; PANNU et al. 2003). Cardiac CT largely faces the same constraints as MR imaging for studying the coronary arteries (see Sect. 14.3). The strategies used to improve the depiction of the coronary arteries with MR imaging (see Sect. 14.5) can to a large extent also be applied to coronary CT angiography. However, there are several problems that are specific to coronary CT angiography. The issue of motion remains a potential problem even with the newer generation of CT scanners. Acquisition windows have been shortened due to faster rotation times and improved multi-sector acquisitions in patient with fast heart rates. However, current available acquisition windows may still be too long to image fast-moving coronary artery segments such as the RCA (Fig. 14.42) (ACHENBACH 2004). Segmented data acquisition in two (or eventually three) heartbeats is feasible as long as the patient has a regular heart rhythm. Breath-hold duration has been considerably shortened with the 16-slice MSCT scanners. A single, 20-s breath-hold is feasible for most patients, especially when an oxygen mask is applied. Spatial resolution is currently superior for CT (e.g. 0.6×0.6×1.0 mm for a 16 slice MSCT) than for MR angiography. Sub-millimetre, nearly isotropic, volumetric data acquisition enables visualization of almost the entire epicardial coronary artery system. However, the current

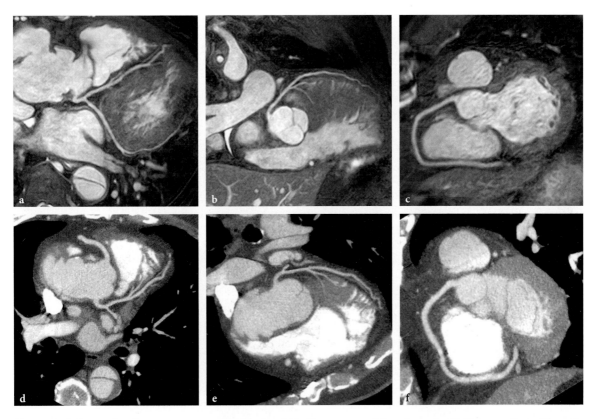

Fig. 14.41a-f. Comparison between coronary MR (**a–c**) and 16-slice coronary CT angiography (**d–f**), in a patient with previous surgery for aortic dissection (type A Stanford) who presented with several pseudoaneurysms in the ascending aorta. The information and image quality obtained by both techniques is quite similar in this patient. No evidence of CAD. All images are reconstructed with the Soap-Bubble analysis program (Philips Medical Systems, Best, The Netherlands)

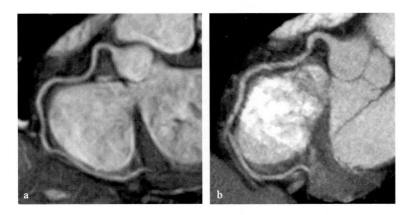

Fig. 14.42a,b. Comparison between coronary MR (**a**) and 16-slice coronary CT angiography (**b**) of the RCA in a patient suspected for CAD. While the image quality on coronary MR angiography is high, the image quality on coronary CT angiography is degraded by motion artefacts and artefacts caused by the high contrast in the right atrium. No evidence of CAD. Both images are reconstructed with the Soap-Bubble analysis program (Philips Medical Systems, Best, The Netherlands)

achievable spatial resolution is likely still insufficient to determine the degree of coronary artery stenoses (BECKER et al. 2002; ACHENBACH 2004) (Fig. 14.43).

Another important issue for CT angiography is the influence of calcium deposition in the coronary wall, which may restrict adequate imaging of the underlying vessel lumen (Fig. 14.43). Two other important issues, which only CT has to face, are the necessity to administer iodinated contrast and the high radiation doses that are currently used in coronary CT angiography. Thus, CT should be considered as being a minimally invasive rather than non-invasive technique.

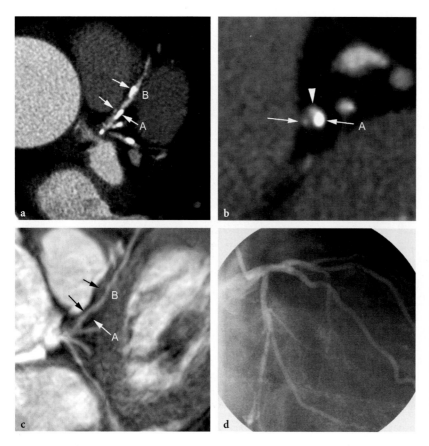

Fig. 14.43a-d. Influence of CA calcifications and CA calibre in the detection of CA stenoses. Comparison between 16-slice coronary CT (**a**, **b**) and coronary MR angiography (**c**). Reference technique is X-ray coronary angiography (**d**). Coronary artery calcifications (*arrows*) may seriously hamper the detection of underlying CA stenosis on coronary CT angiography. In this patient the proximal and mid LAD are not evaluable on coronary CT angiography. In contrast, coronary MR angiography is much less influenced by atherosclerotic calcifications (*arrows*) (**c**). A cross-sectional reconstruction through *A* (**b**) shows a peripheral calcification; the CA lumen is indicated by an arrowhead. Taken into account the normal findings on X-ray coronary angiography (**d**), the latter probably represents a plaque with positive remodelling. (X-ray coronary angiography, courtesy of Walter Desmet, Dept of Cardiology, UZ Leuven, Leuven, Belgium)

The main advantages of CT are simultaneous quantification of the amount of calcium deposition in the coronary arteries – "coronary calcium scoring" – and CT angiography (BECKER et al. 2000). Though, it must be stressed that the role of coronary calcium scoring for assessing the severity of coronary artery disease and in predicting future cardiac events is still a controversial subject in the literature.

Finally, a possible important role for CT is in the characterization of atherosclerotic plaque composition, assessment of coronary remodelling, and definition of the factors contributing to plaque rupture and cardiac events; and further research is required in this domain (KOPP et al. 2002; ACHENBACH et al. 2004a, 2004b).

To date, we do not know whether CT or MR provides the best non-invasive imaging modality for assessing the coronary artery lumen and vessel wall, particularly as neither provides a valuable alternative to conventional X-ray coronary angiography (VAN GEUNS et al. 2002). Both techniques are still emerging and have great potential to become an alternative or complimentary technique for coronary artery imaging.

14.13
Key Points

- Early detection and adequate treatment of CAD is one of the major challenges in current medicine.
- Non-invasive imaging techniques will have a crucial role in determining the "vulnerability index" of atherosclerotic plaques.
- MR imaging has the intrinsic strengths to fulfil this role.
- Coronary artery imaging with MR has become feasible on routine MR scanners equipped with commercially available cardiac MR hardware and software.
- Several approaches for coronary MR angiography are currently available. At present, none of them can be considered as being ideal.
- Coronary MR angiography is a perfect example of trading between different parameters that influence image quality.
- Large parts of the coronary artery tree can be visualized in a reliable fashion, allowing determination of the origin and course of the epicardial

coronary arteries and several of their branches.

- Detection of CA stenoses is closely linked to the image quality. Grading of CA stenoses, however, is hampered by the current lack of spatial resolution.
- Coronary artery wall imaging and plaque characterization with MR is promising, but these techniques are not yet available for routine clinical applications.
- There is close competition between CT and MR in the field of CA imaging. Although promising results can be found in literature for both techniques, they are yet not capable of replacing catheter-based X-ray coronary angiography.

Acknowledgements: the authors would like to thank Mark Kouwenhoven, MSc (Philips Medical Systems, Best, The Netherlands), for the collaboration and his expertise in the exciting field of coronary MR angiography.

References

Achenbach S (2004) Detection of coronary stenoses by multidetector computed tomography: it's all about resolution. J Am Coll Cardiol 43:840–841

Achenbach S, Ropers D, Holle J, Muschiol G, Daniel WG, Moshage W (2000) In-plane coronary arterial motion velocity: measurement with electron-beam CT. Radiology 216:457–463

Achenbach S, Moselewski F, Ropers D et al (2004a) Detection of calcified and noncalcified coronary atherosclerotic plaque by contrast-enhanced, sub-millimetre multidetector spiral computed tomography. A segment-based comparison with intravascular ultrasound. Circulation 109:14–17

Achenbach S, Ropers S, Hoffmann U et al (2004b) Assessment of coronary remodelling in stenotic and nonstenotic coronary atherosclerotic lesions by multidetector spiral computed tomography. J Am Coll Cardiol 43:842–847

Angelini P (1989) Normal and anomalous coronary arteries: definitions and classification. Am Heart J 117:418–434

Anné W, Bogaert J, van de Werf F (2000) A case report of a patient with a large aneurysmatic coronary artery fistula. Acta Cardiol 55:307–310

Atkinson D, Edelman R (1991) Cineangiography of the heart in a single breathhold with a segmented TurboFLASH sequence. Radiology 178:359–362

Aurigemma GP, Reichek N, Axel L, Schiebler M, Harris C, Kressel HY (1989) Noninvasive determination of coronary artery bypass graft patency by cine magnetic resonance imaging. Circulation 80:1595–1602

Austen WG, Edwards JE, Frye RL et al (1975) A reporting system on patients evaluated for coronary artery disease: report of the Ad Hoc Committee for Grading of Coronary Artery Disease, Council in Cardiovascular Surgery, American Heart Association. Circulation 51:5–40

Azhari H, McKenzie CA, Edelman RR (2001) MR angiography using spin-lock flow tagging. Magn Reson Med 46:1041–1044

Balaban RS, Chesnick S, Hedges K, Samaha F, Heineman FW (1991) Magnetization transfer contrast in MR imaging of the heart. Radiology 180:671–675

Becker CR, Knez A, Ohnesorge B et al (2000) Visualization and quantification of coronary calcifications with electron beam and spiral computed tomography. Eur Radiol 10:629–635

Becker CR, Knez A, Leber A et al (2002) Detection of coronary artery stenoses with multi-slice helical CT angiography. J Comput Assist Tomogr 26:750–755

Bedaux WL, Hofman MBM, Visser CA, van Rossum AC (2001) Simultaneous noninvasive measurement of blood flow in the great cardiac vein and left anterior descending artery. J Cardiovasc Magn Reson 3:227–235

Bedaux WL, Hofman MB, Wielopolski PA et al (2002a) Three-dimensional magnetic resonance coronary angiography using a new blood pool contrast agent: initial experience. J Cardiovasc Magn Reson 4:273–282

Bedaux WL, Hofman MBM, Vyt SLA, Bronzwaer JGF, Visser CA, van Rossum AC (2002b) Assessment of coronary artery bypass graft disease using cardiovascular magnetic resonance determination of flow reserve. J Am Coll Cardiol 40:1848–1855

Bogaert J, Duerinckx A (1995) Appearance of the normal pericardium on coronary MR angiograms. J Magn Reson 5:579–587

Bogaert J, Kuzo S, Dymarkowski S, Becker R, Piessens J, Rademakers FE (2003) Coronary artery imaging using real-time navigator 3D Turbo-field-echo MR coronary angiography technique. Initial experience. Radiology 226:707–716

Börnert P, Jensen D (1995) Coronary artery imaging at 0.5T using segmented 3D echo planar imaging. Magn Reson Med 34:779–785

Börnert P, Aldefeld B, Nehrke K (2001a) Improved 3D spiral imaging for coronary MR angiography. Magn Reson Med 45:172–175

Börnert P, Stuber M, Botnar RM et al (2001b) Direct comparison of 3D spiral vs Cartesian gradient-echo coronary magnetic resonance angiography. Magn Reson Med 46:789–794

Börnert P, Stuber M, Botnar RM, Kissinger KV, Manning WJ (2002) Comparison of fat suppression strategies in 3D spiral coronary magnetic resonance angiography. J Magn Reson Imaging 15:462–466

Botnar RM, Stuber M, Danias PG, Kissinger KV, Manning WJ (1999a) Improved coronary artery definition with T2-weighted free-breathing, three-dimensional coronary MRA. Circulation 99:3139–3148

Botnar RM, Stuber M, Danias PG, Kissinger KV, Manning WJ (1999b) A fast 3D approach for coronary MRA. J Magn Reson Imaging 10:821–825

Botnar RM, Stuber M, Kissinger KV, Manning WJ (2000a) Free-breathing 3D coronary MRA: the impact of "isotropic" image resolution. J Magn Reson Imaging 11:389–393

Botnar RM, Stuber M, Kissinger KV, Kim WY, Spuentrup E, Manning WJ (2000b) Noninvasive coronary vessel wall and plaque imaging with magnetic resonance imaging. Circulation 102:2582–2587

Botnar RM, Kim WY, Börnert P, Stuber M, Spuentrup E, Manning WJ (2001) 3D Coronary vessel wall imaging utilizing a local inversion technique with spiral image acquisition. Magn Reson Med 46:848–854

Botnar RM, Stuber M, Lamericks R et al (2003) Initial experiences with in vivo RCA human MR vessel wall imaging at 3 Tesla. J Cardiovasc Magn Reson 5:589–594

Bourassa MG (1994) Long-term vein graft patency. Curr Opin Cardiol 9:685–691

Brittain JH, Hu BS, Wright GA, Meyer CH, Macovski A, Nishimura DG (1995) Coronary angiography with magnetization-prepared T2 contrast. Magn Reson Med 33:689–696

Budoff MJ, Achenbach S, Duerinckx A (2003) Clinical utility of computed tomography and magnetic resonance techniques for noninvasive coronary angiography. J Am Coll Cardiol 42:1867–1878

Bunce NH, Pennell DJ (1999) Coronary MRA – a clinical experience in Europe. J Magn Reson Imag 10:721–727

Bunce NH, Jhooti P, Keegan J et al (2001a) Evaluation of free-breathing three-dimensional magnetic resonance coronary angiography with hybrid ordered phase encoding (HOPE) for the detection of proximal coronary artery stenosis. J Magn Reson Imaging 14:677–684

Bunce NH, Rahman SL, Keegan J, Gatehouse PD, Lorenz CH, Pennell DJ (2001b) Anomalous coronary arteries: anatomic and functional assessment by coronary and perfusion cardiovascular magnetic resonance in three sisters. J Cardiovasc Magn Reson 3:361–369

Bunce NH, Lorenz CH, John AS, Lesser JR, Mohiaddin RH, Pennell D (2003a) Coronary artery bypass graft patency: assessment with true fast imaging with steady-state precession versus Gadolinium-enhanced MR angiography. Radiology 227:440–446

Bunce NH, Lorenz CH, Keegan J et al (2003b) Coronary artery anomalies: assessment with free-breathing three-dimensional coronary MR angiography. Radiology 227:201–208

Burstein D (1991) MR imaging of coronary artery flow in isolated and in-vivo hearts. J Magn Reson Imaging 1:337–346

Butts K, Riederer SJ (1992) Analysis of flow effects in echo-planar imaging. J Magn Reson Imaging 1:643–650

Carr J, Simonetti O, Bundy J, Li D, Pereles S, Finn JP (2001) Cine MR angiography of the heart with segmented true fast imaging with steady-state precession. Radiology 219:828–834

Celermajer DS (1998) Noninvasive detection of atherosclerosis. N Engl J Med 339:2014–2015

Click RL, Holmes DR, Vliestra RE, Kosinski A, Kronmal RA (1989) Anomalous coronary arteries: location, degree of atherosclerosis and effect on survival – a report from the coronary artery surgery study. J Am Coll Cardiol 13:531–537

Chuang ML, Chen MH, Khasgiwala VC, McConnell MV, Edelman RR, Manning WJ (1997) Adaptive correction of imaging plane position in segmented κ-space cine cardiac MRI. J Magn Reson Imaging 7:811–814

Danias PG, McConnell MV, Khasgiwala VC, Chuang ML, Edelman RR, Manning WJ (1997) Prospective navigator correction of image position for coronary MR angiography. Radiology 203:733–736

Davies MJ (1996) Stability and instability: two faces of coronary atheromatosis. Circulation 94:2013–2020

Davis JA, Cecchin F, Jones TK, Portman MA (2001) Major coronary artery anomalies in a pediatric population: incidence and clinical importance. J Am Coll Cardiol 37:593–597

Deshpande VS, Li D (2003) Contrast-enhanced coronary artery imaging using 3D trueFISP. Magn Reson Med 50:570–577

Deshpande VS, Wielopolski PA, Shea SM, Carr J, Zheng J, Li D (2001a) Coronary artery imaging using contrast-enhanced 3D segmented EPI. J Magn Reson Imaging 13:676–681

Deshpande VX, Shea SM, Laub G, Simonetti OP, Finn JP, Li D (2001b) 3D Magnetization-prepared true-FISP: a new technique for imaging coronary arteries. Magn Reson Med 46:494–502

Deshpande VS, Chung Y-C, Zhang Q, Shea SM, Li D (2003) Reduction of transient signal oscillations in true-FISP using a linear flip angle series magnetization preparation. Magn Reson Med 49:151–157

Desmet W, Vanhaecke J, Vrolix M et al (1992) Isolated single coronary artery: a review of 50000 consecutive coronary angiographies. Eur Heart J 13:1637–1640

Dirksen MS, Lamb HJ, Doornbos J, Bax JJ, Jukema KW, de Roos A (2003) Coronary magnetic resonance angiography: technical developments and clinical applications. J Cardiovasc Magn Reson 5:365–386

Douard H, Barat JL, Mora B, Baudet E, Broustet JP (1988) Magnetic resonance imaging of an anomalous origin of the LCA from the pulmonary artery. Eur Heart J 9:1356–1360

Doyle M, Scheidegger MB, de Graaf RG, Vermeulen J, Pohost GM (1993) Coronary artery imaging in multiple 1-sec breath holds. Magn Reson Imaging 11:3–6

Du YP, Parker DL, Davis WL et al (1994) Reduction of partial-volume artefacts with zero-filling interpolation in three-dimensional MR angiography. J Magn Reson Imaging 4:733–741

Duerinckx AJ, Urman M (1994) Two-dimensional coronary MR angiography: analysis of initial clinical results. Radiology 193:731–738

Duerinckx AJ, Bogaert J, Jiang H, Lewis BS (1995) Anomalous origin of the LCA: diagnosis by coronary MR angiography. AJR Am J Roentgenol 164:1095–1096

Duerinckx AJ, Troutman B, Allada V et al (1997) Coronary MR angiography in Kawasaki disease. AJR Am J Roentgenol 168:114–116

Duerinckx AJ, Atkinson D, Hurwitz R (1998) Assessment of coronary artery patency after stent placement using magnetic resonance angiography. J Magn Reson Imaging 8:896–902

Duerinckx AJ, Perloff JK, Currier JW (1999) Arteriovenous fistulas of the circumflex and right coronary arteries with drainage into an aneurysmal coronary sinus. Circulation 99:2827–2828

Duerinckx AJ, Shaaban, Lewis, A, Perloff J, Laks H (2000) 3D MR imaging of coronary arteriovenous fistulas. Eur Rad 10:1459–1463

Duerinckx AJ (ed) (2002) Coronary magnetic resonance angiography. Springer, Berlin Heidelberg New York

Edelman R, Manning W, Burstein D, Paulin S (1991) Coronary arteries: breath-hold MR angiography. Radiology 181:641–643

Edelman RR, Manning WJ, Gervino E, Li W (1993) Flow velocity quantification in human coronary arteries with fast breath-hold MR angiography. J Magn Reson Imaging 3:699–703

Ehman RL, Felmlee JP (1989) Adaptive technique for high-definition MR imaging of moving structures. Radiology 173:255–263

Etienne A, Botnar RM, van Muiswinkel AMC, Boesiger P, Manning WJ, Stuber M (2002) "Soap-Bubble" visualization and quantitative analysis of 3D coronary magnetic resonance angiograms. Magn Reson Med 48:658–666

Faulkner K, Lover HG, Sweeney JK, Bardsley RA (1986) Radiation doses and somatic risk to patients during cardiac radiological procedures. Br J Radiol 59:359–363

Fayad ZA, Fuster V, Fallon JT et al (2000) Noninvasive in vivo human coronary artery lumen and wall imaging using black-blood magnetic resonance imaging. Circulation 102:506–510

Fayad ZA, Fuster V, Nikolaou K, Becker C (2002) Computed tomography and magnetic resonance imaging for noninvasive coronary angiography and plaque imaging. Current and potential future concepts. Circulation 106:2026–2034

Ferrigno M, Hickey DD, Liner MH, Lundgren CEG (1986) Cardiac performance in humans during breath-holding. J Appl Physiol 60:1871–1877

Firmin D, Keegan J (2001) Navigator echoes in cardiac magnetic resonance. J Cardiovasc Magn Reson 3:183–193

Fischer SE, Wickline SA, Lorenz CH (1999) Novel real-time R-wave detection algorithm based on the vectorcardiogram for accurate gate magnetic resonance acquisitions. Magn Reson Med 42:361–370

Flacke S, Setser RM, Barger P et al (2000) Coronary aneurysms in Kawasaki's disease detected by magnetic resonance coronary angiography. Circulation 101:E516–E517

Fleckenstein JL, Archer BT, Barker BA, Vaughan JT, Parkey RW, Peshock RM (1991) Fast short-tau inversion-recovery MR imaging. Radiology 179:499–504

Foo TKF, Perman WH, Poon CSO, Cusma JT, Sandstorm JC (1989) Projection flow imaging by bolus tracking using stimulated echoes. Magn Reson Med 9:203–218

Foo TKF, Ho VB, Hood MN (2000) Vessel tracking: prospective adjustment of section-selective MR angiographic locations for improved coronary artery visualization over the cardiac cycle. Radiology 214:283–289

Furber AP, Lethimonnier F, Le Jeun JJ et al (1999) Noninvasive assessment of the infarct-related coronary artery blood flow velocity using phase-contrast magnetic resonance imaging after coronary angioplasty. Am J Cardiol 84:24–30

Fuster V (1994) Lewis A. Conner memorial lecture: mechanisms leading to myocardial infarction: insights from studies of vascular biology. Circulation 90:2126–2142

Fuster V, Gotto AM (2000) Risk reduction. Circulation 102: IV94–IV102

Fuster V, Fayad ZA, Badimon JJ (1999) Acute coronary syndromes: biology. Lancet 353:SII5–SII9

Galjee MA, van Rossum AC, Doesburg T, van Eenige MJ, Visser CA (1996) Value of magnetic resonance imaging in assessing patency and function of coronary artery bypass grafts. Circulation 93:660–666

Garg N, Tewari S, Kapoor A, Gupta DK, Sinha N (2000) Primary congenital anomalies of the coronary arteries: a coronary arteriographic study. Int J Cardiol 74:39–46

Gerber TC, Fasseas P, Lennon RJ et al (2003a) Clinical safety of magnetic resonance imaging early after coronary artery stent placement. J Am Coll Cardiol 42:1295–1298

Gerber TC, Kuzo RS, Lane GE et al (2003b) Image quality in a standardized algorithm for minimally invasive coronary angiography with multislice spiral computed tomography. J Comput Assist Tomogr 27:62–69

Giesler T, Baum U, Ropers D et al (2002) Noninvasive visualization of coronary arteries using contrast-enhanced multidetector CT: influence of heart rate on image quality and stenosis detection. AJR Am J Roentgenol 170:911–916

Giorgi B, Dymarkowski S, Maes F, Kouwenhoven M, Bogaert J (2002a) Improved visualization of coronary arteries using a new three-dimensional submillimetre MR coronary angiography sequence with balanced gradients. AJR Am J Roentgenol 179:901–910

Giorgi B, Dymarkowski S, Rademakers F, Lebrun F, Bogaert J (2002b) Single coronary artery as cause of acute myocardial infarction in a 12-year-old girl: a comprehensive approach with MRI. AJR-Am J Roentgenol 179:1535–1537

Glagov S, Weisenberg E, Zarins CK et al (1987) Compensatory enlargement of human atherosclerotic coronary arteries. N Engl J Med 316:1371–1375

Goldfarb JW, Edelman RR (1998) Coronary arteries: breath-hold gadolinium-enhanced, three-dimensional MR angiography. Radiology 206:830–834

Gomes A, Lois J, Drinkwater D, Corday S (1987) Coronary artery bypass grafts: visualization with MR imaging. Radiology 162:175–179

Gould KL, Lipscomb K, Hamilton GW (1974) Physiologic basis for assessing critical coronary stenosis: instantaneous flow response and regional distribution during coronary hyperemia as measures of coronary flow reserve. Am J Cardiol 33:87–94

Green JD, Omary RA, Finn JP et al (2003) Two-and three-dimensional MR coronary angiography with intraarterial injections of contrast agents in dogs: a feasibility study. Radiology 226:272–277

Greil GF, Stuber M, Botnar RM et al (2002) Coronary magnetic resonance angiography in adolescents and young adults with Kawasaki disease. Circulation 105:908–911

Grundy SM, Pasternak R, Greenland P, Smith S, Fuster V (1999) Assessment of cardiovascular risk by use of multiple-risk-factor assessment equations. A statement for healthcare professionals from the American Heart Association and the American College of Cardiology. Circulation 100:1481–1492

Haase A, Frahm J, Hänicke W, Matthaei D (1985) 1H NMR chemical shift selective (CHESS) imaging. Phys Med Biol 4:341–344

Hardy CJ, Cline HE (1989) Broadband nuclear magnetic resonance pulses with two-dimensional spatial selectivity. J Appl Phys 66:1513–1520

Herborn CU, Barkhausen J, Paetsch I et al (2003) Coronary arteries: contrast-enhanced MR imaging with SH L 643A – experience in 12 volunteers. Radiology 229:217–223

Ho VB, Foo TKF, Arai AE, Wolff SD (2001) Gadolinium-enhanced, vessel-tracking, two-dimensional coronary MR angiography: single-dose arterial-phase vs. delayed phase imaging. J Magn Reson Imaging 13:682–689

Hofman MBM, Paschal CB, Li D,Haacke M, van Rossum AC, Sprenger M (1995a) MRI of coronary arteries: 2D breath-hold vs 3D respiratory-gated acquisition. J Comput Assist Tomogr 19:56–62

Hofman MBM, Visser FC, van Rossum AC, Vink GQM, Sprenger M, Westerhof N (1995b) In vivo validation of magnetic resonance volume flow measurements with limited spatial resolution in small vessels. Magn Reson Med 33:778–784

Hofman MB, van Rossum AC, Sprenger M, Westerhof N (1996) Assessment of flow in the right human coronary artery by magnetic resonance phase contrast velocity measurement: effects of cardiac and respiratory motion. Magn Reson Med 35:521–531

Hofman MB, Wickline SA, Lorenz CH (1998) Quantification of in-plane motion of the coronary arteries during the cardiac cycle: implication for acquisition window duration for MR flow quantification. J Magn Reson Imaging 8:568–576

Hofman MB, Henson RE, Kovacs SJ et al (1999) Blood pool contrast agent strongly improves 3D magnetic resonance coronary angiography using an inversion prepulse. Magn Reson Med 41:360–367

Holland AE, Goldfarb JW, Edelman RR (1998) Diaphragmatic and cardiac motion during suspended breathing: preliminary experience and implications for breath-hold MR imaging. Radiology 209:483–489

Holsinger AE, Riederer SJ (1990) The importance of phase encoding order in ultra-short TR snapshot MR imaging. Magn Reson Med 16:481–488

Huber A, Nikolaou K, Gonschior P, Knez A, Stehling M, Reiser M (1999) Navigator echo-based respiratory gating for three-dimensional MR coronary angiography: results from healthy volunteers and patients with proximal coronary artery stenoses. AJR Am J Roentgenol 173:95–101

Huber ME, Hengesbach D, Botnar RM et al (2001) Motion artefact reduction and vessel enhancement for free-breathing navigator-gated coronary MRA using 3D κ-space reordering. Magn Reson Med 45:645–652

Hug J, Nagel E, Bornstedt A, Schnackenburg B, Oswald H, Fleck E (2000) Coronary arterial stents: safety and artefacts during MR imaging. Radiology 216:781–787

Hundley WG, Hillis LD, Hamilton CA et al (2000) Assessment of coronary arterial stenosis with phase-contrast magnetic resonance imaging measurements of coronary flow reserve. Circulation 101:2375–2381

Hwang K-P, Green JD, Li D et al (2002) Minimizing contrast agent dose during intraarterial gadolinium-enhanced MR angiography: in vitro assessment. J Magn Reson Imaging 15:55–61

Ishida N, Sakuma H, Cruz BP et al (2001) MR flow measurement in the internal mammary artery-to-coronary artery bypass graft: comparison with graft stenosis at radiographic angiography. Radiology 220:441–447

Jhooti P, Keegan J, Gatehouse PD et al (1999) 3D Coronary artery imaging with phase reordering for improved scan efficiency. Magn Reson Med 41:555–562

Johansson LO, Fischer SE. Lorenz CH (1999) Benefit of T1 reduction for magnetic resonance coronary angiography: a numerical simulation and phantom study. J Magn Reson Imaging 9:552–556

Joyce JD, Schulman DS, Lasorda D et al (1994) Intracoronary

Doppler guide wire versus stress single-photon emission computed tomography thallium-201 imaging in assessment of intermediate coronary stenoses. J Am Coll Cardiol 24:940–947

Kalden P, Kreitner KF, Wittlinger T et al (1999) Assessment of coronary artery bypass grafts: value of different breath-hold MR imaging techniques. AJR Am J Roentgenol 172:1359–1364

Kato H, Sugimura T, Akagi T et al (1996) Long-term consequences of Kawasaki disease. A 10- to 21-year follow-up study of 594 patients. Circulation 94:1379–1385

Keegan J, Gatehouse PD, Taylor AM, Yang GZ, Jhooti P, Firmin DN (1999) Coronary artery imaging in a 0.5 Tesla scanner: implementation of real-time navigator echo controlled segmented κ-space FLASH and interleaved spiral sequences. Magn Reson Med 41:392–399

Keegan J, Gatehause P, Yang G-Z, Firmin D (2002) Coronary artery motion with the respiratory cycle during breath-holding and free-breathing: implications for slice-followed coronary artery imaging. Magn Reson Med 47:476–481

Keegan J, Gatehouse PD, Mohiaddin RH, Yang HZ, Firmin DN (2004) Comparison of spiral and FLASH phase velocity mapping, with and without breath-holding, for the assessment of left and RCA blood flow velocity. J Magn Reson Imaging 19:40–49

Kessler W, Laub G, Achenbach S, Ropers D, Moshage W, Daniel WG (1999) Coronary arteries: MR angiography with fast contrast-enhanced three-dimensional breath-hold imaging – initial experience. Radiology 210:566–572

Kim WY, Stuber M, Kissinger KV, Andersen NT, Manning WJ, Botnar RM (2001a) Impact of bulk cardiac motion on right coronary MR angiography and vessel wall imaging. J Magn Reson Imaging 14:383–390

Kim WY, Danias PG, Stuber M et al (2001b) Coronary magnetic resonance angiography for the detection of coronary stenoses. N Engl J Med 345:1863–1869

Kim WY, Stuber M, Börnert P, Kissinger KV, Manning WJ, Botnar RM (2002) Three-dimensional black-blood cardiac magnetic resonance coronary vessel wall imaging detects positive arterial remodelling in patients with nonsignificant coronary artery disease. Circulation 106:296–299

Klein C, Nagel E, Schnackenburg B et al (2000) The intravascular contrast agent Clariscan (NC 100150 injection) for 3D coronary angiography in patients with coronary artery disease. MAGMA 11:65–67

Kooi ME, Cappendijk VC, Cleutjens KBJM et al (2003) Accumulation of ultrasmall superparamagnetic particles of iron oxide in human atherosclerotic plaques can be detected by in vivo magnetic resonance imaging. Circulation 107:2453–2458

Kopp AF, Küttner A, Heuschmid M, Schröder S, Ohnesorge B, Claussen CD (2002) Multidetector-row CT cardiac imaging with 4 and 16 slices for coronary CTA and imaging of atherosclerotic plaques. Eur Radiol 12:S17–S24

Koskenvuo JW, Hartiala JJ, Knuuti J et al (2001) Assessing coronary sinus flow blood in patients with coronary artery disease: a comparison of phase-contrast MR imaging with positron emission tomography. Am J Roentgenol AJR 177:1161–166

Kragel AH, Gertz SD, Roberts WC (1991) Morphologic comparison of frequency and types of acute lesions in the major epicardial coronary arteries in unstable angina pectoris, sudden coronary death and acute myocardial infarction. J Am Coll Cardiol 18:801–808

Kuettner A, Kopp AF, Schroeder S et al (2004) Diagnostic accuracy of multidetector computed tomography coronary angiography in patients with angiographically proven coronary artery disease. J Am Coll Cardiol 43:831–839

Langerak SE, Kunz P, Vliegen HW et al (2001) Improved MR flow mapping in coronary artery bypass graft during adenosine-induced stress. Radiology 218:540–547

Langerak SE, Vliegen HW, de Roos A et al (2002) Detection of vein graft disease using high-resolution magnetic resonance angiography. Circulation 105:328–333

Langerak SE, Vliegen JW, Zwinderman AH et al (2003a) Vein graft function improvement after percutaneous intervention: evaluation with MR flow mapping. Radiology 228:834–841

Langerak SE, Vliegen HW, Jukema JW et al (2003b) Value of magnetic resonance imaging for the noninvasive detection of stenosis in coronary artery bypass grafts and recipient coronary arteries. Circulation 107:1502–1508

Leberthson RR, Dinsmore RR, Bharati S et al (1974) Aberrant coronary artery origin from the aorta: diagnosis and clinical significance. Circulation 50:774–779

Lenz GW, Haacke EM, White RD (1989) Retrospective cardiac gating: a review of technical aspects and future directions. Magn Reson Med 7:445–455

Lethimonnier F, Furber A, Morel O et al (1999) Three-dimensional coronary artery MR imaging using prospective real-time respiratory navigator and linear phase shift processing: comparison with conventional coronary angiography. Magn Reson Imaging 17:1111–1120

Li D, Paschal CB, Haacke EM, Adler LP (1993) Coronary arteries: three-dimensional MR imaging with fat saturation and magnetization transfer contrast. Radiology 187:401–406

Li D, Kaushikkar S, Haacke EM et al (1996) Coronary arteries: three-dimensional MR imaging with retrospective respiratory gating. Radiology 201:857–863

Li D, Dolan RP, Walovitch RC, Lauffer RB (1998) Three-dimensional MRI of coronary arteries using an intravascular contrast agent. Magn Reson Med 39:1014–1018

Li D, Carr JC, Shea SM, Zheng J, Deshpande VS, Wielopolski PA, Finn JP (2001a) Coronary arteries: magnetization-prepared contrast-enhanced three-dimensional volume targeted breath-hold MR angiography. Radiology 219:270–277

Li D, Zheng J, Weinmann H-J (2001b) Contrast-enhanced MR imaging of coronary arteries: comparison of intra- and extravascular contrast agents in Swine. Radiology 218:670–678

Lipton MJ, Barry WH, Obrez I, Silverman JF, Wexler L (1979) Isolated single coronary artery: diagnosis, angiographic classification, and clinical significance. Radiology 130:39–47

Lorenz CH, Johansson LO (1999) Contrast-enhanced coronary MRA. J Magn Reson Imaging 10:703–708

Lund GK, Wendland MF, Shimakawa A et al (2000) Coronary sinus flow measurement by means of velocity-encoded cine MR imaging: validation by using flow probes in dogs. Radiology 217:487–493

Maintz D, Botnar RM, Fischbach R, Heindel W, Manning WJ, Stuber M (2002) Coronary magnetic resonance angiography for assessment of the stent lumen: a phantom study. J Cardiovasc Magn Reson 4:359–367

Malik IS, Harare O Al-Nahhas A, Beatt K, Mason J (2003) Takayasu's arteritis: management of left main stem stenosis. Heart 89:e9–e12

Manke D, Börnert P, Nehrke K, Nagel E, Dössel O (2001) Accelerated coronary MRA by simultaneous acquisition of multiple 3D stacks. J Magn Reson Imaging 14:478–483

Manke D, Nehrke K, Börnert P, Rosch P, Dossel P (2002) Respiratory motion in coronary magnetic resonance angiography: a comparison of different motion models. J Magn Reson Imaging 15:661–671

Manning WJ, Li W, Boyle NG, Edelman RR (1993a) Fat-suppressed breath-hold magnetic resonance coronary angiography. Circulation 87:94–104

Manning WJ, Li W, Edelman RR (1993b) A preliminary report comparing magnetic resonance coronary angiography with conventional angiography. N Engl J Med 328:828–832

Manning WJ, Li W, Cohen SI, Johnson RG, Edelman RR (1995) Improved definition of anomalous LCA by magnetic resonance coronary angiography. Am Heart J 130:615–617

Marcus ML, Skorton DJ, Johnson MR et al (1988) Visual estimates of percent diameter coronary stenosis: a battered gold standard. J Am Coll Cardiol 11:882–885

Marcus JT, Smeenk HG, Kuijer JPA, van der Geest RJ, Heethaar RM, van Rossum AC (1999) Flow profiles in the left anterior descending and the RCA assessed by MR velocity quantification: effects of through-plane and in-plane motion of the heart. J Comput Assist Tomogr 4:567–576

Marks B, Mitchell DG, Simelaro JP (1997) Breath-holding in healthy and pulmonary-compromised populations: effect of hyperventilation and oxygen inspiration. J Magn Reson Imaging 7:595–597

McCarthy RM, Shea SM, Deshpande VS et al (2003) Coronary MR angiography: true FISP imaging improved by prolonging breath holds with preoxygenation in healthy volunteers. Radiology 227:283–288

McConnell MV, Ganz P, Selwyn AP, Li W, Edelman RR, Manning WJ (1995) Identification of anomalous coronary arteries and their anatomci course by magnetic resonance coronary angiography. Circulation 92:3158–3162

McConnell MV, Khasgiwala VC, Savord BJ et al (1997a) Prospective adaptive navigator correction for breath-hold MR coronary angiography. Magn Reson Med 37:148–152

McConnell MV, Khasgiwala VC, Savord BJ, Chen MH, Chuang ML, Edelman RR, Manning WJ (1997b) Comparison of respiratory suppression methods and navigator locations for MR coronary angiography. AJR Am J Roentgenol 168:1369–1375

McConnell MV, Stuber M, Manning WJ (2000) Clinical role of coronary magnetic resonance angiography in the diagnosis of anomalous coronary arteries. J Cardiovasc Magn Reson 2:217–224

Meyer CH, Pauly JM, Macovski A, Mishimura DG (1990) Simultaneous spatial and spectral selective excitation. Magn Reson Med 15:287–304

Miller S, Scheule AM, Hahn U et al (1999) MR angiography

and flow quantification of the internal mammary artery graft after minimally invasive direct coronary artery bypass. AJR Am J Roentgenol 172:1365–1369

Mohiaddin RH, Bogren HG, Lazim F et al (1996) Magnetic resonance coronary angiography in heart transplant recipients. Coron Art Dis 7:591–597

Möhlenkamp S, Hort W, Ge J, Erbel R (2002) Update on myocardial bridging. Circulation 106:2616–2622

Molinari G, Sardanelli F, Zandrino F et al (2000) Coronary aneurysms and stenosis detected with magnetic resonance coronary angiography in a patient with Kawasaki disease. Ital Heart J 1:368–371

Myers WO, Blackstone EH, Davis K, Foster ED, Kaiser GC (1999) CASS Registry long term surgical survival: Coronary Artery Surgery Study. J Am Coll Cardiol 33:488–498

Nagel E, Bornstedt A, Hug J, Schnackenburg B, Wellnhofer E, Fleck E (1999) Noninvasive determination of coronary blood flow velocity with magnetic resonance imaging: comparison of breath-hold and navigator techniques with intravascular ultrasound. Magn Reson Med 41:544–549

Nagel E, Thouet T, Klein C et al (2003) Noninvasive determination of coronary blood flow velocity with cardiovascular magnetic resonance in patients with stent deployment. Circulation 107:1738–1743

Naghavi M, Libby P, Falk E et al (2003a) From vulnerable plaque to vulnerable patient. A call for nex definitions and risk assessment strategies: part 1. Circulation 108:1664–1672

Naghavi M, Libby P, Falk E et al (2003b) From vulnerable plaque to vulnerable patient. A call for nex definitions and risk assessment strategies, part 1. Circulation 108:1772–1778

Nguyen TD, Nuval A, Mulukutla S, Wang Y (2003) Direct monitoring of coronary artery motion with cardiac fat navigator echoes. Magn Reson Med 50:235–241

Nieman K, Rensing BJ, van Geuns RJM et al (2002a) Noninvasive coronary angiography with multislice spiral computed tomography: impact of heart rate. Heart 88:470–474

Nieman K, Cademartiri F, Lemos PA, Raaijmakers R, Pattynama PMT, de Feyter PJ (2002b) Reliable noninvasive coronary angiography with fast submillimetre spiral computed tomography. Circulation 106:2051–2054

Nishimura DG, Macovski A, Pauly JM (1988) Considerations of magnetic resonance angiography by selective inversion recovery. Magn Reson Med 7:472–484

Nitatori T, Hanaoka H, Yoshino A et al (1995) Clinical application of magnetic resonance angiography for coronary arteries: correlation with conventional angiography and evaluation of imaging time. Nippon Acta Radiol 55:670–676

Omary RA, Green J, Finn JP, Li D (2002a) Catheter-directed gadolinium-enhanced MR angiography. Radiol Clin North Am 40:953–963

Omary RA, Henseler KP, Unal O et al (2002b) Validation of injection parameters for catheter-directed intraarterial gadolinium-enhanced MR angiography. Acad Radiol 9:172–185

Pannu HK, Flohr TG, Corl FM, Fishman EK (2003) Current concepts in multi-detector row CT evaluation of the coronary arteries: principles, techniques, and anatomy. RadioGraphics 23:S111–S125

Paulin S, von Schulthess GK, Fossel E, Krayenbuehl HP (1987) MR imaging of the aortic root and proximal coronary arteries. AJR Am J Roentgenol 148:665–670

Paschal CB, Haacke EM, Adler LP (1993) Three-dimensional MR imaging of the coronary arteries: preliminary clinical experience. J Magn Reson Imaging 3:491–501

Pelliccia A (2001) Congenital coronary artery anomalies in young patients. New perspectives for timely identification. J Am Coll Cardiol 37:598–600

Pennell DJ, Keegan J, Firmin DN, Gatehouse PD, Underwood SR, Longmore DB (1993) Magnetic resonance imaging of the coronary arteries: technique and preliminary results. Br Heart J 70:315–326

Pepine C, Holmes DR, Block PC et al (1996) ACC expert consens document. Coronary artery stents. J Am Coll Cardiol 28:782–794

Plein S, Ridgway JP, Jones TR, Bloomer TN, Sivananthan MU (2002) Coronary artery disease: assessment with a comprehensive MR imaging protocol – initial results. Radiology 225:300–307

Plein S, Bulugahapitiya S, Jones TR, Bainbridge GJ, Ridgway JP, Sivnananthan MU (2003a) Cardiac MR imaging with external respirator: synchronizing cardiac and respiratory motion – feasibility study. Radiology 227:877–882

Plein S, Jones TR, Ridgway JP, Sivananthan MU (2003b) Three-dimensional coronary MR angiography performed with subject-specific cardiac acquisition windows and motion-adapted respiratory gating. Am J Roentgenol AJR 180:505–512

Post JC, van Rossum AC, Bronzwaer JGF et al (1995) Magnetic resonance angiography of anomalous coronary arteries. A new gold standard for delineating the proximal course? Circulation 92:3163–3173

Post JC, van Rossum AC, Hofman MBM, Valk J, Visser CA (1996) Three-dimensional respiratory-gated MR angiography of coronary arteries: comparison with conventional contrast coronary angiography. AJR Am J Roentgenol 166:426–433

Post JC, van Rossum AC, Hofman MB, de Cock CC, Valk J, Visser CA (1997) Clinical utility of two-dimensional magnetic resonance angiography in detecting coronary artery disease. Eur Heart J 18:426–433

Prêtre R, Tamisier D, Bonhoeffer P et al (2001) Results of the arterial switch operation in neonates with transposed great arteries. Lancet 35:1826–1830

Prince MR (1994) Gadolinium-enhanced MR aortography. Radiology 191:155–164

Pruessmann KP, Weiger M, Boesiger P (2001) Sensitivity encoded cardiac MRI. J Cardiovasc Magn Reson 3:1–9

Quick H, Ladd M, Nanz D, Mikolajczyk K, Debatin J (1999) Vascular stents af RF antennas for intravascular MR guidance and imaging. Magn Reson Med 42:738–745

Quick H, Kuehl H, Kaiser G, Bosk S, Debatin JF, Ladd ME (2002) Inductively coupled stent antennas in MRI. Magn Reson Med 48:781–790

Reddy KS, Yusuf S (1998) Emerging epidemic of cardiovascular disease in developing countries. Circulation 97:596–601

Regenfus M, Ropers D, Achenbach S et al (2000) Noninvasive detection of coronary artery stenosis using breath-hold enhanced three-dimensional breath-hold magnetic resonance coronary angiography. J Am Coll Cardiol 36:44–50

Regenfus M, Ropers D, Achenbach S et al (2002) Comparison of contrast-enhanced breath-hold and free-breathing respiratory-gated imaging in three-dimensional magnetic resonance coronary angiography. Am J Cardiol 90:725–730

Regenfus M, Roper D, Achenbach S et al (2003) Diagnostic value of maximum intensity projections versus source images for assessment of contrast-enhanced tree-dimensional breath-hold magnetic resonance coronary angiography. Invest Radiol 38:200–206

Rubinstein RI, Askenase AD, Thickman D, Feldman MS, Agarwal JB, Helfant RH (1987) Magnetic resonance imaging to evaluate patency of aortocoronary bypass grafts. Circulation 76:786–791

Saito Y, Sakuma H, Shibata M et al (2001) Assessment of coronary flow velocity reserve using fast velocity-encoded cine MRI for noninvasive detection of restenosis after coronary stent implantation. J Cardiovasc Magn Reson 3:209–214

Sakuma H, Kawada N, Takeda K, Higgins CB (1999) MR measurment of coronary blood flow. J Magn Reson Imaging 10:728–733

Sandstede JJ, Pabst T, Beer M, Geis N, Kenn W, Neubauer S, Hahn D (1999) Three-dimensional MR coronary angiography using the navigator technique compared with conventional coronary angiography. AJR Am J Roentgenol 172:135–139

Sardanelli F, Molinari G, Zandrino F, Balbi M (2000) Three-dimensional, navigator-echo MR coronary angiography in detecting stenoses of the major epicardial vessels, with conventional coronary angiography as the standard of reference. Radiology 214:808–814

Sardanelli F, Zandrino F, Molinari G, Iozzelli A, Balbi M, Barsotti A (2002) MR evaluation of coronary stents with navigator echo and breath-hold cine gradient-echo techniques. Eur Radiol 12:193–200

Schär M, Kim WY, Stuber M et al (2002) The impact of spatial resolution and respiratory motion on magnetic resonance plaque characterization. J Cardiovasc Magn Reson 4:73–74

Schär M, Kim WY, Stuber M, Boesiger P, Manning WJ, Botnar RM (2003) The impact of spatial resolution and respiratory motion on MR imaging of atherosclerotic plaque. J Magn Reson Imaging 17:538–544

Scheidegger MB, Müller R, Boesiger P (1994) Magnetic resonance angiography: methods and its applications to the coronary arteries. Technol Health Care 2:255–265

Scheidegger MB, Stuber M, Boesiger P, Hess OM (1996) Coronary artery imaging by magnetic resonance. Herz 21:90–96

Schroeder AP, Houlind K, Pedersen AM, Thuesen L, Nielsen TT, Egeblad H (2000) Magnetic resonance imaging seems safe in patients with intracoronary stents. J Cardiovasc Magn Reson 2:43–49

Schwitter J, DeMarco T, Kneifel S et al (2000) Magnetic resonance-based assessment of global coronary flow and flow reserve and its relation to left ventricular functional parameters. A comparison with positron emission tomography. Circulation 101:2696–2702

Scott N, Pettigrew R (1994) Absence of movement of coronary stents after placement in a magnetic resonance imaging field. Am J Cardiol 73:900–901

Serruys PW, de Jaegere P, Kiemeneij F et al (1994) A comparison of balloon-expandable-stent implantation with balloon angioplasty in patients with coronary artery disease. N Engl J Med 331:489–495

Shea SM, Kroeker RM, Deshpande V et al (2001) Coronary artery imaging: 3D segmented κ-space data acquisition with multiple breath-holds and real-time slab following. J Magn Reson Imaging 13:301–307

Shea SM, Deshpande VS, Chung Y-C, Li D (2002) Three-dimensional true-FISP imaging of the coronary arteries: improved contrast with T2-preparation. J Magn Reson Imaging 15:597–602

Simonetti OP, Finn JP, White RD, Laub G, Henry DA (1996) "Black blood" T2-weighted inversion-recovery MR imaging of the heart. Radiology 199:49–57

Sinkus R, Börnert P (1999) Motion pattern adapted real-time respiratory gating. Magn Reson Med 41:148–155

Slavin GS, Riederer SJ, Ehman RL (1998) Two-dimensional multishot echo-planar coronary angiography. Magn Reson Med 40:883–889

Sohn S, Kim HS, Lee SW (200) Multidetector row computed tomography for follow-up of patients with coronary artery aneurysms due to Kawasaki disease. Pediatr Cardiol 25:35–39

Sommer T, Hofer U, Hackenbroch M et al (2002) Submillimeter 3D coronary MR angiography with real-time navigator correction in 107 patients with suspected coronary artery disease. Röfo Fortschr Röntgenstr 174:459–466

Spuentrup E, Stuber M, Botnar RM, Manning WJ (2001) The impact of navigator timing parameters and navigator spatial resolution on 3D coronary magnetic resonance angiography. J Magn Reson Imaging 14:311–318

Spuentrup E, Buecker A, Karassimos E, Günter RW, Stuber M (2002a) Navigator-gated and real-time motion corrected free-breathing MR imaging of myocardial late enhancement. Röfo Fortschr Röntgenstr 174:562–567

Spuentrup E, Manning WJ, Botnar RM, Kissinger KV, Stuber M (2002b) Impact of navigator timing on free-breathing submillimetre 3D coronary magnetic resonance angiography. Magn Reson Med 47:196–201

Spuentrup E, Bornert P, Botnar RM, Groen JP, Manning WJ, Stuber M (2002c) Navigator-gated free-breathing three-dimensional balanced fast field echo (TrueFISP) coronary magnetic resonance angiography. Invest Radiol 37:637–642

Spuentrup E, Katoh M, Stuber M, Botnar R, Schaeffter T, Buecker A, Gunther RW (2003) Coronary MR imaging using free-breathing 3D steady-state free precession with radial κ-space sampling. Röfo Fortschr Röntgenstr 175:1330–1334

Spuentrup E, Katoh M, Buecker A et al (2004) Free-breathing 3D steady-state free-precession coronary MR angiography using radial κ-space sampling: comparison to Cartesian κ-space sampling and Cartesian T2-prepared gradient-echo coronary MR angiography – a pilot study. Radiology

Stary HC, Blankenhorn DH, Chandler AB et al (1992) A definition of the intima of human arteries and of its atherosclerosis-prone regions: a report from the Committee on Vascular Lesions of the Council on Arteriosclerosis, American Heart Association. Special report. Circulation 85:391–405

Stary HC, Chandler AB, Dinsmore RE et al (1995) A definition of advanced types of atherosclerotic lesions and a histological classification of atherosclerosis. Circulation 92:1355–1374

Strohm O, Kivelitz D, Gross W et al (1999) Safety of implantable coronary stents during ^{1}H-magnetic resonance imaging at 1.0 and 1.5 T. J Cardiovasc Magn Reson 3:239–245

Strong JP, Malcolm GT, Oalmann MC et al (1997) The PDAY study: natural history, risk factors, and pathobiology: pathobiological determinants of atherosclerosis in youth. Ann NY Acad Sci 811:226–237

Stuber M, Botnar RM, Danias PG et al (1999a) Contrast agent-enhanced, free-breathing, three-dimensional coronary magnetic resonance angiography. J Magn Reson Imaging 10:790–799

Stuber M, Botnar RM, Danias PG et al (1999b) Double-oblique free-breathing high resolution three-dimensional coronary magnetic resonance angiography. J Am Coll Cardiol 34:524–531

Stuber M, Botnar RM, Danias PG, Kissinger KV, Manning WJ (1999c) Submillimeter three-dimensional coronary MR angiography with real-time navigator correction: comparison of navigator locations. Radiology 212:579–587

Stuber M, Botnar RM, Danias PG, Kissinger KV, Manning WJ (1999d) Breathhold three-dimensional coronary magnetic resonance angiography using real-time navigator technology. J Cardiovasc Magn Reson 1:233–238

Stuber M, Botnar RM, Spuentrup E, Kissinger KV, Manning WJ (2001a) Three-dimensional high-resolution fast spin-echo coronary magnetic resonance angiography. Magn Reson Med 45:206–211

Stuber M, Botnar RM, Kissinger KV, Manning WJ (2001b) Free-breathing black-blood coronary MR angiography: initials results. Radiology 219:278–283

Stuber M, Danias PG, Botnar RM, Sodickson DK, Kissinger KV, Manning WJ (2001c) Superiority of prone position in free-breathing 3D coronary MRA in patients with coronary disease. J Magn Reson Imaging 13:185–191

Stuber M, Börnert P, Spuentrup E, Botnar RM, Manning WJ (2002a) Selective three-dimensional visualization of the coronary arterial lumen using arterial spin tagging. Magn Reson Med 47:322–329

Stuber M, Botnar RM, Fischer SE et al (2002b) Preliminary report on in vivo coronary MRA at 3 Tesla in humans. Magn Reson Med 48:425–429

Tang C, Blatter DD, Parker DL (1993) Accuracy of phase-contrast flow measurements in the presence of partial-volume effects. J Magn Reson Imaging 3:377–385

Taupitz M, Schnorr J, Wagner S et al (2001) Coronary magnetic resonance angiography: experimental evaluation of the new rapid clearance blood pool contrast agent medium P 792. Magn Reson Med 46:932–938

Taupitz M, Schnorr J, Wagner S et al (2002) Coronary MR angiography: experimental results with a monomer-stabilized blood pool contrast medium. Radiology 222:120–126

Taylor AM, Jhooti P, Wiesmann F et al (1997) MR navigator-echo monitoring of temporal changes in diaphragm position: implications for MR coronary angiography. J Magn Reson Imaging 7:629–636

Taylor AM, Panting JR, Keegan J et al (1999) Safety and preliminary findings with the intravascular contrast agent NC100150 injection for MR coronary angiography. J Magn Reson Imaging 9:220–227

Taylor AM, Keegan J, Jhooti P, Gatehouse PD, Firmin DN, Pennell DJ (2000a) A comparison between segmented κ-space FLASH and interleaved spiral MR coronary angiography sequences. J Magn Reson Imaging 11:394–400

Taylor AM, Thorne SA, Rubens MB et al (2000b) Coronary artery imaging in grown up congenital heart disease. Complementary role of magnetic resonance and X-ray coronary angiography. Circulation 101:1670–1678

Taylor AM, Dymarkowski S, Haemaekers P et al Magnetic resonance coronary angiography and late-enhancement myocardial imaging in children with arterial switch operation for transposition of the great arteries. Radiology (in press)

Thedens DR, Irarrazaval P, Sachs TS, Meyer CH, Nishimura DG (1999) Fast magnetic resonance coronary angiography with a three-dimensional stack of spiral trajectory. Magn Reson Med 41:1170–1179

Van den Brink J, Watanabe Y, Kuhl CK et al (2003) Implications of SENSE MR in routine clinical practice. Eur J Radiol 46:3–27

Van Geuns RJM, de Bruin HG, Rensing BJWM Rensing et al (1999) Magnetic resonance imaging of the coronary arteries: clinical results from three dimensional evaluation of a respiratory gated technique. Heart 82:515–519

Van Geuns RJM, Wielopolski PA, de Bruin HG et al (2000) MR coronary angiography with breath-hold targeted volumes: preliminary clinical results. Radiology 217:270–277

Van Geuns RJM, Oudkerk M, Rensing BJVM et al (2002) Comparison of coronary imaging between magnetic resonance imaging and electron beam computed tomography. Am J Cardiol 90:58–63

Van Ooijen PMA, van Geuns RJM, Rensing BJWM, Bongaerts AHH, de Feyter PJ, Oudkerk (2003) Noninvasive coronary imaging using electron beam CT: surface rendering versus volume rendering. AJR Am J Roentgenol 180:223–226

Van Rossum AC, Galjee MA, Post JC, Visser CA (1997) A practical approach to MRI of coronary artery bypass graft patency and flow. Int J Cardiac Imaging 13:199–204

Vick GW III, Muthupillai R, Su JT, Kovalchin JP, Chung T (2003) Magnetic resonance angiography of coronary arteries and peripheral arteries in infants and young children with Kawasaki disease. J Am Coll Cardiol 495A

Vitiello R, McCrindle BW, Nykanen D et al (1998) Complications associated with pediatric cardiac catheterization. J Am Coll Cardiol 32:1433–1440

Vrachliotis TG, Bis KG, Aliabadi D, Shetty AN, Safian R, Simonetti O (1997) Contrast-enhanced breath-hold MR angiography for evaluating patency of coronary artery bypass graft. Am J Roentgenol 168:1073–1080

Walker F, Webb G (2001) Congenital coronary artery anomalies: the adult perspective. Cor Art Dis 12:599–604

Wang Y, Ehman RL (2000) Retrospective adaptive motion correction of navigator-gated 3D coronary MR angiography. J Magn Reson Imaging 11:208–214

Wang Y, Riederer SJ, Ehman RL (1995) Respiratory motion of the heart: kinematics and the implications for the spatial resolution of coronary MR imaging. Magn Reson Med 33:713–719

Wang Y, Rossman PJ, Grimm RC, Riederer SJ, Ehman RL (1996) Navigator-echo-based real-time respiratory gating and triggering for reduction of respiration effects in three-dimensional coronary MR angiography. Radiology 198:55–60

Wang Y, Vidan E, Bergman GW (1999) Cardiac motion of coronary arteries: variability in the rest period and implications for coronary MR angiography. Radiology 213:751–758

Wang Y, Winchester PA, Yu L et al (2000) Breath-hold three-dimensional contrast-enhance coronary MR angiography: motion-matched κ-space sampling for reducing cardiac motion effects. Radiology 215:600–607

Wang Y, Watts R, Mitchell IR et al (2001) Coronary MR angiography: selection of acquisition window of minimal cardiac motion with electrocardiography-triggered navigator cardiac motion prescanning – initial results. Radiology 218:580–585

Weber C, Steiner P, Sinkus R, Dill T, Börnert P, Adam G (2002) Correlation of 3D MR coronary angiography with selective coronary angiography: feasibility of the motion-adapted gating technique. Eur Rad 122:718–726

Weber O, Martin AJ, Higgins CB (2003) Whole-heart steady-state free precession coronary artery magnetic resonance angiography. Magn Reson Med 50:1223–1228

Weiger M, Börnert P, Proksa R, Schaffter T, Haase A (1997) Motion-adapted gating based on κ-space weighting for reduction of respiratory motion artefacts. Magn Reson Med 38:322–333

Weissler AM, Harris WS, Schoenfeld CD (1968) Systolic time intervals in heart failure in man. Circulation 37:149–159

White CW, Wright CB, Doty DB et al (1984) Does visual interpretation of the coronary angiogram predict the physiological importance of a coronary stenosis? N Engl J Med 310:819–824

White CW (1993) Clinical applications of Doppler coronary flow reserve measurements. Am J Cardiol 71:10D–16D

White RD, Caputo GR, Mark AS, Modin GW, Higgins CB (1987) Coronary artery bypass graft patency: noninvasive evaluation with MR imaging. Radiology 164:681–686

White CS, Laskey WK, Stafford JL, NessAiver M (1999) Coronary MRA: use in assessing anomalies of coronary artery origin. J Comput Assist Tomogr 23:203–207

Wielopolski PA, Manning WJ, Edelman RE (1995) Single breath-hold volumetric imaging of the heart using magnetization-prepared 3-dimensional segmented echo-planar imaging. J Magn Res Imaging 5:403–409

Wielopolski PA, van Geuns RJM, de Feyter PJ, Oudkerk M (1998) Breath-hold coronary MR angiography with volume targeted imaging. Radiology 209:209–219

Wielopolski PA, van Geuns RJM, de Feyter PJ, Oudkerk M (2000) Coronary Arteries. Review article. Eur Radiol 10:12–35

Wintersperger BJ, Engelmann MG, von Smekal A et al (1998) Patency of coronary bypass grafts: assessment with breath-hold contrast-enhanced MR angiography – value of a non-electrocardiographically triggered technique. Radiology 208:345–351

Wolff SD, Balaban RS (1989) Magnetization transfer contrast (MTC) and tissue water proton relaxation in vivo. Magn Reson Med 10:135–144

Wolff SD, Eng J, Balaban RS (1991) Magnetization transfer contrast: method for improving contrast in gradient-recalled images. Radiology 179:133–137

Worthley SG, Helft G, Valentin F et al (2000a) Noninvasive in vivo magnetic resonance imaging of experimental coronary artery lesions in a porcine model. Circulation 101:2956–2961

Worthley SG, Helft G, Fuster F et al (2000b) High resolution ex vivo magnetic resonance imaging of in situ coronary and aortic atherosclerotic plaque in a porcine model. Atherosclerosis 150:321–329

Worthley SG, Helft G, Fayad ZA et al (2001) Cardiac gated breath-hold black blood MRI of the coronary artery wall: an in vivo and ex vivo comparison. Int J Cardiovasc Imaging 17:195–201

Worthley SG, Helft G, Fuster V et al (2003) A novel non-obstructive intravascular MRI coil. In vivo imaging of experimental atherosclerosis. Arterioscler Vasc Biol 23:346–350

Yang, GZ, Gatehouse PD, Keegan J, Mohiaddin RH, Firmin DN (1998) Three-dimensional coronary MR angiography using zonal echo planar imaging. Magn Reson Med 39:833–842

Yoshino H, Nitatori T, Kachi E et al (1997) Directed proximal magnetic resonance coronary angiography compared with conventional contrast coronary angiography. Am J Cardiol 80:514–518

Zaman AG, Helft G, Worthley SG, Badimon JJ (2000) The role of plaque rupture and thrombosis in coronary artery disease. Atherosclerosis 149:251–266

Zheng J, Li D, Cavagna FM et al (2001) Contrast-enhanced coronary MR angiography: relationship between coronary artery delineation and blood T1. J Magn Reson Imaging 14:348–354

15 Congenital Heart Disease

Vivek Muthurangu, Reza Razavi, Jan Bogaert, and Andrew M. Taylor

CONTENTS

V. Muthurangu, BSc, MBChB, MRCPCH
R. Razavi, MBBS, MRCP, MRCPCH
Division of Imaging Science, King's College London, Guy's
Hospital Campus, London Bridge, London SE1 9RT, UK
J. Bogaert, MD, PhD
Department of Radiology, Gasthuisberg University Hospital,
Catholic University of Leuven, Herestraat 49, 3000 Leuven,
Belgium
A. M. Taylor, MD, MRCP, FRCR
Cardiothoracic Unit, Institute of Child Health and Great
Ormond Street Hospital for Children, London WC1N 3JH,
UK

15.1 Introduction

Congenital heart disease has an incidence of 6–8 per 1000 in neonates (Hoffman and Kaplan 2002). Improvements in diagnosis and treatment have led to more patients surviving to adulthood, increasing prevalence in the general population. Management of these patients relies heavily on imaging, with echocardiography remaining the most common tool for diagnosis and follow-up. Echocardiography combines the benefit of being able to accurately assess anatomy and function with portability and ease of use. However, echocardiography is limited by acoustic windows, provides poor images of the distal vasculature, and is user-dependent. For more detailed anatomical and functional assessment, X-ray-guided cardiac catheterization remains important. Cardiac catheterization is not without risks due to the invasive nature of the procedure and the exposure to X-radiation. In addition, X-ray fluoroscopy provides a projection image and has only limited three-dimensional (3D) capabilities. Cardiovascular magnetic resonance imaging (MRI) is now an important tool for diagnosis and follow-up of adolescent and adult patients (grown-up congenital heart disease, GUCH) with congenital heart disease (Higgins et al. 1984; Task force of the European Society of Cardiology 1998; British Cardiac Society Working Party 2002; Deanfield et al. 2003), and has become more widely used in neonates and younger children (Razavi and Bakeret al. 1999; Razavi et al. 2003b). Cardiovascular MR provides the capability of imaging in any plane irrespective of body habitus. In addition, the development of 3D MR techniques opens up the possibility of improved visualization of cardiac anatomy without the requirement for expert planning. In this chapter, the use of MR in the diagnosis of congenital heart disease is discussed with reference to specific congenital heart defects.

15.2
Techniques

15.2.1
Spin-Echo Imaging

The earliest MR images of congenital heart disease were acquired using spin-echo "black-blood" sequences (HIGGINS et al. 1984; FLETCHER et al. 1984; JACOBSTEIN et al. 1984). Although other sequences are increasingly being used in cardiovascular MR, the spin-echo black-blood sequence is still important, particularly for accurate delineation of great-vessel anatomy. As the name suggests, blood appears black, due to the moving spins in the blood producing a signal void. This allows delineation between the blood pool and either vessel wall or myocardium. The use of multiple signal averages allows high through- and in-plane spatial resolution, and makes it particularly useful for anatomical delineation. Most spin-echo sequences now acquire multiple-echo trains for each set of radiofrequency pulses (e.g., turbo spin-echo), enabling images to be acquired in a single breath-hold and not over several minutes (HIGGINS et al. 1984) (Fig. 15.1). A further advantage is that phase artifacts related to respiratory motion are also reduced.

The main benefit of spin-echo black blood sequences is that contrast improves when the blood flow velocity is high. Thus, it is a particularly useful technique when imaging vascular obstructions and valvular stenoses because, unlike gradient-echo and angiographic sequences, it performs better in these situations. Black-blood sequences have been used to successfully image valvular stenosis (GREENBERG et al. 1997), conduit stenosis (MARTINEZ et al. 1992), and baffle obstruction (SAMPSON et al. 1994). It should be noted, however, that signal loss due to conduit and baffle calcification can lead to underestimation of stenosis (MARTINEZ et al. 1992).

Black-blood images are also useful when imaging vessels after metallic stent insertion. The majority of stents are safe to image (SHELLOCK and SHELLOCK 1999) but cause marked artifacts on gradient-echo sequences (cine imaging and MR angiography), secondary to T2* field inhomogeneity. Due to the refocusing pulse, spin-echo sequences are not as susceptible to these phenomena, and imaging of the vessel within the stent can be achieved (see Fig. 16.22).

15.2.2
Gradient-Echo Imaging

Gradient-echo imaging is becoming increasingly important in cardiovascular MR. Gradient-echo sequences have shorter repeat times and therefore have higher temporal resolution. Fast acquisition enables multiple phases of the cardiac cycle to be acquired, which can be reconstructed into a cine MR image representing one full cardiac cycle. Gradient-echo imaging has revolutionized cardiovascular MR as it allows dynamic imaging of cardiac anatomy. Recently, balanced steady-state free precession (b-SSFP) sequences have become available, giving improved blood-pool homogeneity throughout the cardiac cycle and faster acquisition times. Gradient-

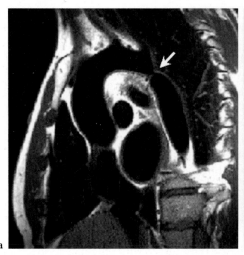
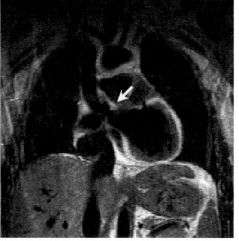

a   b

Fig. 15.1a,b. "Black-blood" turbo-spin-echo images of: **a** an aortic coarctation membrane (*arrow*), and **b** a narrowed superior vena caval pathway in a patient following a Senning operation for transposition of the great arteries (*arrow*)

echo sequences have various roles in cardiac imaging, as set out below.

15.2.2.1
Two-dimensional Balanced-SSFP Imaging

Two-dimensional b-SSFP imaging has become widely used in cardiac imaging. Single-slice imaging allows qualitative assessment of all cardiac chambers (the 4-chamber view), valvular dysfunction, and dynamic vascular anatomy. It proves particularly useful when planning interventions, because accurate measurements, i.e., of vessel diameter, can be made over the whole cardiac cycle (RAZAVI et al. 2004). Unlike older gradient-echo cine sequences, b-SSFP is partially flow compensated and thus the blood-pool signal is homogenous (Fig. 15.2). However, high-velocity blood flow will lead to signal loss, allowing qualitative analysis of blood flow jets.

Multi-slice, two-dimensional (2D) gradient-echo imaging represents the best available in vivo test for ventricular volumetry (BELLENGER et al. 2002; GROTHUES et al. 2002), as it is not reliant on complex geometric models. Currently ventricular function is assessed using b-SSFP sequences, which have the benefit of good blood-pool/myocardial contrast and relatively fast acquisition times. Although b-SSFP sequences allow high spatiotemporal resolution imaging of the ventricles, they do require multiple breath holds. This may not be tolerated in patients, particularly children, with cardiac disease. In such cases, the use of respiratory navigators may obviate the need for breath holds, although acquisition times increase significantly. In children less than 8 years of age, general anesthesia can be used to guarantee no patient movement and enable multiple scans.

Recently, real-time b-SSFP sequences have been developed that allow imaging of the whole ventricle in a single breath-hold (LEE et al. 2002; BARKHAUSEN et al. 2002). However, this is at the expense of spatiotemporal resolution, which has an effect on accuracy (LEE et al. 2002), although in children improved compliance with scanning compensates for the reduced accuracy.

15.2.2.2
Three-dimensional Balanced-SSFP Imaging

The development of 3D cardiac MR acquisition techniques opens up the possibility of improved visualization of cardiac anatomy without the requirement for expert planning. The benefit of axial multi-slice gradient-echo acquisition in delineating complex anatomy without expert planning has been shown in the assessment of congenital heart disease (MIQUEL et al. 2003). This technique enables both slice-by-slice examination and reconstruction and visualization of the cardiac volume. Recently 3D b-SSFP techniques have been developed that allow fast imaging of the entire cardiac volume (RAZAVI et al. 2003b). The improved contrast and resolution of this b-SSFP technique allows simpler volume rendering based on thresholding techniques. In addition, reconstructed voxel size is almost isotropic, allowing accurate multi-planar reformatting (RAZAVI et al. 2003b). This is particularly

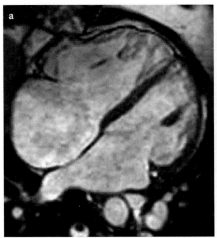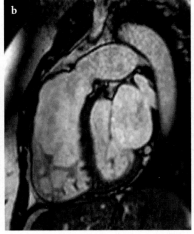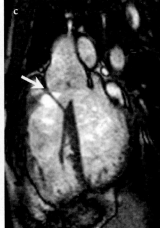

Fig. 15.2a-c. Balanced steady-state free precession (b-SSFP) images. **a** Four-chamber image showing right ventricular and right atrial dilation. **b** Oblique sagittal view of right ventricular outflow tract in a patient with mixed pulmonary valve disease. **c** Balanced-SSFP image of the left ventricular outflow tract in a patient with repaired tetralogy of Fallot; note the ventricular septal defect patch (*arrow*)

useful in the assessment of complex congenital heart disease as it allows offline reconstruction of the often-difficult anatomy (see Fig. 17.7). This technique can also allow assessment of global and regional wall motion of the heart, as volume data is acquired in up to 10 phases of the cardiac cycle.

15.2.2.3
Velocity-Encoded Phase-Contrast MR

Quantification of blood flow and velocity is an important tool in the management of congenital heart disease. Quantification of pulmonary to systemic blood flow ratio (Qp:Qs), valvular regurgitation fraction or vascular stenosis is used to assess disease progression, suitability for surgery, and timing of surgery. Traditionally, blood flow has been invasively quantified using indicator dilution methods (i.e., invasive oximetry or thermodilution) (MUTHURANGU et al. 2004). Invasive catheterization is associated with known morbidity and mortality and thus noninvasive methods of flow quantification are appealing. In addition, invasive methods are less reliable in patients with large intracardiac shunts or valvular regurgitation. Velocity-encoded phase-contrast magnetic resonance (MR) enables noninvasive quantification of blood flow in major vessels. Cardiac output and the pulmonary-to-systemic flow ratio (Qp:Qs) measured using this technique have been shown to be accurate when compared with invasive oximetry (BEERBAUM et al. 2001). In addition, phase-contrast MR has been validated in numerous phantom experiments (BEERBAUM et al. 2001; HUNDLEY et al. 1995) (Fig. 15.3).

Velocity-encoded phase-contrast MR also allows an estimation of pressure gradients across stenoses and has been shown to compare well with Doppler echocardiography and catheter data (HOLMQVIST et al. 2001). This technique is particularly useful in the assessment of the functional significance of an obstruction. The quantification of valvular regurgitation is also an important use of this technique (REBERGEN et al. 1993; KANG et al. 2003). This technique has been internally validated against ventricular volumetry (REBERGEN et al. 1993) and is superior to echocardiography in its ability to quantify regurgitant volume.

15.2.2.4
Gadolinium Contrast-Enhanced MR Angiography

Gadolinium-enhanced MR angiography (Gd-MRA) relies on the T1-shortening effect of dilute gado-

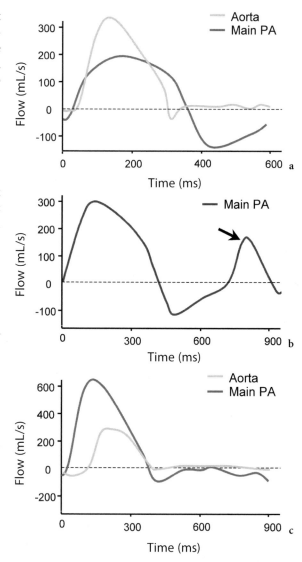

Fig. 15.3a-c. Plots of instantaneous flow (measured by velocity-encoded phase-contrast MR) as a function of time, – **a** pulmonary regurgitation, **b** restrictive right ventricular physiology, note forward flow in diastole (*arrow*), **c** left-to-right shunting, note greater pulmonary blood flow

linium and it has been shown to be useful in delineating thoracic vascular anatomy. More recently, improved gadolinium imaging allows volume scans to be obtained within a breath hold, reducing respiratory artifact. Gd-MRA is also useful in identifying stenotic vessels and has been shown to compare well with X-ray angiography and surgical findings (TAYLOR et al. 2004a). Care should be taken when measuring dimensions from 3D MRA, as the images are not ECG-gated and are thus an average of the dimensions throughout the cardiac cycle.

The major drawback of Gd-MRA, usually performed without cardiac synchronization, is image blurring due to cardiac motion (Razavi et al. 2003b). This affects the ability of this technique to visualize intracardiac anatomy and, to a lesser extent, large vessels such as the proximal pulmonary artery (PA) and aorta. In addition, in the presence of fast-moving blood, signal dropout occurs in Gd-MRA images, which can lead to overestimation of stenoses.

15.3
Sequential Segmental Analysis

The nomenclature of complex congenital heart disease is based on segmental analysis. This requires description of atrial situs, atrioventricular connections, and ventriculoarterial connections, and other associated lesions (Tynan et al. 1979). Transthoracic and transesophageal echocardiography is of proven benefit when establishing cardiac diagnosis based on segmental analysis (Rigby and Redington 1989). However, in some cases invasive cardiac catheterization is required to fully establish a diagnosis. Cardiovascular MR represents a noninvasive method of establishing a cardiac diagnosis when there is uncertainty in the echocardiographic diagnosis.

15.3.1
Step 1 – Atrial Situs

In the normal heart, the morphological right atrium is located to the right of the morphological left atrium (situs solitus). Abnormalities in the atrial situs are often associated with major cardiac malformations and abnormal abdominal and thoracic anatomy. In situs solitus, the inferior vena cava (IVC) is to the right of the abdominal aorta, with a right-sided liver and left-sided spleen. In addition, the right-sided bronchus is shorter than the left-sided bronchus. In situs inversus, the mirror image of the normal anatomy is present and is usually easily demonstrated with echocardiography. In situs ambiguous, atrial situs is uncertain. The most common lesions are right or left isomerism. In isomeric lesions, there are often endocardial cushion defects with varying degrees of atrioventricular septal defect (AVSD).

The atrial appendages are the best method of determining atrial configuration. The right atrial appendage is triangular with a wide base, whilst the left atrial appendage is a tubular structure. The presence of the terminal crest and pectinate muscle in the appendage are more specific internal characteristics of the right atrium and its appendage. Right isomerism is usually associated with bilateral right bronchi and right atrial appendages, asplenia, and a midline liver. Left isomerism is usually associated with bilateral left bronchi and left atrial appendages, polysplenia, and IVC interruption. All of these abnormalities can be determined with MR, particularly 3D b-SSFP techniques (Razavi et al. 2003b). Both right- and left-sided isomerism are associated with gut malrotation.

15.3.2
Step 2 – Ventricular Morphology

Determination of ventricular morphology allows analysis of atrioventricular and ventriculoarterial concordance. Irrespective of atrioventricular concordance, the atrioventricular valve (AV valve) is concordant with the ventricle, i.e., the tricuspid valve connects to the right ventricle, and the mitral valve connects to the left ventricle. The septal insertion of the tricuspid valve is more apical than that of the mitral valve and allows determination of the ventricular morphology. The muscular structure of the ventricles also differs, the right ventricle (RV) being more trabeculated than the left ventricle (LV), with a muscular infundibulum and mid-ventricular "moderator band." The size and shape of the ventricles, although different in normal subjects, is not a good indicator of ventricular origin as it is dependent on load effects.

15.3.3
Step 3 – Ventriculoarterial Connection

Description of ventriculoarterial connections represents the final element of sequential segmental analysis. The aorta and pulmonary arteries are defined by their typical branching patterns. 3D b-SSFP and Gd-MRA techniques are particularly useful in determining the arrangement of the great vessels and the connections with their respective ventricles.

15.3.4
Step 4 – Identification of Other Abnormalities

Other abnormalities to be considered include: abnormal venous connections, atrial septal defects

(ASD), ventricular septal defects (VSD), AVSD, and valve abnormalities.

In general, in congenital heart disease, most abnormalities are single lesions that are easily described. However, almost any combination of abnormalities and connections can occur, and, using the sequential segmental analysis method, the description of all conceivable combinations and diagnoses is possible.

The above is not a comprehensive description of the sequential segmental analysis algorithm for congenital heart disease, and a more complete explanation can be found in Professor Anderson and colleagues' book (ANDERSON 2001).

15.4
Acyanotic Heart Disease

15.4.1
Atrial Septal Defect

Atrial septal defects are the most common congenital heart defects detected in adults, with an incidence of 941 per million live births (HOFFMAN and KAPLAN 2002). Irrespective of their type and location, they cause left-to-right shunting at the atrial level. This leads to atrial dilation, predisposing to tachyarrhythmias, and biventricular volume overload. The presence of an ASD is also an independent risk factor for thromboembolic stroke. This is due to the ability of thromboemboli, originating either in the right atrium or venous vasculature, to pass through the ASD into the systemic circulation (MOHR and HOMMA 2003).

Atrial septal defects are an anatomically and developmentally heterogeneous group of lesions. The exact nature of the ASD has an effect on the natural history and management of this disease. Ostium secundum defects make up 80% of ASDs and are located in the fossa ovalis. These defects are due to failure of the septum secundum to close the ostium secundum. The ostium primum defect, although previously thought of as an ASD, is actually a partial AVSD, usually with some degree of AV valve abnormality. Finally the sinus venosus defect is found at the junction of either one of the caval veins and the right atrium. This type of ASD is rare and is often associated with partial anomalous pulmonary venous drainage.

Management for ASDs has changed in recent years, particularly with the increasing use of trans-

catheter ASD closure devices. Previously surgical closure was only considered when a large left-to-right shunt led to RV overload, atrial dilation, and symptoms. However, with the advent of transcatheter techniques, management has become more aggressive (FISCHER et al. 1999, 2003). Transcatheter techniques are only viable in patients with small- to medium-sized ostium secundum defects (FISCHER et al. 2003), and ASD closure is often done prior to the developments of cardiac failure or atrial dilation. Deficiency of the anterior or posteroinferior rim of the defect precludes transcatheter closure. Patients with large ostium secundum defects and sinus venosus lesions also require operative repair. Timing of surgery depends on the hemodynamic status of the patient. Thus, evaluation of ASDs requires definition of type and location of the defect, quantification of the shunt, detection of any intra-atrial thrombus, assessment of RV function, and visualization of the pulmonary venous anatomy. Furthermore, in patients with ostium secundum defects, special attention must be given to delineating the anatomy of the septal defect rim as this is important in planning invasive management.

Transthoracic echocardiography has a limited ability to visualize small ostium secundum and sinus venosus defects. In addition, detection of pulmonary venous abnormalities is difficult with the transthoracic approach. Transesophageal echocardiography has become the main imaging technique used to assess ASDs (HAUSMANN et al. 1992a, 1992b; GNANAPRAGASAM et al. 1991), and can be used to accurately assess ASD anatomy. However, it cannot be used to quantify the shunt ($Qp:Q_s$) accurately, and it can be difficult to delineate pulmonary venous anatomy. Cardiovascular MR has a significant role to play in the diagnosis and preinterventional assessment of ASDs (Fig. 15.4). Two-dimensional spin-echo black-blood sequences and gradient-echo sequences can be used to accurately define ASD anatomy (TAYLOR et al. 1999; LANGE et al. 1997; MIQUEL et al. 2003) and the results compare well with operative findings (LANGE et al. 1997). Multi-slice 2D gradient-echo techniques can be used to assess the dynamic 3D anatomy of the defect. Multi-slice techniques allow multi-planar reformatting of the data to produce image planes that are useful in planning interventional procedures (MIQUEL et al. 2003). However, multi-slice techniques suffer from poor through-plane resolution, which has an effect on the quality of the multi-plane reformatted image (RAZAVI et al. 2003b). Newer 3D b-SSFP techniques with isotropic resolution allow accurate multi-plane

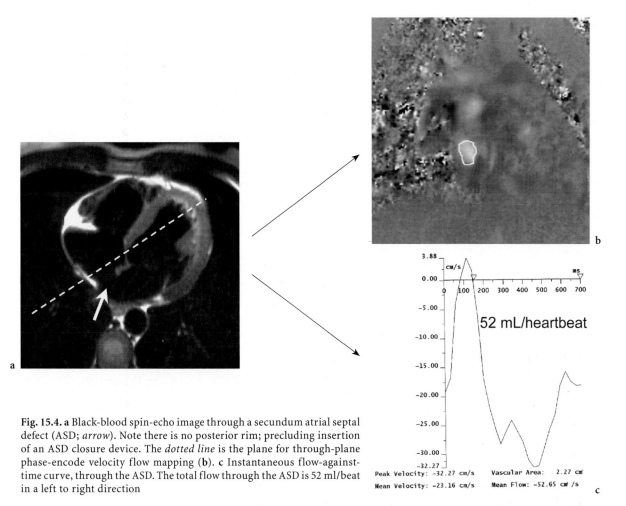

Fig. 15.4. a Black-blood spin-echo image through a secundum atrial septal defect (ASD; *arrow*). Note there is no posterior rim; precluding insertion of an ASD closure device. The *dotted line* is the plane for through-plane phase-encode velocity flow mapping (**b**). **c** Instantaneous flow-against-time curve, through the ASD. The total flow through the ASD is 52 ml/beat in a left to right direction

reformatted images to be produced with no loss of resolution and 3D rendering of the atrial anatomy (RAZAVI et al. 2003b). These techniques are particularly useful in assessment of the anatomy of ASD. Transcatheter ASD closure is dependent on the size of the defect, and measurements made using gradient-echo techniques compare well with both operative and transthoracic echocardiography (TTE) findings (BEERBAUM et al. 2003). It has been shown that MR findings are more powerful predictors of successful catheter closure than TTE or transesophageal-echocardiographic findings (DURONGPISITKUL et al. 2004).

Sinus venosus defects are often associated with pulmonary venous abnormalities. Gd-MRA is a sensitive method for detecting pulmonary venous abnormalities (PUVANESWARY et al. 2003) and can be useful prior to surgical intervention for sinus venosus defects (Fig. 15.5). Hemodynamic assessment is also an important part of the evaluation of ASDs. Invasive catheterization has previously been used to

accurately quantify left-to-right shunts (BEERBAUM et al. 2001). Quantification of left-to-right shunts using velocity-encoded phase-contrast MR compares well with invasive catheterization results (BEERBAUM et al. 2001); it has the benefit of being noninvasive and does not require exposure to ionizing radiation. Furthermore, there is some evidence that in certain situations phase-contrast MR is more accurate than invasive catheterization (MUTHURANGU et al. 2004). Ventricular overload can also be accurately assessed using multi-slice SSFP short-axis imaging (BELLENGER et al. 2002; FOGEL and RYCHIKet al. 1998) and can give important information regarding the timing of invasive intervention.

15.4.2
Atrioventricular Septal Defect

Atrioventricular septal defects are caused by abnormalities of the endocardial cushion and can

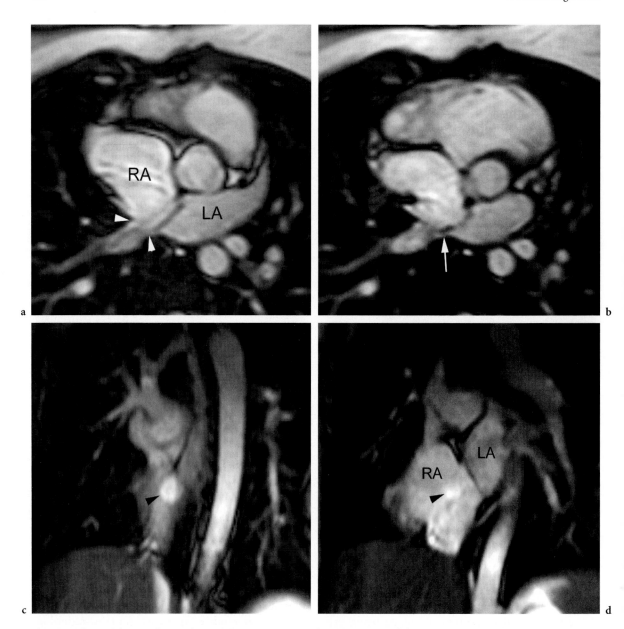

Fig. 15.5a-d. Partial anomalous pulmonary venous return with sinus venosus defect. **a, b** Horizontal long-axis b-SSFP image at two different time points during the cardiac cycle. **c, d** Short-axis b-SSFP image through the base of the atria. The anomalous connection of the right lower pulmonary artery to the right atrium as well as the relation of the atrial septum to the pulmonary vein is clearly visible (**a, b**). Although most of the venous blood from the right lower lobe drains into the right atrium, causing a right heart overload, probably a small amount of blood still goes to the left atrium (*arrow*) (**b**). On the short-axis, the anomalous entrance of the right lower pulmonary vein to the right of the atrial septum is clearly seen (*arrowhead*). *LA* left atrium, *RA* right atrium

be categorized into partial, with a defect of the atrial septum alone (previously described as "primum ASDs"), or complete, with defects of both the atrial and the ventricular septums (Fig. 15.6a). In all AVSDs there are abnormalities of the AV valves, which no longer maintain the form of the tricuspid and mitral valves, and are referred to as the right and left AV valves, respectively. There are typically five valve leaflets: Superior bridging, right anterosuperior, right mural, inferior bridging, and left mural leaflets. AVSDs can further be divided into balanced (relatively equal sized AV valves and ventricles) or unbalanced, when inflow through the AV valves is predominantly into one of the ventricles.

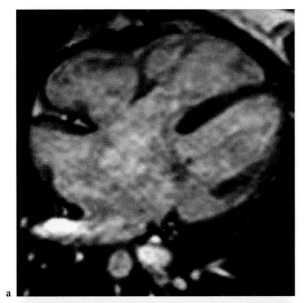

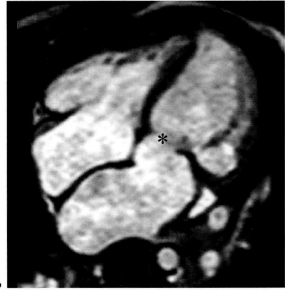

Fig. 15.6. a Balanced-SSFP four-chamber view of a complete AVSD. **b** Balanced-SSFP four-chamber view of repaired, complete AVSD. There is mild left AV valve stenosis (*asterisk*)

Atrioventricular septal defects are relatively complex lesions and, although they are listed as an acyanotic condition, AVSDs are associated with other complex congenital heart anomalies (e.g., isomerism and double-outlet right ventricle). There is also a high incidence of AVSDs in patients with Down syndrome (trisomy 21).

Surgical intervention with closure of the septal defects and repair of the AV valves is possible (Fig. 15.6b), though some patients with unbalanced AVSDs may be better served with surgical treatment

along the single-ventricle Fontan operative pathway (see Sect. 15.5.6)

Preoperative assessment of AVSDs with MR is limited, though MR can sometimes be useful for defining ventricular size to determine whether single or biventricular strategies of surgical treatment are possible.

15.4.3
Ventricular Septal Defect

VSDs are the most common congenital heart lesions, with an incidence of 3,570 per million live births (HOFFMAN and KAPLAN 2002). VSDs are a heterogeneous group of lesions that have a common physiological result of shunting at the ventricular level. The hemodynamic effect of VSDs is dependent on the shunt volume and can vary from insignificant to left-sided heart failure and pulmonary vascular disease. It is this hemodynamic effect that controls the type and timing of treatment. Invasive catheterization has previously been used to accurately quantify left-to-right shunts (BEERBAUM et al. 2001). Quantification of left-to-right shunts using velocity-encoded phase-contrast MR compares well with invasive catheterization results (BEERBAUM et al. 2001) and has the benefit of being noninvasive. Invasive catheterization is also used to quantify pulmonary vascular resistance to exclude pulmonary hypertensive disease prior to defect closure (BERGER 2000). There is some evidence that in certain situations combining phase-contrast MR and invasive pressure measurements is more accurate than traditional methods that rely on the Fick principle (MUTHURANGU et al. 2004). Cardiovascular MR can therefore play an important role in the hemodynamic assessment of VSDs.

The ventricular septum is a complex, helical 3D structure (ACAR et al. 2002). It is commonly divided into membranous, muscular, and apical portions (Fig. 15.7). The location of the VSD controls the natural history of the lesion and the optimum therapy. Perimembranous lesions make up 80% of all VSDs and are characterized by the relationship with ventricular inlet or outlet. The majority of perimembranous VSDs will close spontaneously. Large perimembranous VSDs are unlikely to close and lead to the development of pulmonary vascular disease. In these patients, the VSD must be closed. Operative closure with septal augmentation is the accepted treatment for significant perimembranous VSDs and is associated with low mortality and resid-

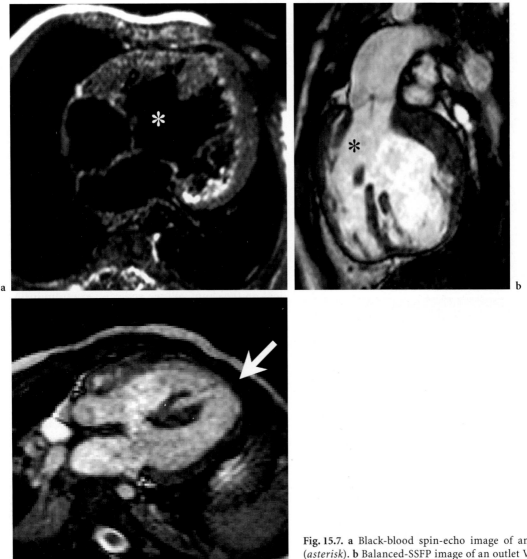

Fig. 15.7. a Black-blood spin-echo image of an inlet VSD (*asterisk*). **b** Balanced-SSFP image of an outlet VSD with an overriding aorta. **c** Balanced-SSFP image of a muscular apical VSD (*arrow*) and an inlet VSD

ual shunting (THANOPOULOS et al. 2003a). However, transcatheter techniques are becoming increasingly relied on due to their reduced postoperative morbidity (THANOPOULOS et al. 2003a). Transcatheter perimembranous VSD closure is not indicated in patients with multiple defects, defects larger than 12 mm, or defects less than 5 mm away from the aortic or mitral valve (THANOPOULOS et al. 2003b; ACAR et al. 2002). TTE is used to assess suitability for operative or transcatheter closure (PUCHALSKI et al. 2002; ACAR et al. 2002); however, TTE is associated with interoperator variability and difficulties in assessing the 3D structure (ACAR et al. 2002). Cardiovascular MR can provide accurate 2D

and 3D images of the defect. Multi-slice 2D gradient-echo techniques can be used to assess the dynamic 3D anatomy of the defect. In addition, multi-slice techniques allow multi-planar reformatting of the data to produce image planes that are useful in planning interventional procedures (MIQUEL et al. 2003). However, multi-slice techniques suffer from poor through-plane resolution, which has an effect on the use of the multi-plane reformatted image (RAZAVI et al. 2003b). Newer, 3D b-SSFP techniques with isotropic resolution allow accurate multi-plane reformatted images to be produced with no loss of resolution and 3D rendering of the ventricular anatomy (RAZAVI et al. 2003b). These techniques are particularly useful in assessment of the anatomy of a VSD. Furthermore, the relationship of the VSD and valvular structures can be accurately demonstrated, which is important when deciding on transcatheter closure.

Between 5% and 20% of VSDs occur in the muscular septum. Muscular VSDs are an extremely heterogeneous group of lesions that can be difficult to close surgically (THOMPSON et al. 2000). Transcatheter techniques have been used in the closure of muscular VSDs with some success (THOMPSON et al. 2000; CHESSA et al. 2002; CHAUDHARI et al. 2001). Optimum treatment (either operative or transcatheter) depends on accurate demonstration of the VSD anatomy (SIVAKUMAR et al. 2003). Muscular defects often have complex 3D structure with multiple defects (Swiss cheese appearance), which can be difficult to assess with TTE. As explained above, cardiovascular MR can give accurate representations of 3D anatomy and this information may be particularly useful when planning interventions.

The management of multiple VSDs can be difficult, as operative and transcatheter closure can leave residual defects (SEDDIO et al. 1999). In such situations palliation with PA banding is indicated. Assessment of PA band adequacy relies on demonstration of a significant pressure gradient across the band using TTE. Gradient-echo cine MR has been used to assess band adequacy (SIMPSON et al. 1993) and has been shown to compare well with surgical and catheter findings. Furthermore, accurate assessment of the Qp:Qs ratio can be obtained which represents the best way to assess band adequacy.

Approximately 50% of patients with a VSD have an associated cardiac abnormality. Coarctation of the aorta and aortic stenosis are particularly important and are associated with posterior malalignment of the VSD. Cardiovascular MR is a useful imaging modality in the assessment of valvular stenosis and coarctation, and these subjects are dealt with in more detail in the chapters on valvular heart disease (see Chap. 13) and imaging of great vessels (see Chap. 16), respectively.

15.4.3
Congenital Aortic Supravalvular Stenosis

Congenital supravalvular aortic stenosis is a rare congenital heart defect that is often associated with Williams syndrome (WILLIAMS et al. 1961). The stenosis is due to thickening of the proximal ascending aortic wall and three types have been described: an hourglass type, a membranous type, and a diffuse type. Over time there is progression of the supravalvular stenosis, possibly due to failure of growth of the sinotubular junction (KIM et al. 1999). This progression seems to be worse in patients with an initial gradient across the stenosis of more than 20 mmHg (WESSEL et al. 1994). In 1966, Rastelli described the first successful repair of supravalvular aortic stenosis using a pericardial patch augmentation of the aorta (RASTELLI et al. 1966). For the diffuse type of supravalvular stenosis, a more extensive repair is required, involving augmentation of the aorta with a pantaloon-shaped Dacron patch (DOTY et al. 1977). Both procedures have a good surgical outcome (BROWN et al. 2002; ENGLISH et al. 2003), although approximately 14% of patients undergo reoperation (BROWN et al. 2002).

X-ray angiography can be associated with severe complications, secondary to vessel spasm in the region of the aortic narrowing. Noninvasive assessment is thus important. The main roles of cardiovascular MR are preoperative anatomical and functional assessment of the stenosis and assessment of re-stenosis (Fig. 15.8). Gd-MRA is an accurate method of assessing the type and severity of the defect as well as its relationship to the aortic valve. However, if stenosis is severe signal loss in the Gd-MRA may lead to overestimation of the severity of the stenosis. In these situations, 2D black-blood imaging is useful in assessing both the external and internal diameter of the stenotic region of the aorta. Exact measurement of the extent of the lesion using either Gd-MRA or 2D black-blood imaging allows better preoperative decision-making regarding the type of surgery. Velocity-encoded phase-contrast MR can be used to measure peak velocities at the level of the supravalvular aortic obstruction. The pressure gradient gives some indication of the functional significance of a stenosis and is particularly important in deciding the type and timing of any intervention.

15.4.4
Congenital Anomalies of the Aorta

Congenital anomalies of the aorta are covered in Chap. 16.4.1.1.

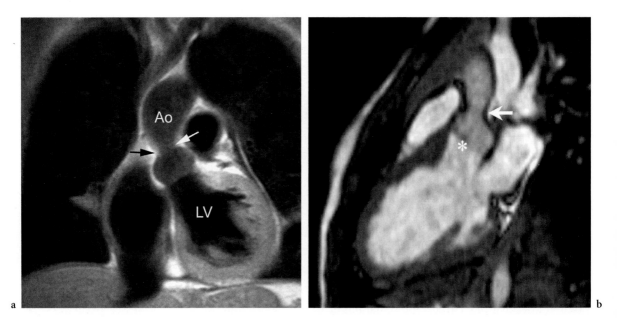

Fig. 15.8. a Black-blood spin-echo left ventricular outflow tract view of supravalvular aortic stenosis (*arrows*). **b** Balanced-SSFP inflow/outflow view of the left ventricle showing supravalvular aortic stenosis (*arrow*) in relation to the position of the aortic valve (*asterisk*)

15.5
Cyanotic Heart Disease

15.5.1
Tetralogy of Fallot

Tetralogy of Fallot (ToF) is the most common cyanotic congenital heart defect, with an incidence of approximately 420 per million live births (Hoffman and Kaplan 2002). It is caused by malalignment of the infundibular septum, which leads to right ventricular outflow (RVOT) obstruction, a subaortic VSD with aortic override, and right ventricular hypertrophy (Fig. 15.9). Treatment for this condition was revolutionized by the introduction of the Blalock and Tausig shunt in the late 1940s (Fig. 15.10). Current management consists of early single-stage reconstructive surgery (Lillehei et al. 1986). This procedure has the benefit of leaving the patient acyanotic and has good survival rates (Nollert et al. 1997a, 1997b). Staged reconstruction is still required if there is significant hypoplasia of the central pulmonary arteries (Marshall et al. 2003). TTE is the imaging modality of choice for initial diagnosis and assessment (Tworetzky et al. 1999).

MR imaging does have a role in delineating PA anatomy, which is particularly important when deciding between single- and multi-stage recon-structive surgery. It has been shown that PA Gd-MR angiographic findings compare well with both operative and X-ray angiographic findings (Beekman et al. 1997; Holmqvist et al. 2001). MR may in fact be more powerful than X-ray angiography in defining the central PA structure (Beekman et al. 1997). MR can also be used to accurately assess the 3D orientation of the VSD and the degree of aortic override (Beekman et al. 1997).

The main role of MR in patients with ToF is assessment of postoperative complications. Operative repair of ToF consists of resection of the infundibular stenosis, enlargement of the pulmonary valve/annulus and closure of the VSD. The most common late postoperative complication is pulmonary regurgitation (Nollert et al. 1997a, 1997b), which leads to right ventricular dysfunction. This is secondary to transannular patch reconstruction of the RVOT/pulmonary annulus and is often associated with aneurismal dilation of the RVOT (Fig. 15.11). Surgical or transcatheter valve replacement is the current method of managing patients with severe pulmonary regurgitation (Bonehoffer et al. 2002). Accurate quantification of regurgitation and definition of RVOT anatomy is particularly important in deciding the type and timing of procedures. Velocity-encoded phase-contrast MR has been shown to accurately quantify pulmonary regurgitation and has been internally validated

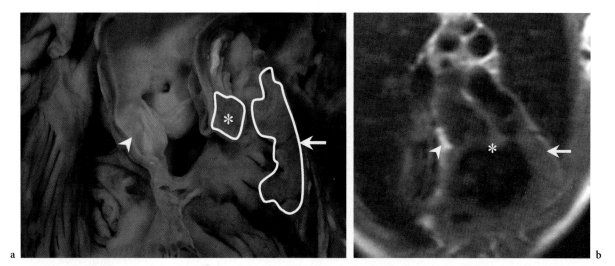

Fig. 15.9a,b. Right ventricular outflow tract coronal view of tetralogy of Fallot. Corresponding morphological (**a**) and black-blood spin-echo images (**b**) – the deviated outlet septum (*asterisk*), aortic root (*arrowhead*), and hypertrophied septoparietal trabeculations (*arrow*) are shown

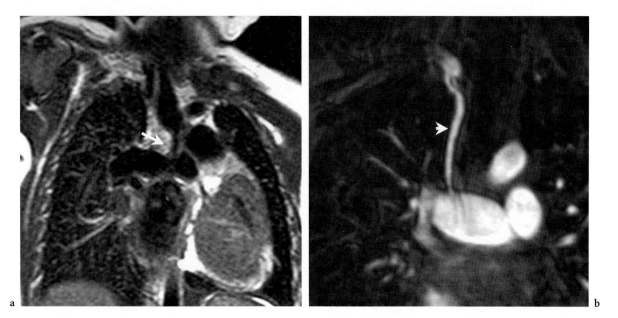

Fig. 15.10a,b. Modified Blalock-Taussig (BT) shunts. **a** Black-blood spin-echo image of a right modified BT shunt (*arrow*). **b** Maximum-intensity projection image from a gadolinium-enhanced MR angiogram of a right modified BT shunt. The distal insertion into the right pulmonary artery is narrowed

against MR ventricular volumetry in patients with ToF (REBERGEN et al. 1993) (Fig. 15.12). It has also been shown that phase-contrast MR can accurately assess differential regurgitation in the branch pulmonary arteries (KANG et al. 2003). This may be important as there is some evidence that transcatheter valve placement in the regurgitant branch PA may obviate the need for pulmonary valve replacement (KANG et al. 2003). Although regurgitation can be

qualitatively assessed using TTE or transesophageal echocardiography, the ability of MR to quantify regurgitant volume makes it a superior technique.

Pulmonary regurgitation is often associated with anatomical abnormalities of the RVOT and main PAs. Delineation of RVOT anatomy is important for planning surgical or interventional valve replacement (BONEHOFFER et al. 2004) (Fig. 15.13). 2D spin-echo black blood and SSFP sequences can be used

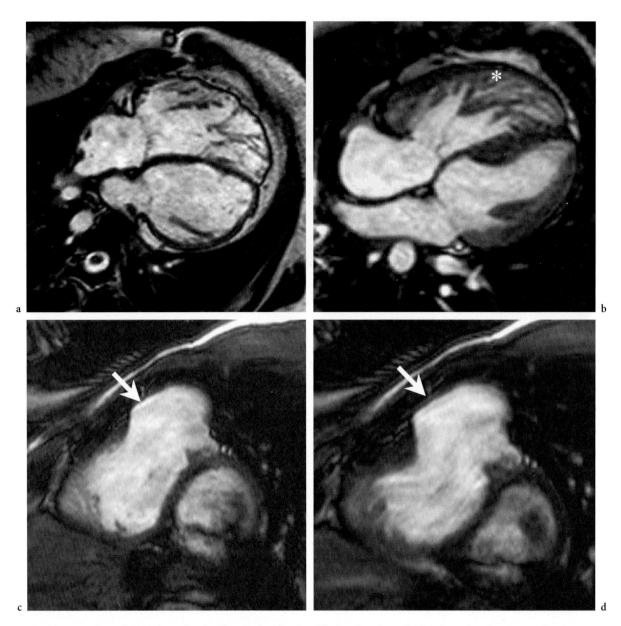

Fig. 15.11. a Balanced-SSFP four-chamber image showing RV dilation. **b** Balanced-SSFP four-chamber image showing RV hypertrophy (*asterisk*). **c, d** Balanced-SSFP oblique sagittal view of RVOT aneurysm (*arrow*) in diastole (**c**) and systole (**d**)

to delineate RVOT anatomy and quantitatively assess RVOT dilation or stenosis, and measurements made from MR data compare favorably with-echocardiography and X-ray angiography (GREENBERG et al. 1997). Furthermore, velocity-encoded phase-contrast MR can be used to measure peak velocities at the level of RVOT obstruction; pressure gradients calculated from MR peak velocities compare well with catheter pressure gradients (HOLMVQUIST et al. 2001). The pressure gradient gives some indication of the functional significance of a stenosis and

is particularly important in deciding the type and timing of any intervention.

Branch pulmonary stenosis may also be present in this patient group, which is often difficult to evaluate with-echocardiography. It is important to detect any branch PA narrowings, as these can contribute to RV dysfunction, and significant obstructions should be repaired at the same time as valve replacement (Fig. 15.14). It has been shown that MRA is more sensitive than-echocardiography in anatomically detecting branch PA stenoses, and

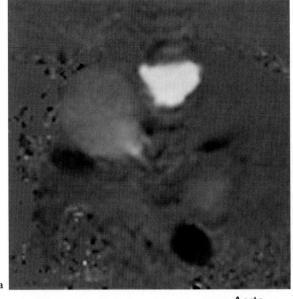
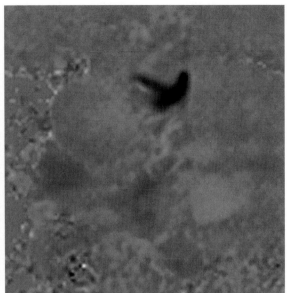

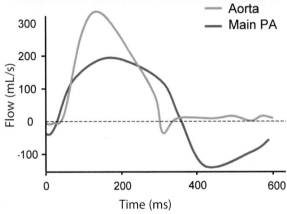

Fig. 15.12a-c. Magnetic resonance phase-contrast flow images through the pulmonary artery (*PA*): **a** systole – forward flow shown as *white*; **b** diastole – reverse flow shown as *black*. **c** Flow plotted against time for the aorta and pulmonary artery, demonstrating pulmonary incompetence (regurgitant fraction = 30%)

MR findings compare well with operative findings (GREENBERG et al. 1997). Velocity-encoded phase-contrast MR can be used to measure peak velocities at the level of obstruction, giving some indication of the functional significance of any stenosis. Anatomical and functional information concerning RVOT and branch PA stenosis can be obtained using a combination of TTE and X-ray angiography: however, the ability to obtain this data noninvasively and in one sitting makes MR a useful technique.

The final role of MR is in evaluating right ventricular function. This is important for timing of invasive therapeutic measures. Measuring ventricular function is also important when evaluating the effect of any invasive procedure (VLIEGEN et al. 2002; RAZAVI et al. 2004). Multi-slice short-axis b-SSFP imaging has been shown to be the most powerful method of ventricular function quantification (BELLENGER et al. 2002). It has been shown that, using a combination of MR ventricular volumetry and tricuspid and pulmonary flow maps, precise information about global and diastolic ventricular function can be assessed in patients with repaired ToF (HELBING et al. 1996).

In patients with ToF, 3D MRA can be used to delineate PA anatomy (pre- and postoperatively), spin-echo and gradient-echo sequences to delineate RVOT anatomy, b-SSFP cine-imaging to quantify ventricular function, and phase-contrast velocity mapping to quantify pulmonary regurgitation.

15.5.2
Pulmonary Atresia

Pulmonary atresia is defined as a lack of continuity between the RVOT and the central pulmonary arteries, with a variable degree of hypoplasia of these

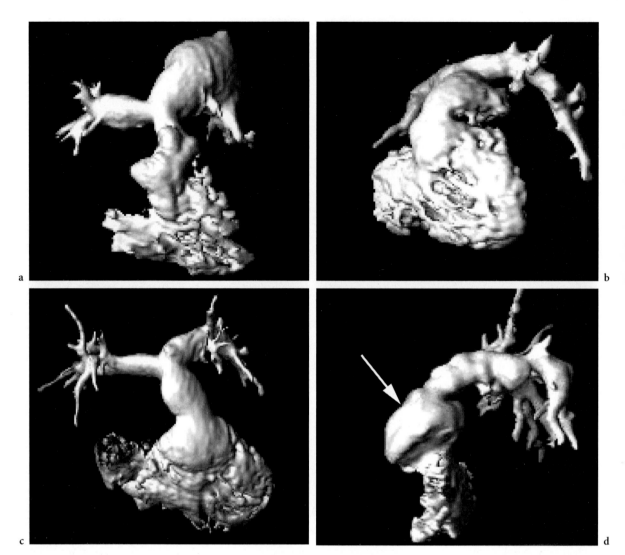

Fig. 15.13a-d. Volume-rendered 3D reconstruction from gadolinium-enhanced MR angiograms of the right ventricular outflow tract (RVOT) and proximal pulmonary arteries: **a-d** anatomical variations. In **d** a large RVOT aneurysm is seen at the site of previous transannular patch repair (*arrow*)

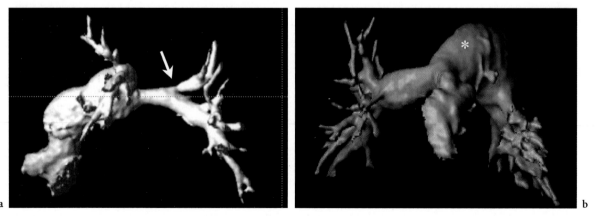

Fig. 15.14a,b. Volume-rendered 3D reconstruction from gadolinium-enhanced MR angiograms of the pulmonary arteries: **a** Right pulmonary artery hypoplasia and a discrete right upper pulmonary branch stenosis (*arrow*). **b** Marked pulmonary artery dilation in a patient with absent pulmonary valve syndrome. Severely dilated left pulmonary artery (*asterisk*)

structures. Pulmonary atresia can be separated into two groups depending on the presence of a VSD. As the diagnosis and subsequent management of these two groups is different, it is useful to consider them separately.

Pulmonary atresia with a VSD is the most common variant and is considered by some to be a severe form of ToF, with a subaortic VSD, overriding aorta, and often major aortopulmonary collaterals (MAPCAs). Surgical therapy has evolved in recent years and there is now a move toward one-stage unifocalization of MAPCAs, establishment of RVOT to PA continuity, with a homograft, and intracardiac repair of the VSD (REDDY et al. 1997; MURTHY et al. 1999). Success of this one-stage procedure is dependent on accurate anatomical definition of the "true" central pulmonary arteries and detection of all MAPCAs. Gd-MR angiography has a role in preoperative assessment and has been shown to be an excellent method of delineating central pulmonary arteries and MAPCAs (GEVA et al. 2002). In addition, the 3D visualization provided by Gd-MR angiograms, rather than the projection visualization provided by X-ray angiography, allows improved surgical or interventional planning (Fig. 15.15).

As with ToF, the main role of MR in patients with pulmonary atresia and a VSD is assessment of postoperative complications. The most common long-term complication is homograft failure, usually mixed stenosis (Fig. 15.16) and regurgitation leading to RV dysfunction. This is secondary to valvular degeneration and the patient "out-growing" the nonviable homograft. Current management consists of either homograft replacement or some form of valved stent placement and is dependent on the amount of stenosis and regurgitation and the anatomy of the homograft (RAZAVI et al. 2004). As with ToF, velocity-encoded phase-contrast MR is useful in quantifying regurgitation, particularly as Doppler-echocardiography of conduits is difficult. Velocity-encoded phase-contrast MR can be used to measure peak velocities at the level of the conduit obstruction. Pressure gradients calculated from MR peak velocities compare well with catheter pressure gradients and give some indication of the functional significance of any stenosis (HOLMQVIST et al. 2001). Such functional data (including ventricular volumetry) is useful in deciding the timing of any invasive procedures. The type of repair undertaken is very dependent on the anatomy of the homograft (RAZAVI et al. 2004). Due to the high velocity of blood through most stenosed conduits, spin-echo black-blood sequences are the most useful technique for accurate

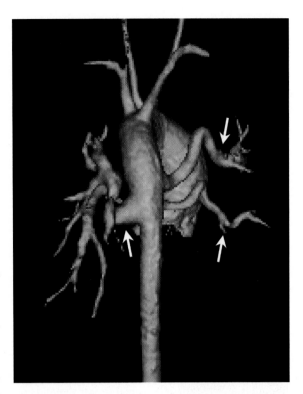

Fig. 15.15. Volume-rendered 3D reconstruction from gadolinium-enhanced MR angiogram of the aorta in a patient with pulmonary atresia/VSD, showing three large major aortopulmonary collateral arteries (MAPCAs) supplying the lungs (*arrows*)

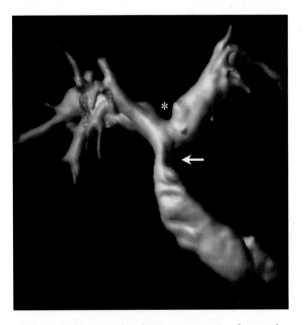

Fig. 15.16. Volume-rendered 3D reconstruction from gadolinium-enhanced MR angiogram of the pulmonary arteries in a patient with a pulmonary conduit showing severe conduit stenosis (*arrow*) and mild narrowing of the left pulmonary artery origin (*asterisk*)

measurement of conduit obstruction, as they are less susceptible to flow artifacts (Martinez et al. 1992). Unfortunately, conduit stenosis is often secondary to calcification of the nonviable homograft, and calcified tissue is difficult to visualize using spin-echo black-blood imaging. Failure to detect intraluminal calcium can lead to underreporting of obstruction (Martinez et al. 1992). Gd-MRA is also useful in assessment of the homograft, with the often-complex 3D anatomy of the conduit better appreciated with 3D MR angiograms (Razavi et al. 2004). One limitation of both these techniques is the inability to assess the dynamic anatomy of the conduit. Two-dimensional b-SSFP techniques are very useful in assessing the change in conduit architecture during the cardiac cycle, changes which may have a significant effect on the success of interventional procedures (Razavi et al. 2004). Other long-term complications are similar to those found in patients with ToF and have been discussed in the previous section.

Pulmonary atresia with intact ventricular septum is the less common variant of pulmonary atresia and is associated with a variable degree of RV hypoplasia. The type of surgical repair depends on the size and shape of the RV cavity (Shimpo et al. 2000). The presence of an RV infundibulum allows a biventricular repair (Sano et al. 2000). Thus, preoperative assessment of the RV cavity is vital. Spin-echo sequences, b-SSFP sequences, and MRA can all be used to assess the RV cavity. However, no formal trials have yet been done to assess the role of MR in preoperative management. The complications of biventricular repair are similar to those in repair of pulmonary atresia and a ventricular septal defect. If the RV cavity is small then single ventricular physiology is established. The MR assessment of such patients is considered in the section on hypoplastic left heart syndrome.

15.5.3
Transposition of the Great Arteries

Transposition of the great arteries (TGA) is the second-commonest cyanotic congenital heart disease in the first year of life, with an incidence of 315 per million live births (Hoffman and Kaplan 2002). It is defined as ventriculoarterial discordance with an anterior aorta arising from the RV, and the PA arising from the LV (Fig. 15.17). Forty-percent of patients with TGA have a VSD and 30% of these patients have subpulmonary stenosis (Park et al. 1978). Surgical therapy for this condition was revolutionized in 1958

with the introduction of the Senning procedure, in which an intra-atrial baffle was used to divert blood from the right atrium to the left ventricle, and the left atrium to the right ventricle (Senning 1975). A further variation was the Mustard procedure, in which a pericardial patch was used to construct the intra-atrial baffle (Mustard 1968). Both procedures produced a physiologically normal but an anatomically abnormal circulation (systemic venous return to the left atrium, LV, and then PA; pulmonary venous return to the right atrium, RV, and then aorta). In 1975, Jatene performed the first arterial switch operation. This had the benefit of producing both a physiological and anatomically normal circulation (Jatene et al. 1976). For this reason, the arterial switch operation has become the procedure of choice for TGA (Fig. 15.18). In cases of TGA associated with a VSD and sub-pulmonary stenosis, the Rastelli procedure is preferred (Rastelli et al. 1969).

Currently TTE is the imaging modality of choice for preoperative diagnosis and assessment. The role of MR is mainly in diagnosis of postoperative complications, particularly those that develop as the child grows older.

The main complications of the arterial switch operation are RVOT or branch PA obstruction (Haas et al. 1999; Gutberlet et al. 2000). The RVOT obstruction is thought to be due to poor growth of the reconstructed PA and may be associated with fibrous tissue formation at the suture lines (Haas et al. 1999). RVOT obstruction may also be due to compression of the PA between the aorta and the sternum secondary to the Lecompte maneuver; and branch PA stenosis is often secondary to compression by the posterior aorta. Due to the unusual position of the pulmonary arteries immediately behind the sternum, TTE is poor at detecting these lesions. Cardiovascular MR is not constrained by the intrathoracic position of vessels and is ideal for imaging the RVOT and branch pulmonary arteries in this group of patients (Fig. 15.19). Furthermore, as the narrowing causes compression on the branch pulmonary arteries in the anteroposterior plane, X-ray angiography lateral and anterior views may not clearly depict such findings. Gd-MRA is used to visualize the 3D anatomy, particularly the relationship between the pulmonary arteries and the aorta, while spin-echo sequences are used to accurately assess the degree of stenosis. It has been shown that a combination of these techniques is superior to-echocardiography in detecting these lesions (Hardy et al. 1994). In addition, MR compares favorably with X-ray angiography findings. Velocity-encoded phase-

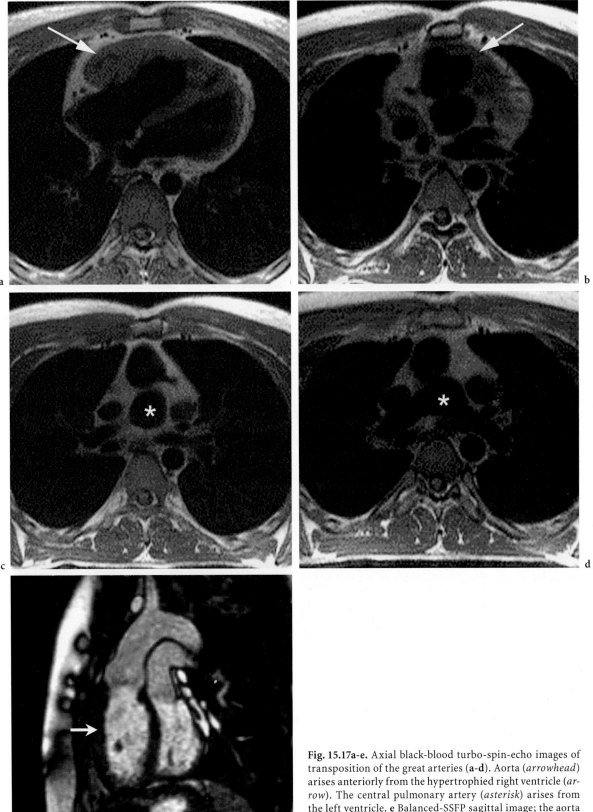

Fig. 15.17a-e. Axial black-blood turbo-spin-echo images of transposition of the great arteries (**a-d**). Aorta (*arrowhead*) arises anteriorly from the hypertrophied right ventricle (*arrow*). The central pulmonary artery (*asterisk*) arises from the left ventricle. **e** Balanced-SSFP sagittal image; the aorta arises from the hypertrophied right ventricle (*arrow*), posterior pulmonary artery

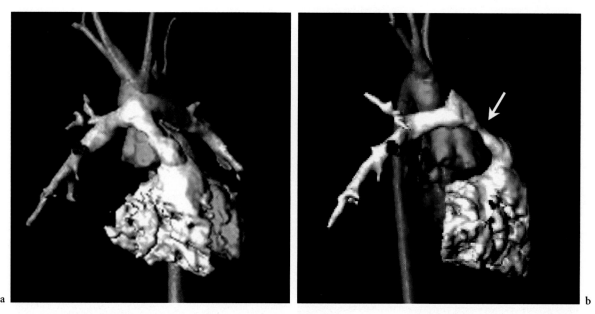

Fig. 15.18a,b. Volume-rendered 3D reconstruction from gadolinium-enhanced MR angiogram of the aorta (*red*) and pulmonary arteries (*white*) after the arterial switch operation, showing the classic configuration after the Lecompte maneuver: **a** anterior view, **b** right anterior oblique view. Note that there is mild supravalvular pulmonary narrowing (*arrow*)

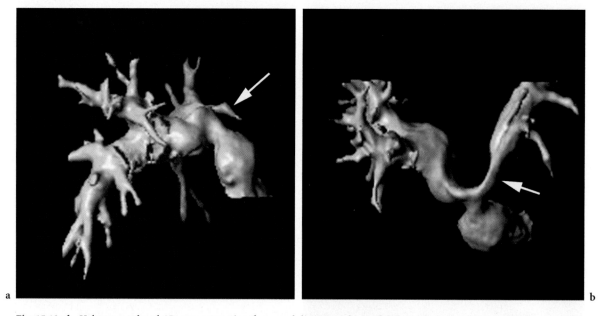

Fig. 15.19a,b. Volume-rendered 3D reconstruction from gadolinium-enhanced MR angiogram of the pulmonary arteries after the arterial switch operation. **a** Right lateral view showing some supravalvular pulmonary narrowing (*arrow*), but narrowings of the branch pulmonary arteries are difficult to perceive. **b** However, the compression of the branch pulmonary arteries [left (*arrowhead*) greater than right] as they pass around the ascending aorta (not shown) are clearly seen when the MR angiogram is viewed from above

contrast MR can be used to measure peak velocities at the level of the obstruction and calculate pressure gradients. It has been shown that there is greater agreement between MR-derived pressure gradients and invasive pressure measurements than between Doppler ultrasound pressure gradients and invasive measures (GUTBERLET et al. 2000). Using such structural and functional information, improved management decisions can be made without resorting to invasive diagnostic procedures.

RVOT/branch PA narrowing maybe associated with pulmonary regurgitation and RV dysfunction. As already stated in the previous sections, MR represents the imaging modality of choice for quantifications of these parameters.

A less common complication of the arterial switch operation is coronary stenosis secondary to the re-implantation procedure. Although the majority of coronary complications cause early postoperative mortality, a sub-set of patients suffer from late coronary events (LEGENDRE et al. 2003). In this group, X-ray coronary angiography probably represents the modality of choice for investigation. However, coronary MR angiography is a useful noninvasive method for investigating coronary arteries, particularly the proximal segments (TAYLOR et al. 2004b) (Fig. 15.20).

Although intra-atrial repair has been superseded by the arterial switch operation, there is a sizeable population who have undergone either a Senning or Mustard operation. The most common complications of intra-atrial repair are baffle obstruction or leak, arrhythmias, and RV dysfunction. Baffle obstruction is more common in the Mustard operation (SARKAR et al. 1999), probably due to calcification and poor growth of the pericardial tissue used to construct the baffle. The venous pathways have a complex 3D structure and are difficult to accurately assess with TTE. It has been shown that Gd-MRA can fully demonstrate the 3D anatomy of the Senning–Mustard anatomy and detect any luminal narrowing (FOGEL et al. 2001, 2002). Unfortunately, this is flow-sensitive, nongated sequence imaging and is susceptible to signal dropout. Spin-echo sequences are useful in accurately measuring static baffle obstruction (SAMPSON et al. 1994), while 2D and 3D b-SSFP sequences are able to accurately delineate the dynamic anatomy of intra-atrial baffles and qualitatively assess flow (SAMPSON et al. 1994). A combination of all these MR techniques allows comprehensive assessment of intra-atrial baffles (Fig. 15.21).

The etiology of RV dysfunction in patients with intra-atrial baffles is complex. Deranged AV valve coupling may be important, and repair of baffle obstruction or regurgitant AV valves does improve RV function. However, in a significant group, RV dysfunction is present without abnormal AV valve coupling and is thought to be due to the systemic nature of the RV (DERRICK et al. 2000, 2001). RV function has been assessed in patients with intra-atrial repair of TGA using multi-slice b-SSFP sequences (LORENZ et al. 1995; TULEVSKI et al. 2002), and it has been shown that RV ejection fraction and end-systolic volume are lower than in matched controls (TULEVSKI et al. 2002). In addition, these patients also show a reduced response to dobutamine stress that may be secondary to abnormal AV coupling (TULEVSKI et al. 2000).

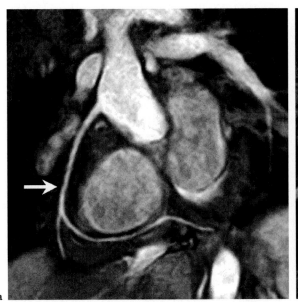
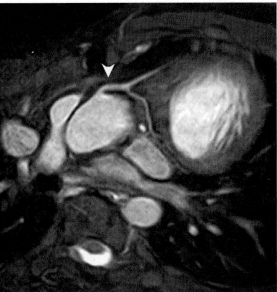

a   b

Fig. 15.20a,b. Normal MR coronary angiogram in a patient with arterial switch operation for transposition of the great arteries: **a** oblique sagittal view of right coronary artery (*arrow*), **b** oblique axial view of the left coronary artery system, left main (*arrowhead*)

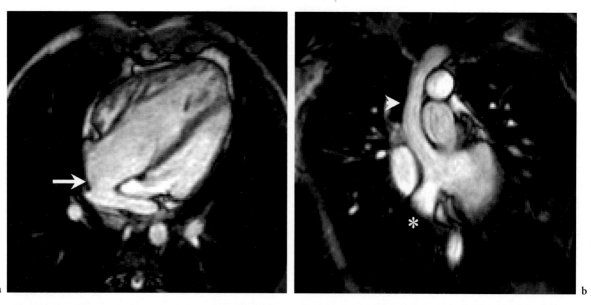

Fig. 15.21a,b. Balanced-SSFP images of intra-atrial baffles in a patient who has undergone the atrial switch Senning operation: **a** Baffle taking pulmonary venous blood into the right atrium (*arrow*), **b** baffles taking systemic venous blood into the left atrium, superior pathway (*arrowhead*), inferior pathway (*asterisk*)

In cases of TGA with sub-pulmonary stenosis, the Rastelli procedure is usually preferred. This involves construction of an intracardiac tunnel through the VSD, which directs flow from the LV to the aorta. Pulmonary blood flow is completed with the placement of an RV-to-PA conduit. The most common complication is conduit stenosis, and the role of MR in assessment of this problem has already been discussed. Less common is LVOT obstruction due to the VSD becoming restrictive. MR does have a role to play in assessment of LVOT obstruction, particularly Gd-MRA and 3D b-SSFP techniques, which allow assessment of the 3D structure of the tunnel. Spin-echo and gradient-echo sequences also have a role to play in accurate measurement of luminal obstruction.

Congenitally corrected transposition (CCTGA) is a rare disorder characterized by atrioventricular and ventricle-arterial discordance (right atrium to left ventricle to PA, and left atrium to right ventricle to aorta). Thus, although the heart is anatomically abnormal, it is physiologically normal in terms of the pulmonary and systemic circuits. This disease is not cyanotic; however, many of the problems are similar to those experienced by patients with TGA. CCTGA may be asymptomatic and in some patients is an incidental finding (Fig. 15.22); however, the majority of patients with CCTGA have associated cardiac lesions (BJARKE and KIDD 1976). The most common associated lesion is a ventricular septal de-

fect. Pulmonary stenosis is present in approximately 50% of cases, and tricuspid valve abnormalities (i.e., Ebstein's abnormality) are found in 20% of cases (BJARKE and KIDD 1976). Even without associated abnormalities, the majority of patients with CCTGA develop systemic ventricular failure over time (CONNELLY et al. 1996), which may be due to the inability of the right ventricle to cope with systemic afterload. The main role of MR is in evaluation of associated lesions, quantification of ventricular function, and assessment of postoperative complications. The assessment of VSDs and pulmonary stenosis has been dealt with previously in this chapter. Valve abnormalities are dealt with in the chapter on valvular heart disease (Chap. 13). RV function has been assessed in patients with CCTGA multi-slice SSFP sequences (DODGE-KHATAMI et al. 2002; TULEVSKI et al. 2002), and it has been shown that RV ejection fraction, end-systolic volume, and response to dobutamine stress are lower than in matched controls (DODGE-KHATAMI et al. 2002; TULEVSKI et al. 2002). Late failure of the systemic right ventricle has led to the increasing use of anatomical repair in CCTGA. This involves either an atrial and arterial switch (LANGLEY et al. 2003) or, in the case of CCTGA with an associated VSD, a Rastelli procedure with an atrial switch (BRAWN and BARRON 2003). The complications of these operative procedures and the role of MR in investigating them have been described in the previous section.

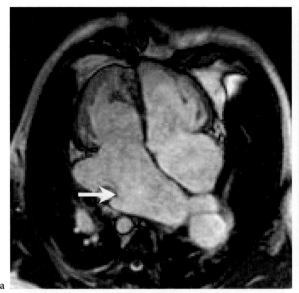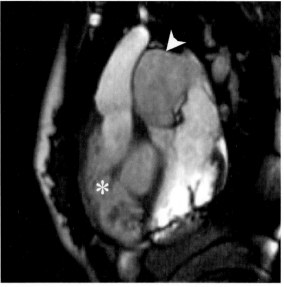

a   b

Fig. 15.22a,b. Balanced-SSFP image of a patient with congenitally corrected transposition of the great arteries. a Axial 4-chamber view – left atrium (*arrow*) connecting to right ventricle. b Oblique sagittal view – hypertrophied right ventricle (*asterisk*) connecting to anterior aorta; posterior pulmonary artery shown (*arrowhead*)

15.5.4
Double-Outlet Right Ventricle

In double-outlet right ventricle, both great vessels emerge from the right ventricle, with the left ventricle emptying through a VSD. The clinical picture and type of surgical correction depend on the arrangement of the great vessels and the anatomy of the VSD. The most common variant is normal arrangement of the great vessels and a sub-aortic VSD. This variant is often referred to as the Fallot type, as it is often associated with pulmonary stenosis and has a similar presentation. Double-outlet right ventricle can also be associated with an anterior aorta and a sub-pulmonary VSD, known as the Taussig-Bing anomaly. This presents in a similar manner to TGA with VSD. Rarer are the variants with doubly committed or noncommitted VSDs. These patients present with cardiac failure and some degree of cyanosis. Surgical correction for the Fallot-type variant consists of patch closure of the VSD, which redirects blood to the aorta, and correction of any pulmonary stenosis (BROWN et al. 2001). For the Taussig-Bing anomaly, surgery depends on the presence of the pulmonary obstruction. In the absence of pulmonary obstruction, correction consists of patch closure of the VSD and arterial switch (MASUDA et al. 1999). In the presence of obstruction, LV flow is tunnelled through the VSD to the aorta, and a RV-PA pathway is established (WU et al. 2003). The role of MR

in the assessment of postoperative complications of the Fallot-type repair, the arterial switch, and the Rastelli procedure have been discussed in previous sections. However, MR can also play an important role in preoperative assessment in this group of patients. The anatomy of the VSD and the arrangement of the great vessels are particularly important when deciding the type of surgery. Spin-echo black-blood imaging of the VSD has been shown to compare well with surgical findings and is able to predict the type of repair finally done (BEEKMAN et al. 2000). 3D b-SSFP and 2D b-SSFP cine techniques are also useful as they give both anatomical and functional information (KILNER et al. 2002). Finally MRA is useful in delineating great-vessel arrangement and the 3D anatomy of the VSD.

15.5.5
Common Arterial Trunk

Common arterial trunk (truncus arteriosis) is defined as a single arterial trunk arising from both ventricles, which overrides a large, malaligned VSD. The pulmonary, systemic, and coronary vessels originate from the single common arterial trunk. The classification of common arterial trunk relies on the branching pattern of the PA. In type I, a short main PA arises from the common trunk and subsequently divides. In type II, the RPA and LPA originate from the posterior wall of the common trunk; and, in type III, the RPA and LPA emerge from the lateral wall of the common trunk. The truncal valve is often abnormal, with varying degrees of stenosis and insufficiency. Surgical repair consists of reconstruction of the trunk to produce a systemic vessel from the LV, patch closure of the VSD, and establishment of a RV-to-PA conduit. The main role of MR is in assessment of postoperative complications, though MRA can be used to better delineate the vascular anatomy (RAZAVI et al. 2004), which maybe useful in surgical planning.

The main complications of truncal repair are homograft failure, truncal insufficiency, and VSD patch leak. The role of MR in the assessment of these problems has been discussed previously.

15.5.6
Hypoplastic Left Heart Syndrome

Hypoplastic left heart syndrome (HLHS) is the fourth commonest cardiac malformation to present in the 1st year of life, with an incidence of approximately 266 per million live births (HOFFMAN and KAPLAN 2002). HLHS constitutes a spectrum of congenital heart disease with hypoplasia or atresia of the left-sided heart components and normal relation of the great vessels. At birth, the right ventricle supplies both the systemic and pulmonary circulations via a patent ductus arteriosus (PDA). After birth, closure of the PDA and the presence of a restrictive patent foramen ovale lead to increasing cyanosis and heart failure. Surgical treatment has been revolutionized by the introduction of the Norwood procedure in 1980 (NORWOOD et al. 1980) with subsequent conversion to a total cavopulmonary connection (TCPC). The Norwood procedure is performed in the 1st week of life and involves the anastomosis of the main PA to the hypoplastic aorta augmented with a patch of homograft tissue. Pulmonary blood supply is maintained by a modified Blalock-Taussig (BT) shunt from the innominate artery to the proximal right PA (Fig. 15.23). The atrial septum is excised to enable nonrestricted pulmonary venous return to the right atrium via the left atrium. A recent development is the modified Norwood procedure (PIZARRO et al. 2003), in which an RV conduit is used rather than a BT shunt. This is thought to reduce diastolic runoff, thus improving coronary perfusion (PIZARRO et al. 2003). Prior to staged conversion to a TCPC circulation, preoperative invasive catheterization is performed to

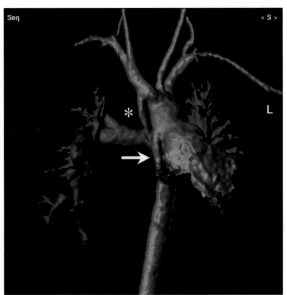

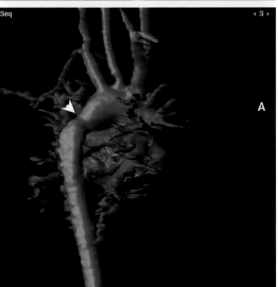

Fig. 15.23a,b. Volume-rendered 3D reconstruction from gadolinium-enhanced MR angiogram in hypoplastic left heart syndrome (HLHS) following the Norwood stage 1 operation. **a** Anterior view, **b** right posterior oblique view. The hypoplastic native aorta (*arrow*), the neoaorta, aortic arch, descending aorta, and aortopulmonary shunt (*asterisk*) are shown in *red*. Note there is a very mild narrowing at the junction of the reconstructed aortic arch and the native descending aorta (**b**) (*arrowhead*). The pulmonary arteries are shown in *blue* and are not narrowed in this patient. Color-coding is for ease of visualization and is not related to blood saturation, which will be the same for both circulations

identify any complications that may require repair; branch PA stenosis, aortic arch obstruction, tricuspid regurgitation, and systemic/pulmonary shunt obstruction. Branch PA stenosis is common post-

Norwood procedure and is often associated with the BT shunt. Gd-MRA can give excellent 3D images of any obstruction, although spin-echo images are better for accurate measurement of stenosis (TAYLOR et al. 2004a). Neoaortic arch obstruction is also a recognized problem in this group of patients (CHESSA et al. 2000) and is a significant cause of morbidity and mortality. Preoperative (stage II) detection of neoaortic obstruction is vital, as aortic angioplasty prior to further repair, or aortic reconstruction can be done at the same time as conversion of a bidirectional Glenn shunt. Gd-MRA is the modality of choice for imaging the often-complex 3D arch obstructions present (TAYLOR et al. 2004a).

Velocity-encoded phase-contrast MR can also be used to quantify the pressure gradient across any obstruction. The use of MR to detect great vessel stenosis been shown to be a good alternative to invasive cardiac catheterization in pre-stage II patients , and results compare well with operative findings (TAYLOR et al. 2004a) (Fig. 15.24). Obstruction of the BT shunt is another serious complication with significant mortality. BT shunt visualization can be difficult with-echocardiography, and routine inva-

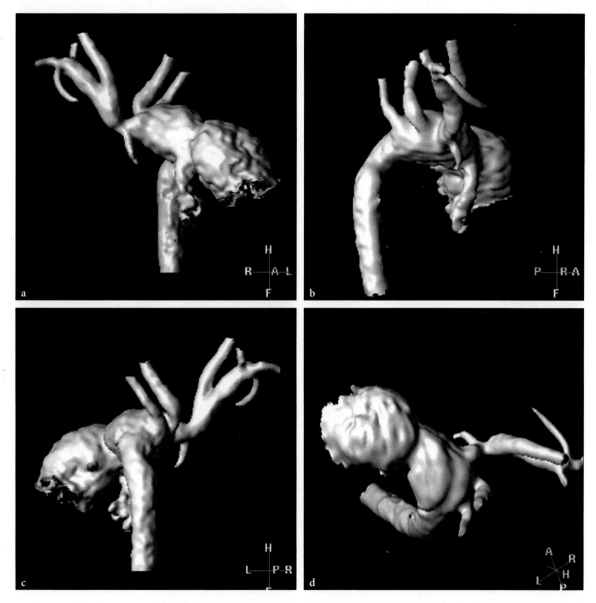

Fig. 15.24a-d. Aortic-arch 3D volume-rendered reconstruction from the MR angiogram raw data showing kinked head and neck vessel origins: **a** right anterior oblique, **b** right posterior oblique, **c** left posterior oblique, and **d** left superior oblique views. Note that there are no discrete head and neck vessel narrowings despite the vessel kinking

sive catheterization may fail to detect some stenosis (VINCENT et al. 2000). In addition, invasive selective catheterization of the shunt is associated with some risk. The use of spin-echo and MR angiographic sequences has allowed accurate, noninvasive visualization of the shunt, and results compare well with X-ray angiography and operative findings (ICHIDA et al. 1992; TAYLOR et al. 2004a). Tricuspid regurgitation is often present in patients post-Norwood procedure; however, in a small proportion, severe tricuspid regurgitation leads to RV failure. This requires annuloplasty usually during the stage II or III operation. Doppler-echocardiography is able to detect valvular incompetence; however, with velocity-encoded phase-contrast MR, the volume regurgitation and any associated RV dysfunction can be accurately quantified (TAYLOR et al. 2004a).

At 3–9 months of age, a stage II (hemi-Fontan, bidirectional Glenn) operation is performed with a side-to-side anastomosis between the superior vena cava (SVC) and pulmonary arteries, a patch dividing the SVC from the right atrium, and the removal of the innominate/PA shunt. The main complication following stage II is branch PA narrowing, either due to compression by other vascular structures or fibrosis and scarring. Visualization of the Glenn shunt is very difficult with-echocardiography, and routine assessment with invasive X-ray catheterization is necessary. In addition, before stage III, it is important to detect any pulmonary venous obstructions, because they lead to failure of the Fontan circuit. MRA can give excellent 3D images of the Glenn shunt and pulmonary venous anatomy and has been shown to compare well with X-ray angiography and operative findings (JULSRUD et al. 1989) (Fig. 15.25). However, one must remember, as the Glenn circuit contains slow-flowing blood, and if normal concentrations of gadolinium are used, signal dropout will occur due to the T2* effect. Thus, one must either dilute the gadolinium (10%) and administer it slowly (1 ml/s) or image the gadolinium bolus on the 2nd recirculation through the vasculature. For Glenn imaging, 3D b-SSFP imaging may have some benefits over MRA as the slow flow of blood improves blood-pool contrast. The final stage III (total cavopulmonary anatomosis, Fontan) operation is usually performed at 2–3 years of age and consists of either anastomsosis of the right atrium to the Glenn shunt or creation of a lateral or extracardiac tunnel between the IVC and the Glenn shunt. The Fontan operation was originally designed for treatment of tricuspid atresia (FONTAN and BAUDET 1971), although its use was extended to other single ventricu-

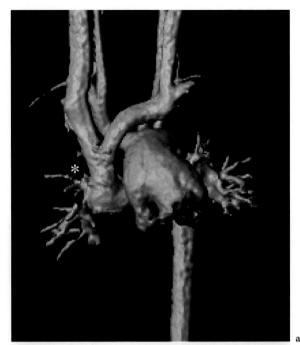

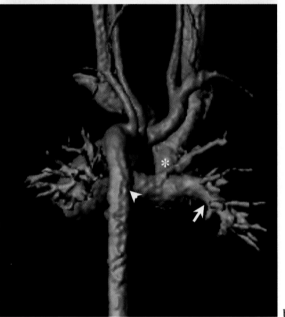

Fig. 15.25a,b. Volume-rendered 3D reconstruction from gadolinium-enhanced MR angiogram of a bidirectional Glenn shunt (*blue*) in a patient with HLHS (i.e., post-stage 2 operation). **a** Anterior view, **b** posterior view: right pulmonary artery (*arrow*), superior caval vein (*asterisk*), and descending aorta (*arrowhead*)

lar morphology lesions, including HLHS. Although long-term results have been good (DE VIVIE et al. 1981), increased right atrial pressure leads to atrial dilation and predisposes to atrial tachyarrhythmias (GATES et al. 1997). The modified Fontan procedure with either an extracardiac (LASCHINGER et al. 1996) or lateral tunnel (DE LEVAL et al. 1988) between the IVC and Glenn shunt was proposed. These procedures have a lower complication rates than the classic Fontan and have become the procedures of choice for the stage III operation in HLHS.

There is, however, a sizeable population with a standard Fontan circulation who require diagnostic assessment. Right atrial dilation is the major complication of the Fontan procedure and, using MR (either MRA or 3D b-SSFP), the 3D anatomy of the atrium can be delineated (Fig. 15.26). Right atrial dilation can cause pulmonary vein compression, which can lead to failure of the Fontan circulation (CONTE et al. 1999; HEGDE et al. 2004). 3D MRA has been shown to be useful in assessing pulmonary vein obstruction (PILLEUL and MERCHANT 2000) and it is therefore a useful modality in the assessment of the Fontan circulation. MR also has a role to play in the assessment of the modified Fontan procedures, particularly assessment of the branch pulmonary arteries and tunnels (FOGEL et al. 2001) (Fig. 15.27). Finally, MR can be used to accurately assess ventricular function. It has been demonstrated that ventricular function is lower in patients with Fontan circulation (FOGEL and RYCHIN 1998); in addition ventricular dysfunction may require cardiac transplantation. Multi-slice b-SSFP imaging of the ventricle is the most accurate method of assessing global ventricular function and is invaluable in this group of patients (FOGEL and RYCHIN 1998).

The above description of MR assessment of stage II and III operations for HLHS holds true for the MR assessment of other univentricular hearts (e.g., tricuspid atresia), or where a single ventricle surgical strategy has been followed (bidirectional Glenn, classic Fontan, and TCPC circulations).

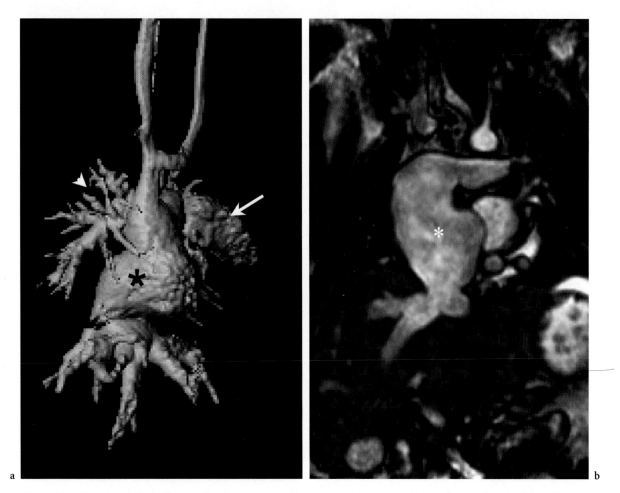

a   b

Fig. 15.26. a Volume-rendered 3D reconstruction from gadolinium-enhanced MR angiogram of a classic Fontan circulation showing severe right atrial dilation (*asterisk*): right pulmonary artery (*arrowhead*), right atrial appendage (*arrow*). **b** Balanced-SSFP coronal view through the right atrium (*asterisk*)

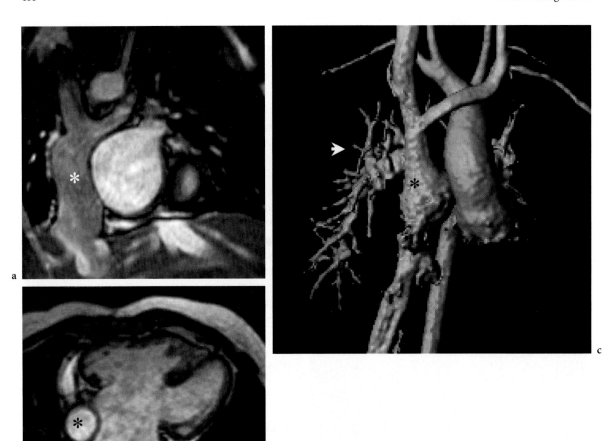

Fig. 15.27. a, b Balanced-SSFP coronal and axial images through the lateral tunnel (*asterisk*): **a** coronal view, **b** axial view. Note how the lateral tunnel is separated from the remainder of the right and left atriums. **c** Volume-rendered 3D reconstruction from gadolinium-enhanced MR angiogram of a total caval pulmonary connection (TCPC) lateral tunnel Fontan circulation: lateral tunnel (*asterisk*), right pulmonary artery (*arrowhead*)

15.6
Coronary Arteries

15.6.1
Kawasaki Disease

Kawaski disease is an acute vasculitis that usually occurs in children under 5 years of age (see also Sect. 14.11.2). These children develop acute myocarditis and pericarditis. Most morbidity is due to the medium-term development of coronary artery aneurysms, which occur in approximately 20% of patients (PARK et al. 2002). Coronary aneurysms predispose the patient to the development of myocardial ischemia and infarction (BURNS et al. 1996). Thus, long-term follow-up into adulthood is important in the management of this condition (BURNS et al. 1996). X-ray coronary angiography has been considered the gold standard in following up coronary abnormalities in Kawasaki disease. Unfortunately it is invasive and exposes the patient to ionizing radiation, which limits its usefulness (GREIL et al. 2002). Echocardiography is also useful in the assessment of coronary vascular abnormalities; however, it is more difficult in older children and adolescents (GREIL et al. 2002). Three-dimensional gradient-echo angiography can be used to delineate coronary abnormalities in Kawasaki disease. It has been shown that MR angiography findings compare well with X-ray angiography findings in both children (MAVORGENI et al. 2004) and young adults (GREIL et al. 2002) (Fig. 15.28). Furthermore, cardiovascular MR can be used to assess perfusion and infarct (FUJIWARA et al. 2001).

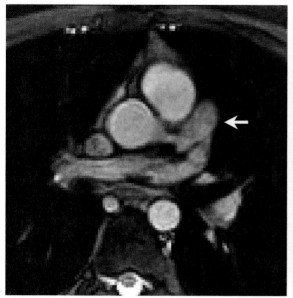
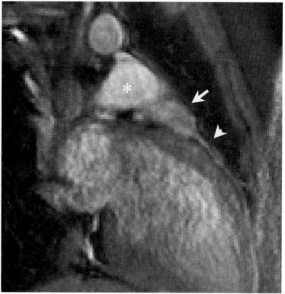

a   b

Fig. 15.28a,b. MR coronary angiography in a patient with Kawasaki's disease. **a** Oblique axial image of the left main stem (LMS) bifurcation. **b** Oblique coronal image of the left anterior descending (LAD) artery: pulmonary trunk (*asterisk*). There is a large aneurysm of the proximal LAD artery (*arrow*), which commences at the bifurcation of the LMS. The inflow into the aneurysm and outflow from the aneurysm (*arrowhead*) are patent

15.6.2
Anomalous Coronary Artery

Anomalous coronary artery origin and proximal course is a recognized cause of myocardial ischemia and sudden death (TAYLOR et al. 1997) (see also Sect. 14.11.1). Conventionally, the origin and proximal course of the coronary arteries has been assessed by TTE (PLEHN et al. 1988), transesophageal echocardiography (GIANNOCCARO et al. 1993), and X-ray angiography (POST et al. 1995). Echocardiography has some limitations, particularly in older children and adults, due to poor echo windows (POST et al. 1995). X-ray angiography has been considered the gold standard for evaluation of anomalous coronary arteries. However, there are risks attached to cardiac catheterization in addition to the exposure to X-radiation (RAZAVI et al. 2003a). Early studies using black-blood imaging demonstrated that MR was a viable option for imaging anomalous coronary arteries (DOUARD et al. 1988). Recently, b-SSFP techniques have been used to delineate coronary artery anatomy (GIORGI et al. 2002). MR coronary angiography compares well with results from X-ray angiography (MCCONNELL et al. 1995; TAYLOR et al. 2000) and in some, results in improved delineation of coronary anatomy (POST et al. 1995) (Fig. 15.29). Cardiovascular MR can also be used to assess perfusion and infarct size (GIORGI et al. 2002), which is useful in determining prognosis.

15.7
An MR Imaging Protocol for Congenital Heart Disease

The protocol below is a general protocol for imaging of congenital heart disease. It should be altered to answer clinical questions depending on patient anatomy.

1. Scouts and reference scans (parallel imaging)

2. Balanced-SSFP 3D volume (or conventional black-blood axial imaging if not available)

3. Interactive imaging for acquisition of scan plane geometries
   a. Four-chamber view
   b. RVOT view in two planes
   c. LVOT view in two planes
   d. Short-axis plane
   e. Pulmonary trunk through-plane
   f. Aorta through-plane
   g. Branch pulmonary arteries

4. 2D single-slice b-SSFP cine images
   a. Four-chamber view
   b. RVOT in both planes
   c. LVOT

5. 2D multi-slice b-SSFP cine images
   a. Whole ventricle in short-axis plane

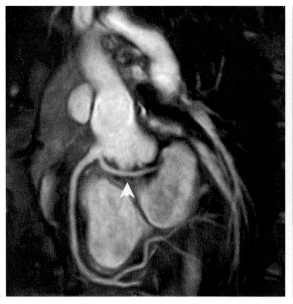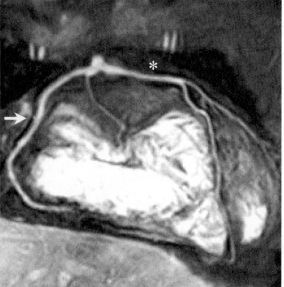

a   b

Fig. 15.29a,b. Maximum intensity projection (MIP) images reconstructed from the 3D MR coronary angiograms using Pride Workstation and Soap Bubble software (both, Philips Medical Systems, Best, the Netherlands). **a** Oblique sagittal view demonstrating an anomalous origin of the left circumflex (*arrowhead*) from the RCA. **b** Coronal view demonstrating an anomalous accessory left anterior descending artery (*asterisk*) arising from the same ostia as the RCA (*arrow*). No ostial stenoses or proximal coronary artery kinking are seen

6. 2D single-slice black-blood imaging
   a. Branch pulmonary arteries
   b. Aortic arch
   c. Vascular stenosis
7. Phase-contrast velocity mapping
   a. Main PA through-plane
   b. Ascending aorta through-plane
   c. Vascular stenosis in-plane
8. 3D contrast-enhanced MRA of the thoracic great vessels

15.8
Conclusion

Cardiovascular imaging is becoming an important tool for diagnosis and follow-up of children and adult patients with congenital heart disease. Its main role is as an adjunct to echocardiography, rather than a replacement. In situations where echocardiography cannot answer all the clinical questions, cardiovascular MR can provide an accurate, noninvasive method of imaging patients with congenital heart disease. It represents a viable alternative to X-ray angiography and in some situations performs better than traditional angiography. Cardiovascular MR

also represents the best available in vivo method for quantifications of ventricular function and vascular flow. The use of velocity-encoded phase-contrast MR allows accurate, noninvasive quantification of blood flow and pressure gradients. Finally, although less common in congenital heart disease patients, MR allows assessment of coronary anatomy, perfusion, and scar. Thus MR provides a "one-stop" imaging modality, allowing assessment of anatomy, function, and perfusion.

15.8.1
Future Direction

New techniques in cardiovascular MR may have major ramifications for the assessment of congenital heart disease. MR-guided cardiac catheterizations allow the simultaneous acquisition of MR flow data and invasive pressure measurements and thus accurate measurement of pulmonary vascular resistance (MUTHURANGU et al. 2004) (see Chap. 17). In the future, interventions (i.e., ASD closure) may be performed under MR guidance and will benefit from the extra anatomical information provided by this imaging modality. New, fast imaging techniques will allow shorter scan times, which will improve scan compliance, particularly in the pediatric population. Finally, high field-strength magnets (3T) with multiple channels and fast gradients will allow better imaging in smaller patients.

15.9
Key Points

- Imaging method of choice for grown-up congenital heart disease
- One stop imaging modality for assessment of form and function
- Accurate 3D assessment of anatomy
- Accurate quantification of Qp:Qs
- Ability to derive pressure gradients from velocity data
- Best available in vivo method for ventricular volumetry (in particular for assessment of the right ventricle)
- Increasing ability of MR to assess myocardial perfusion and coronary artery anatomy

Acknowledgements
We would like to acknowledge the following for their help and support with cardiovascular MR. From Great Ormond Street Hospital for Children, London, UK: Professor John Deanfield and Professor Philipp Bonhoeffer of the Cardiothoracic Unit; Dr. Cathy Owens, Rod Jones, Wendy Norman, and Clare Thompson of the Department of Radiology; and Dr. Angus McEwan of the Anaesthetic Department. From Guy's Hospital, London, UK: Dr.Derek Hill, Dr. Steve Keevil, Dr. Marc Miquel, Dr.Kawal Rhodes, Rado Andriantsimiavona, Redha Boubertakh, Maxime Sermesant, and Professor David Hawkes of the Division of Imaging Sciences; Dr.Shakeel Quresh and Dr. Edward Baker of the Department of Paediatric Cardiology; Dr. Michael Barnet of the Anaesthetic Department; and John Spence, Stephen Sinclear, Rebeca Lund, and other staff of the Radiology Department.

References

Acar P, Abdel-Massih T, Douste-Blazy MY, et al (2002) Assessment of muscular ventricular septal defect closure by transcatheter or surgical approach: a three-dimensional-echocardiographic study. Eur J Echocardiogr 3:185–191

Anderson RH (2001) Terminology. In: Anderson RH, Baker EJ, Macarthy FJ et al (eds) Paediatric cardiology. Churchill Livingstone, London, pp 19–36

Barkhausen J, Goyen M, Ruhm SG, et al (2002) Assessment of ventricular function with single breath-hold real-time steady-state free precession cine MR imaging. AJR Am J Roentengol178:731–735

Beekman RP, Beek FJ, Meijboom EJ (1997) Usefulness of MRI for the pre-operative evaluation of the pulmonary arteries in tetralogy of Fallot. Magn Reson Imaging 15:1005–1015

Beekman RP, Roest AA, Helbing WA (2000) Spin echo MRI in the evaluation of hearts with a double outlet right ventricle: usefulness and limitations. Magn Reson Imaging 18:245–253

Beerbaum P, Korperich H, Barth P, et al (2001) Noninvasive quantification of left-to-right shunt in pediatric patients: phase-contrast cine magnetic resonance imaging compared with invasive oximetry. Circulation 103:2476–2482

Beerbaum P, Korperich H, Esdorn H (2003) Atrial septal defects in pediatric patients: noninvasive sizing with cardiovascular MR imaging. Radiology 228:361–369

Bellenger NG, Marcus NJ, Rajappan K, et al (2002) Comparison of techniques for the measurement of left ventricular function following cardiac transplantation. J Cardiovasc Magn Reson 4:255–263

Berger RM (2000) Possibilities and impossibilities in the evaluation of pulmonary vascular disease in congenital heart defects. Eur Heart J 21:17–27

Bjarke BB, Kidd BS (1976) Congenitally corrected transposition of the great arteries. A clinical study of 101 cases. Acta Paediatr Scand 65:153–160

Bonhoeffer P, Boudjemline Y, Qureshi SA, et al (2002) Percutaneous insertion of the pulmonary valve. J Am Coll Cardiol 39:1664–1669

Brawn WJ, Barron DJ (2003) Technical aspects of the Rastelli and atrial switch procedure for congenitally corrected transposition of the great arteries with ventricular septal defect and pulmonary stenosis or atresia: results of therapy. Semin Thorac Cardiovasc Surg Pediatr Card Surg Annu 6:4–8

Brown JW, Ruzmetov M, Okada Y, Vijay P, Turrentine MW (2001) Surgical results in patients with double outlet right ventricle: a 20-year experience. Ann Thorac Surg 72:1630–1635

Brown JW, Ruzmetov M, Vijay P, Turrentine MW (2002) Surgical repair of congenital supravalvular aortic stenosis in children. Eur J Cardiothorac Surg 21:50–56

Burns JC, Shike H, Gordon JB (1996) Sequelae of Kawasaki disease in adolescents and young adults. J Am Coll Cardiol 28:253–257

Chaudhari M, Chessa M, Stumper O, Giovanni JV de (2001) Transcatheter coil closure of muscular ventricular septal defects. J Interv Cardiol 14:165–168

Chessa M, Dindar A, Vettukattil JJ et al (2000) Balloon angioplasty in infants with aortic obstruction after the modified stage I Norwood procedure. Am Heart J 140:227–231

Chessa M, Carminati M, Cao QL et al (2002) Transcatheter closure of congenital and acquired muscular ventricular septal defects using the Amplatzer device. J Invasive Cardiol 14:322–327

Connelly MS, Liu PP, Williams WG, et al (1996) Congenitally

corrected transposition of the great arteries in the adult: functional status and complications. J Am Coll Cardiol 27:1238–1243

Conte S, Gewillig M, Eyskens B, Dumoulin M, Daenen W (1999) Management of late complications after classic Fontan procedure by conversion to total cavopulmonary connection. Cardiovasc Surg 7:651–655

Deanfield J, Thaulow E, Warnes C, et al (2003) Task Force on the Management of Grown Up Congenital Heart Disease, European Society of Cardiology; ESC Committee for Practice Guidelines. Management of grown up congenital heart disease. Eur Heart J 24:1035–1084

De Leval MR, Kilner P, Gewillig M, Bull C (1988) Total cavopulmonary connection: a logical alternative to atriopulmonary connection for complex Fontan operations. Experimental studies and early clinical experience. J Thorac Cardiovasc Surg 96:682–695

Derrick GP, Narang I, White PA et al (2000) Failure of stroke volume augmentation during exercise and dobutamine stress is unrelated to load-independent indexes of right ventricular performance after the Mustard operation. Circulation [Suppl 3] 102:154–159

Derrick GP, Josen M, Vogel M, et al (2001) Abnormalities of right ventricular long axis function after atrial repair of transposition of the great arteries. Heart 86:203–206

De Vivie ER, Ruschewski W, Koveker G, et al (1981) Fontan procedure - indication and clinical results. Thorac Cardiovasc Surg 29:348–354

Dodge-Khatami A, Tulevski II, Bennink GB et al (2002) Comparable systemic ventricular function in healthy adults and patients with unoperated congenitally corrected transposition using MRI dobutamine stress testing. Ann Thorac Surg 73:1759–1764

Doty DB, Polansky DB, Jenson CB (1977) Supravalvular aortic stenosis. Repair by extended aortoplasty. J Thorac Cardiovasc Surg 74:362–371

Douard H, Barat JL, Laurent F, et al (1988) Magnetic resonance imaging of an anomalous origin of the left coronary artery from the pulmonary artery. Eur Heart J 9:1356–1360

Durongpisitkul K, Tang NL, Soongswang J, Laohaprasitiporn D, Nanal A (2004) Predictors of successful transcatheter closure of atrial septal defect by cardiac magnetic resonance imaging. Pediatr Cardiol 25:124–130

English RF, Colan SD, Kanani PM, Ettedgui JA (2003) Growth of the aorta in children with Williams syndrome: does surgery make a difference? Pediatr Cardiol 24:566–568

Fischer G, Kramer HH, Stieh J, Harding P, Jung O (1999) Transcatheter closure of secundum atrial septal defects with the new self-centering Amplatzer septal occluder. Eur Heart J 20:541–549

Fischer G, Stieh J, Uebing A, et al (2003) Experience with transcatheter closure of secundum atrial septal defects using the Amplatzer septal occluder: a single centre study in 236 consecutive patients. Heart 89:199–204

Fletcher BD, Jacobstein MD, Nelson AD, Riemenschneider TA, Alfidi RJ (1984) Gated magnetic resonance imaging of congenital cardiac malformations. Radiology 150:137–140

Fogel MA, Rychik J (1998) Right ventricular function in congenital heart disease: pressure and volume overload lesions. Prog Cardiovasc Dis 40:343–356

Fogel MA, Hubbard A, Weinberg PM (2001) A simplified approach for assessment of intracardiac baffles and extracardiac conduits in congenital heart surgery with two- and three-dimensional magnetic resonance imaging. Am Heart J 142:1028–1036

Fogel MA, Hubbard A, Weinberg PM (2002) Mid-term follow-up of patients with transposition of the great arteries after atrial inversion operation using two- and three-dimensional magnetic resonance imaging. Pediatr Radiol 32:440–446

Fontan F, Baudet E (1971) Surgical repair of tricuspid atresia. Thorax 26:240–248

Fujiwara M, Yamada TN, Ono Y, et al (2001) Magnetic resonance imaging of old myocardial infarction in young patients with a history of Kawasaki disease. Clin Cardiol 24:247–252

Gates RN, Laks H, Drinkwater DC Jr et al (1997) The Fontan procedure in adults. Ann Thorac Surg 63:1085–1090

Geva T, Greil GF, Marshall AC, Landzberg M, Powell AJ (2002) Gadolinium-enhanced 3-dimensional magnetic resonance angiography of pulmonary blood supply in patients with complex pulmonary stenosis or atresia: comparison with x-ray angiography. Circulation 106:473–478

Giannoccaro PJ, Sochowski RA, Morton BC, Chan KL (1993) Complementary role of transoesophageal echocardiography to coronary angiography in the assessment of coronary artery anomalies. Br Heart J 70:70–74

Giorgi B, Dymarkowski S, Rademakers FE, Lebrun F, Bogaert J (2002) Single coronary artery as cause of acute myocardial infarction in a 12-year-old girl: a comprehensive approach with MR imaging. AJR Am J Roentgenol 179:1535–1537

Gnanapragasam JP, Houston AB, Northridge DB, Jamieson MP, Pollock JC (1991) Transoesophageal echocardiographic assessment of primum, secundum and sinus venosus atrial septal defects. Int J Cardiol 31:167–174

Greenberg SB, Crisci KL, Koenig P, et al (1997) Magnetic resonance imaging compared with echocardiography in the evaluation of pulmonary artery abnormalities in children with tetralogy of Fallot following palliative and corrective surgery. Pediatr Radiol 27:932–935

Greil GF, Stuber M, Botnar RM, et al (2002) Coronary magnetic resonance angiography in adolescents and young adults with Kawasaki disease. Circulation 105:908–911

British Cardiac Society Working Party (2002) Grown-up congenital heart (GUCH) disease: current needs and provision of service for adolescents and adults with congenital heart disease in the UK. Report of the British Cardiac Society Working Party. Heart (Suppl I) 88:1–14

Grothues F, Smith GC, Moon JC et al (2002) Comparison of interstudy reproducibility of cardiovascular magnetic resonance with two-dimensional echocardiography in normal subjects and in patients with heart failure or left ventricular hypertrophy. Am J Cardiol 90:29–34

Gutberlet M, Boeckel T, Hosten N et al (2000) Arterial switch procedure for D-transposition of the great arteries: quantitative midterm evaluation of hemodynamic changes with cine MR imaging and phase-shift velocity mapping-initial experience. Radiology 214:467–475

Haas F, Wottke M, Poppert H, Meisner H (1999) Long-term survival and functional follow-up in patients after the arterial switch operation. Ann Thorac Surg 68:1692–1697

Hardy CE, Helton GJ, Kondo C, et al (1994) Usefulness of magnetic resonance imaging for evaluating great-vessel anatomy after arterial switch operation for D-transposition of the great arteries. Am Heart J 128:326–332

Hausmann D, Daniel WG, Mugge A, Ziemer G, Pearlman AS (1992a) Value of transesophageal color Doppler echocardiography for detection of different types of atrial septal defect in adults. J Am Soc Echocardiogr 5:481–488

Hausmann D, Mugge A, Becht I, Daniel WG (1992b) Diagnosis of patent foramen ovale by transesophageal echocardiography and association with cerebral and peripheral embolic events. Am J Cardiol 70:668–672

Hegde S, Taylor AM, Miquel M, et al (2004) MRI is a useful tool to detect pulmonary vein compression in patients with Fontan circulation (abstract). Eur Congr Radiol 244:B–531

Helbing WA, Niezen RA, Le Cessie S, et al (1996) Right ventricular diastolic function in children with pulmonary regurgitation after repair of tetralogy of Fallot: volumetric evaluation by magnetic resonance velocity mapping. J Am Coll Cardiol 28:1827–1835

Higgins CB, Byrd BF 3rd, Farmer DW, et al (1984) Magnetic resonance imaging in patients with congenital heart disease. Circulation 70:851–860

Hoffman JI, Kaplan S (2002) The incidence of congenital heart disease. J Am Coll Cardiol 39:1890–1900

Holmqvist C, Hochbergs P, Bjorkhem G, Brockstedt S, Laurin S (2001) Pre-operative evaluation with MR in tetralogy of fallot and pulmonary atresia with ventricular septal defect. Acta Radiol 42:63–69

Hundley WG, Li HF, Hillis LD, Meshack BM et al (1995) Quantitation of cardiac output with velocity-encoded, phase-difference magnetic resonance imaging. Am J Cardiol 75:1250–1255

Ichida,F, Hashimoto I, Miyazaki A et al (1992) Magnetic resonance imaging: evaluation of the Blalock-Taussig shunts and anatomy of the pulmonary artery. J Cardiol 22:669–678

Jacobstein MD, Fletcher BD, Nelson AD, et al (1984) ECG-gated nuclear magnetic resonance imaging: appearance of the congenitally malformed heart. Am Heart J 107:1014–1020

Jatene AD, Fontes VF, Paulista PP et al (1976) Anatomic correction of transposition of the great vessels. J Thorac Cardiovasc Surg 72:364–370

Julsrud PR, Ehman RL, Hagler DJ, Ilstrup DM (1989) Extracardiac vasculature in candidates for Fontan surgery: MR imaging. Radiology 173:503–506

Kang IS, Redington AN, Benson LN et al (2003) Differential regurgitation in branch pulmonary arteries after repair of tetralogy of Fallot: a phase-contrast cine magnetic resonance study. Circulation 107:2938–2943

Kilner PJ, Sievers B, Meyer GP, Ho SY et al (2002) Double-chambered right ventricle or sub-infundibular stenosis assessed by cardiovascular magnetic resonance. J Cardiovasc Magn Reson 4:373–379

Kim YM, Yoo SJ, Choi JY, et al (1999) Natural course of supravalvar aortic stenosis and peripheral pulmonary arterial stenosis in Williams' syndrome. Cardiol Young 9:37–41

Lange A, Walayat M, Turnbull CM et al (1997) Assessment of atrial septal defect morphology by transthoracic three dimensional echocardiography using standard grey scale and Doppler myocardial imaging techniques: comparison with magnetic resonance imaging and intraoperative findings. Heart 78:382–389

Langley SM, Winlaw DS, Stumper O et al (2003) Midterm results after restoration of the morphologically left ventricle to the systemic circulation in patients with congenitally corrected transposition of the great arteries. J Thorac Cardiovasc Surg 125:1229–1241

Laschinger JC, Redmond JM, Cameron DE, Kan JS, Ringel RE (1996) Intermediate results of the extracardiac Fontan procedure. Ann Thorac Surg 62:1261–1267; discussion 1266–1267

Lee VS, Resnick D, Bundy JM, et al (2002) Cardiac function: MR evaluation in one breath hold with real-time true fast imaging with steady-state precession. Radiology 222:835–842

Legendre A, Losay J, Touchot-Kone A et al (2003) Coronary events after arterial switch operation for transposition of the great arteries. Circulation [Suppl 1] 108:186–190

Lillehei CW, Varco RL, Cohen M et al (1986) The first open heart corrections of tetralogy of Fallot. A 26–31 year follow-up of 106 patients. Ann Surg 204:490–502

Lorenz CH, Walker ES, Graham TP Jr, Powers TA (1995) Right ventricular performance and mass by use of cine MRI late after atrial repair of transposition of the great arteries. Circulation 92:233–239

Marshall AC, Love BA, Lang P et al (2003) Staged repair of tetralogy of Fallot and diminutive pulmonary arteries with a fenestrated ventricular septal defect patch. J Thorac Cardiovasc Surg 126:1427–1433

Martinez JE, Mohiaddin RH, Kilner PJ et al (1992) Obstruction in extracardiac ventriculopulmonary conduits: value of nuclear magnetic resonance imaging with velocity mapping and Doppler echocardiography. J Am Coll Cardiol 20:338–344

Masuda M, Kado H, Shiokawa Y et al (1999) Clinical results of arterial switch operation for double-outlet right ventricle with subpulmonary VSD: Eur J Cardiothorac Surg 15:283–288

Mavrogeni S, Papadopoulos G, Douskou M et al (2004) Magnetic resonance angiography is equivalent to X-ray coronary angiography for the evaluation of coronary arteries in Kawasaki disease. J Am Coll Cardiol 43:649–652

McConnell MV, Ganz P, Selwyn AP, et al (1995) Identification of anomalous coronary arteries and their anatomic course by magnetic resonance coronary angiography. Circulation 92:3158–3162

Miquel ME, Hill DL, Baker EJ et al (2003) Three- and four-dimensional reconstruction of intra-cardiac anatomy from two-dimensional magnetic resonance images. Int J Cardiovasc Imaging 19:239–254; discussion 255–256

Mohr JP, Homma S (2003) Patent cardiac foramen ovale: stroke risk and closure. Ann Intern Med 139:787–788

Muthurangu V, Taylor AM, Andriantsimiavona R et al (2004) A novel method of quantifying pulmonary vascular resistance utilizing simultaneous invasive pressure monitoring and phase contrast MR flow. Circulation (in press)

Murthy KS, Rao SG, Naik SK, et al (1999) Evolving surgical management for ventricular septal defect, pulmonary atresia, and major aortopulmonary collateral arteries. Ann Thorac Surg 67:760–764

Mustard WT (1968) Recent experiences with surgical management of transposition of the great arteries. J Cardiovasc Surg (Torino) 9:532–536

Nollert G, Fischlein T, Bouterwek S et al (1997a) Long-term results of total repair of tetralogy of Fallot in adulthood: 35 years follow-up in 104 patients corrected at the age of 18 or older. Thorac Cardiovasc Surg 45:178–181

Nollert G, Fischlein T, Bouterwek S, et al (1997b) Long-term survival in patients with repair of tetralogy of Fallot: 36-year follow-up of 490 survivors of the first year after surgical repair. J Am Coll Cardiol 30:1374–1383

Norwood WI, Kirklin JK, Sanders SP (1980) Hypoplastic left heart syndrome: experience with palliative surgery. Am J Cardiol 45:87–91

Park SC, Neches WH., Zuberbuhler JR, et al (1978) Echocardiographic and hemodynamic correlation in transposition of the great arteries. Circulation 57:291–298

Park YW, Park IS, Kim CH et al (2002) Epidemiologic study of Kawasaki disease in Korea, 1997–1999: comparison with previous studies during 1991–1996. J Korean Med Sci 17:453–456

Pilleul F, Merchant N (2000) MRI of the pulmonary veins: comparison between 3D MR angiography and T1-weighted spin echo. J Comput Assist Tomogr 24:683–687

Pizarro C, Malec E, Maher KO et al (2003) Right ventricle to pulmonary artery conduit improves outcome after stage I Norwood for hypoplastic left heart syndrome. Circulation [Suppl 1] 108:155–160

Plehn JF, Ruggie N, Liebson PR, Messer JV (1988) Visualization of an anomalous left main coronary artery with two-dimensional-echocardiography. Am Heart J 115:468–470

Post JC, Rossum AC van, Bronzwaer JG et al (1995) Magnetic resonance angiography of anomalous coronary arteries. A new gold standard for delineating the proximal course? Circulation 92:3163–3171

Puchalski MD, Brook MM, Silverman NH (2002) Simplified echocardiographic criteria for decision making in perimembranous ventricular septal defect in childhood. Am J Cardiol 90:569–571

Puvaneswary M, Leitch J, Chard RB (2003) MRI of partial anomalous pulmonary venous return (scimitar syndrome): Australas Radiol 47:92–93

Rastelli GC, McGoon DC, Ongley PA, Mankin HT, Kirklin JW (1966) Surgical treatment of supravalvular aortic stenosis. Report of 16 cases and review of literature. J Thorac Cardiovasc Surg 51:873–882

Rastelli GC, McGoon DC, Wallace RB (1969) Anatomic correction of transposition of the great arteries with ventricular septal defect and subpulmonary stenosis. J Thorac Cardiovasc Surg 58:545–552

Razavi R, Baker E (1999) Magnetic resonance imaging comes of age. Cardiol Young 9:529–538

Razavi R, Hill DL, Keevil SF et al (2003a) Cardiac catheterisation guided by MRI in children and adults with congenital heart disease: Lancet 362:1877–1882

Razavi RS, Hill DL, Muthurangu V et al (2003b) Three-dimensional magnetic resonance imaging of congenital cardiac anomalies. Cardiol Young 13:461–465

Razavi R, Miquel M, Baker E (2004) Diagnosis of hemi-truncus arteriosis by three-dimensional magnetic resonance angiography. Circulation 109:E15–E16

Rebergen SA, Chin JG, Ottenkamp J, Wall EE van der, Roos A de (1993) Pulmonary regurgitation in the late postoperative follow-up of tetralogy of Fallot. Volumetric quantitation by nuclear magnetic resonance velocity mapping: Circulation 88:2257–2266

Reddy VM, Petrossian E, McElhinney DB, et al (1997) One-stage complete unifocalization in infants: when should the ventricular septal defect be closed? J Thorac Cardiovasc Surg 113:858–866; discussion 866–868

Rigby ML, Redington AN (1989) Cross-sectional echocardiography. Br Med Bull 45:1036–1060

Sampson C, Kilner PJ, Hirsch R, et al (1994) Venoatrial pathways after the Mustard operation for transposition of the great arteries: anatomic and functional MR imaging. Radiology 193:211–217

Sano S, Ishino K, Kawada M, et al (2000) Staged biventricular repair of pulmonary atresia or stenosis with intact ventricular septum. Ann Thorac Surg 70:1501–1506

Sarkar D, Bull C, Yates R et al (1999) Comparison of long-term outcomes of atrial repair of simple transposition with implications for a late arterial switch strategy. Circulation 100:II176–II181

Seddio F, Reddy VM, McElhinney DB, et al (1999) Multiple ventricular septal defects: how and when should they be repaired? J Thorac Cardiovasc Surg 117:134–139; discussion 39–40

Senning A (1975) Correction of the transposition of the great arteries. Ann Surg 182:287–292

Shellock FG, Shellock VJ (1999) Metallic stents: evaluation of MR imaging safety. AJR Am J Roentgenol 173:543–547

Shimpo H, Hayakawa H, Miyake Y, Takabayashi S, Yada I (2000) Strategy for pulmonary atresia and intact ventricular septum. Ann Thorac Surg 70:287–289

Simpson IA, Valdes-Cruz LM, Berthoty DP (1993) Cine magnetic resonance imaging and color Doppler flow mapping in infants and children with pulmonary artery bands. Am J Cardiol 71:1419–1426

Sivakumar K, Anil SR, Rao SG, Shivaprakash K, Kumar RK (2003) Closure of muscular ventricular septal defects guided by en face reconstruction and pictorial representation. Ann Thorac Surg 76:158–166

Task Force of the European Society of Cardiology/Association of European Paediatric Cardiologists (1998) Eur Heart J 19:19–39

Taylor AJ, Byers JP, Cheitlin MD, Virmani R (1997) Anomalous right or left coronary artery from the contralateral coronary sinus: "high-risk" abnormalities in the initial coronary artery course and heterogeneous clinical outcomes. Am Heart J 133:428–435

Taylor AM, Stables RH, Poole-Wilson PA, Pennell DJ (1999) Definitive clinical assessment of atrial septal defect by magnetic resonance imaging. J Cardiovasc Magn Reson 1:43–47

Taylor AM, Thorne SA, Rubens MB et al (2000) Coronary artery imaging in congenital heart disease: complementary role of magnetic resonance and X-ray coronary angiography. Circulation 101:1670–1678

Taylor AM, Muthurangu V, Hegde SR, et al (2004a) Magnetic resonance imaging for hypoplastic left heart syndrome following the Norwood stage 1 operation (abstract). J Cardiovasc Magn Reson 6:407

Taylor AM, Dymarkowski S, Hamaekers P et al (2004b) Magnetic resonance coronary angiography and late-enhancement myocardial imaging in children with arterial switch operation for transposition of the great arteries. Radiology (in press)

Thanopoulos BD, Karanassios E, Tsaousis G, Papadopoulos GS, Stefanadis C (2003a) Catheter closure of congenital/acquired muscular VSDs and perimembranous VSDs using the Amplatzer devices. J Interv Cardiol 16:399–407

Thanopoulos BD, Tsaousis GS, Karanasios E, Eleftherakis NG, Paphitis C (2003b) Transcatheter closure of perimembranous ventricular septal defects with the Amplatzer asymmetric ventricular septal defect occluder: preliminary experience in children. Heart 89:918–922

Thomson JD, Gibbs JL, Doorn C van (2000) Cardiac catheter guided surgical closure of an apical ventricular septal defect. Ann Thorac Surg 70:1402–1404

Tulevski II, Lee PL, Groenink M et al (2000) Dobutamine-induced increase of right ventricular contractility without increased stroke volume in adolescent patients with transposition of the great arteries: evaluation with magnetic resonance imaging. Int J Card Imaging 16:471–478

Tulevski II, Wall EE van der, Groenink M et al (2002) Usefulness of magnetic resonance imaging dobutamine stress in asymptomatic and minimally symptomatic patients with decreased cardiac reserve from congenital heart disease (complete and corrected transposition of the great arteries and subpulmonic obstruction). Am J Cardiol 89:1077–1081

Tworetzky W, McElhinney DB, Brook MM, et al (1999) Echocardiographic diagnosis alone for the complete repair of major congenital heart defects. J Am Coll Cardiol 33:228–233

Tynan MJ, Becker AE, Macartney FJ, et al (1979) Nomenclature and classification of congenital heart disease. Br Heart J 41:544–553

Vincent RN, Porter AG, Tam VK, Kanter KR (2000) Diagnosis and catheter treatment of innominate artery stenosis following stage I Norwood procedure. Catheter Cardiovasc Interv 49:415–418

Vliegen HW, Straten A van, Roos A de, et al (2002) Magnetic resonance imaging to assess the hemodynamic effects of pulmonary valve replacement in adults late after repair of tetralogy of fallot. Circulation 106:1703–1707

Wessel A, Pankau R, Kececioglu D, Ruschewski W, Bursch JH (1994) Three decades of follow-up of aortic and pulmonary vascular lesions in the Williams-Beuren syndrome. Am J Med Genet 52:297–301

Williams JC, Barratt-Boyes BG, Lowe JB (1961) Supravalvular aortic stenosis. Circulation 24:1311–1318

Wu Q, Yu Q, Yang X (2003) Modified Rastelli procedure for double outlet right ventricle with left-malposition of the great arteries: report of 9 cases. Ann Thorac Surg 75:138–142

16 Imaging of Great Vessels

Sanjeet R. Hegde, Reza Razavi, Jan Bogaert, and Andrew M. Taylor

S. R. Hegde, MD
Division of Imaging Science, King's College London, Guy's Hospital Campus, London Bridge, London SE1 9RT, UK
R. Razavi, MBBS, MRCP, MRCPCH
Division of Imaging Science, King's College London, Guy's Hospital Campus, London Bridge, London SE1 9RT, UK
J. Bogaert MD, PhD
Department of Radiology, Gasthuisberg University Hospital, Catholic University of Leuven, Herestraat 49, 3000 Leuven, Belgium
A.M. Taylor MD, MRCP, FRCR
Cardiothoracic Unit, Institute of Child Health and Great Ormond Street Hospital for Children, London WC1N 3JH, UK

16.1 Introduction

In an era where there is a quest for an imaging modality that is noninvasive, has multi-planar capability, and does not use ionizing radiation, magnetic resonance imaging (MRI) has established itself as a powerful imaging tool (Pettigrew et al. 1999). Faster gradients have resulted in shorter repetition times, thereby increasing the acquisition speed of MRI. Newer pulse sequences and ultrafast MR angiography techniques have pushed the field even further (Lardo 2000). MRI is therefore fast becoming the modality of choice for imaging the pathological entities that affect the great vessels (Marchal and Bogaert 1998).

Conventional ECG gated spin-echo (SE) imaging and cine gradient-echo (GE) techniques have earned MRI the reputation of being the ideal tool for evaluating the great vessels of the chest, in particular the aorta (Hartnell et al. 1994; Amparo et al. 1985; Nienaber et al. 1993). The lack of signal from blood on "black-blood" SE pulse sequences or enhanced signal intensity from blood on "bright-blood" GE sequences provides a high natural contrast between intracardiac/intravascular blood pools and the surrounding cardiac and vascular structures. However, motion artifacts due to the pulsatile nature of flowing blood and respiratory motion, in combination with poor vessel-to-background contrast, in patients with reduced cardiac function, have been perceived as limiting factors for cardiovascular MR. More recently, this perception has changed with the advent of turbo-SE (TSE) or fast-SE imaging (Simonetti et al. 1996), MR angiography, especially contrast-enhanced 3D MR angiography (Prince et al. 1993), and bright-blood balanced steady-state free precession imaging (b-SSFP) techniques (Oppelt et al. 1986; Scheffler and Lehnhardt 2003).

Contrast-enhanced (CE) 3D MR angiography allows rapid acquisition and multi-planar imaging with minimal dephasing artifacts (Hartnell et al. 1995). This technique is diagnostic and provides accurate assessment of the great vessels based on data acquired in a comfortable breath-hold interval without the need for ECG gating (LEUNG and DEBATIN 1997). b-SSFP cine imaging (CARR et al. 2001) and 3D b-SSFP volume acquisition techniques (RAZAVI et al. 2003) are also extremely useful for morphological and functional evaluation of congenital heart disease. Phase-contrast imaging is another technique that has broken new ground, enabling the evaluation of flow in the great vessels with accurate quantification of peak velocity, and forward and regurgitant flow (NAYLER et al. 1986; MARKL et al. 2003b).

MRI of pulmonary arteries, pulmonary veins (PVs), and systemic veins can also now be performed to diagnostic standards (HERNANDEZ 2002; POWELL et al. 2000; VOGT et al. 2003). Faster and stronger gradients and more complex pulse sequences allow dedicated cardiovascular MR examinations with detailed morphological imaging and information on flow and function that can be applied to pre- and postoperative evaluation of congenital heart diseases (HIGGINS and CAPUTO 1993; CHUNG 2000; VAN DER WALL et al. 1997).

Finally, an important research tool in great vessel imaging is the study of the arterial wall and the characterization of atheromatous plaque formation (FAYAD 2003). MRI combines high spatial-resolution imaging (less than 500 µm) with unrivalled spatial resolution. Using a combination of MR sequences, the different components of the plaques can be mapped. Contrast agents with high affinity for certain plaque components are utilized to study the plaque vulnerability, and, because of its noninvasive nature, MRI is the ideal technique to follow up the plaque evolution under therapy.

16.2
MRI Techniques

16.2.1
Balanced Steady-State Free Precession Imaging

b-SSFP is a recently developed, T2-weighted GE technique that is now widely used for cine imaging of the heart (OPPELT et al. 1986; CARR et al. 2001). It is an exciting new technique that provides excellent contrast between blood and surrounding tissue without the use of contrast agents. Contrast to noise depends on T2/T1 differences, which, at

short repetition times (TR), are high for blood and soft tissues. A prerequisite for artifact-free b-SSFP imaging is a short TR; thus b-SSFP sequences can only be successfully performed on scanners with high-performance gradients. The typical TR is 2.8 ms, with an echo time (TE) of 1.4 ms and flip-angles between 50 and 60°. b-SSFP can be implemented as either a single-shot or cine technique for imaging the thoracic aorta (PERELES et al. 2001).

The single-shot technique is an ECG-triggered, two-dimensional (2D) acquisition and is essentially independent of respiratory motion artifact. Imaging can therefore be successfully carried out without breath-holding, which is particularly advantageous in critically ill patients. Often a trigger delay of 400–600 ms can be used to push the acquisition further into diastole, adjusted to the RR interval. Cine b-SSFP is a breath-hold ECG-triggered segmented κ-space acquisition technique with an average imaging time of 7–9 s/slice. These cine images can be acquired at selected anatomical levels and orientations. A sagittal oblique image through the upper chest is particularly useful for demonstrating the aortic arch (CARR and FINN 2003) (Fig. 16.1).

An alternative cine technique in patients who cannot hold their breath is real-time b-SSFP, as it does not require breath-holding or ECG triggering (LEE et al. 2002) (see Fig. 17.10). Diagnostic images of the thoracic aorta and aortic valve can usually be obtained at reduced spatial and temporal resolution. 3D b-SSFP volume scans can also be acquired using a multi-chunk, multi-breath-hold, multi-phase technique. TR is typically is 3–4.5 ms, TE is approx. 1.5–2 ms, with a flip angle of 40–50° and an image matrix of approximately 160 pixels by 256 pixels. The volume is acquired in multiple phases of the cardiac cycle and the scan divided into 8–14 smaller chunks with each chunk acquired as a single breath-hold of 10–20 s. The scan is acquired in the axial plane and therefore requires no complex planning. High-resolution images are reconstructed from the raw data, with a resolution of 1.3×1.3×1 mm in any image plane (see Fig. 17.9). To prevent misalignment of volumes in nonventilated patients, respiratory navigator techniques can be used (RAZAVI et al. 2003).

A new technique under development is phase-contrast steady-state free precession (PC-SSFP), which provides unbiased velocity measurement with high signal-to-noise ratio (SNR) at short TRs by using a refocused b-SSFP pulse sequence (MARKL et al. 2003a).

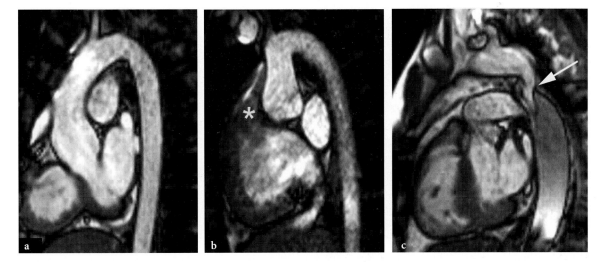

Fig. 16.1a-c. Oblique sagittal balanced steady-state free precession images through the aorta: **a** normal aorta; **b** normal aortic anatomy in transposition of great arteries after arterial switch operation. The anterior pulmonary trunk is labeled (*asterisk*); **c** turbulent streaming of flow through a tortuous coarctation repair (*arrow*)

16.2.2
Black-Blood Imaging

Black-blood pulse sequences remain an essential component of aortic imaging for evaluation of mural disease and of the mediastinum (STEMERMAN et al. 1999).

ECG-triggered, breath-hold, black-blood TSE has been the cornerstone of black-blood MRI for aortic disease (SIMONETTI et al. 1996). A double inversion-recovery technique is used to null the blood signal. The first 180° inversion-recovery pulse is non-slice-selective and occurs at the R-wave trigger and inverts the magnetization in the entire tissue volume. A slice-selective 180° pulse follows, which restores magnetization in the slice to be imaged. The black-blood appearance is the result of nulling of the blood flowing into the slice by the first 180° inversion pulse at a specific inversion time (TI). A TSE readout (series of 180° pulses) is then used to acquire κ-space lines in a segmented fashion, with the center of κ-space acquired at the TI. Imaging occurs during mid to late diastole and the entire image is acquired over several heartbeats (CARR and FINN 2003). Typical imaging parameters are; TR RR interval, TE 80 ms, flip angle 90°, slice thickness 6 mm, number of signal averages 3–4, matrix 256×256 (Fig. 16.2).

ECG-triggered, black-blood, half-Fourier acquisition single-shot TSE (HASTE) uses a black-blood preparation to null signal from blood (STEHLING et al. 1996) and allows acquisition of an entire image in a single heartbeat; particularly useful in patients who cannot hold their breath (CARR and FINN 2003).

16.2.3
Magnetic Resonance Angiography

Magnetic resonance angiography is fast emerging as a valuable technique for imaging vascular disease as a result of significant improvement in acquisition strategies (KRINSKY et al. 1997; MASUI et al. 2000) and MR contrast agents (GOYEN et al. 2000). It is now widely regarded as an accurate, noninvasive alternative for the diagnostic evaluation of intrathoracic vessels (LEUNG and DEBATIN 1997; DYMARKOWSKI et al. 1999; RAZAVI and BAKER 1999).

However, when imaging the great vessels, it is essential to use more than one imaging sequence. In particular, if only MR angiography is used important pathology will be missed. In our own practice, MR angiography and at least one other sequence are performed (usually a black-blood TSE sequence), to ensure that a complete assessment has been performed.

16.2.3.1
Contrast-Enhanced MR Angiography

CE MR angiography (CE-MRA) is the most widely accepted method for comprehensive evaluation of the thoracic aorta (ARPASI et al. 2000). Conventional CE-MRA provides good spatial resolution and therefore is suitable for the depiction of abnormalities such as penetrating atherosclerotic ulcers, dissection, coarctation, and aneurysm (Table 16.1). It is less useful for assessing the ascending thoracic aorta, which is affected by motion artifact from

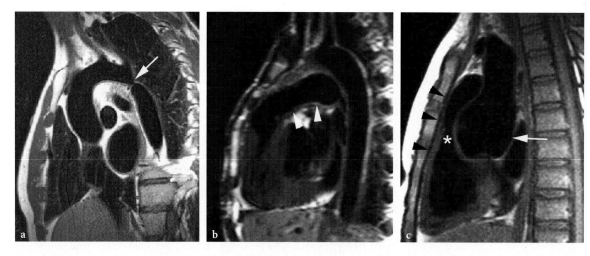

Fig. 16.2a-c. Turbo-spin-echo "black-blood" images. **a** Oblique sagittal image through the aorta showing a coarctation membrane (*arrow*). It was possible to pass a guide wire through the membrane and perform balloon angioplasty to dilate the lesion. **b** Sagittal image through the pulmonary trunk after insertion of percutaneous pulmonary valve stent for pulmonary homograft stenosis. The stent is widely patent, and the proximal and distal ends of the stent can be seen on the inferior aspect of the pulmonary trunk wall (*arrowheads*). **c** Oblique sagittal view through an aortic root dilatation (*arrow*) in a patient with transposition of the great arteries and the arterial switch operation. The aortic root dilatation is secondary to severe neoaortic valve incompetence, and compressed the anterior pulmonary trunk (*asterisk*) against the posterior sternum (*black arrowheads*)

Table 16.1. Indications for contrast-enhanced MR angiography

Aortic aneurysm
Aortic dissection
Congenital anomalies of great vessels
Vasculitis evaluation
Central thoracic veins
Pulmonary artery anatomy
Postsurgical follow-up
Contraindications to computed tomography

cardiac pulsation or obscured by overlapping vascular structures. This region is better evaluated on the time-resolved CE-MRA, which is essentially free from motion artifact.

The basic pulse sequence for conventional CE-MRA is a standard 3D GE acquisition (PRINCE et al. 1996), with typical TR of 4.5 ms, TE 1.5 ms, flip-angle 40°, slice thickness 0.6–1.2 mm, and matrix 240×512. By using a gadolinium chelate contrast agent (0.2 ml/kg) the T1 (longitudinal relaxation) of blood is shortened so that the blood appears bright irrespective of flow patterns or velocities (PRINCE 1994).

As the time between intravenous injection and the arrival of the contrast bolus in the vessel can vary between different patients, and even within a single patient, the correct timing of imaging is important to ensure synchronization between the transit of contrast material and scanning (FRANCOIS

et al. 2003). The "bolus-track" (real-time method for fluoroscopic triggering of the arrival of contrast agent) technique is now recognized as the optimal solution, with reliability of 98.5% for bolus detection (RIEDERER et al. 2000) (Fig. 16.3). Other timing methods commonly used include using a test bolus (EARLS et al. 1996) and moving-table MRA (HO et al. 1999). An automated bolus detection algorithm has also been developed for optimization of gadolinium-enhanced MRA (HO and FOO 1998).

Using bolus-track, the 3D MRA scan is synchronized to the arterial arrival of an intravenously injected bolus of contrast agent by means of a 2D fluoroscopic preview scan which displays the bolus arrival in real time. Using a suitable MR-compatible injector, 20–40 ml of gadolinium (0.2–0.4 ml/kg) is injected at 2–4 ml/s by way of a cannula placed in the right antecubital vein. The bolus-track technique should be combined with a centric-order, phase-encode MRA sequence, such that low-frequency phase-encode steps that encode for bulk contrast are acquired first, and higher-frequency phase-encode steps that encode for edge definition are acquired at the end of the sequence. Not only does this enable high contrast to be ensured, but also, if the patient is unable to maintain the breath-hold for the entire scan duration, image blurring should be kept to a minimum. Thus, with a centric-ordered phase-encode MRA sequence, the scan is triggered when the contrast is seen to arrive in the vessel that needs

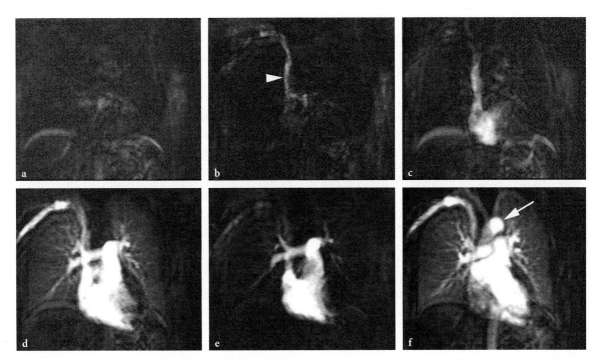

Fig. 16.3a-f. Selected coronal 2D "bolus-track" images from a 20-s (20-image) sequence. **a** Image before gadolinium contrast administration; **b** contrast arriving in the superior vena cava (*arrowhead*); **c** contrast in the right atrium; **d** contrast in the pulmonary trunk (trigger MR pulmonary angiogram at this time point); **e** contrast passing through the pulmonary parenchyma; **f** contrast reaching the aortic arch (*arrow*) (trigger MR aortic angiogram at this time point)

Fig. 16.4a-d. Triggers for pulmonary (**a**) and aortic (**b**) MR angiograms. Coronal pulmonary (**c**) and systemic (**d**) arterial maximum-intensity projection images viewed from anterior

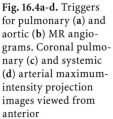

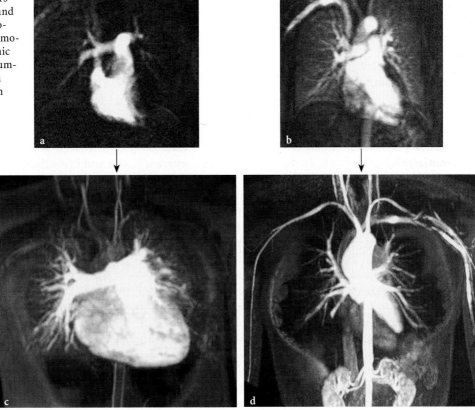

imaging (Fig. 16.4). It should be noted that, on most scanners, there is a small delay when switching from the 2D bolus track sequence to the MRA sequence, and this should be taken into account for optimal MRA imaging.

It is difficult to use the bolus-track technique in combination with a conventional κ-space filling algorithm, as the imager needs to predict when the contrast will arrive at the vessel of choice (half the MRA sequence acquisition time), such that the center of κ-space coincides with the peak signal intensity of contrast arrival.

With newer scanner hardware, MRA images can be acquired in approximately 10–14 s (using parallel imaging techniques; see Chap. 1), and thus multiple MR angiograms can be acquired in a single, 20-s breath-hold. In our own experience, this enables the acquisition of an optimal pulmonary MRA (triggered as contrast enters the main pulmonary artery), and an optimal aortic MRA, which is acquired after the transit of contrast through the pulmonary vasculature.

Postprocessing algorithms (e.g., maximum-intensity projection, MIP) can be used to create 3D images, though these should be interpreted in conjunction with the raw data. Additional postprocessing by way of surface and volume rendering and curved multi-planar reformation provide very useful images that help to delineate and better understand complex vascular anatomy (Fig. 16.5).

16.2.3.2
Time-Resolved Contrast-Enhanced MR Angiography

A 3D MR angiogram with sub-second temporal resolution is now possible due to shorter TRs from recent advances in gradient strength. This is advantageous in the thoracic aorta, where high temporal resolution is useful for evaluating high-flow vascular abnormalities such as dissections and shunts, and also in evaluating patients with aortic stent-graft endoleaks (KOROSEC et al. 1996; FINN et al. 2002). The need for contrast bolus timing is eliminated.

The pulse sequence is similar to a conventional CE-MRA (3D GE acquisition with typical TR 1.6 ms and TE 0.8 ms), but asymmetric κ-space scanning in all three axes, view sharing, temporal interpolation, and zero filling are all used to further shorten the acquisition time (VOGT et al. 2003). The rapid frame rates mean there is no appreciable reduction in image quality in patients who cannot hold their breath for very long and hence this scanning method

is suitable for scanning critically ill patients (CARR and FINN 2003).

16.2.3.3
Phase-Contrast MR Angiography

Phase-contrast MR angiography (PC-MRA) is based on the principle that changes in the phase of flowing spins along a magnetic gradient, relative to stationary spins, are proportional to the velocity of flow. By applying magnetic field, gradients of opposite polarity phase shifts for moving spins are generated. The sequence can be either ECG triggered or retrospectively gated. It is important that the 2D slice is oriented perpendicular to the vessel of interest and that the region of interest is positioned in the center of the magnetic field to avoid artifact from eddy currents. The velocity-encoding (VENC) value controls the amplitude of the magnetic gradient and is typically 100–200 cm/s for normal aortic and main pulmonary artery flow. If the VENC is too low, aliasing will occur, resulting in mismapping or signal dropout from the center of the lumen. Two images are reconstructed; the "magnitude" image that provides anatomical information, and the velocity map that is derived from the phase data that provides flow velocity information. PC-MRA is useful when CE-MRA shows an aortic narrowing or when an aortic valve stenosis is suspected, and for measuring through-plane flow for quantification of valvular regurgitation (see Chap. 13.3.2) and quantification of collateral flow in aortic coarctation.

From the PC-MRA data, peak velocity, regurgitant flow, and forward flow can be calculated, as every pixel in the phase image is linearly related to the velocity. The analysis of curve shape and slope can also help determine whether stenoses are significant (CARR and FINN 2003). However, image artifacts from complex flow patterns, including slow flow, re-circulation zone, and pulsatile flow, can adversely affect accuracy of results (FATOURAEE and AMINI 2003).

16.3
Other Imaging Techniques

Conventional X-ray angiography has traditionally been the gold standard for imaging great vessels, but the lack of multi-planar capability and use of ionizing radiation are major drawbacks. Computed tomography (CT) is quick, has multi-planar capa-

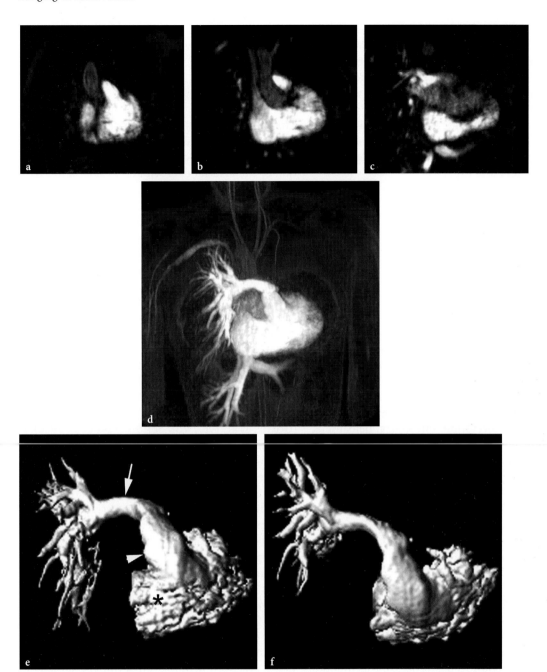

Fig. 16.5a-f. Reconstruction of MR angiographic data. **a-c** Selected coronal pulmonary MR angiography raw data (3 of 64 images). **d** Maximum-intensity projection (MIP) reconstruction of all the MR raw data viewed from anterior. **e, f** Volume-rendered 3D reconstruction of the right ventricle (*star*), pulmonary trunk (*arrowhead*), and right pulmonary artery (*arrow*): **e** anterior view, and **f** superior right anterior oblique view

bility with good diagnostic accuracy, and is readily available in most hospitals; but, like X-ray angiography, it employs ionizing radiation and potentially nephrotoxic contrast agents. Transesophageal echocardiography (TEE) is relatively invasive, with limited coverage of large vessels and greater operator dependence, but its bedside availability is a redeeming feature. In general, the image modality of choice for assessing great vessel pathology will depend on local availability and expertise.

16.4
Disease of the Great Vessels

16.4.1
Aorta

The noninvasive and multi-planar nature of MRI is well suited for evaluation of congenital cardiovascular malformations of the aorta, which include coarctation and vascular rings (Table 16.2). MRI is now also recommended for the evaluation of the acquired anomalies of the aorta, including dissection, aneurysm, ulceration, intramural hematoma, and trauma.

Table 16.2. Aortic arch anomalies

Right aortic arch
• Aberrant left subclavian artery
• Mirror-image branching
• Isolated left subclavian artery
Left aortic arch
• Aberrant right subclavian artery
• Right descending aorta
Double aortic arch
Cervical aortic arch

All of these conditions are best assessed using CE-MRA (CARR and FINN 2003; SOLER et al. 1998; BOGAERT et al. 2000). 3D postprocessing techniques can be used to great effect, allowing the abnormalities to be viewed from different orientations. However, as stressed above, 3D MRA should be combined with at least one other MRI sequence of the same area. This is particularly important when assessing aortic dissection and aortic trauma. Thus, CE-MRA is usually preceded by 3D b-SSFP volume scans and/or black-blood TSE imaging in the axial and sagittal oblique planes. Cine imaging of the heart should always accompany an assessment for congenital abnormalities of the aorta, to detect accompanying lesions in the heart (HIGGINS and SAKUMA 1996).

16.4.1.1
Congenital Anomalies of the Aorta

16.4.1.1.1
Aortic Coarctation

Coarctation accounts for 6–8% of live births with congenital heart disease and refers to an area of narrowing of the thoracic aorta in the region of insertion of the arterial duct with or without additional abnormalities of the aortic arch (BRIERLEY et al. 2001).

Coarctation was believed to be a simple, surgically correctable lesion since the first operative correction in 1944 (CRAFOORD 1980), but, more recently, studies have shown that a third of patients remain or become hypertensive despite corrective surgery. There is also an increased risk of atherosclerosis and end-organ damage, with recoarctation occurring in 3–35% of patients (ROOS-HESSELINK et al. 2003; DIETL et al. 1992).

Angiography has been the gold standard for diagnosis of coarctation, but MRI has been shown to be diagnostic and well suited for both pre- and postoperative evaluation of aortic coarctation (Fig. 16.6) (GOMES et al. 1987; VON SCHULTHESS et al. 1986). It is crucial for management decisions to establish the location and degree of stenosis, length of coarctation segment, associated aortic arch involvement (such as tubular hypoplasia), the collateral pathways (internal mammary and posterior mediastinal arteries), relationship to aberrant subclavian artery, poststenotic dilatation, and left ventricular (LV) hypertrophy.

SE imaging in the sagittal and oblique-sagittal planes provides excellent information of stenotic areas and even collateral pathways (HOLMQVIST et al. 2002). 3D CE-MRA can display the severity and extent of involvement without spin dephasing artifacts and partial volume errors (DEBATIN and HANY 1998). MR flow mapping can define the severity of the stenosis by measuring velocity jets at the level of coarctation (MOHIADDIN et al. 1993; FATTORI and NIENABER 1999). On cine GE images, the stenotic jets appear as an area of signal dropout; this is less marked with b-SSFP sequences with short echo times (TE). However, in tortuous coarctation segments, estimation of the velocity may be difficult. An estimation of the collateral circulation can also be carried out by measuring flow (HOLMQVIST et al. 2002) in the proximal and descending aorta (SZOLAR et al. 1996). Reassessment of collateral flow following treatment can be used to assess the

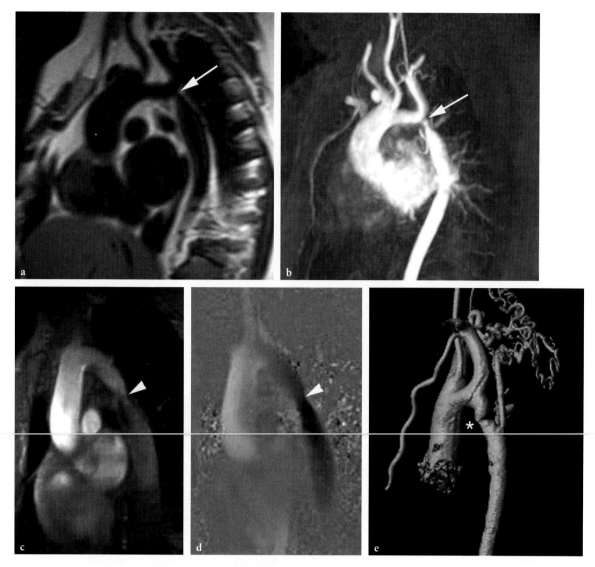

Fig. 16.6a-e. MRI of aortic coarctation. Images from various subjects. **a** Black-blood turbo-spin-echo oblique sagittal image through the aorta showing a tight discrete aortic coarctation at the aortic isthmus (*arrow*). **b** Maximum-intensity projection image from gadolinium MR angiography, showing the coarctation in the same subject. **c, d** Magnitude (**c**) and velocity map (**d**) images of a more distal moderate coarctation (*arrowhead*) – different subject to **a** and **b**. **e** Volume-rendered 3D reconstruction of contrast-enhanced MR angiography data in a third subject, showing severe coarctation (*asterisk*) and multiple collateral vessels

success of the treatment option (ARAOZ et al. 2003) (Fig. 16.7).

MRI can also be used to assess secondary pathology in patients with coarctation, including: assessment of the aortic root for dilatation secondary to a bicuspid aortic valve – frequency in coarctation of 15% (ROOS-HESSELINK et al. 2003); assessment of aortic incompetence and aortic stenosis (see Chap. 13 Valvular Heart Disease); and an assessment of ventricular function and LV mass (an indirect indicator of increased LV afterload secondary to either the coarctation obstruction itself or associated hypertension).

Discrete, localized stenoses are generally thought to be amenable to balloon dilatation, whereas long transverse arch or isthmal tubular stenoses are typically referred for surgical repair. High-resolution MRI of the aortic arch therefore may help define the most appropriate treatment algorithm. MRI is very useful for noninvasive follow-up after surgical repair (BOGAERT et al. 2000, 2001), in particular in the evaluation of recoarctation, residual stenosis,

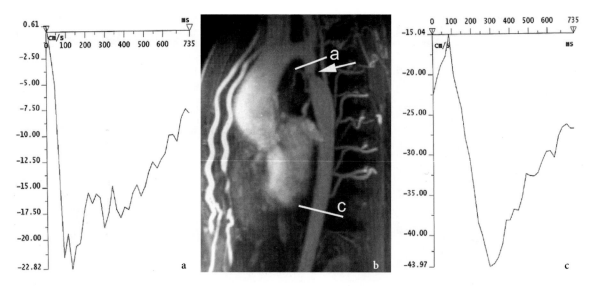

Fig. 16.7a-c. Collateral flow assessment in aortic coarctation. Flow is measured just prior to the coarctation (**a**) and in the descending aorta at the level of the diaphragm (**c**). Planes prescribed from an oblique sagittal maximum-intensity projection image from a contrast-enhanced MR angiogram (**b**). The coarctation is in the usual position (*arrow*). Flow in **c** is higher than that in **a**, indicating extensive collateral flow to the descending aorta, and a significant coarctation. The "saw-toothed" appearance to flow in **a** is quite typical. This method is best used for follow-up of treated aorta coarctation to assess the success (reduced collateral flow) in individual subjects

persistence of aortic arch hypoplasia (Fig. 16.8), and false aneurysm at the level of repair (Fig. 16.9) (Bogaert et al. 1995; Kaemmerer et al. 1993).

16.4.1.1.2
Interrupted Aortic Arch

A structural discontinuity between the ascending and descending aorta is described as an interrupted aortic arch. The site of interruption relative to the brachiocephalic arteries is the basis of classification (Table 16.3).

The site and length of interruption and any associated anomalies can be demonstrated well by MRI. 3D CE-MRA is the most useful technique (Roche et al. 1999). SE imaging in the sagittal and oblique-sagittal planes provides additional useful information (Fig. 16.10).

16.4.1.1.3
Anomalies of the Aortic Arch

Embryologically, the left aortic arch persists and right arch involutes except the proximal segment, which forms the proximal right subclavian artery (Edwards 1948). Any deviation from this developmental process will result in various arch anomalies. Understanding of double-arch anatomy and the various potential anomalies that can occur is

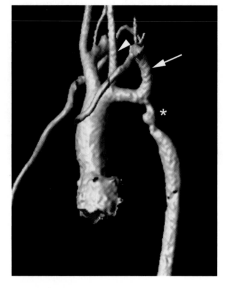

Fig. 16.8. Volume-rendered 3D reconstruction from contrast-enhanced MR angiogram of severe complex recoarctation (sagittal view), after a previous end-to-end anastomosis. This is further complicated by a hypoplastic arch between the origin of the left common carotid (*arrowhead*) and left subclavian (*arrow*) arteries

based on Edward's embryonic hypothetical double aortic arch schema (Fig. 16.11). This model should be borne in mind when considering congenital anomalies of the aortic arch, as atretic segments may persist (including right and left arterial ducts),

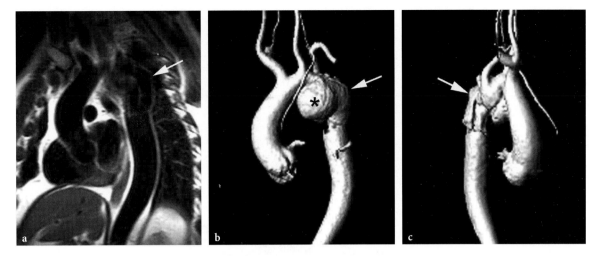

Fig. 16.9a-c. Large proximal descending aorta pseudoaneurysm, complicating a previous end-to-end coarctation repair. **a** Black-blood turbo-spin-echo oblique sagittal view through the aorta, showing a complex lesion at the site of previous surgery. The 3D nature of the lesion is difficult to appreciate completely on this 2D image. **b, c** Volume-rendered 3D reconstruction from contrast-enhanced-MR angiography, showing a large pseudoaneurysm, which is compressing the posterior aorta, to create a narrow posterior channel (*white arrows*). This can now be appreciated on the black-blood image in **a**

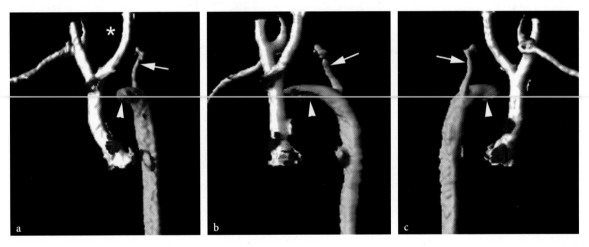

Fig. 16.10a-c. Interrupted aortic arch. Volume-rendered 3D reconstruction from contrast-enhanced-MR angiography of a type-B aortic arch interruption between the left common carotid (*star*) and the left subclavian arteries (*arrow*). The left subclavian artery and the descending aorta (*pale blue*) are supplied via the patent arterial duct (*arrowhead*, pulmonary circulation not shown). The ascending aorta is shown in *white*. The first branch is the innominate artery

Table 16.3. Classification of interrupted aortic arch (VAN PRAAGH et al. 1971)

Type A (44%)
- Discontinuity of the aortic arch distal to the left subclavian artery

Type B (55%)
- Discontinuity between the left subclavian and the left common carotid arteries

Type C (5%)
- Interruption between the left common carotid and the innominate arteries

which may not be visualized on imaging, and which may have the potential to cause complete vascular rings (Table 16.4).

Imaging with MR is considered to be the modality of choice for identifying arch anomalies (KERSTING-SOMMERHOFF et al. 1987a). SE imaging in axial, coronal, and oblique sagittal planes followed by 3D CE-MRA provides comprehensive and adequate information to make a diagnosis. Newer techniques such as 3D b-SSFP volume imaging are also being shown to be very useful. However, careful consideration needs to be made about the need for assessing

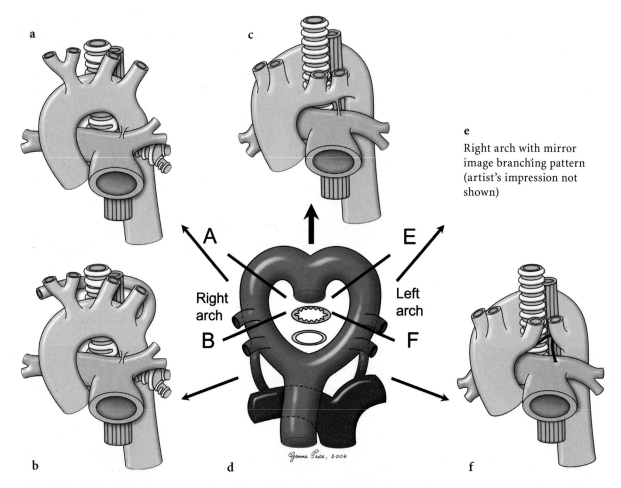

e

Right arch with mirror
image branching pattern
(artist's impression not
shown)

Fig 16.11 a-e. d A schematic representation of Edward's hypothetical double aortic arch, showing right and left aortic arches and bilateral arterial ducts. Image (**c**) shows an artist's impression of a double arch with the ringed trachea and striated esophagus within the vascular ring. Division of the double arch along the line *A* gives (**a**), an artist's impression of a normal left-sided arch; ringed trachea and striated esophagus posteriorly. Division of the double arch along the line *B* gives (**b**), artist's impression of left aortic arch with aberrant, retro-esophageal right subclavian artery. Division along the line *E*, would give a right-sided aortic arch, with mirror image branching; artist's impression not shown. Division along the line *F* gives (**f**), an artist's impression of a right arch with aberrant retro-esophageal left subclavian artery. In the artist's impression shown, the descending thoracic aorta is retroesophageal and the black lines represent potential complete vascular rings of an atretic left arch (*superior line*) and a fibrotic left arterial duct (*inferior line*). [All images reproduced with permission of Professor Robert H Anderson, Dr. Andrew C Cook and Gemma Price, Cardiac Unit, Institute of Child Health, who also retain full copyright.]'

the main airways in children with suspected arch anomalies. If airway imaging is important, we currently use spiral CT angiography through the chest, in combination with dynamic contrast bronchography. The appropriately windowed images of the airways currently give more reliable airway definition than MR in our experience (Fig. 16.12).

In double aortic arch, the right arch is usually larger than the left, which may be atretic or hypoplastic (Fig. 16.13). This, along with the ascending aorta, can result in the formation of a vascular ring, which may compress the trachea and esopha-

gus. The arterial duct is usually left sided, but can be right sided or even bilateral and worsen the degree of compression on the trachea and esophagus. Often the atretic fibrous left arch will not be visualized on the MR images; however, the overall configuration of the arch will be suggestive of a double-aortic arch. The surgeon can thus be asked to operate with a high degree of certainty, identifying and transecting the fibrous connection at operation, with immediate relief of the vascular ring. When two arches are not clearly seen, a high degree of suspicion for a vascular ring with an atretic seg-

Table 16.4. Vascular rings

Usually symptomatic lesions
1. Double aortic arch
2. Right aortic arch with right descending aorta + aberrant left subclavian artery + persistent left arterial duct
3. Left aortic arch with right descending aorta + right arterial ductus
4. Left pulmonary artery sling

Occasionally symptomatic
1. Anomalous right innominate artery
2. Anomalous left common carotid artery
3. Right aortic arch with left descending aorta + left ductus

Usually asymptomatic
1. Left aortic arch + aberrant right subclavian artery
2. Left aortic arch with right descending aorta
3. Right aortic arch with right descending aorta + mirror-image branching
4. Right aortic arch with right descending aorta + left aberrant subclavian artery
5. Right aortic arch with right descending aorta + isolation of left subclavian artery

ment of aorta should be considered in symptomatic subjects if there is:

1. A Kommerel's diverticulum: this represents the distal remnant of the second, non-patent arch (Fig. 16.14)
2. The proximal descending aorta has a retroesophageal course: a right arch with a left-sided proximal descending aorta, or a left arch with a right-sided proximal descending aorta (Fig. 16.15)

In our own experience, the two are usually seen in association (Figs. 16.14 and 16.15).

It should also be borne in mind that there may in fact be two vascular rings in the same patient. Thus, in the case of a left aortic arch, retroesophageal proximal descending aorta, Kommerel's diverticulum, and right descending aorta (Fig. 16.15), there is potentially an atretic right arch, completing one ring, and a fibrotic right arterial duct, completing a second ring (see Fig. 16.16).

Two further potential vascular rings can occur: the left pulmonary artery sling (see Sect. 16.4.2), and a right aortic arch, aberrant left subclavian artery, connected to the fibrosed left arterial duct.

A right-side aortic arch can have either a mirror-image branching pattern, which, in isolation, is not

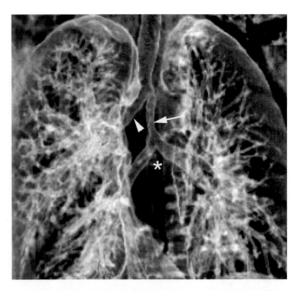

Fig. 16.12. Volume-rendered 3D reconstruction from a 16-slice multi-detector computed tomography scan through the chest of the proximal airways in a patient with pulmonary artery sling (see Fig. 16.31). The image shows an accessory right upper lobe '"pig" bronchus (*arrowhead*), and a narrowed "stove pipe" distal trachea (*arrow*) prior to the carina (*asterisk*). This tracheobronchial anatomy is associated with the left pulmonary artery sling. Care should be taken when bronchoscopy is performed in such patients, as it is often mistaken that the carina has been visualized, when in fact the first bifurcation is at the origin of the accessory right upper lobe bronchus. (Figure courtesy of Dr. Cathy Owens, Department of Clinical Radiology, Great Ormond Street Hospital for Children, who retains copyright)

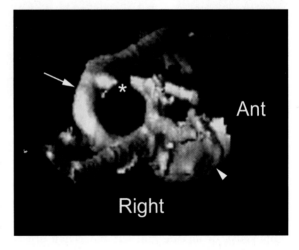

Fig. 16.13. Volume-rendered 3D reconstruction from contrast-enhanced-MR angiogram of a potential double aortic arch. The aorta is viewed from above; the anterior ascending aorta (*arrowhead*) is on the *right* of the image. There is a complete right aortic arch (*arrow*); there is a near-complete left arch. At surgery, a band of fibrous tissue was found completing the left arch (*asterisk*). Division of this band resulted in release of the compressive vascular ring

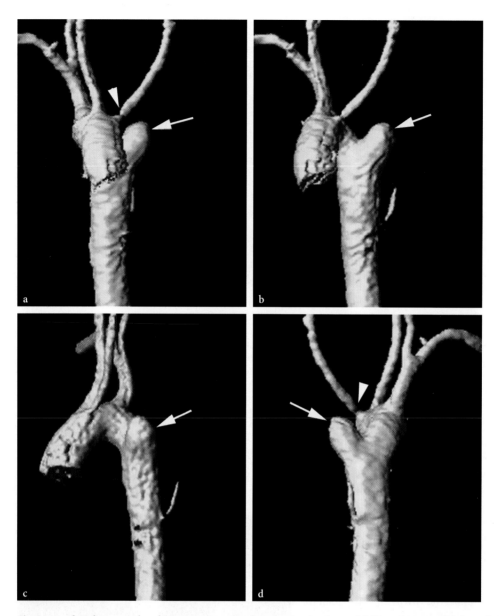

Fig. 16.14a-d. Volume-rendered 3D reconstruction from contrast-enhanced-MR angiogram of right arch with mirror-image branching head and neck vessels, but a left-sided descending aorta and a Kommerel's diverticulum (*arrow*). **a** anterior view, **b** left anterior oblique view, **c** left lateral view, **d** posterior view. At surgery, two fibrotic bands were found, one completing an atretic left arch, and one from the fibrosed left arterial duct. Narrowing at the origin of the left common carotid artery (*arrowhead*). Left subclavian artery not seen

usually associated with vascular ring compression of the central mediastinal structures (trachea and esophagus), or an aberrant left subclavian artery (last branch of the aortic arch). The presence of a subclavian artery in this setting can result in posterior esophageal compression and, a complete vascular ring can occur with a right arch with a left-sided duct remnant.

A final very rare anomaly associated with a right aortic arch is an isolated left subclavian artery,

which is supplied retrogradely via the left vertebral artery, and can cause vertebral steal syndrome (Fig. 16.17) (van Grimberge et al. 2000).

It should be noted that a right aberrant subclavian artery from a left arch does not usually cause a complete vascular ring (though it is theoretically possible for a right fibrosed arterial duct to be present and complete a vascular ring); posterior esophageal compression may cause dysphagia (Fig. 16.18).

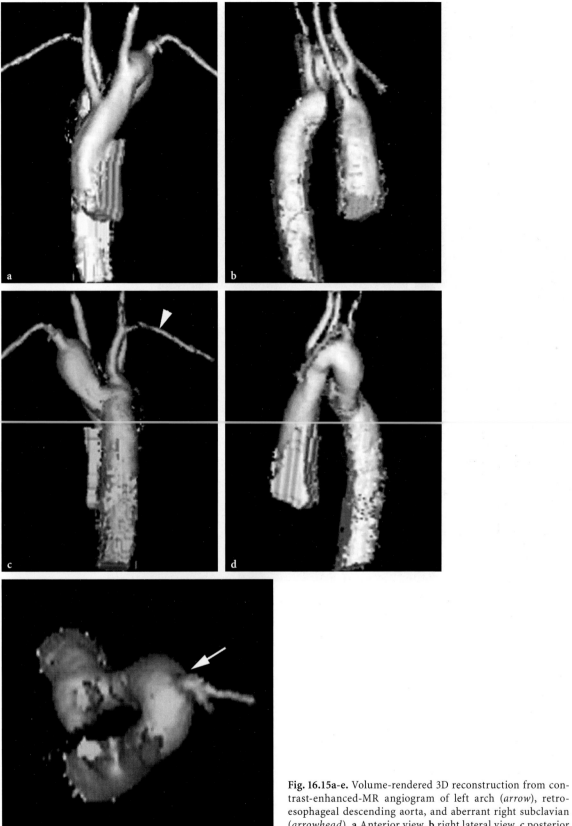

Fig. 16.15a-e. Volume-rendered 3D reconstruction from contrast-enhanced-MR angiogram of left arch (*arrow*), retroesophageal descending aorta, and aberrant right subclavian (*arrowhead*). **a** Anterior view, **b** right lateral view, **c** posterior view, **d** left lateral view, **e** viewed from above

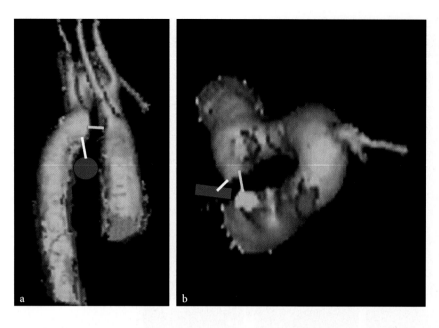

Fig. 16.16a,b. Potential vascular rings in the aortic arch from Fig. 16.15. Schematic position of the right pulmonary artery is indicated (*blue*). Potential vascular rings are completed by an atretic right arch (*yellow line*) and (2) a fibrosed right arterial duct (*white line*)

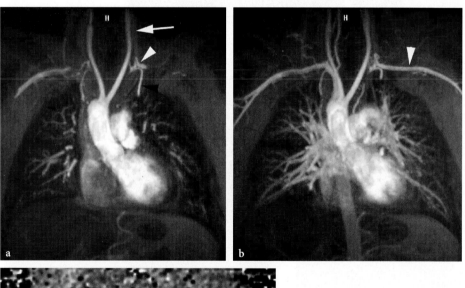

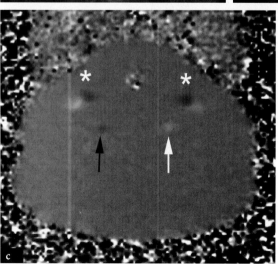

Fig. 16.17a-c. Right aortic arch with isolated left subclavian artery. **a** Coronal maximum-intensity projection (MIP) of early phase of a contrast-enhanced-MR angiogram (CE-MRA). The proximal left subclavian is seen (*white arrowhead*), but is not directly connected to the aortic arch. The left subclavian is supplied by the left vertebral artery (*white arrow*) and a large inferior collateral (*black arrowhead*). **b** Coronal MIP of late phase of a CE-MRA. The left subclavian artery is now completely filled with contrast (*arrowhead*). **c** Phase-contrast of arterial flow in the neck; *black* is flow to the head in both carotid arteries (*star*) and the right vertebral artery (*black arrow*), and *white* is retrograde flow from the left vertebral artery to the left subclavian artery. This raises the potential for a subclavian steal syndrome

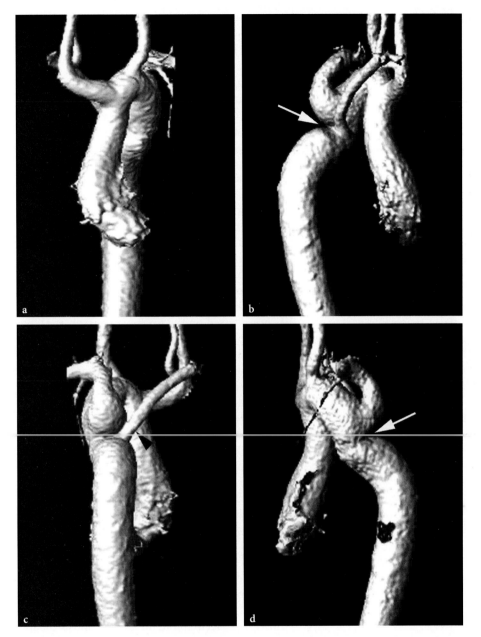

Fig. 16.18a-d. Volume-rendered 3D reconstruction from CE-MRA of left arch with an aberrant right subclavian (*black arrowhead*). Note the aberrant right subclavian originates from beyond an aortic coarctation (*arrow*). **a** anterior view, **b** right lateral view, **c** posterior view, **d** left lateral view

16.4.1.2
Aortic Aneurysm

An aortic aneurysm is defined as a localized or diffuse dilatation involving all layers of the aortic wall and exceeding the expected aortic diameter by a factor of 1.5 or more (FATTORI and NIENABER 1999). Aneurysms of the thoracic aorta are common and are important because of their potentially reversible lethal consequences (Table 16.5) (PITT and BONSER 1997).

Evaluation of the size and location of the aneurismal segment is critical. Optimal imaging therefore should include the involved aortic segments for quantification of transluminal diameter and comparison with uninvolved segments (Fig. 16.19). To produce consistent results, vessel dimensions should be measured at the same anatomical loca-

Table 16.5. Causes of aortic aneurysm

Atherosclerosis
Marfan syndrome
Ehlers-Danlos syndrome
Syphilis
Infectious aortitis
Giant cell arteritis
Aortic trauma
Aortic dissection
Secondary to aortic valve pathology (stenosis or
    regurgitation)
Postoperative

tions each time. The multi-planar ability of MRI and the availability of multiple-pulse sequences is ideal for evaluation of aneurysms and provides a better understanding of pathology (SCHMIDTA et al. 2000). 3D CE-MRA is most useful for depicting location, extent, and exact diameter. It is important to remember that MIP images represent a cast of the lumen; therefore, measurements should be obtained from source images where the vessel wall is visible. Standard SE sequences are also helpful in the evaluation of changes to the aortic wall and periaortic space (Fig. 16.20).

MRI is very useful for the detection of the characteristic morphology of aneurysms such as annuloaortic ectasia of aortic root due to cystic medial necrosis (e.g., Ehlers-Danlos syndrome, Marfan syndrome), fusiform aneurysm of descending aortic segment due to atherosclerosis and saccular

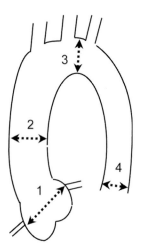

Figure 16.19. Schema for normal aortic dimensions; left anterior oblique orientation. Normal diameters measured perpendicular to the vessel: (*1*) sinus of Valsalva, 3.3 cm, (*2*) mid-ascending aorta, 3.0 cm, (*3*) aortic arch, 2.7 cm, (*4*) distal descending thoracic aorta, 2.4 cm

out-pouching of under surface of aortic isthmus due to posttraumatic pseudoaneurysm formation. (Fig. 16.21).

MRI is frequently used as a follow-up tool for monitoring the progression of disease. Where aneurysms involve the ascending aorta or sinuses of Valsalva, concomitant aortic valve disease can be evaluated using cine imaging of the heart.

16.4.1.3
Aortic Dissection

Aortic wall dissection is diagnosed if two separate lumens, the true and a false lumen separated by an intimal flap, are identifiable (Table 16.6) (NIENABER et al. 1993). Classification of aortic dissections has been based traditionally on anatomical location (Stanford or De Bakey) and time from onset (Table 16.7, Fig. 16.21). Recently, a new classification based on the work of Svensson et al. has been proposed (SVENSSON et al. 1999; ERBEL et al. 2001). This new classification includes also intramural hemorrhage or hematoma, and aortic ulcers, since these may be signs of evolving dissections or dissection subtypes (see Sect. 16.4.1.5). The 14-day period after onset has been designated as the acute phase, because morbidity and mortality (15–25%) rates are highest and surviving patients typically stabilize during this period. Early diagnosis is crucial, as the clinical features are diverse and serious complications occur rapidly (HAGAN et al. 2000). While TEE and multi-slice spiral CT have traditionally been used for imaging aortic dissection, MRI with its high sensitivity and specificity (TEE has comparable sensitivity and specificity) is now increasingly regarded as the best available method for imaging this abnormality (Table 16.8) (Figs. 16.22 and 16.23).

MRI has been found to be the most reliable method of avoiding false-positive findings while providing comprehensive information of clinically important complications of dissections such as aortic valve insufficiency, myocardial infarction from coronary artery compromise, aortic wall rupture, and arterial branch vessel dissection or occlusion (SUMMERS et al. 1996; NIENABER et al. 1993; ACR PRACTICE GUIDELINES 2003). Single-shot b-SSFP, with its inherent high SNR from blood, allows accurate delineation of true and false lumen and therefore is very useful for the classification and diagnosis of aortic dissection (PERELES et al. 2001). Note that, in the early stages of aortic dissection, the true lumen is most often the smaller of the

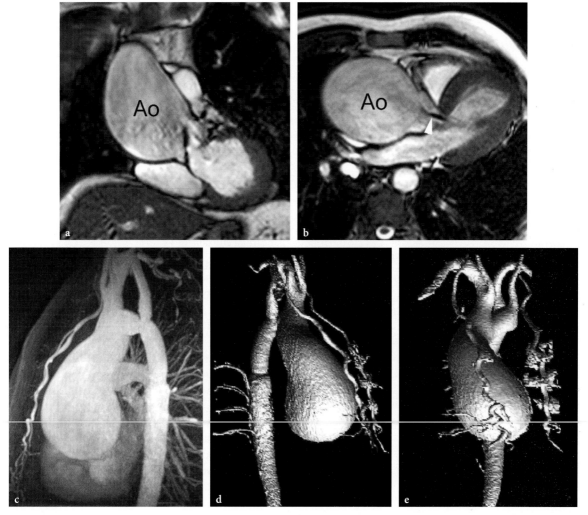

Fig. 16.20a-e. Aneurysm of the ascending aorta in a 42-year-old man with history of previous surgical correction for aortic coarctation, and concomitant bicuspid aortic valve. **a-e** Balanced steady-state free precession in the coronal view (**a**) and LV outflow tract view (**b**). CE-MRA MIP view (**c**) and volume-rendered view (**d, e**). A huge, fusiform aneurysm (85 mm) of the ascending aorta is clearly visible. The 3D geometry can be best appreciated on the 3D volume-rendered views. On cine MRI (**a, b**) an important aortic regurgitation is shown (*arrowhead*). Note also the contour abnormalities of the aortic isthmus and proximal descending aorta from the previous surgical repair of the aortic coarctation

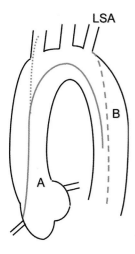

Fig. 16.21. Schema for origin and type of aortic dissection; left anterior oblique orientation. Type A (*red line*): (60%) originate a few centimeters above the aortic valve, along the right anterolateral aspect of the aorta, where hydrodynamic and torsional forces are greatest. The dissection may extend into the head and neck vessels (*dotted red line*) or extend into the descending aorta (*solid red line*). Type B (*striped red line*): (40%) originate in the descending thoracic aorta just beyond the insertion of the ligamentum arteriosum (anchorage of the relative mobile arch to the thoracic cage)

Table 16.6. Causes of aortic dissection

Hypertension
Coarctation
Iatrogenic injury
Valvular disease
Marfan syndrome

Table 16.8. Aortic dissection

	Angio	CT	TTE	TEE	MRI
Invasive	+++	0	0	++	0
Contrast	+	+	0	0	(±)
Sensitivity	++	++(+)	+	+++	+++
Specificity	+++	+++	+	++	+++
Site of intimal tear	++	+	+	++	+++
Extension					
Coronaries	++	+(+)	(+)	++	? (+)
Side branches	+++	+	(+)	+	++(+)
Abdominal	++	++	0	0	++
Thrombus	+++	++	+	+	+++
Ao insufficiency	+++	0	++	+++	++
Pericardial effusion	+++	0	++	+++	+++

Angio angiography, *CT* computed tomography,
TTE transthoracic echocardiography, *TEE* transesophageal
echocardiography, *MRI* magnetic resonance imaging

Table 16.7. Classification of aortic dissection

DE BAKEY et al. (1965)

> *Type I[a]*
> Intimal tear in ascending aorta; terminates distal to
> innominate artery
>
> *Type II[a]*
> Intimal tear in ascending aorta; terminates proximal to
> innominate artery
>
> *Type III[b]*
> Intimal tear at or distal to left subclavian artery with
> extension of intimal tear in descending aorta
>
> *Reversed Type III*
> Intimal tear at or distal to left sublavian artery with
> proximal extension of intimal flap

STANFORD

> *Type A[a]*
> Involves ascending aorta + descending aorta; needs
> immediate surgery
>
> *Type B[b]*
> Involves descending aorta only

SVENSSON et al. (1999)

> *Class 1*
> Classic aortic dissection with an intimal flap between
> true and false lumen
>
> *Class 2*
> Medial disruption with formation of intramural
> hematoma/hemorrhage
>
> *Class 3*
> Discrete/subtle dissection without hematoma eccentric
> bulge at tear site
>
> *Class 4*
> Plaque rupture leading to aortic ulceration, penetrating
> aortic atherosclerotic ulcer with surrounding hematoma,
> usually subadventitial
>
> *Class 5*
> Iatrogenic and traumatic dissection

[a]Requires urgent surgery
[b]Can be treated medically if uncomplicated

two lumens seen on MR images (see Fig. 16.23). It is also possible to accurately demonstrate dissections and postoperative complications such as development of false channels, anastomotic aneurysms, and dilatation of the residual aorta with conventional ECG-gated SE (Fig. 16.24) (HARTNELL et al. 1994; HARTNELL 2001). By using GE and/or phase-contrast techniques, it is possible to distinguish thrombosis of the false lumen from slow flow (BOGAERT et al. 1997). A slight thickening around the graft due to perigraft fibrosis is a common finding (GAUBERT et al. 1995), but large or asymmetric thickening suggests localized hematoma due to an anastomotic leakage (FATTORI and NIENABER 1999).

Along with non-ECG-triggered real-time b-SSFP, single-shot b-SSFP imaging is ideally suited for critically ill patients who cannot hold their breath (LEE et al. 2002). It may be difficult to distinguish intramural hematoma from a thrombosed false lumen of an aortic dissection.

CE-MRA is also accurate in diagnosing aortic dissections, though the diagnosis is usually made on the b-SSFP images. CE-MRA is useful for assessing the proximal and distal extent of the dissection and its involvement of branch vessels. A separate CE-MRA study of the abdomen may be required to assess distal dissections extending into the abdominal aorta (CARR and FINN 2003).

As a noninvasive, safe and increasingly fast technique, MRI is well suited for the follow-up of both

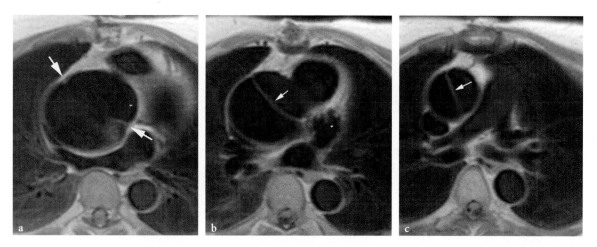

Fig. 16.22a-c. Type II De Bakey aortic dissection in a patient with an aneurysm of the ascending aorta. Turbo-spin-echo black-blood axial images from foot (**a**) to head (**c**). The aortic dissection flap is restricted to the ascending aorta (*arrow*). Careful analysis of aneurysms of the ascending aorta not infrequently shows underlying dissections limited to the aneurysm (SVENSSON et al. 1999)

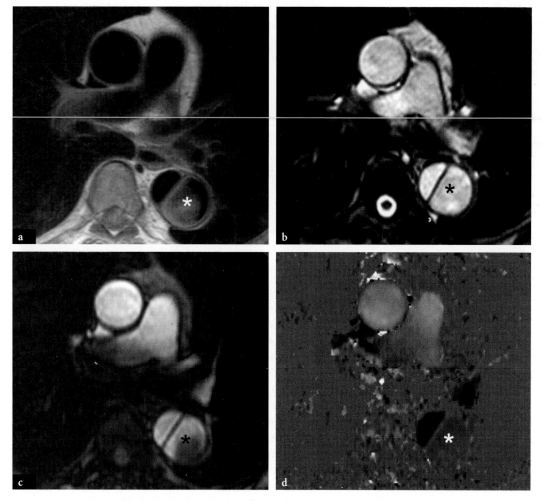

Fig. 16.23a-d. Type B Stanford aortic dissection. Axial images in the same plane with: **a** turbo-spin-echo black-blood sequence, **b** Balanced steady-state free precession sequence, and phase-contrast velocity mapping, **c** magnitude image, **d** velocity map. The false lumen (*star*) is the large lumen, and has less flow within it on the velocity map

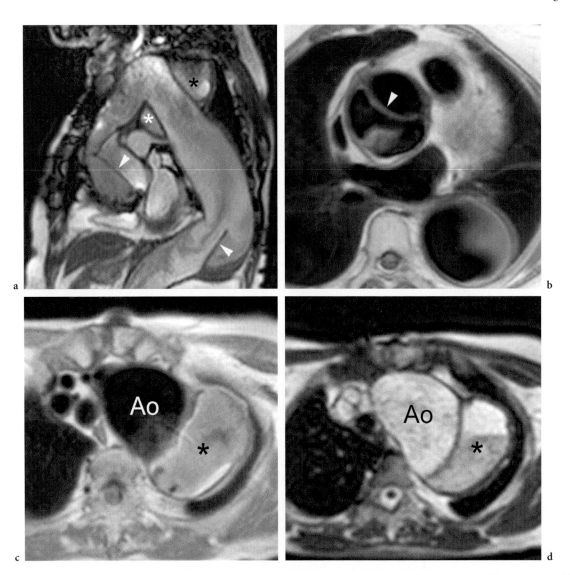

Fig. 16.24a-d. Residual aortic dissection with multiple large pseudoaneurysms in a patients post-Bentall operation. **a** Oblique sagittal balanced steady-state free precession (b-SSFP) image through the aorta, showing ascending and descending aorta dissection flaps (*white arrowheads*), and several pseudoaneurysms (*star*). **b** Turbo-spin-echo (TSE) black-blood axial image through the ascending aorta showing a dissection flap (*white arrowhead*). Axial TSE black-blood (**c**) and b-SSFP (**d**) images in the same plane at the level of the aortic arch showing a large psuedoaneurysm (*black asterisk*)

surgically (usually Stanford type A) and medically (usually Stanford type B) treated patients. MRI will help evaluate recurrence of dissection, aneurysm formation, aortic regurgitation, partial or complete thrombosis of the false lumen, the degree of compression of the true lumen by the false channel, and the distal extension of the dissection (BOGAERT et al. 1997).

In Stanford type A aneurysms, extension into the aortic root may be complicated by aortic incompetence, coronary artery compromise, and pericardial effusion, and these can be assessed by cardiovascular MRI.

16.4.1.4
Marfan Syndrome

Aortic dilatation and/or dissection are the major criteria in the cardiovascular system for diagnosis of Marfan syndrome (Ghent diagnostic nosology). MRI provides definitive measurements of aortic dimensions, which are essential for the diagnosis of aortic involvement and monitoring the course of aortic enlargement in Marfan patients (KERSTING-SOMMERHOFF et al. 1987b). The dilatation usually starts at the sinuses of Valsalva, and hence this measurement is critical in monitoring the early evolution of this condition (Fig. 16.25). Diameters must, however, be related to normal values for age and body surface area (ROMAN et al. 1987; MOHIADDIN et al. 1990).

MRI also enables the assessment of aortic biophysical properties in the majority of patients with Marfan syndrome (GROENINK et al. 2001; FATTORI

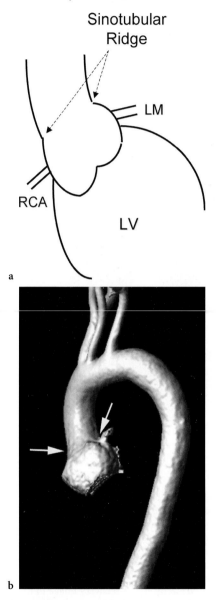

Fig. 16.25. a Schematic of the aortic root showing the sinotibular junction. **b** Volume-rendered 3D reconstruction from CE-MRA of the aorta in a Marfan subject; sagittal view. In Marfan syndrome, dilatation usually starts at the sinuses of Valsalva, so this measurement is critical for follow-up. Effacement of the sinotubular ridge occurs in Marfan syndrome, annuloaortic ectasia, and syphilis, but not in post-stenotic dilatation secondary to aortic stenosis. *RCA*, right coronary artery; *LV*, left ventricle; *LM*, left main stem coronary artery

et al. 2000). A number of studies have shown that significantly decreased aortic distensibility and increased flow wave velocity can be detected in undilated aorta distal to the aortic root in these patients. Dilatation of the pulmonary artery in patients below the age of 40 years should also be evaluated (NOLLEN et al. 2003).

16.4.1.5
Aortic Ulceration and Intramural Hematoma

Intramural hematoma accounts for 10–30% of all acute aortic syndromes. It results from either spontaneous rupture of the aortic wall vasa vasorum or from a penetrating atherosclerotic ulcer (EVANGELISTA et al. 2002). The major risk of intramural hematoma is that it may evolve into an overt aortic dissection (VON KODOLITSCH et al. 2003). Moreover, the outcome is similar to that for aortic dissection. Therefore, intramural hematoma is classified, and should be treated in a similar fashion to aortic dissection (see Svensson Classification, Table 16.7). This means (urgent) surgery for type A intramural hematoma, and medical treatment for type B hematoma (NIENABER et al. 2004).

Intramural hematoma appears as smooth, often circumferential thickening of the aortic wall that can be associated with infiltration of the adjacent mediastinal fat and/or pericardial effusion, caused by leakage of blood. Because of the short T1-relaxation time of fresh blood, differentiation from the adjacent mediastinal fat may be difficult. Intramural blood can be best detected on fat-saturated T1-weighted GE or black-blood techniques. CE-MRA (MOHIADDIN et al. 2001) or conventional cine MRA are required to differentiate hematoma from dissection (Fig. 16.26) (SONNABEND et al. 1990).

Aortic ulcer is characterized by rupture of an atheromatous plaque disrupting the internal elastic lamina, which can evolve to saccular pseudoaneurysm formation or intramural hematoma. Aortic ulcers occur almost exclusively in the descending aorta, but involvement of the aortic arch or the ascending aorta has also been reported (Fig. 16.27). The visualization of a crater-like ulcer on axial and sagittal SE images helps in diagnosis, but, unlike CT, MRI cannot detect dislodgement of the intimal calcification (FATTORI and NIENABER 1999). There is considerable clinical and imaging overlap between intramural hematoma, thrombosed false lumen in a localized dissection, and penetrating atherosclerotic ulcer (SOLOMON et al. 1990; YUCEL et al. 1990; WOLFF et al. 1991). A thrombosed false lumen in

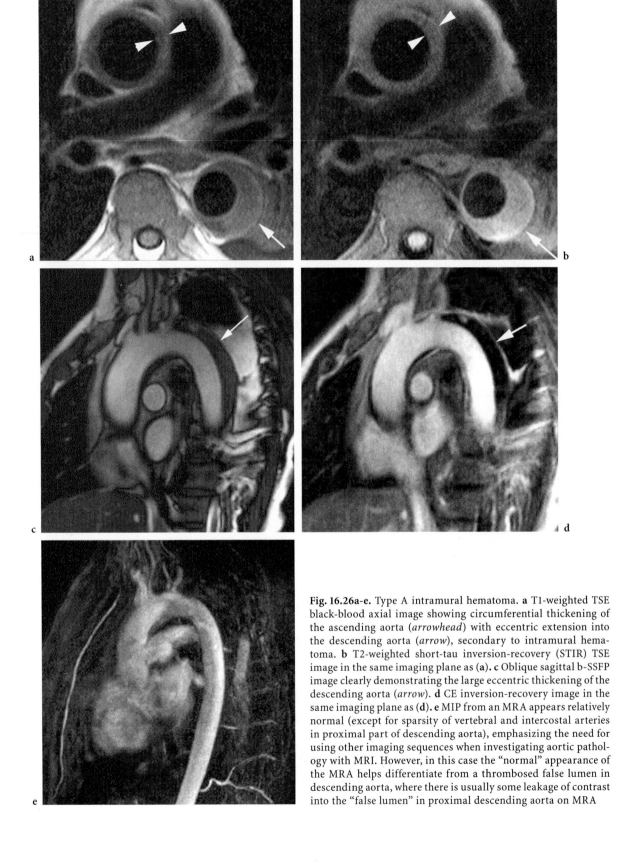

Fig. 16.26a-e. Type A intramural hematoma. **a** T1-weighted TSE black-blood axial image showing circumferential thickening of the ascending aorta (*arrowhead*) with eccentric extension into the descending aorta (*arrow*), secondary to intramural hematoma. **b** T2-weighted short-tau inversion-recovery (STIR) TSE image in the same imaging plane as (**a**). **c** Oblique sagittal b-SSFP image clearly demonstrating the large eccentric thickening of the descending aorta (*arrow*). **d** CE inversion-recovery image in the same imaging plane as (**d**). **e** MIP from an MRA appears relatively normal (except for sparsity of vertebral and intercostal arteries in proximal part of descending aorta), emphasizing the need for using other imaging sequences when investigating aortic pathology with MRI. However, in this case the "normal" appearance of the MRA helps differentiate from a thrombosed false lumen in descending aorta, where there is usually some leakage of contrast into the "false lumen" in proximal descending aorta on MRA

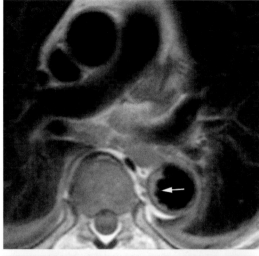

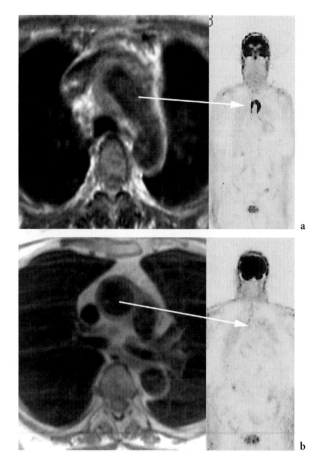

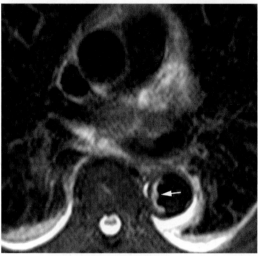

Fig. 16.27a,b. Extensive atherosclerotic disease of the descending aorta. Axial T1-weighted TSE (**a**) and T2-weighted STIR TSE (**b**) shows irregular centrally ulcerated plaque (thickness 5 mm) along the medial border of the descending aorta (*arrow*). Further ulceration may evolve toward a penetrating ulcer when the entire aortic wall is ulcerated

Fig. 16.28a,b. Giant cell aortitis in a 62-year-old woman. Axial T1-weighted SE MR image after administration of gadolinium-diethylene triamine penta-acetic acid (*left*) and coronal FDG positron-emission tomography (PET; *right*) at initial presentation (**a**) and after 6 weeks of corticosteroid treatment (**b**). Strong enhancement is found in the thickened wall of the ascending aorta. This inflamed thickened aortic wall shows high glucose metabolism on FDG-PET (**a**). After corticosteroid treatment (**b**), wall thickness has nearly normalized, and no abnormal glucose metabolism is found on FDG-PET

an aortic dissection often has a more eccentric or asymmetrical appearance, while the spread of blood in an intramural hematoma has a tendency to affect the aortic wall more circumferentially.

16.4.1.6
Inflammation and Infection

Inflammatory aortitis syndromes (Table 16.9) can be imaged with MR especially in patients where conventional contrast angiography can be harmful (Fig. 16.28). In Takayasu's disease, the aorta and its major branches and the pulmonary artery can

Table 16.9. Causes of aortic inflammation

Syphilitic aortitis
Rheumatic aortitis
   Rheumatoid arthritis
   Ankylosing spondylitis
   Psoriatic arthritis
   Reiter's syndrome
   Behçet's syndrome
   Relapsing polychondritis
   Inflammatory bowel disease
Takayasu's arteritis
Giant cell arteritis
Atherosclerosis

be affected (Fig. 16.29). Isolated mural thickening of the aorta, or thickening associated with either constriction or aneurismal dilatation can be detected on MR images. The response to treatment with steroids can also be monitored (Fig. 16.28). The MRI protocol should consist of SE sequences before and after contrast administration to evaluate vessel wall thickness and to assess the extent of inflammation; and CE-MRA to better evaluate aneurysm

formation and/or stenosis formation. There may be a role too for CE inversion-recovery MRI in assessing (peri)vessel inflammation.

While MRI is not recommended as the investigation of choice in patients with infective endocarditis, it is useful for demonstrating perivalvular infectious pseudoaneurysms complicating cardiac surgery (WINKLER and HIGGINS 1986; AKINS et al. 1991).

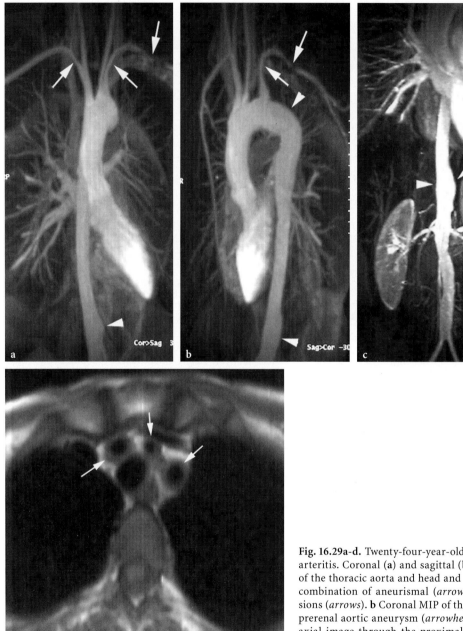

Fig. 16.29a-d. Twenty-four-year-old woman with Takayasu arteritis. Coronal (**a**) and sagittal (**b**) MIP from a CE-MRA of the thoracic aorta and head and neck vessels, showing a combination of aneurismal (*arrowheads*) and stenotic lesions (*arrows*). **b** Coronal MIP of the entire aorta showing a prerenal aortic aneurysm (*arrowheads*). **c** TSE black-blood axial image through the proximal head and neck vessels (*arrows*) showing arterial wall thickening, secondary to arteritis

16.4.1.7
Aortic Trauma

Aortic rupture or transection occurs following major trauma such as road traffic accidents and is associated with a significant mortality. Any delay in diagnosis and treatment can lead to death. The most common site of aortic rupture is the region just beyond the isthmus where the relatively mobile thoracic aorta is joined by the ligamentum arteriosus; the site of greatest strain. In one study, MRI demonstrated 100% accuracy for detecting traumatic lesions, compared with 84% for X-ray angiography and 69% for standard CT (FATTORI et al. 1996). MRI can detect the hemorrhagic component of the lesion by the high signal intensity, with SE imaging of the aorta in the sagittal plane helping to prognosticate by differentiating between partial and complete lesions (FATTORI and NIENABER 1999). In all forms of imaging, care should be taken not to interpret a prominent ampulla (site of previous ligamentum arteriosus insertion) as an aortic transection. However, despite the high accuracy of MRI, its usefulness in assessing these acute patients is usually limited, mainly due to restricted 24-h access to the magnet and for safety reasons.

Some of these aortic lesions, however, may not manifest themselves immediately after the trauma. Often, these patients may present many years later with symptoms that are caused by complications of a previous, often forgotten chest trauma. The most frequent delayed complication of the thoracic aorta is a chronic saccular pseudoaneurysm originating from the distal aortic arch. The size of the pseudoaneurysm is consistent and about 3–5 cm. The most common site of disease is the isthmus just distal to the left subclavian artery at the attachment of the ligamentum arteriosum medial and anterior to the aortic isthmus. This is related to different shear forces during rapid deceleration between the somewhat fixed descending aorta and relatively mobile heart and aortic arch (SEVITT 1977). A distinction has to be made between the immediately fatal rupture of the posterolateral wall of the isthmus and the disruption at the anteromedial wall. Gundry and colleagues have stated that the expanding hematoma from a medial tear could be contained by the pulmonary artery and the left main stem bronchus inferiorly (GUNDRY et al. 1984). The adherence of the mediastinal parietal pleura to these structures may limit expansion of the hematoma laterally. Because of the medial tear, the pseudoaneurysm typically forms in a saccular configuration adjacent to the descending aorta and the rest of a normal arch.

Compression of the pseudoaneurysm on the airways or recurrent laryngeal nerve will cause symptoms of dyspnea or hoarseness, but pseudoaneurysms are often an incidental finding on routine X-ray chest films. Because the exact time required for the acute lesion to convert into a pseudoaneurysm is not known, a chronic traumatic pseudoaneurysm is defined as existing 3 months or more after the injury. MRI should be considered one of the preferred imaging techniques to confirm the presence of and to evaluate the precise location and extent of a pseudoaneurysm. Also the presence of a mural thrombus partially, or rarely completely, obliterating the aneurismal lumen can be depicted. Imaging with MR may be helpful for demonstrating the relationship of the saccular pseudoaneurysm to the aorta and to the origin of the left subclavian artery. This is of great importance for the operative procedure, as clamping of the left subclavian artery should be avoided during the repair of the pseudoaneurysm, or prior to an aortic stent placement. A combination of SE and 3D CE MR angiography is the best strategy to study chronic posttraumatic aneurysms.

16.4.1.8
Aortic Stent and Stent-Graft Imaging

Increasingly, patients with aortic pathology are being treated with aortic stents (aortic coarctation; HAMDAN et al. 2001) and aortic stent-grafts (aortic aneurysms; DAKE et al. 1998). These metallic implants are safe to image under MR, and safety evaluation for various stents/stent-grafts has been carried out with some shown to be safe for in vivo diagnostic MRI (HILFIKER et al. 1999; ENGELLAU et al. 2000). Cardiovascular MR is important in the assessment of these interventions; however, GE sequences are prone to the field inhomogeneity caused by these metallic implants (secondary to T2* effects). Black-blood imaging provides the solution to this, with the T2* effects compensated for by the 180° refocusing pulse. Thus, patients with stents in situ can still be assessed by MR, and restenosis or inadequate stent placement can be analyzed (Fig. 16.30).

MRI in patients with stent-grafts will help in evaluating the morphology of the stent-graft (i.e., the position and configuration of the metallic frames, kinking or rotation, and irregularity of aortic profile), the state of the aneurismal sac, aneurysm dimension, and the diameter and wall morphology of the proximal and distal neck (FATTORI et al. 2003).

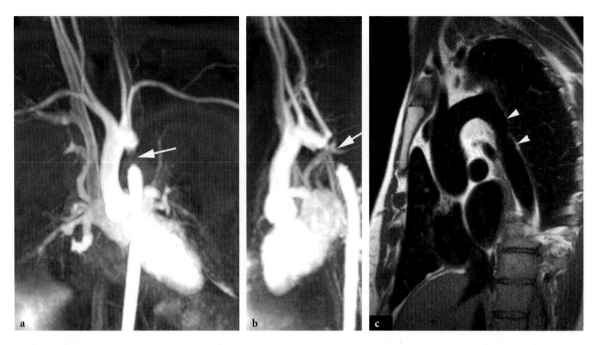

Fig. 16.30a-c. Aortic coarctation stent imaging. **a** Coronal and **b** sagittal MIPs from an aortic CE-MRA showing signal loss at the site of a proximal descending aorta metallic stent (*arrow*). **c** Oblique sagittal TSE black-blood image in the same patient clearly demonstrates that the stent is widely patent. The length of the stent is indicated by the *arrowheads*

16.4.2
Pulmonary Arteries

Imaging of pulmonary artery anatomy is crucial for surgical planning and follow-up in patients with complex congenital heart disease (see Chap. 15). Imaging of the branch pulmonary arteries can be difficult on echocardiograms, in particular in older patients and postsurgical patients, and MRI can provide a noninvasive alternative to X-ray cardiac catheterization for the assessment of the pulmonary arteries (CANTER et al. 1989). MRI can define the size, patency, confluence, and character of the extraparenchymal pulmonary arteries and has been shown to be 100% sensitive and specific for the diagnosis of main and branch pulmonary artery hypoplasia or stenosis, as well as discontinuous or absent branch pulmonary arteries (POWELL et al. 2000).

While 2D SE and cine GE imaging techniques may suffice for delineating central pulmonary arteries, CE-3D MRA is essential to adequately evaluate the hilar and intrapulmonary segments of the central pulmonary arteries and aortopulmonary collaterals (WANG et al. 1996). In patients with respiratory distress, time-resolved 3D MRA may be more suitable (VOGT et al. 2003). Aortopulmonary collateral vessels may originate from brachiocephalic arteries, from the descending thoracic aorta, or from the subdia-

phragmatic aorta (see Fig. 15.15) (HERNANDEZ 2002). The central pulmonary arteries in cases of right ventricular outflow obstruction may be hypoplastic or, if atretic, not identifiable. Focal branch stenosis proximal to the pulmonary hila may be identified directly. In cases of supravalvular pulmonary stenosis, the main and central pulmonary arteries (as an isolated lesion or in association with Williams or Noonan's syndromes) exhibit diffuse or focal wall thickening. Similarly, pulmonary arterial banding results in focal pulmonary artery narrowing.

MRI can also be useful in the assessment of hypoplastic lung syndrome, demonstrating reduced lung volume, and identifying of any of the known associations: hypoplastic supplying pulmonary artery; partial anomalous pulmonary venous drainage (Scimitar vein); and pulmonary sequestration.

Pulmonary arterial anomalies such as pulmonary artery sling and origin of the pulmonary artery from the ductus arteriosus can be characterized explicitly on MR images (BEEKMAN et al. 1998) (Fig. 16.31). An aberrant or anomalous left pulmonary artery is commonly referred to as a pulmonary sling. If the anomalous pulmonary artery is associated with long-segment tracheal stenosis then it can be fatal, and therefore early and accurate diagnosis will aid prompt treatment with better outcome (see Fig. 16.12) (BERDON 2000).

Dilatation of the main pulmonary artery, with or without associated left or right pulmonary arterial enlargement, may be seen in patients with valvular pulmonary stenosis. Aneurysmal dilatation of the pulmonary arterial tree may be found in patients with chronic, mild valvular pulmonary stenosis or pulmonary insufficiency. Aneurysmal dilatation of the main and mediastinal branch pulmonary arteries along with absent or rudimentary pulmonary valve tissue and severe pulmonary regurgitation is characteristic of tetralogy of Fallot with absent pulmonary valve syndrome (Fig. 16.32). The resulting tracheobronchial compression by the grossly dilated pulmonary arteries and occasionally aortopulmonary collaterals (KNAUTH et al. 2004) can be a cause of significant morbidity and mortality. While the pulmonary arterial anatomy is better defined by MR, CT is often more useful to assess the tracheobronchial tree.

Diagnosis of pulmonary embolism using breath-hold CE 3D MR angiography is now possible, but it is crucial to acquire the data in a reasonably short breath-hold, as most patients with pulmonary embolism tend to be dyspneic. One study has revealed 100% diagnostic accuracy (GRIST et al. 1993; VAN BEEK et al. 2003). In patients with difficulty in breath-holding, half-κ-space sampling in the phase-encode direction or reducing the spatial resolution by acquiring fewer sections may be required. Another major advantage is that MRA of the pulmonary vasculature can be complemented by MR venography of the pelvic and femoral veins (CARPENTER et al. 1993). Despite these studies, the wide availability and ease of use of pulmonary CT angiography means that CT is currently the imaging modality of choice for direct visualization of the pulmonary vasculature in suspected pulmonary embolus (KANNE and LALANI 2004).

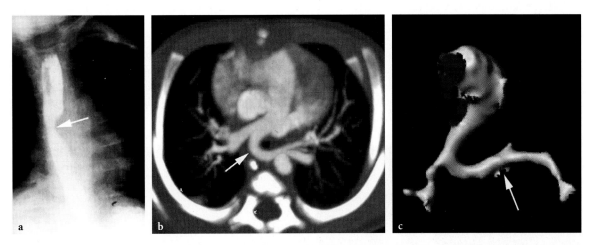

Fig. 16.31a-c. Left pulmonary artery sling. **a** Right anterior oblique projection from a barium swallow showing anterior esophageal indentation (*arrow*). **b** Axial image from a postcontrast multi-slice CT scan showing the left pulmonary artery sling, originating from the mid-portion of the right pulmonary artery and passing behind the trachea (*arrow*). **c** Volume-rendered 3D reconstruction from CE-MRA of left pulmonary artery sling (*arrow*) viewed from below. (**a** and **b** courtesy of Dr. Cathy Owens, Department of Clinical Radiology, Great Ormond Street Hospital for Children, whom retains copyright)

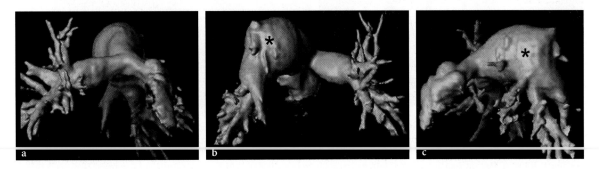

Fig. 16.32a-c. Volume-rendered 3D reconstruction from CE-MRA of massively dilated pulmonary arteries in a patient with absent pulmonary valve syndrome. **a** Right anterior oblique view; **b** posterior view; **c** left lateral view; *star* left pulmonary artery

16.4.3
Pulmonary Veins

MRI can help evaluate the course of the PVs for differentiation between forms of partial anomalous pulmonary venous return (e.g., right upper PV to superior vena cava (SVC) in association with atrial septal defect, ASD) (PRASAD et al. 2004) and total anomalous pulmonary venous return [Darling's classification type I (supracardiac), type II (cardiac), and type III (infracardiac)]. While 3D b-SSFP volume and 3D MRA (PILLEUL and MERCHANT 2000; GREIL et al. 2002) are most useful, axial SE acquisitions (MASUI et al. 1991) and axial GE imaging (WHITE et al. 1998) can also be used to evaluate pulmonary venous anomalies. Pulmonary venous varix may appear as a dilated tubular structure confluent with the left atrium (LA) (WILDENHAIN and BOUREKAS 1991).

MR can help identify the site and degree of narrowing by optimal imaging of the involved PV segment for quantification of reduction in transluminal diameter. PV compression by dilated right atrium in Fontan patients (MCELHINNEY et al. 1996; HEGDE et al. 2004) and dilated LA and descending aorta (O'DONNELL et al. 2003) can be detected on MR images. 3D b-SSFP volume and 3D MRA should be performed to evaluate pulmonary venous narrowings and obstruction. Recently, MR phase-shift velocity mapping has been shown to be helpful in delineating the site and hemodynamic severity of pulmonary venous obstruction in patients with congenital heart disease (VIDELEFSKY et al. 2001).

Cardiovascular MRI of PVs in children should be performed with caution, as the surgeon often wants to know the extent of the PV narrowing, and our own experience is that stenosis length can be overestimated on MR images (Fig. 16.33).

16.4.4
Systemic Veins

MRI is superior to echocardiography in its ability to delineate systemic venous structures and therefore is very useful in the anatomical and hemodynamic evaluation of cardiac heterotaxia in infants and children (WHITE 2000).

Systemic venous abnormalities that can be diagnosed and should be looked for on MR images include anomalous left innominate vein, left inferior vena cava, duplication of the inferior vena cava, persistence of left SVC (Fig. 16.34) and thrombosis of the superior caval vein (HERNANDEZ 2002). The

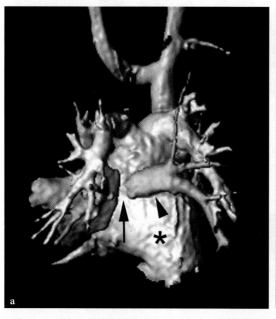
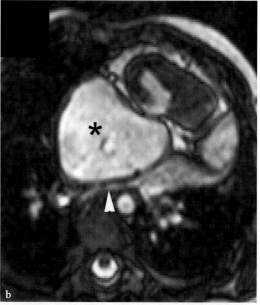

Fig. 16.33a,b. An example of overestimation of pulmonary venous narrowing on MR angiograms. **a** Volume-rendered 3D reconstruction from CE-MRA of pulmonary venous return (*red*) in a patient with a Fontan circulation for tricuspid atresia, posterior view. The right pulmonary vein (*black arrowhead*) is compressed behind the dilated right atrium (*asterisk*), with the impression of discontinuation of the right pulmonary vein as it enters the left atrium (*black arrow*). However, this is not the case, as in **b**, an axial b-SSFP image, the right pulmonary vein is seen to be compressed behind the right atrium, but patent throughout its length (*white arrowhead*)

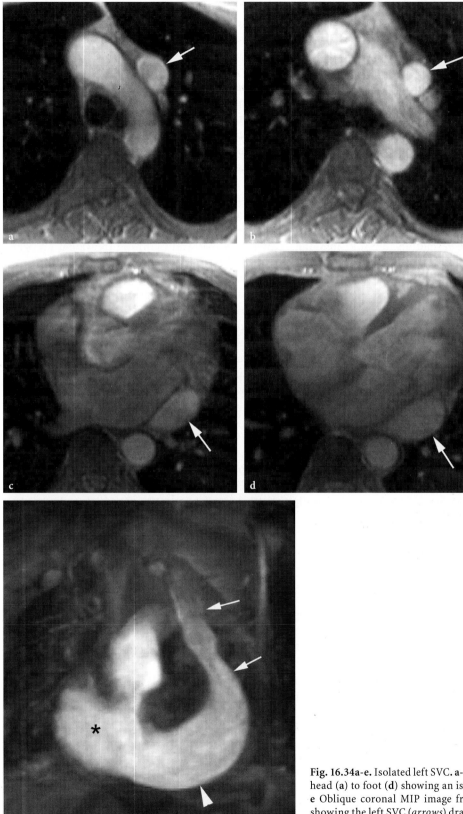

Fig. 16.34a-e. Isolated left SVC. **a-d** Axial GE images from head (**a**) to foot (**d**) showing an isolated left SVC (*arrow*). **e** Oblique coronal MIP image from an MR angiogram, showing the left SVC (*arrows*) draining into a dilated coronary sinus (*arrowhead*) and then into the right atrium (*star*)

innominate vein coursing posterior to the aorta can sometimes be mistaken for the right pulmonary artery (DIDIER et al. 1999). 3D b-SSFP volume (RAZAVI et al. 2003) and 3D MRA will help in comprehensive evaluation of systemic venous abnormalities. The demonstration of a left SVC as well as azygos continuation is of importance in surgical planning, particularly in cases of functional single ventricle in which cavopulmonary shunts (Fontan operation) may be required (see Chap. 15.5.6).

A significant cause of morbidity and mortality in patients with indwelling catheters, malignancy, and hematologic disease is thrombosis of systemic veins. Two-dimensional time-of-flight MRI (HARTNELL et al. 1995), 3D CE-MRA (LEBOWITZ et al. 1997) and, more recently, high-resolution b-SSFP imaging (SPUENTRUP et al. 2001) have all been shown to be very useful for venography.

16.5
Conclusion

The value of MRI is now well recognized as the optimal imaging modality for assessing and monitoring a wide variety of diseases of the great vessels and surrounding structures. However, the imaging modality of choice may vary between centers and is influenced by local availability and expertise. A variety of new techniques and faster pulse sequences have made cardiovascular MRI appealing to both cardiologists and radiologists, especially for the assessment of great vessels of the chest.

Parallel imaging techniques such as simultaneous acquisition of spatial harmonics (SMASH) (SODICKSON and MANNING 1997; SODICKSON et al. 2000) and sensitivity-encoding (SENSE) (WEIGER et al. 2000a, 2000b) have enabled improvements in temporal and/or spatial resolution by changing the way data is acquired and processed. Improvements in temporal resolution in combination with conventional 3D CE-MRA and b-SSFP cine imaging will enable more dynamic imaging of the great vessels to be performed.

16.5.1
Future Directions

MRI is increasingly being used to evaluate atherosclerosis plaques. In vivo characterisation of atherosclerosis plaque components in human

aorta is now possible (TOUSSAINT 2002). Good correlation has also been found between multicontrast MRI and TEE for aortic plaque quantification and characterization (FAYAD 2003). There is growing interest in developing contrast agents that specifically target and identify components of vulnerable plaque (FLACKE et al. 2001). The progression of atherosclerosis especially by positive arterial remodeling has been demonstrated in transgenic mouse models (CHOUDHURY et al. 2002). Angiogenesis is thought to be a critical feature of plaque development in atherosclerosis and therefore a molecular imaging approach to detect and characterize early angiogenesis might prove very useful both in understanding the evolution of atherosclerosis and planning treatment (WINTER et al. 2003).

The high spatial resolution of MRI and improved contrast agents is giving MRI the edge over positron-emission tomography (PET), other nuclear techniques, and CT in the field of molecular imaging. MRI, therefore, holds the promise of becoming a valuable tool to image the presence or activity of specific molecules in vivo (WEISSLEDER and MAHMOOD 2001).

16.6
Key Points

- When available, MRI is the noninvasive method of choice for assessing the great vessels of the thorax.
- Imaging with gadolinium contrast-enhanced MR angiography provides exquisite 3D imaging, but should always be combined with at least one other MRI sequence to ensure that pathology is not overlooked.
- A combination of bright-blood and black-blood MRI is the best strategy to assess vessel lumen, vessel wall, and surrounding structures.
- Assessment of ventricular function and intracardiac anatomy may be important in a variety of vascular diseases and should be performed when necessary.
- The decision whether or not a patient with an aortic dissection will need surgery is primarily determined by the involvement or not of the ascending aorta.
- An aneurysm of the ascending aorta may develop a concomitant aortic dissection (usually type II DeBakey).

- The classification, treatment, and prognosis for intramural hematoma is the same as for an overt aortic dissection.
- Imaging protocols for the great vessels are outlined in Tables 16.10–16.12

Table 16.10. Cardiovascular MRI protocol for the aorta

1. 3D balanced steady-state free precession (b-SSFP) volume
2. b-SSFP cines of: 4-chamber, LV outflow tract, and aorta-in-plane
3. b-SSFP short-axis quantification of LV function and mass
4. "Black-blood" turbo-spin-echo images of the aorta in-plane (oblique sagittal 3-point view)
5. Phase-contrast velocity mapping, both through-plane and in-plane at the site of any narrowings, and in the aortic root to assess for aortic valvular disease
6. 3D contrast-enhanced MR angiography

Table 16.11. Cardiovascular MRI protocol for the pulmonary arteries

1. 3D b-SSFP volume
2. Balanced SSFP cines of: 4-chamber and RVOT in two planes
3. Balanced SSFP short-axis quantification of RV function
4. Black-blood turbo-spin-echo images of the pulmonary trunk and branch pulmonary arteries (especially if stents are in situ)
5. Phase-contrast velocity mapping through any narrowings (in-plane, through-plane), across the proximal pulmonary trunk to assess pulmonary valvular function, and across the branch pulmonary arteries to assess differential pulmonary blood flow
6. 3D contrast-enhanced MR angiography

Table 16.12. Cardiovascular MRI protocol for the systemic and pulmonary veins

1. 3D b-SSFP volume
2. b-SSFP cines of left atrium, if pulmonary venous ostial stenosis a possibility
3. Black-blood turbo-spin-echo images through any narrowings
4. 3D MR angiography (often delayed imaging is required to ensure that the venous system is completely filled)

Acknowledgements

We would like to acknowledge the following for their help and support with cardiovascular MR. From Great Ormond Street Hospital for Children, London, UK: Professor John Deanfield and Professor Philipp Bonhoeffer of the Cardiothoracic Unit; Dr. Cathy Owens, Rod Jones, Wendy Norman, and Clare Thompson of the Department of Radiology; and Dr. Angus McEwan of the Anesthetic Department. From the MR Unit, Guy's Hospital, London, UK: Dr. Vivek Muthurangu, Dr. Derek Hill, Dr. Steve Keevil, Dr. Marc Miquel, Dr.Kawal Rhodes, Rado Andriantsimiavona, Redha Boubertakh, Maxime Sermesant, and Professor David Hawkes of the Division of Imaging Sciences.

References

ACR Practice Guideline for the Performance of Cardiovascular Magnetic Resonance Imaging (MRI) (2003)

Akins EW, Slone RM, Wiechmann BN, et al (1991) Perivalvular pseudoaneurysm complicating bacterial endocarditis: MR detection in five cases. AJR Am J Roentgenol 156:1155–1158

Amparo EG, Higgins CB, Hricak H, Sollitto R (1985) Aortic dissection: magnetic resonance imaging. Radiology 155:399–406

Araoz PA, Reddy GP, Tarnoff H, Roge CL, Higgins CB (2003) MR findings of collateral circulation are more accurate measures of hemodynamic significance than arm-leg blood pressure gradient after repair of coarctation of the aorta. J Magn Reson Imaging 17:177–183

Arpasi PJ, Bis KG, Shetty AN, White RD, Simonetti OP (2000) MR angiography of the thoracic aorta with an electrocardiographically triggered breath-hold contrast-enhanced sequence. Radiographics 20:107–120

Beekman RP, Hazekamp MG, Sobotka MA et al (1998) A new diagnostic approach to vascular rings and pulmonary slings: the role of MRI. Magn Reson Imaging 16:137–145

Berdon WE (2000) Rings, slings, and other things: vascular compression of the infant trachea updated from the midcentury to the millennium – the legacy of Robert E. Gross, MD, and Edward B. D. Neuhauser, MD. Radiology 216:624–632

Bogaert J, Gewillig M, Rademakers F et al (1995) Transverse arch hypoplasia predisposes to aneurysm formation at the repair site after patch angioplasty for coarctation of the aorta. J Am Coll Cardiol 26:521–527

Bogaert J, Meyns B, Rademakers F et al (1997) Aortic dissection: contribution of MR angiography for evaluation of the abdominal aorta and its branches. Eur Radiol 7:695–702

Bogaert J, Kuzo R, Dymarkowski S et al (2000) Follow-up of patients with previous treatment for coarctation of the thoracic aorta: comparison between contrast-enhanced MR angiography and fast SE MR imaging. Eur Radiol 10:1847–1854

Bogaert J Dymarkowski S, Budts W, Daenen W, Gewillig M (2001) Graft dilatation after redo surgery for aneurysm formation following patch angioplasty for coarctation of the aorta. Eur J Thorac Cardiovasc Surg 19: 274–278

Brierley J, Redington AN, Anderson RH, et al (2001) Paediatric cardiology, 2nd edn, chap 56. Churchill Livingstone, Edinburgh, pp 1523–1551

Canter CE, Gutierrez FR, Mirowitz SA, Martin TC, Hartmann AF Jr (1989) Evaluation of pulmonary arterial morphology in cyanotic congenital heart disease by magnetic resonance imaging. Am Heart J 118:347–354

Carpenter JP, Holland GA, Baum RA, et al (1993) Magnetic resonance venography for the detection of deep venous thrombosis: comparison with contrast venography and duplex Doppler ultrasonography. J Vasc Surg 18:734–741

Carr J, Finn JP (2003) MR imaging of the thoracic aorta. Magn Reson Imaging Clin North Am 11:135–148

Carr J, Simonetti O, Bundy J et al (2001) Cine MR angiography of the heart with segmented true fast imaging with steady-state precession. Radiology 219:828–834

Choudhury RP, Fuster V, Badimon JJ, Fisher EA, Fayad ZA (2002) MRI and characterization of atherosclerotic plaque: emerging applications and molecular imaging. Arterioscler Thromb Vasc Biol 22:1065–1074

Chung T (2000) Assessment of cardiovascular anatomy in patients with congenital heart disease by magnetic resonance imaging. Pediatr Cardiol 21:18–26

Crafoord C (1980) Classics in thoracic surgery. Correction of aortic coarctation. Ann Thorac Surg 30:300–302

Dake MD, Miller DC, Mitchell RS, et al (1998) The "first generation" of endovascular stent-grafts for patients with aneurysms of the descending thoracic aorta. J Thorac Cardiovasc Surg 116:689–704

DeBakey ME, Henly WS, Cooley DA et al (1965) Surgical management of dissecting aneurysms of the aorta. J Thorac Cardiovasc Surg 49:130–148

Debatin JF, Hany TF (1998) MR-based assessment of vascular morphology and function. Eur Radiol 8:528–539.

Didier D, Ratib O, Beghetti M, Oberhaensli I, Friedli B (1999) Morphologic and functional evaluation of congenital heart disease by magnetic resonance imaging. J Magn Reson Imaging 10:639–655

Dietl CA, Torres AR, Favaloro RG, Fessler CL, Grunkemeier GL (1992) Risk of recoarctation in neonates and infants after repair with patch aortoplasty, subclavian flap, and the combined resection-flap procedure. J Thorac Cardiovasc Surg 103:724–732

Dymarkowski S, Bosmans H, Marchal G, Bogaert J (1999) 3D MR angiography of thoracic outlet. Am J Roentgenol 173:1005–1008

Earls JP, Rofsky NM, DeCorato DR, Krinsky GA, Weinreb JC (1996) Breath-hold single-dose gadolinium-enhanced three-dimensional MR aortography: usefulness of a timing examination and MR power injector. Radiology 201:705–710

Edwards JE (1948) Anomalies of the derivatives of the aortic arch system. Med Clin North Am 33:925–949

Engellau L, Olsrud J, Brockstedt S et al (2000) MR evaluation ex vivo and in vivo of a covered stent-graft for abdominal aortic aneurysms: ferromagnetism, heating, artifacts, and velocity mapping. J Magn Reson Imaging 12:112–121

Erbel R, Alfonso F, Boileau C et al (2001) Diagnosis and management of aortic dissection. Recommendations of the Task Force on Aortic Dissection, European Society of Cardiology. Eur Heart J 22:1642–1681

Evangelista A, Avegliano G, Elorz C, et al (2002) Transesophageal echocardiography in the diagnosis of acute aortic syndrome. J Card Surg 17:95–106

Fatouraee N, Amini AA (2003) Regularization of flow streamlines in multislice phase-contrast MR imaging. IEEE Trans Med Imaging 22:699–709

Fattori R, Nienaber CA (1999) MRI of acute and chronic aortic pathology: pre-operative and post-operative evaluation. J Magn Reson Imaging 10:741–750

Fattori R, Celletti F, Bertaccini P et al (1996) Delayed surgery of traumatic aortic rupture. Role of magnetic resonance imaging. Circulation 94:2865–2870

Fattori R, Bacchi Reggiani L, Pepe G et al (2000) Magnetic resonance imaging evaluation of aortic elastic properties as early expression of Marfan syndrome. J Cardiovasc Magn Reson 2:251–256

Fattori R, Napoli G, Lovato L et al (2003) Descending thoracic aortic diseases: stent-graft repair. Radiology 229:176–183

Fayad ZA (2003) MR imaging for the noninvasive assessment of atherothrombotic plaques. Magn Reson Imaging Clin North Am 11:101–113

Finn JP, Baskaran V, Carr JC et al (2002) Thorax: low-dose contrast-enhanced three-dimensional MR angiography with subsecond temporal resolution – initial results. Radiology 224:896–904

Flacke S, Fischer S, Scott MJ et al (2001) Novel MRI contrast agent for molecular imaging of fibrin: implications for detecting vulnerable plaques. Circulation 104:1280–1285

Francois CJ, Shors SM, Bonow RO, Finn JP (2003) Analysis of cardiopulmonary transit times at contrast material-enhanced MR imaging in patients with heart disease. Radiology 227:447–452

Gaubert JY, Moulin G, Mesana T et al (1995) Type A dissection of the thoracic aorta: use of MR imaging for long-term follow-up. Radiology 196:363–369

Gomes AS, Lois JF, George B, Alpan G, Williams RG (1987) Congenital abnormalities of the aortic arch: MR imaging. Radiology 165:691–695

Goyen M, Ruehm SG, Debatin JF (2000) MR-angiography: the role of contrast agents. Eur J Radiol 34:247–256

Greil GF, Powell AJ, Gildein HP, Geva T (2002) Gadolinium-enhanced three-dimensional magnetic resonance angiography of pulmonary and systemic venous anomalies. J Am Coll Cardiol 39:335–341

Grist TM, Sostman HD, MacFall JR et al (1993) Pulmonary angiography with MR imaging: preliminary clinical experience. Radiology 189:523–530

Groenink M, Roos A de, Mulder BJ et al (2001) Biophysical properties of the normal-sized aorta in patients with Marfan syndrome: evaluation with MR flow mapping. Radiology 219:535–540

Gundry SR, Burney RE, Mackenzie JR, et al (1984) Traumatic pseudoaneurysms of the thoracic aorta. Anatomic and radiologic correlations. Arch Surg 119:1055–1060

Hagan PG, Nienaber CA, Isselbacher EM et al (2000) The International Registry of Acute Aortic Dissection (IRAD): new insights into an old disease. JAMA 283:897–903

Hamdan MA, Maheshwari S, Fahey JT, Hellenbrand WE (2001) Endovascular stents for coarctation of the aorta: initial results and intermediate-term follow-up. J Am Coll Cardiol 38:1518–1523

Hartnell GG (2001) Imaging of aortic aneurysms and dissections: CT and MRI. J Thorac Imaging 16:35–46

Hartnell GG, Finn JP, Zenni M et al (1994) MR imaging of the thoracic aorta: comparison of spin-echo, angiographic, and breath-hold techniques. Radiology 191:697–704

Hartnell GG, Hughes LA, Finn JP, Longmaid HE 3rd (1995)

Magnetic resonance angiography of the central chest veins. A new gold standard? Chest 107:1053–1057

Hegde SR, Taylor AM, Muthurangu VM, Miquel ME, Razavi R (2004) The use of MRI in detecting pulmonary vein compression in patients with Fontan circulation. ECR Conf Proc [Suppl 2] 14:B-531

Hernandez RJ (2002) Magnetic resonance imaging of mediastinal vessels. Magn Reson Imaging Clin North Am 10:237–251

Higgins CB, Caputo GR (1993) Role of MR imaging in acquired and congenital cardiovascular disease. AJR Am J Roentgenol 161:13–22

Higgins CB, Sakuma H (1996) Heart disease: functional evaluation with MR imaging. Radiology 199:307–315

Hilfiker PR, Quick HH, Pfammatter T, Schmidt M, Debatin JF (1999) Three-dimensional MR angiography of a nitinol-based abdominal aortic stent graft: assessment of heating and imaging characteristics. Eur Radiol 9:1775–1780

Ho VB, Foo TK (1998) Optimization of gadolinium-enhanced magnetic resonance angiography using an automated bolus-detection algorithm (MR SmartPrep). Original investigation. Invest Radiol 33:515–523

Ho VB, Choyke PL, Foo TK et al (1999) Automated bolus chase peripheral MR angiography: initial practical experiences and future directions of this work-in-progress. J Magn Reson Imaging 10:376–388

Holmqvist C, Stahlberg F, Hanseus K et al (2002) Collateral flow in coarctation of the aorta with magnetic resonance velocity mapping: correlation to morphological imaging of collateral vessels. J Magn Reson Imaging 15:39–46

Kaemmerer H, Theissen P, Konig U, Sechtem U, Vivie ER de (1993) Follow-up using magnetic resonance imaging in adult patients after surgery for aortic coarctation. Thorac Cardiovasc Surg 41:107–111

Kanne JP, Lalani TA (2004) Role of computed tomography and magnetic resonance imaging for deep venous thrombosis and pulmonary embolism. Circulation [Suppl 1] 109:15–21

Kersting-Sommerhoff BA, Sechtem UP, Fisher MR, Higgins CB (1987a) MR imaging of congenital anomalies of the aortic arch. AJR Am J Roentgenol 149:9–13

Kersting-Sommerhoff BA, Sechtem UP, Schiller NB, Lipton MJ, Higgins CB (1987b) MR imaging of the thoracic aorta in Marfan patients. J Comput Assist Tomogr 11:633–639

Knauth AL, Marshall AC, Geva T, Jonas RA, Marx GR (2004) Respiratory symptoms secondary to aortopulmonary collateral vessels in tetralogy of Fallot absent pulmonary valve syndrome. Am J Cardiol 93:503–505

Korosec FR, Grist TM, Mistretta CA (1996) Time-resolved contrast-enhanced 3D MR angiography. Magn Reson Med 36:345–351

Krinsky GA, Rofsky NM, DeCorato DR et al (1997) Thoracic aorta: comparison of gadolinium-enhanced three-dimensional MR angiography with conventional MR imaging. Radiology 202:183–193

Lardo AC (2000) Real-time magnetic resonance imaging: diagnostic and interventional applications. Pediatr Cardiol 21:80–98

Lebowitz JA, Rofsky NM, Krinsky GA, Weinreb JC (1997) Gadolinium-enhanced body MR venography with subtraction technique. AJR Am J Roentgenol 169:755–758

Lee VS, Resnick D, Bundy JM et al (2002) Cardiac function: MR evaluation in one breath hold with real-time true fast imaging with steady state precession. Radiology 222:835–842

Leung DA, Debatin JF (1997) Three-dimensional contrast-enhanced magnetic resonance angiography of the thoracic vasculature. Eur Radiol 7:981–989

Marchal G, Bogaert J (1998) Non-invasive imaging of the great vessels of the chest. Eur Radiol 8:1099–1105

Markl M, Alley MT, Pelc NJ (2003a) Balanced phase-contrast steady-state free precession (PC-SSFP): a novel technique for velocity encoding by gradient inversion. Magn Reson Med 49:945–952

Markl M, Chan FP, Alley MT et al (2003b) Time-resolved three-dimensional phase-contrast MRI. J Magn Reson Imaging 17:499–506

Masui T, Seelos KC, Kersting-Sommerhoff BA, Higgins CB (1991) Abnormalities of the pulmonary veins: evaluation with MR imaging and comparison with cardiac angiography and echocardiography. Radiology 181:645–649

Masui T, Katayama M, Kobayashi S et al (2000) Gadolinium-enhanced MR angiography in the evaluation of congenital cardiovascular disease pre- and postoperative states in infants and children. J Magn Reson Imaging 12:1034–1042

McElhinney DB, Reddy VM, Moore P, Hanley FL (1996) Revision of previous Fontan connections to extracardiac or intraatrial conduit cavopulmonary anastomosis. Ann Thorac Surg 62:1276–1283

Mohiaddin RH, Schoser K, Amanuma M, Burman ED, Longmore DB (1990) MR imaging of age-related dimensional changes of thoracic aorta. J Comput Assist Tomogr 14:748–752

Mohiaddin RH, Kilner PJ, Rees S et al (1993) Magnetic resonance volume flow and jet velocity mapping in aortic coarctation. J Am Coll Cardiol 22:1515–1521

Mohiaddin RH, McCrohon J, Francis JM et al (2001) Contrast-enhanced magnetic resonance angiogram of penetrating aortic ulcer. Circulation 103:18–19

Nayler GL, Firmin DN, Longmore DB (1986) Blood flow imaging by cine magnetic resonance. J Comput Assist Tomogr 10:715–722

Nienaber CA, Con Kodolitsch Y, Nicolas V et al (1993) The diagnosis of aortic dissection by non-invasive imaging procedures. N Engl J Med 328:1–9

Nienaber CA, Richartz BM, Rehders T, Ince H, Petzsch M (2004) Aortic intramural haematoma: natural history and predictive factors for complications. Heart 90:372–374

Nollen GJ, Schijndel KE van, Timmermans J et al (2003) Magnetic resonance imaging of the main pulmonary artery: reliable assessment of dimensions in Marfan patients on a simple axial spin echo image. Int J Cardiovasc Imaging 19:141–147

O'Donnell CP, Lock JE, Powell AJ, Perry SB (2003) Compression of pulmonary veins between the left atrium and the descending aorta. Am J Cardiol 91:248–251

Oppelt A, Graumann R, Barfuss H (1986) FISP – a new fast MRI sequence. Electromedica 54:15–18

Pereles FS, Kapoor V, Carr JC et al (2001) Usefulness of segmented trueFISP cardiac pulse sequence in evaluation of congenital and acquired adult cardiac abnormalities. AJR Am J Roentgenol 177:1155–1160

Pettigrew RI, Oshinski JN, Chatzimavroudis G, Dixon WT (1999) MRI techniques for cardiovascular imaging. J Magn Reson Imaging 10:590–601

Pilleul F, Merchant N (2000) MRI of the pulmonary veins: comparison between 3D MR angiography and T1-weighted spin echo. J Comput Assist Tomogr 24:683–687

Pitt MP, Bonser RS (1997) The natural history of thoracic aortic aneurysm disease: an overview. J Card Surg [Suppl 2] 12:270–278

Powell AJ, Chung T, Landzberg MJ, Geva T (2000) Accuracy of MRI evaluation of pulmonary blood supply in patients with complex pulmonary stenosis or atresia. Int J Card Imaging 16:169–174

Prasad SK, Soukias N, Hornung T et al (2004) Role of magnetic resonance angiography in the diagnosis of major aortopulmonary collateral arteries and partial anomalous pulmonary venous drainage. Circulation 109:207–214

Prince MR (1994) Gadolinium-enhanced MR aortography. Radiology 191:155–164

Prince MR, Yucel EK, Kaufman JA, Harrison DC, Geller SC (1993) Dynamic gadolinium-enhanced three-dimensional abdominal MR arteriography. J Magn Reson Imaging 3:877–381

Prince MR, Narasimham DL, Jacoby WT et al (1996) Three-dimensional gadolinium-enhanced MR angiography of the thoracic aorta. AJR Am J Roentgenol 166:1387–1397

Razavi R, Baker E (1999) Magnetic resonance imaging comes of age. Cardiol Young 9:529–538

Razavi RS, Hill DL, Muthurangu V et al (2003) Three-dimensional magnetic resonance imaging of congenital cardiac anomalies. Cardiol Young 13:461–465

Riederer SJ, Bernstein MA, Breen JF et al (2000) Three-dimensional contrast-enhanced MR angiography with real-time fluoroscopic triggering: design specifications and technical reliability in 330 patient studies. Radiology 215:584–593

Roche KJ, Krinsky G, Lee VS, Rofsky N, Genieser NB (1999) Interrupted aortic arch: diagnosis with gadolinium-enhanced 3D MRA. J Comput Assist Tomogr 23:197–202

Roman MJ, Devereux RB, Niles NW et al (1987) Aortic root dilatation as a cause of isolated, severe aortic regurgitation. Prevalence, clinical and echocardiographic patterns, and relation to left ventricular hypertrophy and function. Ann Intern Med 106:800–807

Roos-Hesselink JW, Scholzel BE, Heijdra RJ et al (2003) Aortic valve and aortic arch pathology after coarctation repair. Heart 89:1074–1077

Scheffler K, Lehnhardt S (2003) Principles and applications of balanced SSFP techniques. Eur Radiol 13:2409–2418

Schmidta M, Theissen P, Klempt G et al (2000) Long-term follow-up of 82 patients with chronic disease of the thoracic aorta using spin-echo and cine gradient magnetic resonance imaging. Magn Reson Imaging 18:795–806

Sevitt S (1977) The mechanisms of traumatic rupture of the thoracic aorta. Br J Surg 64:166–173

Simonetti OP, Finn JP, White RD et al (1996) "Black-blood" T2-weighted inversion-recovery MR imaging of the heart. Radiology 199:49–57

Sodickson DK, Manning WJ (1997) Simultaneous acquisition of spatial harmonics (SMASH): fast imaging with radiofrequency coil arrays. Magn Reson Med 38:591–603

Sodickson DK, McKenzie CA, Li W, Wolff S, Manning WJ, Edelman RR (2000) Contrast-enhanced 3D MR angiography with simultaneous acquisition of spatial harmonics: a pilot study. Radiology 217:284–289

Soler R, Rodriguez E, Requejo I et al (1998) Magnetic reso-nance imaging of congenital abnormalities of the thoracic aorta. Eur Radiol 8:540–546

Solomon SL, Brown JJ, Glazer HS, Mirowitz SA, Lee JK (1990) Thoracic aortic dissection: pitfalls and artifacts in MR imaging. Radiology 177:223–228

Sonnabend SB, Colletti PM, Pentecost MJ (1990) Demonstration of aortic lesions via cine magnetic resonance imaging. Magn Reson Imaging 8:613–618

Spuentrup E, Buecker A, Stuber M, Gunther RW (2001) MR-venography using high resolution True-FISP. Rofo Fortschr Geb Rontgenstr Neuen Bildgeb Verfahr 173:686–690

Stehling MK, Holzknecht NG, Laub G et al (1996) Single-shot T1 and T2 weighted magnetic resonance imaging of the heart with black blood: preliminary experience. MAGMA 4:231–240

Stemerman DH, Krinsky GA, Lee VS, et al (1999) Thoracic aorta: rapid black-blood MR imaging with half-Fourier rapid acquisition with relaxation enhancement with or without electrocardiographic triggering. Radiology 213:185–191

Summers RM, Sostman HD, Spritzer CE, Fidler JL (1996) Fast spoiled gradient-recalled MR imaging of thoracic aortic dissection: preliminary clinical experience at 1.5 T. Magn Reson Imaging 14:1–9

Svensson LG, Labib SB, Eisenhauer AC, Butterly JR (1999) Intimal tear without hematoma. An important variant of aortic dissection that can elude current imaging techniques. Circulation 99:1331–1336

Szolar DH, Sakuma H, Higgins CB (1996) Cardiovascular applications of magnetic resonance flow and velocity measurements. J Magn Reson Imaging 6:78–89

Toussaint JF (2002) MRI characterization of atherosclerotic arteries: diagnosis of plaque rupture. J Neuroradiol 29:223–230

Van Beek EJ, Wild JM, Fink C, et al (2003) MRI for the diagnosis of pulmonary embolism. J Magn Reson Imaging 18:627–640

Van der Wall EE, Rugge FP van, Vliegen HW, et al (1997) Ischemic heart disease: value of MR techniques. Int J Card Imaging 13:179–189

Van Grimberge F, Dymarkowski S, Budts W, Bogaert J (2000) Role of magnetic resonance in the diagnosis of subclavian steal syndrome. J Magn Reson Imaging 12:339–342

Van Praagh R, Bernhard WF, Rosenthal A et al (1971) Interrupted aortic arch: surgical treatment. Am J Cardiol 27:200–211

Videlefsky N, Parks WJ, Oshinski J et al (2001) Magnetic resonance phase-shift velocity mapping in pediatric patients with pulmonary venous obstruction. J Am Coll Cardiol 38:262–267

Vogt FM, Goyen M, Debatin JF (2003) MR angiography of the chest. Radiol Clin North Am 41:29–41

Von Kodolitsch Y, Csosz SK, Koschyk DH et al (2003) Intramural hematoma of the aorta: predictors of progression to dissection and rupture. Circulation 107:1158–1163

Von Schulthess GK, Higashino SM, Higgins SS, et al (1986) Coarctation of the aorta: MR imaging. Radiology 158:469–474

Wang Y, Rossman PJ, Grimm RC, et al (1996) 3D MR angiography of pulmonary arteries using real-time navigator gating and magnetization preparation. Magn Reson Med 36:579–587

Weiger M, Pruessmann KP, Boesiger P (2000a) Cardiac real-time imaging using SENSE. SENSitivity Encoding scheme. Magn Reson Med 43:177–184

Weiger M, Pruessmann KP, Kassner A et al (2000b) Contrast-enhanced 3D MRA using SENSE. J Magn Reson Imaging 12:671–677

Weissleder R, Mahmood U (2001) Molecular imaging. Radiology 219:316–333

White CS (2000) MR imaging of thoracic veins. Magn Reson Imaging Clin North Am 8:17–32

White CS, Baffa JM, Haney PJ, Campbell AB, NessAiver M (1998) Anomalies of pulmonary veins: usefulness of spin-echo and gradient-echo MR images. AJR Am J Roentgenol 170:1365–1368

Wildenhain PM, Bourekas EC (1991) Pulmonary varix: magnetic resonance findings. Cathet Cardiovasc Diagn 24:268–270

Winkler ML, Higgins CB (1986) MRI of perivalvular infectious pseudoaneurysms. AJR Am J Roentgenol 147:253–256

Winter PM, Morawski AM, Caruthers SD et al (2003) Molecular imaging of angiogenesis in early-stage atherosclerosis with alpha(v)beta3-integrin-targeted nanoparticles. Circulation 108:2270–2274

Wolff KA, Herold CJ, Tempany CM, Parravano JG, Zerhouni EA (1991) Aortic dissection: atypical patterns seen at MR imaging. Radiology 181:489–495

Yucel EK, Steinberg FL, Egglin TK et al (1990) Penetrating aortic ulcers: diagnosis with MR imaging. Radiology 177:779–781

17 MR-Guided Cardiac Catheterization

Reza Razavi, Vivek Muthurangu, Sanjeet R. Hegde, and Andrew M. Taylor

CONTENTS

R. Razavi, MBBS, MRCP, MRCPCH
V. Muthurangu, BSc, MBChB, MRCPCH
S. R Hegde, MBBS, MRCPCH
Division of Imaging Science, King's College London, Guy's Hospital Campus, London Bridge, London SE1 9RT, UK
A. M. Taylor, MD, MRCP, FRCR
Cardiothoracic Unit, Institute of Child Health and Great Ormond Street Hospital for Children, London WC1N 3JH, UK

17.1 Introduction

Cardiac catheterization is one of the most important procedures in cardiology for diagnosis (e.g., ischemic and congenital heart disease) and more recently as an effective and less invasive method of performing interventions, replacing cardiac surgery for a number of indications (Pihkala et al. 1999).

There have been a great number of advances in cardiac catheterization since Claude Bernard passed a catheter into the right and left ventricles of a horse in 1844. The advent of X-ray imaging made cardiac catheterization a reality, though, when Werner Forssmann passed a urinary catheter into his own right atrium, via the left antecubital vein, under fluoroscopic guidance and then climbed the stairs to the radiology department to undergo a chest X-ray, he was met with a great deal of skepticism. Other pioneers such as Andre Cournard, Dickenson Richards, and Louis Dexter expanded the work to include the study of cardiac physiology in humans and demonstrated the clinical use of this technique, especially in congenital heart disease. Modern day cardiac catheterization has made great progress from this early days. There have been developments in x-ray technology that enables high frame rates during acquisition (25 frames/s), coupled with better resolution (0.5 mm), biplane imaging, and, most recently, flat-plate technology.

There has also been a great deal of progress made in the design of catheters, guide wires, and devices used during cardiac catheterization. This has allowed a growing number of cardiovascular interventions to be carried out during cardiac catheterization rather than at surgery, including: balloon atrial septostomy; balloon dilation of pulmonary (Rao et al. 1998) and aortic valves (Magee et al. 1997); stent implantation in coronary arteries and aortic coarctation (Magee et al. 1999); and effective closure of atrial septal (Du et al. 2002) and ventricular septal defects (Holzer et al. 2004a,b). Interventional cardiac catheterization has changed the management of patients with cardiovascular disease, and innovative progress in this area continues with, for example, the development and recent clinical use of trans-catheter valve stents for pulmonary valve replacement, heralding a new chapter in the progress of interventional cardiology (BONHOEFFER et al. 2002).

Cardiac catheterization under X-ray guidance is therefore an integral part of the management of patients with cardiovascular disease. However, developments in other areas of cardiovascular imaging (echocardiography, nuclear cardiology, and cardiovascular MR) have changed the clinical practice of cardiac catheterization over time. For example, in many patients with congenital heart disease, diagnostic cardiac catheterization has become a second- or third-line investigation that is reserved for problem solving. This is especially true for neonates, where echocardiography can provide clear diagnostic anatomical information and, in combination with Doppler ultrasonography (Doppler) and color flow Doppler imaging (color Doppler), a reasonable understanding of the physiology of complex abnormalities (SILVERMAN and SCHILLER 1978; SNIDER and SILVERMAN 1981). For some conditions, echocardiography alone can be used to guide further treatment (medical, interventional catheterization, or surgery). Furthermore, where expertise in cardiovascular MRI exists, MRI can be used to provide much of the information that has previously been gleaned from diagnostic cardiac catheterization both in presurgical or interventional planning and in the follow-up of these procedures (RAZAVI and BAKER 1999) (see Chap. 15). There still remains; however, an important role for diagnostic cardiac catheterization where invasive pressures are needed (e.g., measurement of pulmonary vascular resistance) and where other imaging modalities cannot as yet provide good enough image quality (e.g., coronary artery imaging).

Although there has been great progress in the last few years, with many more interventional procedures being performed, correcting lesions that previously would have required surgery, there has been little change in the imaging methods used for cardiac catheterization. The mainstay remains X-ray angiography, although transesophageal echocardiography is used as an adjunct in transcatheter closure of atrial septal defects (MAGNI et al. 1997), and, to a much smaller extent, intracardiac echocardiography (KOENIG et al. 2003).

The limitations of X-ray angiography have become more apparent as more complicated interventional cardiac catheterization procedures (e.g.,

radiofrequency, RF, ablation of tachyarrhythmias) have been attempted. Firstly, these procedures take longer to perform, increasing the X-radiation dose of each procedure. As patients with congenital heart disease now have a much-improved life expectancy, the risk of developing a malignancy in later life is becoming significant. Secondly, these procedures require precise anatomical positioning of catheters or devices, with exact measurement of lesion size, which is crucial for selecting the appropriately sized device; both of which are difficult with X-ray angiography. Finally, physiological measurements are also important and can be less accurate and more difficult to obtain from X-ray-guided cardiac catheterization than from cardiovascular MRI.

17.2
Rationale for MR-Guided Cardiac Catheterization

17.2.1
Reduced X-Ray Exposure

There is increasing concern about the long-term health effects of the X-ray dose following cardiac catheterization (MODAN et al. 2000; BERRINGTON DE GONZALEZ and DARBY 2004; FAULKNER et al. 1986; KOVOOR et al. 1998). In adults, the UK National Radiation Protection Board (NRPB 1999) has calculated the mean risk of developing a solid tumor as a result of a single cardiac catheterization procedure is approximately 1 in 2,500 (NRPB 1999). In children; however, there are three important additional factors. Firstly, the younger the patient the higher this risk becomes. If exposure occurs at 5 years of age, the risk is increased by a factor of 2.3 to approximately 1 in 1000 (median age of patients undergoing X-ray cardiac catheterization in our unit is 7 years) (IRCP 1990). Secondly, the NRPB data relate to an average procedure with a screening time of 21 min; average screening time for patient's in our conventional cardiac catheter laboratory is 22 min (RAZAVI et al. 2003b). Some procedures in patients with congenital heart disease often require longer X-ray exposure. The worst case in the NRPB study was a screening time of 176 min. Finally, the risk is multiplied in patients who have a number of cardiac catheter procedures.

Furthermore, there is also a significant risk from X-ray exposure to the staff in the catheter laboratory during these procedures despite the use of protective shields.

17.2.2
Increased Anatomical Information

Another shortcoming of performing cardiac catheterization under X-ray is the poor contrast of soft tissues such as the heart and great vessels. When positioning guide wires, catheters, balloons, and interventional devices, it is not possible to visualize the relevant structures: The operator has to rely on mental images of the anatomy from previous experience, or on contrast angiographic images acquired earlier in the procedure. This leads to some difficulty and a degree of trial and error, which not only prolongs the procedure, but also has the small risk of perforating the heart or great vessels or other complications. The lack of visualization of the relevant anatomy is particularly a handicap in interventional cardiac catheterization procedures and RF ablation of arrhythmias.

In interventional cardiac catheterization procedures for congenital heart disease, accurate measurement of the size of defects and nearby anatomical structures is crucial, as this determines the selection and deployment of the correct-sized device. Accurate size measurement under X-ray angiography can be difficult. Firstly, it requires some calibration object, such as the catheter, to determine the scale. This calibration object may be small or not exactly in the plane of the area being measured, and this can introduce error. Secondly, the structures of interest are nearly always three-dimensional (3D), and the two-dimensional (2D) X-ray image may not allow full appreciation of the accurate size.

Furthermore, the ability to visualize the surface anatomy of the heart or vessel would be very helpful when positioning catheters (Fig. 17.1) or devices both for RF ablation and interventional cardiac catheterization. Often the difference between a satisfactory or unsatisfactory outcome is malpositioning of the RF ablation catheter by a few centimeters or even millimeters, and exact positioning under X-ray fluoroscopy alone can at times be difficult.

MRI, using the right sequence acquisition, allows accurate measurement of 3D structures as well as accurate rendering of the 3D surface of the heart and vessels.

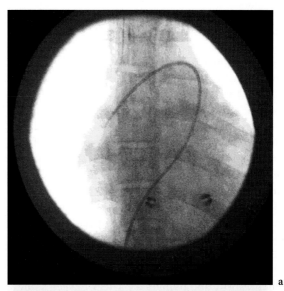

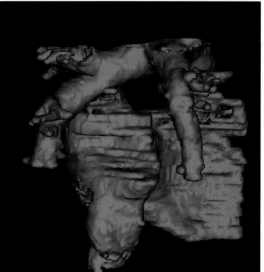

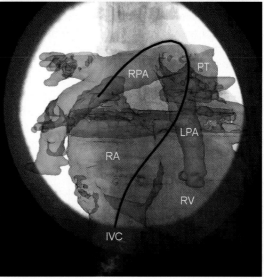

Fig. 17.1. a X-ray cardiac catheterization – projectional image of a cardiac catheter looped through the right side of the heart with its tip lying in the right pulmonary artery. **b** Surface rendering of the right side of the heart derived from the MR images. **c** The MR and X-ray image have been registered, clearly demonstrating the 3D course of the catheter

17.2.3
Increased Functional Information

Cardiac catheterization is used to provide not only anatomical information but also functional information. Invasive pressures and blood gases are used to calculate systemic and pulmonary blood flow and resistance using the Fick principle. Cine angiography is also used to assess global ventricular function as well as regional wall motion abnormalities. The functional information obtained at cardiac catheterization is used alongside the anatomical information to assess the suitability for surgery or interventional cardiac catheterization, or the need for long-term vasodilator therapy in patients with pulmonary vascular disease.

The Fick principle requires measurement of hemoglobin, aortic and pulmonary artery oxygen saturations and partial pressures, and oxygen consumption. This dependency on multiple measurements leads to the accumulation of individual measurement errors and is a considerable source of inaccuracy (HILLIS et al. 1985a; CIGARROA et al. 1989; DHINGRA et al. 2002). The accuracy and precision of the Fick principle is further reduced in patients with large intracardiac shunts and high pulmonary blood flow, due to the reduced pulmonary arteriovenous oxygen content difference (HILLIS et al. 1985a; CIGARROA et al. 1989; DHINGRA et al. 2002). Reliable pulmonary vascular resistance (PVR) quantification is vital in this group of patients, as they are likely to develop pulmonary vascular disease, which will alter their surgical management. The use of high-concentration oxygen, as a pulmonary vasodilator, further reduces the reliability of the Fick principle. This is a severe limitation, because response to vasodilators is important in making management decisions regarding long-term medical therapy (ATZ et al. 1999). Other methods of

invasive flow quantification (e.g., indicator dilution and thermodilution techniques) can be used in patients with congenital heart disease (RAZAVI et al. 2001). However, these techniques also suffer from significantly reduced reliability in the presence of cardiac shunts, especially if there is tricuspid or pulmonary valve regurgitation (RAZAVI et al. 2001).

There is therefore a need for a method of flow quantification that allows accurate and reproducible measurement of PVR. Velocity-encoded phase-contrast MR enables quantification of blood flow in major vessels. Cardiac output and the pulmonary to systemic flow ratio ($Q_p:Q_s$) measured using this technique have been shown to be accurate (HUNDLEY et al. 1995; BEERBAUM et al. 2001). In addition, phase-contrast MR has been validated in numerous phantom experiments (BEERBAUM et al. 2001; ROBERTSON et al. 2001).

Assessment of global and regional ventricular function can also be carried out much more accurately with cine b-SSFP cardiac MR than with X-ray angiography. Using cardiac MR for assessing global ventricular function and regional wall function, there is no need to make assumptions about cardiac geometry that have to be made with X-ray angiography, inductance catheters, and echocardiography (BELLENGER et al. 2002). This is particularly important when assessing right ventricular function (HELBING et al. 1995).

Finally, combining invasive pressure measurement with MR-derived blood flow and ventricular volumes offers a novel method of investigating the pathophysiology of pulmonary vascular compliance and impedance, as well as ventricular pressure volume loops and the parameters that can be derived from these measurements for assessment of load-independent ventricular function (e.g., end-systolic elastance) (Fig. 17.2).

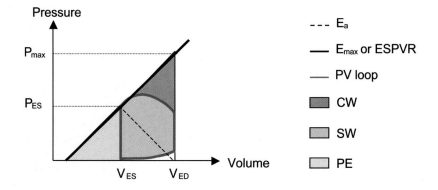

Fig. 17.2. Schematic plot of right ventricular single-beat pressure-volume loop. E_a, arterial elastance; *ESPVR* (E_{max}), end-systolic pressure-volume relation; *CW*, cardiac work; *SW*, stroke work; *PE*, potential energy; P_{ES}, end-systolic pressure; V_{ES}, end-systolic volume; V_{ED}, end-diastolic volume; *PV loop*, pressure-volume loop. Such loops offer the potential to measure load-independent parameters of ventricular function

17.3
Potential Advantages of MR Catheter Guidance

17.3.1
Better Catheter Guidance; Reduced Risks

Guidance of catheter guide wires and devices through the heart and great vessels of patients, especially with complex congenital heart disease, can be challenging. During X-ray fluoroscopy, only the catheters or devices are normally visualized and the heart and vessels are not seen. It can, for example, be difficult to differentiate between a catheter pointing anteriorly or posteriorly when looking from the anterior–posterior (AP) view. In more difficult cases, or with a less experienced operator, there is a risk of perforating the heart or vessel especially in infants and young children. Although previous X-ray angiographic images may help understanding of the anatomy, the inability to visualize the surrounding anatomy during catheter/device manipulation remains a real problem.

MR-guided cardiac catheterization allows visualization of the anatomy during catheter guidance and so has the potential to make more difficult cases safer as well as easier and quicker to perform.

17.3.2
Better Information; More Difficult Interventional Procedures

Over the last few years, many procedures that were previously performed surgically have been carried out with interventional cardiac catheterization in patients with congenital heart disease. In some centers most cases of atrial septal defects, branch pulmonary narrowing, and recoarctation or coarctation in older children and adults are treated with interventional cardiac catheterization. More recently, some ventricular septal defect (HIJAZI et al. 2002; HOLZER et al. 2004a,b) and pulmonary valve replacement (BONHOEFFER et al. 2002) procedures have been performed by interventional cardiac catheterization, though there remain a sizable percentage of these cases that are still repaired surgically.

To be able to perform these more challenging cases under cardiac catheterization, the ability to visualize 3D anatomy during device placement would be helpful. For example, for complex aortic coarctation with transverse arch narrowing, stent positioning needs to be accurate to avoid obstruction of the bra-chiocephalic vessels. In the future, if transcatheter aortic valve replacement becomes a reality, accurate positioning of the aortic valve to avoid the coronary ostia and anterior leaflet of the mitral valve will be necessary. Such accurate placement of devices can be difficult with X-ray fluoroscopy alone, while MR guidance has the potential to help with these procedures and make them possible.

The advantages of visualization of anatomy with MR for interventional cases also apply to difficult cases of RF ablation of arrhythmias. In particular, during ablation of atrial arrhythmias via the pulmonary veins, it can be difficult to judge the exact position of the RF ablation catheter, without superimposed 3D anatomical data.

17.4
MR-Guided Intervention and MR-Guided Cardiac Catheterization

Performing procedures under MR guidance to take advantage of the precise anatomical and functional information has been the subject of extensive research and development over the last 10 years. Originally, it was thought that open, low-field systems would be the way forward, as they provide easy access to the patient (FAHRIG et al. 2001, 2003). However, this is at the expense of the better quality and faster imaging obtained on higher field-strength (1.5 T) systems.

There has been significant progress made with both low-field and high-field systems in MR-guided intervention in the field of neurosurgery (LIU et al. 2000; FAHRIG et al. 2003). However, other applications such as vascular and cardiac imaging, which would also benefit from MR guidance, have been much slower to develop. There have been a number of recent developments that are making MR-guided vascular and cardiac procedures possible. Firstly, it is now possible to acquire reasonable-quality (spatial resolution) images very quickly (high temporal resolution) (BAKKER et al. 1996). From clinical experience and experimental data, MR catheter guidance requires a temporal resolution of at least 10 images per second. Secondly, it is possible to interactively move the imaging plane of the catheter, as it is manipulated in real time (MIQUEL et al. 2004). The temporal and spatial resolution required for this is only possible in a 1.5-T MR scanner.

Visualization of cardiac catheters, guide wires, and devices under MR guidance has also been an area of active research for a number of years. The two main methods of active (LEUNG et al. 1995; OCALI and ATALAR 1997; LADD et al. 1998a) and passive visualization (BAKKER et al. 1997; OMARY et al. 2000; MIQUEL et al. 2004) have distinct advantages and drawbacks. There is also a third method of semiactive visualization, which consists of a microcoil without the wire connections seen in active visualization (KUEHNE et al. 2003a). Although a great deal of phantom and animal experimental work has been carried out, this work has only recently been translated to humans.

17.4.1
Passive Catheter Tracking

Passive catheter visualization relies on either increased signal or, more usually, signal void/artifact for tracking. Unlike active tracking, there are no external connections to the MR scanner or source of electrical energy, and therefore not the same safety concerns as in active tacking. The signal void is secondary to: (1) displacement of fluid and hence water protons by the catheter or device, and (2) differing magnetic susceptibilities between the materials used for passive tracking (dysprosium oxide, gadolinium, or, in our clinical experience, carbon dioxide-filled balloon), and the surrounding tissues cause field inhomogeneity and so shortening of $T2^*$ (BAKKER et al. 1997) (Fig. 17.3). Both of these factors lead to loss of local signal and provide negative contrast within a vessel imaged with "bright-blood" sequences such as b-SSFP. The susceptibility artifact produced by these passive catheter methods is dependent on device shape, orientation to the magnetic field, and the phase-encode and readout directions.

Most catheters used in routine X-ray catheterization are metal braided for extra torque and are therefore not MR compatible. They not only are moved by the MR scanner's magnetic field, but also have the potential to induce current within them and so can experience a temperature rise within the MR scanner.

Currently available guide wires are also not safe to use in the MR environment. Even nonferrous guide wires (e.g., those made from nitinol) can have current induced in them and heat up to over 70°C (KONINGS et al. 2000; NITZ et al. 2001; YEUNG et al. 2002a,b).

There has been much work carried out on passive catheter tracking form a number of groups. In particular, the group at University Hospital, Utrecht, has demonstrated that conventional, nonbraided

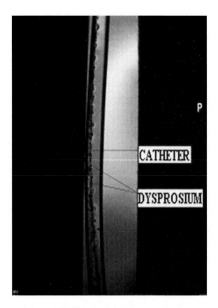

Fig. 17.3. Dysprosium catheter. A dysprosium oxide-impregnated catheter is seen within a static phantom. The catheter is clearly visualized along its full length despite being orientated along B_0 (worst-case visualization conditions for susceptibility techniques). Fast field echo image: TR 23 ms, TE 7.8 ms, flip angle 50°, rectangular FOV 35%, slice thickness 3 mm, matrix 1,024×1,024.

catheters marked with dysprosium rings along their length can be visualized using fast, real-time imaging sequences when the catheter is moved in the vessels in phantoms and experimental animals (BAKKER et al. 1996, 1997). Although nitinol guide wires similarly marked with dysprosium have also been visualized with passive tracking, safety concerns have precluded their use in humans.

Passive catheter tracking using increased signal from the catheter has been more difficult to establish, despite good early work with catheters filled with diluted (4–6%) gadolinium (OMARY et al. 2000). This is mainly because modern, fast, real-time imaging techniques use bright-blood b-SSFP and so a signal void (negative contrast) from the catheter is easier to visualize. Very recently, the use of saturation pulses to reduce background signal has made dilute gadolinium-filled catheter visualization more realistic. However, this has the disadvantage of masking the image of the heart and vessels; one of the main motivations of MR-guided cardiac catheterization.

In our XMR unit at Guy's Hospital, London, we have performed a number of phantom experiments with both high-signal and signal-void passive catheter visualization techniques with a number of different sequences and parameters in a flow phantom setting. We found that optimum passive tracking was achieved using nonbraided routine balloon angiographic catheters (Swan-Ganz catheters). By filling the distal balloon with carbon dioxide, we were able to visualize the signal void at the catheter tip when manipulating the catheter in phantoms and subsequently in human subjects (Fig. 17.4).

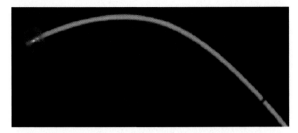

Fig. 17.4. Photograph of an inflated balloon angiographic Bermann catheter (Arrow International, Reading, PA), filled with 0.8 ml of CO_2

17.4.2
Active Catheter Tracking

An active catheter is one that contains a device that is electronically connected to the scanner. One type of active catheter tracking uses the field inhomogeneity caused by running a small amount of DC current in wires running along the length of the catheter (GLOWINSKI et al. 1997). This then provides a susceptibility artifact similar to that seen in passive tracking with dysprosium oxide.

More typical types of active catheters contain a coil or antenna, which receives signal from tissue in its immediate vicinity. These devices do not transmit signal into the patient, but rely on the body coil to transmit to the patient. The signal received by these coils can then be used either to pinpoint their position or for imaging of local tissue or both (LADD et al. 1997, 1998a,b). There are two important types of these active catheters: Those based on small coils positioned, for example, at the end of a catheter; and those based on a loopless antenna that can run along the catheter or be made into a guide wire.

The great advantage of these active systems is that the location of the catheter is unambiguous. Charles DeMoulin, of GE Medical Systems, is widely credited with inventing this approach. He showed that the location of a small resonant coil at the tip of a catheter could be identified by a series of three, 1D projections along each axis (LEUNG et al. 1995). This can be done quickly (in 3 repetition times) and so can be repeated for very fast update of the catheter position, allowing real-time tracking of the catheter. The position of the catheter can then be projected over a previously acquired road map. Similar techniques have been combined with fast, real-time imaging of the heart or vessels using surface coils, and the combined (interleaved) sequence has allowed simultaneous localization of the catheter as well as imaging of the surrounding tissues. Further adaptation of these sequences has allowed automatic imaging plane manipulation to keep track of changes in catheter position (Philips, Hamburg catheter tracking software). More recently, the group at the National Institutes of Health, USA (NIH) has developed a technique that allows real-time visualization of two simultaneously acquired planes, as well as the catheter or device position, thus overcoming the major problem of the catheter moving through-plane when only one imaging plane is visualized (GUTTMAN et al. 2002). This technique has been used to great effect in animal experiments demonstrating the potential of MR-guided cardiac catheterization in targeted intramyocardial injection of progenitor stem cells in myocardial infarction, where the position of the delivery device was visualized using active catheter tracking (HILL et al. 2003).

Active visualization has great potential, as it allows the whole length of the catheter or guide wire to be visualized, the imaging plane to be automatically adapted to the moving catheter, and potentially the ability to acquire high-resolution images of small areas of interest adjacent to the coil, when the coil or antenna is used in its imaging mode (e.g., vessel wall plaque). However, the main disadvantage of active devices is concerns over safety. These devices use intravascular coils as RF antennae that are connected to the external circuits via a long wire, which can possibly induce electrical current and heating within the MR static field (cf. guide wires). There have been developments to overcome these risks, such as electrical decoupling of loopless antennae (OCALI and ATALAR 1997; SERFATY et al. 2000), and the use of optical coupling and long fiber optic connections (WONG et al. 2000; EGGERS et al. 2003). However, further safety testing is required for both active guide wire and the optically coupled system.

17.4.3
Semiactive Catheter Tracking

Semiactive devices incorporate tuned coils, which have no direct connection to the scanner. These devices can be incorporated into fiducial markers by surrounding a small cell containing a short T1 solution surrounded by tuned windings (Fig. 17.5).

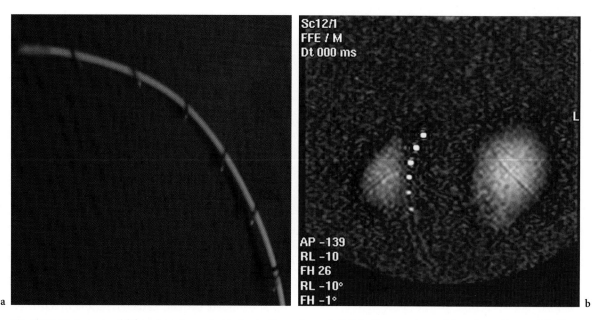

Fig. 17.5. a Six prewound fiducial markers mounted onto the surface of a 5-Fr balloon angiographic catheter (Arrow, Reading, PA) 17 mm apart and aligned 45° to the long axis of the catheter. b The catheter was manipulated in a polyethylene tube of size 20 mm taped on to the chest of a volunteer. A real-time spoiled gradient-echo sequence (fast field echo-FFE: TR 2.3 ms, TE 1.2 ms, flip angle 50°, slice thickness 20 mm) followed by an interactive FFE sequence with interleaving of scans with flip angles of 2° and 50° and a frame rate of 4/s was used. All the six markers are visualized along the length of the catheter

These semiactive devices can also be used to enhance externally applied RF pulses and hence produce a high signal intensity using "flip-angle amplification". The main disadvantage of semiactive devices is that the signal produced is dependent on the device orientation to the main magnetic field, B_0. Recently, these tuned coils have been used in pairs at an angle to each other (quadrature) to overcome this problem and so produce signal enhancement for any catheter orientation (KUEHNE et al. 2003a). This technique looks promising, especially if a number of these coils are attached along the length of the catheter so that a longer segment of the catheter can be visualized.

Semiactive devices do not have the same safety implications as active devices, as there are no long conductors attached to them. A further advantage is the potential for automatic tracking and slice plane following, in a similar fashion to active catheter tracking. However, before these devices can be used in patients, further miniaturization of the capacitors and coils to make the catheters a reasonable diameter, while maintaining the catheter's flexibility and maneuverability, is necessary. It will also be important to have a fault-proof system of securing the capacitors and coils to the catheter so that there is no risk of embolization of the small coils.

17.5
Experience of MR-Guided Cardiac Catheterization in Animals

Over the last few years, there have been a number of studies performed demonstrating the possibility of MR-guided cardiac catheterization in animal models. These include work from centers in San Francisco and Aachen, both of which have XMR (combined MR and X-ray catheterization suites, see Sect. 17.6) cardiac catheterization laboratories.

The group in San Francisco, led by Professor Charles Higgins, have manipulated a homemade pulmonary valve stent into the pulmonary valve of a pig under MR guidance (KUEHNE et al. 2003b). They used a nitinol guide wire to guide the balloon-mounted stent into position. As mentioned above, there are concerns about heating of these wires that precludes their use in patients. The pulmonary valve stent was successfully inserted by using passive visualization and interactive/real-time b-SSFP to guide the stent into position. This study also demonstrated that phase contrast through plane flow in the pulmonary trunk was useful for quantifying the amount of pulmonary incompetence seen before and after device placement.

Higgins and co-workers have also shown the benefits of active catheter (Schalla et al. 2003). Again in an animal model, they have demonstrated that the catheter can be guided to the different chambers of the heart, while the automatic catheter tracking software shows the position of the coil at the tip of the catheter and also automatically changes the imaging plane to keep pace with the catheter position.

The group in Aachen has demonstrated that atrial septal defects can be closed using a homemade device and delivery system in a swine model (Buecker et al. 2002a,b). They used passive visualization though the delivery system was made of nitinol, which is not safe for use in patients. A similar demonstration of ASD closure using a commercially available Amplatzer device has also been performed (Rickers et al. 2003). However, again, the guide wire used for the delivery device is not safe for patient use.

The group in Aachen has also published studies demonstrating coronary stent implantation using passive visualization (Spuentrup et al. 2002), as well as balloon dilation of iliac stenosis in swine models (Buecker et al. 2000).

As mentioned previously, the group at NIH has performed a number of studies demonstrating how active catheters can be used to guide myocardial injection of stem cells (Hill et al. 2003). None of the above studies can currently be translated directly to patients, as there remain safety concerns about guide wires and active devices.

17.6
Introduction to XMR

XMR is the phrase coined to indicate the potential for MR and X-ray imaging to be used in the same facility, with easy transfer between the two imaging modalities. The potential for MR-guided cardiac catheterization is great; however, currently, it remains crucial to have X-ray angiography available as an adjunct. This is mainly due to the fact that the nonbraided catheters available for MR guidance have less torque, and there are instances where a guide wire and/or a braided catheter is required for catheter manipulation. In these cases, it is essential to have X-ray fluoroscopy and angiography available, with easy and safe transfer of patients between the two imaging modalities even when anesthetized. As we gain more experience with MR-guided cardiac catheterization, and especially with the introduction of more MR-compatible catheters and most

importantly guide wires, it may become possible to perform cardiac catheterization under MR guidance alone in the future. However, over the next few years, both practically and ethically it is desirable to have the two imaging modalities side by side.

Importantly, for several indications, MR and X-ray act as complementary tools – e.g., for performing interventional cardiac catheterization and RF ablation procedures. None of the catheters or delivery mechanisms used for these procedures is MR compatible. However, the 3D MR anatomical data is useful for planning and carrying out these procedures. By using registration methods, anatomical information from MR can be combined with the X-ray images of the catheters and devices, so that the exact position of these is visualized in relation to the anatomy (Rhode et al. 2003). This gives some of the advantages of MR without having to compromise on the catheters and devices being used. There are also times when it is useful to relate the device position seen under X-ray to the same anatomical MR coordinates. For example, for relating the position of electrophysiological catheters and thus the electrical map of the heart to the same anatomical coordinates of myocardial motion measured by MR tagging techniques. In theses instances, it appears that XMR has added advantages over X-ray or MR systems in isolation.

17.7
MR Hazards and Safety Issues of XMR

There is a great deal of literature on MR hazards and safety issues, and a comprehensive review and discussion of the subject is outside the scope of this chapter (Shellock 1989; Shellock and Kanal 1991, 1996, 1998, 1999). However, this area is probably one of the most important considerations in setting up a program of MR-guided cardiac catheterization, and we have spent a great deal of time and effort to insure that we minimized the hazards related to the MR scanner, to maintain very high safety standards in our own facility.

Any ferromagnetic object that comes within the MR scanner's magnetic field will be attracted to the scanner. For modern MR scanners, with active shielding, the field is reduced peripherally, thus allowing safe use of ferromagnetic material at distance; however, there is a dramatic increase in this magnetic field over a short distance at close proximity to the magnet bore. Thus, ferromagnetic objects that feel easily controllable at distance can suddenly be pulled with irresistible force into magnets and act as an uncontrollable projectiles, which can potentially cause damage, injury, or even death. All catheterization is therefore done beyond the 5-gauss line.

There are also a number of safety issues that need to be addressed with regard to catheters and devices used during MR-guided cardiac catheterization. Any object that can potentially conduct electricity, and that includes all metals (including nonferromagnetic metals such as nitinol or platinum) can have current induced within them in the MR scanner and therefore can potentially act as an electrical and/or heating hazard. This does not preclude the use of all metals in the MR environment, as of course the imaging coils and wires connecting the electrocardiogram (ECG) signal from patient to the scanner have metal components. However, such leads have been designed to be safe and if used in the correct manner do not provide a significant safety risk. Similarly, there are devices that are implanted into the patient during cardiac catheterization, such as ASD closure devices and stents that are made from metal, but have been found to be safe in the MR environment. When we plan to use any catheters or devices that are a potential safety hazard, we perform extensive testing for hazards before using them in patients. *Thus, we always err on the side of caution, and ensure that nothing is introduced beyond the 5-gauss line that has the slightest potential to be a hazard.*

17.8
Detailed Planning for an XMR Facility

The room design of our XMR facility at Guy's Hospital, London, is outlined in Fig. 17.6. There are many design features that make this room different from standard MRI facilities.

The facility is designed so that half of the room is outside the 5-gauss line (Fig. 17.6) of the magnet, permitting use of traditional instruments and devices, as well as transesophageal echocardiography (TEE) and RF ablation equipment when required. A movable tabletop allows patients to be easily moved between modalities in less than 60 s.

The paramount factor in the design, build, and operation of an XMR facility is safety, and a comprehensive safety protocol has been drawn up to minimize possible hazards. The safety features of our XMR facility include:

- All staff who are involved in XMR procedures undergo compulsory MR safety training prior to performing an XMR case on a patient
- There is clear demarcation of the ferromagnetic safe and unsafe areas by different color floor covering and a movable barrier
- There is restricted entrance to the facility during an XMR procedure. There are two entrances into the room. The large entrance directly into the room is only used to bring large pieces of equipment (such as anesthetic equipment) into the room before proceeding, and for transporting the patient into and out of the room at the beginning and end of the procedure. This entrance is otherwise closed and access to the room during the procedure is via the control room, through the scrub room. This entrance is constantly monitored and admittance is limited to staff who have undergone the appropriate safety training and wear specially designed clothes without pockets, to prevent accidentally carrying unsafe material into the room
- Ferromagnetic equipment is tethered to the walls as an added safety precaution
- There is a designated safety officer in the room throughout the procedure to ensure that the safety protocols are adhered to, especially at the time of patient transfer. All ferromagnetic equipment used is monitored and logged. Prior to transfer of the patient beyond the 5-gauss line, a double check is performed to ensure that all ferromagnetic equipment is accounted for
- A written log is kept of all safety infringements, no matter how minor, and is discussed weekly, with the safety protocol being adapted as necessary. A 3-monthly report of the log and action taken is sent to the Hospital Ethics Committee

Traditionally, MR scans are planned and run from the control room away from the magnet and the patient. However, during MR-guided cardiac catheterization, there is need for real-time changes to the scanning-sequence parameters in order to follow catheter manipulation in the heart and great vessels. Also, the imager needs to have a clear view of the MR images while performing the procedure. There is, therefore, a fully functional set of ceiling-mounted, moveable screens and scanner controls within the MR scanner room, which can be placed at either end of the bore of the scanner in close proximity to the patient.

The XMR suite includes appropriate MR-compatible anesthetic equipment and monitoring

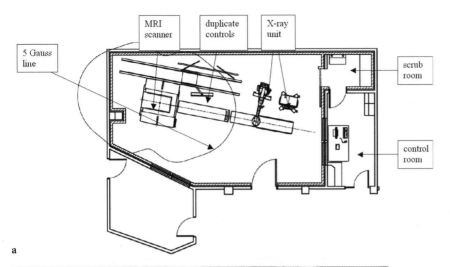

a

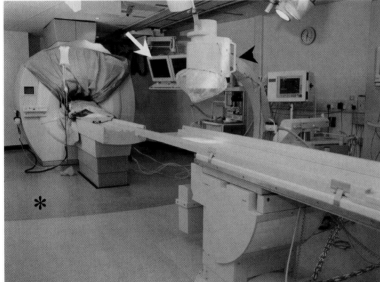

b

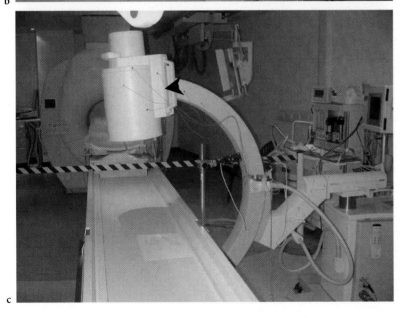

c

Fig. 17.6. a Schematic room plan of our XMR facility. b, c Photographs of the room view from b the side, and c) the end of the X-ray table. The C-arm is seen in the foreground (*arrowhead*), the ceiling-mounted MR monitor and controls are seen in the distance (*arrow*), and the 5-gauss color marking in shown (*asterisk*).

equipment for invasive pressure monitoring via the catheter. A great deal of thought has been given to safety of patients under anesthetic, especially during the transfer between the X-ray and MR tables. All the anesthetic and monitoring tubing and lines are designed with extra length and are secured to the movable tabletop to ensure smooth patient transfer.

The ECG and invasive pressure data is sent from the MR-compatible monitoring equipment via an optical network to a computer in the control room, where the cardiac technician is stationed. The appropriate measurement and recording of the data is made in the usual way. The technician has access to monitors, which show the appropriate X-ray or MR images of the procedure. The imagers in the room can view the MR images and any monitoring data (ECG, invasive pressure data). Blood samples taken during the procedure are labeled in the room and passed to the technician in the control room via a wave-guide.

Another complication of performing cardiac catheterization under MR guidance is the noise generated during scanning. There is a headphone and microphone system in the room that reduces the noise, but allows staff to communicate with each other in both the scanner and control rooms.

Some MR coils have X-ray-visible components and would need to be removed between MR imaging and X-ray imaging of patients. It is therefore necessary to have specifically designed coils that are sufficiently radiotranslucent to be left in place during X-ray imaging without any deterioration of image quality. We use these coils in our procedures so that the patients do not have to be disturbed when moving from one imaging modality to the other.

The XMR suite has positive-pressure air handling and filtration appropriate for a catheterization laboratory. There is a scrub room which is also RF and X-ray shielded and can be accessed both from the XMR suite and control room. This room acts as an RF lock, allowing access to the XMR suite during MR scanning.

From the previous discussion, it is clear that some parts of an MR-guided catheterization will have to be performed under X-ray guidance as the appropriate MR-compatible catheters and devices are still not available. However, it is often useful to have anatomical and functional information from MR images available during X-ray fluoroscopy. Similarly, knowledge of the position of a catheter under X-ray, such as the tip of an ablation catheter following successful RF ablation of an accessory pathway, would

be useful in subsequent MR imaging of the results of the ablation. We therefore have developed a method of registering and overlaying the MR and X-ray images. This requires the tracking of the X-ray table and X-ray C-arm by an optical tracking system, which is positioned at the X-ray end of the room (Fig. 17.7).

17.8.1
Reliable ECG

Reliable and accurate ECG synchronization is essential for cardiovascular MRI and in particular MR-guided cardiac catheterization. When manipulating catheters in the heart, there is the potential to cause arrhythmias (tachyarrhythmias and/or heart block). It is therefore important to perform accurate monitoring of the cardiac rhythm at all times during XMR catheterization. Obtaining a reliable ECG in the magnet, particularly during some MR sequences, can be difficult. The magnetohydrodynamic effect and gradient noise can seriously disturb the ECG signal (Dimick et al. 1987). This interference can reduce trigger signal reliability to less than 40%. Vector electrocardiogram (VCG) is a QRS detection algorithm, which automatically adjusts to the actual electrical axis of the patient's heart and the specific multi-dimensional QRS waveform. In our experience, this greatly improves reliability of R-wave detection to nearly 100%. A reliable R wave, with the P and T waves that are also always clearly seen with the VCG, allow detection of nearly all arrhythmias. Unfortunately, there are no ECG systems that can reliably provide ST segment or T-wave morphological information. In the future, using signal-processing techniques, it may be possible to obtain ECG during MRI scanning that provide ST and T wave information reliably.

17.8.2
Techniques Used in MRI-Guided Cardiac Catheterization

The majority of MR sequences used during an MR-guided cardiac catheterization have been covered in Chap. 1; however, there are two specific sequences – 3D volume b-SSFP and interactive/real time – that are very useful for MR-guided cardiac catheterization, and they will be described in detail in this section.

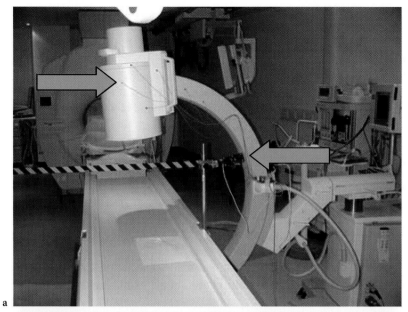

a

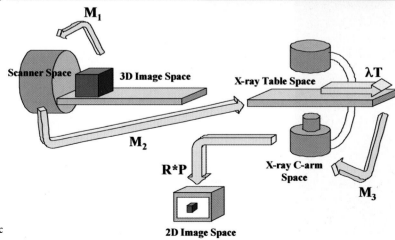

b

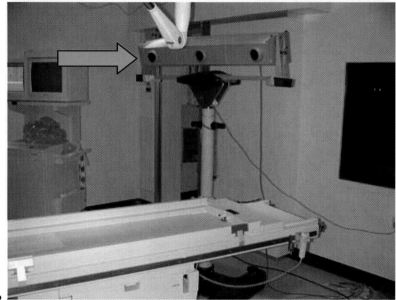

c

Fig. 17.7a-c. To register 3D MR image space to 2D X-ray image space, a combination of system calibration and tracking is required. It is necessary to track the moving components of the XMR system. These comprise the X-ray C-arm (**a**) and the X-ray table (**b**), each of which has six infrared-emitting diodes (IREDS) affixed. These are tracked by a Northern Digital Optotrak 3020 system (NDI, Ontario, Canada). The tabletop is automatically tracked by the MR scanner when docked with the MR table. The relationship between these coordinate systems is shown in **c**

17.8.2.1
Three-dimensional Volume Balanced-SSFP

We have recently described a new 3D b-SSFP sequence in combination with parallel imaging (SENSE factor 2) that allows rapid acquisition of the entire cardiac volume (RAZAVI et al. 2003a). Cardiovascular MR provides the capability of imaging in any plane. This distinguishes it from echocardiography, which is limited by acoustic windows and X-ray angiography, which only provides projectional imaging. Unfortunately, the 3D nature of some congenital cardiac defects is difficult to demonstrate with 2D imaging.

Acquiring 3D anatomical information plays a particularly important part in MR-guided cardiac catheterization in congenital heart disease, as it complements the invasive pressure and physi-

ological measures such as pulmonary blood flow. Gadolinium-enhanced MR angiography is an accurate 3D imaging technique that allows assessment of congenital malformation of vessels such as the aorta, pulmonary arteries, and veins (Fig. 17.8). However, the lack of cardiac synchronization leads to blurring of the image due to cardiac motion, which is particularly problematic when assessing intracardiac anatomy. The 3D b-SSFP sequence has the advantage of providing clear intracardiac images at different points in the cardiac cycle with good contrast and resolution. These 3D data sets are more amenable to visualization techniques based on thresholding, rather than the time-consuming manual segmentation required for older gradient-echo techniques (MIQUEL et al. 2003).

Three-dimensional b-SSFP scans are acquired using a multi-chunk, multi-breath-hold, multi-phase

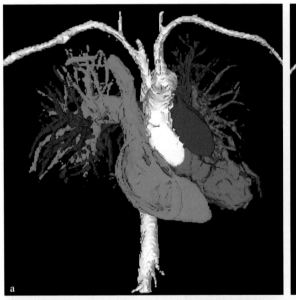

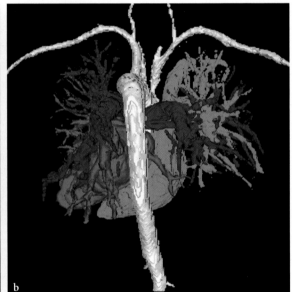

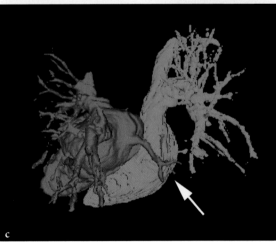

Fig. 17.8a-c. Three-dimensional volume-rendered reconstructions from gadolinium-enhanced MR angiograms in a 46-year-old who presented with shortness of breath on exercise and intermittent atrial tachycardia. The images show partial anomalous pulmonary venous drainage of the right upper and middle lobes into the SVC, with the smaller right lower lobe pulmonary vein draining into the left atrium. a Anterior view, b posterior view: *green*, right atrium and partial anomalous pulmonary venous drainage from the right upper and middle lobes of the right lung; *red*, left atrium, right lower lobe pulmonary vein (*arrow*) and normal left lung pulmonary venous drainage; *white*, aorta; *blue*, pulmonary arteries. c Left and right atrium; left posterior oblique view

technique (TR 4 ms, TE 2 ms, the field of view 300-350 mm, image matrix 192×256 pixels). As imaging the whole cardiac volume is not possible in 1 breath-hold, the scan is divided into 8–12 smaller chunks. Each chunk is acquired as a single breath-hold of 8–15 s. The acquisition time for the whole sequence is between 6–10 min. The scan is acquired in the axial plane and therefore requires no complex planning. High–resolution images are reconstructed with a resolution of approximately 1 mm in all three directions. Typically one volume scan yields 80–144 slices (Fig. 17.9 a–d).

Each volume is also acquired in multiple phases of the cardiac cycle. In most cases delineation of anatomy is the most important consideration and, to keep scan times to a minimum, only 3–7 phases of the cardiac cycle are acquired. However, up to 10 cardiac phases can be obtained, each acquired in approximately 8% of the cardiac cycle to give information about cardiac motion and sharp systolic images. This leads to an increase in scan time to 25–30 s per breath-hold. As the great majority of our patients undergoing MR-guided cardiac catheterization are ventilated, breath-holds are achieved through suspension of ventilation. Therefore the position of the heart is uniformly maintained between chunks, preventing misregistration of volume data.

Images are analyzed offline on a commercial image-analysis workstation (EasyVision 5.1, Philips Medical Systems, Best, The Netherlands). As well as looking through the volume in the original axial slices, multiplanar reformatting, which allows viewing of the volume in any plane, can be used. Volume rendering of the blood pool can also be performed, using an automated segmentation technique in which the user sets a threshold and seeds the structures of interest by clicking on them with the mouse. This enables different structures of the heart to be segmented separately and given different colors in the rendering process (Fig. 17.9e). A rendering of the image is generated on the same workstation and can be visualized from any direction, and movies of the heart rotating can also be generated. In most patients, only the end-diastolic images are segmented, but where there is a clinical interest, the systolic volume can also be rendered. The segmentation and rendering process normally takes between 5 and 10 min.

17.8.2.2
Interactive/Real-Time MRI

One of the major recent developments that has made MR-guided cardiac catheterization possible is the introduction of fast b-SSFP sequences that allow acquisition, rapid reconstruction, and visualization of a slice through the heart and great vessels in around 100 ms (BAKKER et al. 1996). Because of the speed of these sequences, there is no need for ECG gating, with dynamic real–time images acquired at approximately 10 frames per cardiac cycle depending on heart rate. The ability to perform what is in effect MR fluoroscopy means that rapidly changing images of the moving catheter can be seen with very little latency and immediate feedback to the operator who is manipulating the catheter.

The interactive sequence has a number of added functionalities that allow changes in scan geometry and parameters such as slice thickness, field of view, and fold-over (readout) direction on the fly. There are also four viewing windows so that up to three previously acquired images can be seen as well as the active imaging window. This allows the relationship of the active imaging window to the three predetermined imaging planes to be visualized in real time, with the active imaging plane depicted as a line overlaid on the stored images (Fig. 17.10).

The geometry of the active imaging plane can be manipulated in a number of different ways:

- 1. A line in any direction can be drawn on any of the three saved images to determine the active imaging plane
- 2. The three lines on the three stored images can be moved in any direction to change the geometry of the active imaging plane
- 3. The active imaging plane can be "pulled" or "pushed" and so shifted in parallel to the imaging plane by any predetermined amount (as little as 1 mm)

Both the image and the geometry of the active imaging plane can be stored for later reference. The one drawback of this technique is that, because such a large number of images are acquired (more than 1000 every 2 min), images cannot be automatically saved and so specific images of interest have to be saved by the click of the mouse. We have implemented a local solution with a separate computer that grabs the images from the MR console screen, enabling storage of the interactive images as movies. The parameters for the interactive sequence are: TR 2.8 ms, TE 1.4 ms, flip angle of 50°, image matrix 128×128, and a 75% scan percentage. Other parameters, including rectangular field of view, are adjusted for each patient. The minimum frame rate (depending on rectangular field of view) is at least 10 frames/s.

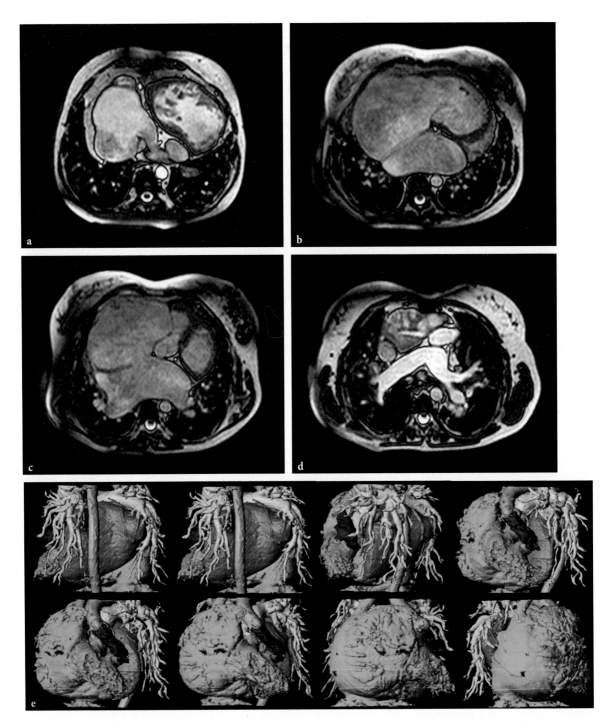

Fig. 17.9a-e. Multi-chunk, multi-breath-hold 3D steady-state free precession (SSFP) axial images (selected images). The images show atrio-ventricular and ventricular-arterial discordance, tricuspid atresia, and right ventricular hypoplasia. **a** Coronary sinus entering right atrium. **b** Right atrium to left ventricle and with left atrium and right ventricle separated by atretic tricuspid valve. **c** Atrial septal defect. **d** Posterior pulmonary arteries and anterior aorta. **e** Three-dimensional volume rendered images created from the multi-chunk, multi-breath-hold 3D balanced-SSFP axial images. 3D volume rotating from posterior to left lateral projection (*top row left to right*), and from anterior to right lateral (*bottom row left to right*). Massively dilated right atrium (*turquoise*) connects to left ventricle (*mid-blue*), connects to pulmonary trunk (*pale blue*); left atrium (*dark red*). Hypoplastic right ventricle (*dark blue*) connects to aorta (*pale red*)

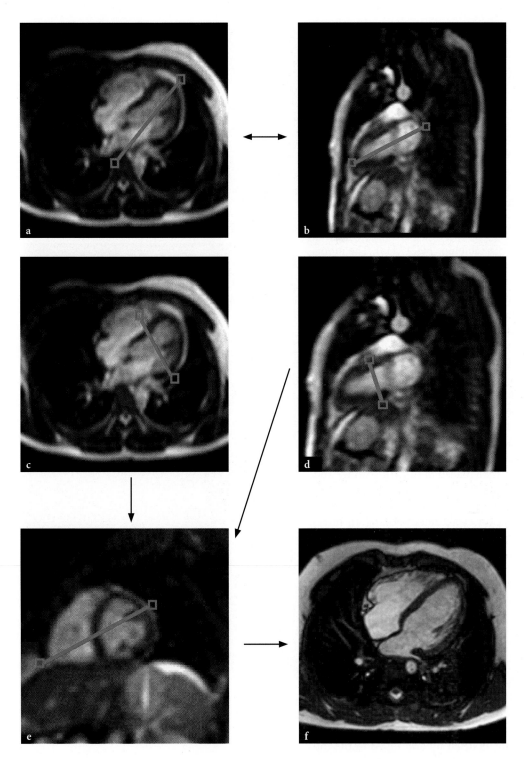

Fig. 17.10a-f. Real time interactive images: TR 2.9 ms, TE 1.45 ms, flip angle 45°, matrix 128×128, FOV 250–350, temporal resolution of 10–14 frames/s. **a** Axial image, with alignment of the vertical long-axis (VLA) through the mitral valve and left ventricular apex to give **b**. Short-axis plane planned on the axial (**c**) and VLA (**d**) images to give **e** mid-ventricular short-axis slice. The four-chamber view is then planned from **e** to yield **f**. **f** High-resolution four-chamber view (diastolic frame of a b-SSFP cine image)

The interactive sequence is used both in determining the likely planes of interest before the MR-guided cardiac catheterization procedure and for catheter tracking during the procedure.

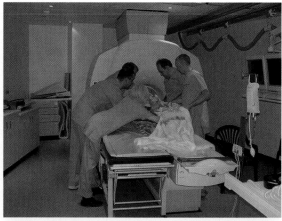

17.9
Performing a Typical Case

A typical MR-guided catheter case is described in the following section (RAZAVI et al. 2003b). Following induction of anesthesia, the patient is transferred to the MR end of the XMR facility and positioned on the MR scanner tabletop (Fig. 17.11a). The monitoring and anesthetic equipment are attached. The patient monitoring includes a 3-lead ECG, separate to the VCG used for ECG triggering/monitoring during MR scanning. The VCG electrodes are placed on the subcostal margin outside the X-ray field of view. An MR-compatible pulse oximeter and noninvasive blood pressure monitoring are also attached. The exhaled anesthetic gases are monitored for end-tidal carbon dioxide as well as the concentration of the volatile anesthetic agents. Flexible phase array coils are used. These coils are relatively X-ray lucent and thus do not need to be removed between MR and X-ray imaging.

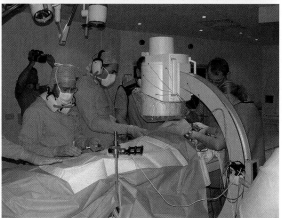

The patient is then placed in the MR scanner and a multi-breath-hold 3D SSFP scan of the heart and great vessels (1.1 mm × 1.1 mm × 1 mm resolution) is obtained (RAZAVI et al. 2003a). Using an interactive SSFP sequence (10 frames/s), with real-time manipulation of scan parameters, the likely imaging planes needed for subsequent catheter tracking, ventricular function, and flow quantification are stored. The patient is then transferred to the X-ray end of the room. Draping and vascular access are carried out as per routine cardiac catheterization (Fig. 17.11b). A second large drape is placed over the patient.

Following safety checks, including an operating theatre-style "ticking off" of all metallic objects on the catheterization trolley or given to the operators, the patient is transferred back to the MR scanner. The second drape is lifted up and taped to the top of the magnet; in effect providing sterile draping of the bore and sides of the magnet (Fig. 17.11c). An end hole, or side-holes balloon angiographic catheter (4F–7F) is placed in the sheath and, with the balloon inflated with CO_2 (Fig. 17.4), the catheter tip is passively visualized using the interactive sequences described above. The previously stored imaging planes

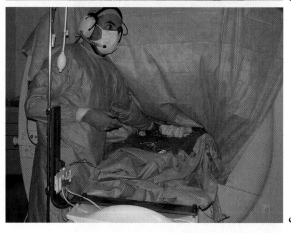

Fig. 17.11a-c. Photographs of XMR facility. **a** Patient being placed on MR tabletop. **b** Patient slid across to the X-ray half of the room for sheath insertion. **c** Passive catheter manipulation under MR guidance

are used, and when necessary, using the interactive positioning, the imaging plane is changed to track the catheter. As only the tip of the catheter is visualized, care is taken not to push the catheter too fast and thus beyond the MR imaging plane. This also ensures that the catheter does not accidentally form loops and possible knots.

During catheter manipulation, the duplicate MR control console is positioned next to the bore of the magnet so that the interactive window can be easily visualized while the catheter is manipulated (Fig. 17.12). This requires two operators; one to move the catheter and one to alter the MR imaging planes to ensure that the catheter tip is tracked, using the real-time interactive sequence.

Once the catheter is positioned in the desired vessel or chamber, the appropriated pressure data and saturation/blood gas samples are obtained as for a routine cardiac catheterization. If necessary, ventricular function (short-axis b-SSFP) and flow (phase contrast) scans can be performed using the appropriate previously stored imaging planes.

If it is not possible to position the catheter into a particular heart chamber or vessel using MR guidance alone, the patient is transferred back to the X-ray end of the room, where the catheterization can be continued under X-ray fluoroscopy (e.g., to use a guide wire or a non–MRI-compatible catheter). Once the catheter is correctly positioned, the patient can be transferred back to the MR scanner for further MR measurements.

In cases where an interventional cardiac catheter or RF ablation of arrhythmias is performed, the main part of the procedure is performed under X-ray fluoroscopy, as the ablation catheters and delivery devices are not MR compatible. Thus, MR imaging is performed at the beginning of the procedure for planning and use in guiding the procedure, and at the end of the procedure for evaluation of the

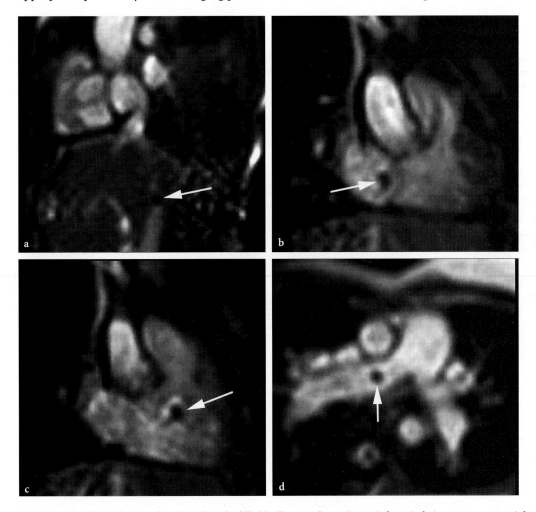

Fig. 17.12a-d. Manipulation of carbon dioxide-filled balloon catheter (*arrow*) from inferior vena cava to right pulmonary artery using solely MR guidance. Real-time interactive images: TR 2.9 ms, TE 1.45 ms, flip angle 45°, matrix 128x128, FOV 250–350, temporal resolution of 10–14 frames/s. *Arrows* show signal void of catheter tip. **a** Sagittal plane – balloon in IVC. **b** Coronal plane – balloon in right atrium, about to cross the tricuspid valve. **c** Coronal plane – balloon in right ventricular outflow tract. **d** Axial plane – balloon in right pulmonary artery

outcome. At the end of the procedure, the vascular sheaths are removed and the patient transferred to the recovery area.

17.10
Current Experience in Humans and Future Directions

17.10.1
Diagnostic XMR Cardiac Catheterization

We performed 30 diagnostic cardiac catheterizations under XMR guidance. Patients ranged in age from 1 month to 42 years of age (RAZAVI et al. 2003b). We performed 10 of these cases without the need for X-ray imaging, and in all other patients a significant portion of the procedures was performed under MR guidance. For all patients, the overall X-ray dose for the XMR procedure was significantly less than for control cases performed under standard X-ray guidance (5.5×10 Gycm^2 vs 35.4×36.7 Gycm^2, respectively). In some cases, we have performed selective

contrast-enhanced (CE) MRA through an injection in the catheter (RAZAVI et al. 2003b). Pulmonary vascular resistance was also assessed in the majority of patients as described in the next section.

17.10.2
Assessment of Pulmonary Vascular Resistance Using XMR

We have used XMR to measure PVR in 24 patients. MR-guided cardiac catheterization was used to acquire simultaneous measurement of invasive pressures and MR flow data. The results were compared with conventional PVR measurements acquired using the Fick calculation, performed during the same procedure (Fig. 17.13).

In this study, we demonstrated moderate/good agreement between Fick- and phase contrast-derived PVR at baseline. This corroborates a number of other studies that have shown reasonable agreement between phase-contrast MR flow and invasive methods of flow quantification (e.g., Fick) (HUNDLEY et al. 1995; BEERBAUM et al. 2001). However, in the pres-

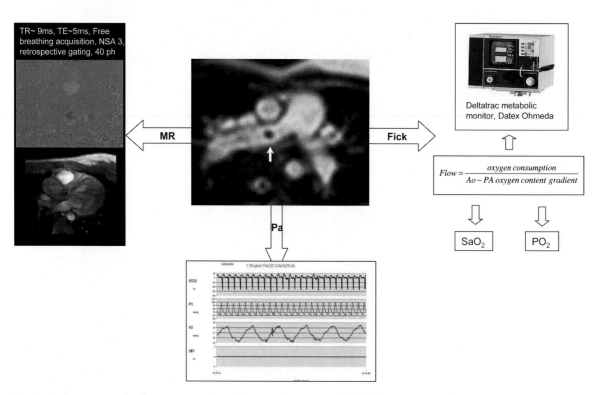

Fig. 17.13. Assessment of pulmonary vascular resistance using MR-guided catheterization, comparison of MR method and conventional Fick method. The *central image* shows the CO_2-filled angiographic balloon catheter tip in the proximal right pulmonary artery (*arrow*). The *right panel* shows the MR flow measurement. The *left panel* shows the equipment used to measure blood oxygen content to calculate flow using the Fick principle. The *lower panel* shows the simultaneous pressure data recorded in the right pulmonary artery (*red*) and the aorta (*green*, catheter not shown)

ence of nitric oxide, used to assess pulmonary vaso-reactivity, there was less agreement between the two methods. In the presence of 100% oxygen and nitric oxide, there was not only worsening agreement, but also a large bias.

The Fick principle is known to be inaccurate and imprecise in the presence of high pulmonary blood flow and high concentrations of oxygen (HILLIS et al. 1985b). We have also demonstrated the in vitro accuracy and precision of phase-contrast MR in our facility using a flow phantom that replicates in vivo conditions more closely than previous studies (MUTHURANGU et al. 2004). In addition, the oxygen content of pulmonary arterial blood at 100% oxygen is similar to the oxygen content of aortic blood at baseline, where it has been shown that phase-contrast MR is accurate (BEERBAUM et al. 2001).

We therefore believe that the worsening agreement between the two methods in response to pulmonary vasodilatation is due to errors in the Fick method rather than phase-contrast MR, and that the Fick method underestimates PVR in the presence of 100% oxygen and 20 ppm of NO. This has important implications for patient management, as response to vasodilators is integral to the assessment of patients with pulmonary hypertension.

Overall, this study demonstrates the feasibility of combining invasive pressure measurements and MR flow data to quantify PVR in humans (MUTHURANGU et al. 2004). This technique raises the possibility of a more accurate method of PVR quantification, leading to better management of patients with pulmonary hypertension. In addition, this technique is straightforward to carry out, leads to reduced exposure to ionizing radiation and can be combined with other MR techniques, allowing comprehensive cardiac assessment.

17.10.3
Planning and Monitoring Device Insertion Using XMR

We have performed MR-guided interventional cardiac catheterization on three patients: ASD device closure (Fig. 17.14), dilatation of a right pulmonary artery stent, and stent implantation of coarctation (Fig. 17.15).

In all these cases, some catheter manipulation was done under MR guidance, but the interventional procedures were performed under X-ray fluoroscopy. The reason for this was the MR-incompatible nature of the catheters and devices. In all three cases, MR

imaging was helpful at the beginning of the procedure for planning the intervention, and at the end of the procedure for evaluating the outcome.

For the aortic coarctation patient, the stent was deployed in the correct position, utilizing both the fluoroscopic images and the XMR images. These were found to be helpful in positioning the stent, particularly in this anatomically difficult case (Fig. 17.15).

These cases demonstrate the feasibility of performing interventional cardiac catheterization procedures under XMR guidance. The XMR images were helpful; however, we will have to perform this in a larger number of patients and compare it to procedures performed in the standard X-ray cardiac

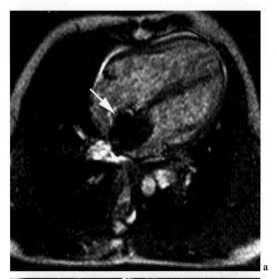

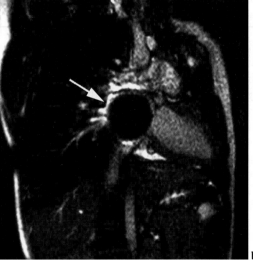

Fig. 17.14a,b. Amplatzer atrial septal defect (ASD) device after implantation in a 7-year-old patient. **a** Diastolic frame of four-chamber and **b** vertical long-axis b-SSFP cine images showing marked artifact from the ASD device (*arrow*)

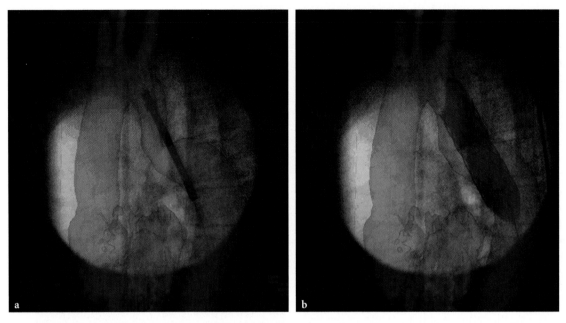

Fig. 17.15a,b. MR angiography image superimposed onto the X-ray cardiac catheter image during stent implantation. The combined images show that the implanted open stent lies in a satisfactory position, distal to the origin of the left subclavian artery, and across the coarctation narrowing. **a** Uninflated stent and guide wire across the coarctation site. **b** Inflated stent. Note stent implantation was performed in the X-ray half of the XMR facility. MRI was used prior to stent insertion to acquire the 3D MRA images, and after the procedure (guide wires removed) to confirm no aortic obstruction and satisfactory stent position

catheterization laboratory to prove the efficacy and benefits of this technique.

17.10.4
Electrophysiological Studies and RF Ablation Using XMR

We have performed ten cases of electrophysiological study and RF ablation in the XMR facility.

Nine of these cases involved RF ablation in the pulmonary veins for patients with atrial fibrillation. Initially, a CE–MRA was performed to acquire the 3D pulmonary venous anatomy. The patients were then returned to the X-ray fluoroscopic area, where a needle atrial septostomy was performed under X-ray guidance. Once in the left atrium, a braided multipurpose catheter was used to identify the pulmonary veins. At this stage the combined MR-derived surface and X-ray fluoroscopic images were used to guide the catheter and steerable long sheath into each pulmonary vein. Iodine-contrast X-ray angiograms were also performed to visualize the pulmonary veins, and this allowed a comparison between the MR and X-ray anatomy. We found in all cases that there was good

registration when comparing the X-ray angiograms and the MR surface-rendered images taking into account different breath-hold positions at the beginning of the case. Once the long sheath was placed into the appropriate pulmonary vein, a T-flex helical ablation catheter (Cardima, Freemont, California, USA) was deployed and positioned so that it sat at the proximal end of the pulmonary vein (Fig. 17.16).

Although we have shown the feasibility of this technique in these nine patients, we still need to study more patients and compare this group with patients undergoing similar procedures under standard X-ray fluoroscopy.

We have also used MR guidance to assist in RF ablation of a right ventricular outflow tract ventricular tachycardia in one patient. The 3D MR volume data was superimposed on the X-ray catheter images of the RF ablation catheters and the constellation catheter (used for mapping electrical activity). The catheters used for these procedures are not MR compatible, as they are comprised of long electrical conductors. The MR to X-ray registration enabled us to relate the position of the measured electrophysiology data from the basket electrode to the 3D cardiac motion. (Fig. 17.17).

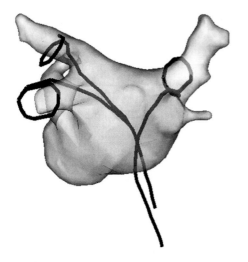

Fig. 17.16. Pulmonary vein ablation. 3D MRA images and T-flex helical catheters superimposed on each other, showing the position of the catheters within the pulmonary vein orifices

17.11 Conclusion

In this chapter, the feasibility of performing cardiac catheterizations under XMR guidance has been outlined. The technique has been shown to be safe with a number of benefits and potential benefits over standard X-ray-guided cardiac catheterization.

There are, however, still a number of issues that need to be improved before MR-guided cardiac catheterization becomes routine practice. These include practical issues such as noise management and communications, improved access to the patient, and improved safety procedures. More importantly, there is a need for catheter and device manufacturers to produce tools specifically for MR-guided cardiac catheterization.

There have been a number of important gains from this new technique. These include the reduc-

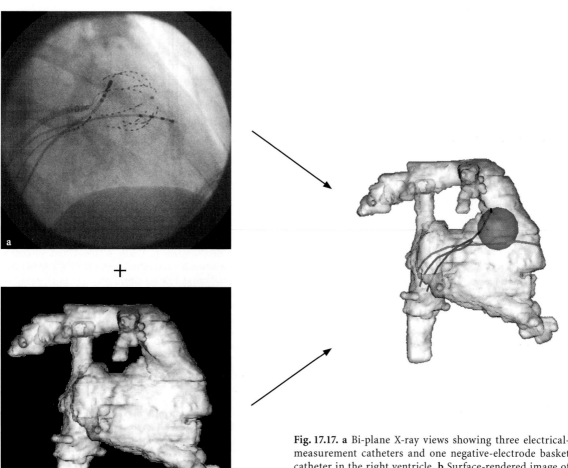

Fig. 17.17. a Bi-plane X-ray views showing three electrical-measurement catheters and one negative-electrode basket catheter in the right ventricle. **b** Surface-rendered image of the 3D MR image data of the right side of the heart. **c** Surface-rendered MR image (oblique view) of the right side of the heart incorporating the superimposed, registered three catheters and constellation catheter basket

tion of X-ray dose, accurate assessment of pulmonary vascular resistance, better visualization of complex anatomy for both diagnostic cardiac catheterization and interventional cardiac catheterization, and radio-frequency ablation of arrhythmias, using XMR images.

In the future, with better catheter visualization and tracking techniques, it should be possible to reduce and even eliminate the X-radiation dose in diagnostic cardiac catheterization and provide more accurate and varied pathophysiological information. Applying the X-ray and MR image registration technique in a larger group of patients should allow the potential benefits of XMR over standard X-ray-guided cardiac catheterization to be established. This may make MR guidance the method of choice for diagnostic cardiac catheterization in congenital heart disease patients, and an important tool in interventional cardiac catheterization and RF ablation of arrhythmias in the future.

17.12
Key Points

- Currently, MR-guided cardiac catheterization can rarely be performed in isolation, and X-ray imaging in close proximity is required for accurate, safe imaging
- Safety is paramount when performing XMR-guided procedures, and strict safety procedures must be developed and adhered to
- MR-guided cardiac catheterization provides additional anatomical and functional information to X-ray cardiac catheterization with no X-ray dose
- Accurate image registration is necessary to perform procedures where 3D MR images are registered onto the X-ray images for accurate placement in catheters
- Reported MR-guided cardiac catheter applications in humans are few. Assessment of pulmonary vascular resistance and RF ablation procedures have been performed using XMR systems
- For MR-guided cardiac catheterization to progress further, the development of MR-compatible catheters, guide wires, and devices that are safe in humans will be essential

Acknowledgements
The work described in this chapter was performed at Guy's Hospital, London, UK, by a team of academic and clinical staff. As well as the authors, particular acknowledgement is due to: Derek Hill, Steve Keevil, Marc Miquel, Kawal Rhodes, Rado Andriantsimiavona, Redha Boubertakh, Maxime Sermesant, and David Hawkes in the Division of Imaging sciences; and Shakeel Quresh, Jas Gill, Eric Rosenthal, Robert Tulloh, and Edward Baker in the Departments of Paediatric and Adult Cardiology. We would also like to acknowledge Michael Barnet and other members of the Anaesthetic Department; and John Spence, Stephen Sinclear, and Rebeca Lund and other staff from the Radiology Department who have provided considerable support.

References

Atz AM, Adatia I, Lock JE, Wessel DL (1999) Combined effects of nitric oxide and oxygen during acute pulmonary vasodilator testing. J Am Coll Cardiol 33:813–819

Bakker CJ, Hoogeveen RM, Weber J et al (1996) Visualization of dedicated catheters using fast scanning techniques with potential for MR-guided vascular interventions. Magn Reson Med 36:816–820

Bakker CJ, Hoogeveen RM, Hurtak WF et al (1997) MR-guided endovascular interventions: susceptibility-based catheter and near-real-time imaging technique. Radiology 202:273–276

Beerbaum P, Korperich H, Barth P, et al (2001) Noninvasive quantification of left-to-right shunt in pediatric patients: phase-contrast cine magnetic resonance imaging compared with invasive oximetry. Circulation 103:2476–2482

Bellenger NG, Marcus NJ, Rajappan K, et al (2002) Comparison of techniques for the measurement of left ventricular function following cardiac transplantation. J Cardiovasc Magn Reson 4:255–263

Berrington de Gonzalez A, Darby S (2004) Risk of cancer from diagnostic X-rays: estimates for the UK and 14 other countries. Lancet 363:345–351

Bonhoeffer P, Boudjemline Y, Qureshi SA et al (2002) Percutaneous insertion of the pulmonary valve. J Am Coll Cardiol 39:1664–1669

Buecker A, Neuerburg JM, Adam GB et al (2000) Real-time MR fluoroscopy for MR-guided iliac artery stent placement. J Magn Reson Imaging 12:616–622

Buecker A, Spuentrup E, Grabitz R et al (2002a) Real-time-MR guidance for placement of a self-made fully MR-compatible atrial septal occluder: in vitro test. Rofo Fortschr Geb Rontgenstr Neuen Bildgeb Verfahr 174:283–285

Buecker A, Spuentrup E, Grabitz R et al (2002b) Magnetic resonance-guided placement of atrial septal closure device in animal model of patent foramen ovale. Circulation 106:511–515

Cigarroa RG, Lange RA, Hillis LD (1989) Oximetric quantitation of intracardiac left-to-right shunting: limitations of the Qp/Qs ratio. Am J Cardiol 64:246–247

Dhingra VK, Fenwick JC, Walley KR, Chittock DR, Ronco

JJ (2002) Lack of agreement between thermodilution and Fick cardiac output in critically ill patients. Chest 122:990–997

Dimick RN, Hedlund LW, Herfkens RJ, Fram EK, Utz J (1987) Optimizing electrocardiograph electrode placement for cardiac-gated magnetic resonance imaging. Invest Radiol 22:17–22

Du ZD, Hijazi ZM, Kleinman CS, et al (2002) Comparison between transcatheter and surgical closure of secundum atrial septal defect in children and adults: results of a multicenter nonrandomized trial. J Am Coll Cardiol 39:1836–1844

Eggers H, Weiss S, Boernert P, Boesiger P (2003) Image-based tracking of optically detunable parallel resonant circuits. Magn Reson Med 49:1163–1174

Fahrig R, Butts K, Wen Z et al (2001) Truly hybrid interventional MR/X-ray system: investigation of in vivo applications. Acad Radiol 8:1200–1207

Fahrig R, Heit G, Wen Z, et al (2003) First use of a truly-hybrid X-ray/MR imaging system for guidance of brain biopsy. Acta Neurochir (Wien) 145:995–997; discussion 997

Faulkner K, Love HG, Sweeney JK, Bardsley RA (1986) Radiation doses and somatic risk to patients during cardiac radiological procedures. Br J Radiol 59:359–363

Glowinski A, Adam G, Bucker A, et al (1997) Catheter visualization using locally induced, actively controlled field inhomogeneities. Magn Reson Med 38:253–258

Guttman MA, Lederman RJ, Sorger JM, McVeigh ER (2002) Real-time volume rendered MRI for interventional guidance. J Cardiovasc Magn Reson 4:431–442; erratum: J Cardiovasc Magn Reson (2003) 5:407

Helbing WA, Rebergen SA, Maliepaard C et al (1995) Quantification of right ventricular function with magnetic resonance imaging in children with normal hearts and with congenital heart disease. Am Heart J 130:828–837

Hijazi ZM, Hakim F, Haweleh A A et al (2002) Catheter closure of perimembranous ventricular septal defects using the new Amplatzer membranous VSD occluder: initial clinical experience. Catheter Cardiovasc Interv 56:508–515

Hill JM, Dick AJ, Raman VK et al (2003) Serial cardiac magnetic resonance imaging of injected mesenchymal stem cells. Circulation 108:1009–1014. Epub 11 Aug 2003

Hillis LD, Winniford MD, Jackson JA, Firth BG (1985a) Measurements of left-to-right intracardiac shunting in adults: oximetric versus indicator dilution techniques. Cathet Cardiovasc Diagn 11:467–472

Hillis LD, Firth BG, Winniford MD (1985b) Analysis of factors affecting the variability of Fick versus indicator dilution measurements of cardiac output. Am J Cardiol 56:764–768

Holzer R, Balzer D, Cao QL, et al (2004a) Device closure of muscular ventricular septal defects using the Amplatzer muscular ventricular septal defect occluder: immediate and mid-term results of a U.S. registry. J Am Coll Cardiol 43:1257–1263

Holzer R, Balzer D, Amin Z et al (2004b) Transcatheter closure of postinfarction ventricular septal defects using the new Amplatzer muscular VSD occluder: results of a US registry. Catheter Cardiovasc Interv 61:196–201

Hundley WG, Li HF, Hillis LD et al (1995) Quantitation of cardiac output with velocity-encoded, phase-difference magnetic resonance imaging. Am J Cardiol 75:1250–1255

ICRP (1990) Recommendations of the International Commission on Radiological Protection. ICRP 60. Ann ICRP 21:1–3

Koenig PR, Abdulla RI, Cao QL, Hijazi ZM (2003) Use of intracardiac echocardiography to guide catheter closure of atrial communications. Echocardiography 20:781–787

Konings MK, Bartels LW, Smits HF, Bakker CJ (2000) Heating around intravascular guide wires by resonating RF waves. J Magn Reson Imaging 12:79–85

Kovoor P, Ricciardello M, Collins L, Uther JB, Ross DL (1998) Risk to patients from radiation associated with radiofrequency ablation for supraventricular tachycardia. Circulation 98:1534–1540

Kuehne T, Fahrig R, Butts K (2003a) Pair of resonant fiducial markers for localization of endovascular catheters at all catheter orientations. J Magn Reson Imaging 17:620–624

Kuehne T, Saeed M, Higgins CB et al (2003b) Endovascular stents in pulmonary valve and artery in swine: feasibility study of MR imaging-guided deployment and postinterventional assessment. Radiology 226:475–481

Ladd ME, Erhart P, Debatin JF et al (1997) Guide wire antennas for MR fluoroscopy. Magn Reson Med 37:891–897

Ladd ME, Zimmermann GG, Quick HH et al (1998a) Active MR visualization of a vascular guide wire in vivo. J Magn Reson Imaging 8:220–225

Ladd ME, Zimmermann GG, McKinnon GC et al (1998b) Visualization of vascular guide wires using MR tracking. J Magn Reson Imaging 8:251–253

Leung DA, Debatin JF, Wildermuth S et al (1995) Intravascular MR tracking catheter: preliminary experimental evaluation. AJR Am J Roentgenol 164:1265–1270

Liu H, Hall WA, Martin AJ, Maxwell RE, Truwit CL (2000) MR-guided and MR-monitored neurosurgical procedures at 1.5 T. J Comput Assist Tomogr 24:909–918

Magee AG, Nykanen D, McCrindle BW, et al (1997) Balloon dilation of severe aortic stenosis in the neonate: comparison of anterograde and retrograde catheter approaches. J Am Coll Cardiol 30:1061–1066

Magee AG, Brzezinska-Rajszys G, Qureshi SA et al (1999) Stent implantation for aortic coarctation and recoarctation. Heart 82:600–606

Magni G, Hijazi ZM, Pandian NG et al (1997) Two- and three-dimensional transesophageal echocardiography in patient selection and assessment of atrial septal defect closure by the new DAS-Angel Wings device: initial clinical experience. Circulation 96:1722–1728

Miquel ME, Hill DL, Baker EJ et al (2003) Three- and four-dimensional reconstruction of intra-cardiac anatomy from two-dimensional magnetic resonance images. Int J Cardiovasc Imaging 19:239–254; discussion 255–256

Miquel ME, Hegde S, Muthurangu V et al (2004) Visualization and tracking of an inflatable balloon catheter using SSFP in a flow phantom and in the heart and great vessels of patients. Magn Reson Med 51:988–995

Modan B, Keinan L, Blumstein T, Sadetzki S (2000) Cancer following cardiac catheterization in childhood. Int J Epidemiol 29:424–428

Muthurangu V, Taylor AM, Andriantsimiavona R et al (2004) A novel method of quantifying pulmonary vascular resistance utilizing simultaneous invasive pressure monitoring and phase-contrast MR flow. Circulation (in press)

Nitz WR, Oppelt A, Renz W, et al (2001) On the heating of linear conductive structures as guide wires and catheters in interventional MRI. J Magn Reson Imaging 13:105–114

NRPB (1999) Guidelines on patient dose to promote the optimisation of protection for diagnostic medical exposures. National Radiation Protection Board 10:1

Ocali O, Atalar E (1997) Intravascular magnetic resonance imaging using a loopless catheter antenna. Magn Reson Med 37:112–118

Omary RA, Unal O, Koscielski DS et al (2000) Real-time MR imaging-guided passive catheter tracking with use of gadolinium-filled catheters. J Vasc Interv Radiol 11:1079–1085

Pihkala J, Nykanen D, Freedom RM, Benson LN (1999) Interventional cardiac catheterization. Pediatr Clin North Am 46:441–464

Rao PS, Galal O, Patnana M, Buck SH, Wilson AD (1998) Results of 3 to 10 year follow up of balloon dilatation of the pulmonary valve. Heart 80:591–595

Razavi R, Baker E (1999) Magnetic resonance imaging comes of age. Cardiol Young 9:529–538

Razavi RS, Baker A, Qureshi SA et al (2001) Hemodynamic response to continuous infusion of dobutamine in Alagille's syndrome. Transplantation 72:823–828

Razavi RS, Hill DL, Muthurangu V et al (2003a) Three-dimensional magnetic resonance imaging of congenital cardiac anomalies. Cardiol Young 13:461–465

Razavi R, Hill DL, Keevil SF et al (2003b) Cardiac catheterisation guided by MRI in children and adults with congenital heart disease. Lancet 362:1877–1882

Rhode KS, Hill DLG, Edwards PJ et al (2003) Registration and tracking to integrate X-ray and MR images in an XMR facility. IEEE Trans Med Imaging 22:1369–1378

Rickers C, Seethamraju RT, Jerosch-Herold M, Wilke NM (2003) Magnetic resonance imaging guided cardiovascular interventions in congenital heart diseases. J Interv Cardiol 16:143–147

Robertson MB, Kohler U, Hoskins PR, Marshall I (2001) Quantitative analysis of PC MRI velocity maps: pulsatile flow in cylindrical vessels. Magn Reson Imaging 19:685–695

Schalla S, Saeed M, Higgins CB, et al (2003) Magnetic resonance-guided cardiac catheterization in a swine model of atrial septal defect. Circulation 108:1865–1870

Serfaty JM, Yang X, Aksit P, et al (2000) Toward MRI-guided coronary catheterization: visualization of guiding catheters, guide wires, and anatomy in real time. J Magn Reson Imaging 12:590–594

Shellock FG (1989) Biological effects and safety aspects of magnetic resonance imaging. Magn Reson Q 5:243–261

Shellock FG, Kanal E (1991) Policies, guidelines, and recommendations for MR imaging safety and patient management. SMRI Safety Committee. J Magn Reson Imaging 1:97–101

Shellock FG, Kanal E (1996) Burns associated with the use of monitoring equipment during MR procedures. J Magn Reson Imaging 6:271–272

Shellock FG, Shellock VJ (1998) Cardiovascular catheters and accessories: ex vivo testing of ferromagnetism, heating, and artifacts associated with MRI. J Magn Reson Imaging 8:1338–1342

Shellock FG, Shellock VJ (1999) Metallic stents: evaluation of MR imaging safety. AJR Am J Roentgenol 173:543–547

Silverman NH, Schiller NB (1978) Apex echocardiography. A two-dimensional technique for evaluating congenital heart disease. Circulation 57:503–511

Snider AR, Silverman NH (1981) Suprasternal notch echocardiography: a two-dimensional technique for evaluating congenital heart disease. Circulation 63:165–173

Spuentrup E, Ruebben A, Schaeffter T, et al (2002) Magnetic resonance-guided coronary artery stent placement in a swine model. Circulation 105:874–879

Wong EY, Zhang Q, Duerk JL, Lewin JS, Wendt M (2000) An optical system for wireless detuning of parallel resonant circuits. J Magn Reson Imaging 12:632–638

Yeung CJ, Susil RC, Atalar E (2002a) RF safety of wires in interventional MRI: using a safety index. Magn Reson Med 47:187–193

Yeung CJ, Susil RC, Atalar E (2002b) RF heating due to conductive wires during MRI depends on the phase distribution of the transmit field. Magn Reson Med 48:1096–1098

18 General Conclusions

Jan Bogaert, Steven Dymarkowski, and Andrew M. Taylor

Imaging has become an essential part of medical decision-making. An arsenal of imaging modalities is currently available, as an extension to the patient's clinical examination. Although for cardiac diseases ultrasound is still the first-line imaging modality, the value of magnetic resonance imaging (MRI) is now widely recognized. As we have shown in the textbook, MRI has evolved over the last two decades to become an important and well-validated clinical imaging technique for the heart and great vessels.

In the early years of MRI in medicine, the heart was unquestionably the most difficult organ to investigate. However improvements in MR hardware (e.g., fast gradients, coil design), MR software (e.g., MR sequence design, navigator echoes), and postprocessing techniques have made of cardiac MRI not just an imaging technique, but one that combines many facets to investigate the cardiovascular system and comes close to the goal of a complete examination with a single technical modality. This property of MRI is not matched by any other technique. Relevant information on all aspects of the heart, including structure, global and regional ventricular function, valve function, flow patterns, myocardial perfusion, myocardial viability, and myocardial metabolism can be obtained in a totally noninvasive manner. The progress in other domains such as coronary artery luminal and wall imaging has been substantial.

In the current climate of rising health care costs, assessment of the cost-effectiveness of cardiac imaging techniques and their effect on diagnosis, diagnostic certainty, and patient management and outcome will be of utmost importance in the coming years. A description of the actual cost of each

J. Bogaert, MD, PhD; S. Dymarkowski, MD, PhD
Department of Radiology, Gasthuisberg University Hospital, Catholic University of Leuven, Herestraat 49, 3000 Leuven, Belgium
A.M. Taylor, MD, MRCP, FRCR
Cardiothoracic Unit, Institute of Child Health and Great Ormond Street Hospital for Children, London, WC1N 3JH, UK

cardiac imaging session is beyond the scope of this book due to the great differences in cost and reimbursement between countries. The cost-effectiveness of MRI as a cardiac imaging technique is under active evaluation and will determine whether MRI results in significant economic benefits in diagnosing cardiac disease.

In Table 18.1 is shown the current clinical position of MRI in comparison to the other cardiac imaging techniques. This table is based on recent literature and, although potentially controversial, it should serve as a guideline for the clinician in choosing the most appropriate diagnostic imaging modality for a particular cardiovascular problem. In our opinion, MRI is the only imaging technique that achieves a satisfactory score for nearly all diagnostic aspects of the heart and great vessels; and, in many respects, MRI can be considered as the gold standard.

General Key Points:

- The key to a successful cardiac MRI examination is a thorough knowledge of cardiac MRI techniques, and of cardiac anatomy and physiology in normal and pathological conditions.
- Patient positioning and adequate ECG triggering are crucial to obtain optimal image quality.
- MRI competes well with other cardiac imaging techniques, and should be included in an integrative approach to the investigation of patients with cardiovascular disease.
- "Black-blood" and "bright-blood" sequences are used in different imaging planes to study cardiac anatomy and function.
- The heart should not be considered as a purely morphological structure, and the impact of a heart disease on cardiac pump activity must always be determined.
- Cardiac pump activity is a repetitive process of ejection and filling. Both processes can be accurately assessed with MRI techniques and should

Table 18.1. Current clinical position of MR among the cardiac imaging modalities

	MRI	Echocardiography		MDCT	Nuclear cardiology	X-ray angiography
		TTE	TEE			
Cardiac anatomy						
Pericardium						
Thickness	+++	+	++	++	0	−
Effusion	+++	++	+++	+++	0	±
Calcifications	+	+	−	+++	0	+
Inflammation	+++	+	−	++	+	0
Myocardium						
Thickness	+++	+	++	+++	−	+
Mass	+++	+	+	+++	0	0
Tissue characterization	++(+)	+	+	+	+	−
Cardiac cavities						
Endoluminal masses	+++	++	+++	++(+)	0	++
Volume quantification	+++	++	++	++(+)	++	++
Cardiac valves						
Number of leaflets	++	++	+++	++	0	++
Valve integrity	+(+)	++	+++	+	0	+
Perivalvular space (e.g., abscess)	++	++	+++	++	0	+
Intra- and extracardiac communications						
Patent foramen ovale	+	+	+++	−	0	0
Patent ductus arteriosus	+(+)	++	++	++	0	++
Atrial septal defect	++	++	+++	+	0	++
Ventricular septal defect	++	++	+++	++	0	+++
Extracardiac spaces	+++	+(+)	+(+)	+++	0	0
Cardiac function						
Systolic function						
Global	+++	++	++	++	++(+)	++
Regional	+++	++	++	+(+)	++	+(+)
Stress imaging	+++	+++	+++	+	++	++
Diastolic function	++(+)	+++	+++	0	+	+
Strain analysis	+++	++[a]	-	0	0	0
Valvular function						
Valve stenosis	++	+++	++(+)	+	0	++(+)
Valve regurgitation	++(+)	++	+++	0	+	++
Myocardial perfusion	++(+)	+(+)	+(+)	+	++(+)	−
Myocardial viability						
Myocardial edema	+++	-	-	-	-	-
Myocardial ischemia	++(+)	++	++	0	++(+)	+
Myocardial stunning	++	++	++	0	++	+
Myocardial hibernation	++(+)	++	++	0	++(+)	+
Myocardial infarction	+++	+	+	+	++	+
Myocardial metabolism	+	0	0	0	+(+)	0
Coronary arteries						
Anatomy	++	+	−	++	0	++(+)
Patency	+	−	−	+(+)	0	+++
Calcifications	−	−	−	+++	0	+

Table 18.1. Current clinical position of MR among the cardiac imaging modalities

	MRI	Echocardiography		MDCT	Nuclear cardiology	X-ray angiography
		TTE	TEE			
Wall imaging and characterization	+	−	−(+++)[b]	+(+)	0	0
Flow and flow reserve	+	−	−(+++)[b]	−	+	+
Great vessels						
Anatomy	+++	+(+)	++(+)	+++	0	+++
Vessel wall						
Thickness	+++	+	++	+++	0	+
Integrity	++(+)	+	++	++	+	−
Vessel lumen	+++	+	++(+)	+++	0	+++
Flow pattern	+++	+	++(+)	+	0	++

+++, Excellent; ++, good; +, average; −, poor; 0, not possible
[a]Tissue Doppler imaging
[b]Intracoronary echo-Doppler
Abbreviations: MDCT, multi-detector computed tomography; MRI, magnetic resonance imaging; TEE, transesophageal echocardiography; TTE, transthoracic echocardiography

be part of a comprehensive functional evaluation.

- Cine-MRI, using the balanced steady-state free-precession (b-SSFP) technique, is currently the gold standard for global and regional functional cardiac analysis, at least if performed and interpreted adequately.
- MRI tagging techniques enable noninvasive tracking of myocardial deformation during the cardiac cycle.
- Real-time cine-MRI techniques have potential to assess the constant hemodynamic variations of the heart.
- Velocity-encoded cine-MRI techniques enable noninvasive quantification of flow velocities and volumes in vessels and through cardiac valves.
- First-pass myocardial stress perfusion imaging and dobutamine stress MRI are able to detect hemodynamically significant stenoses. Their clinical value in assessing coronary artery disease (CAD) patients is currently underestimated.
- T2-weighted, short-tau inversion-recovery (STIR) fast spin-echo MRI is unique in detecting myocardial edema.
- Contrast-enhanced inversion-recovery (CE-IR) MRI with late or delayed imaging is currently the best approach to image myocardial infarction and scarring.

- The same approach can be used to evaluate a variety of nonischemic myocardial diseases (e.g., myocarditis, myocardial fibrosis, infiltrative diseases) and pericardial diseases (e.g., pericardial inflammation).
- Coronary MR angiography is indicated to explore the origin and proximal course of the epicardial coronary arteries. Detection and quantification of coronary artery stenoses, as well as wall imaging and plaque characterization, are possible but as yet unrefined for clinical use.
- Cardiac MRI is a highly valuable technique to study cardiac masses. Cardiac thrombi can be best assessed using a combination of cine-MRI and CE-IR MRI techniques.
- The contribution of MRI in valvular heart disease is three-fold: morphological evaluation, functional evaluation of the severity, and assessment of the impact of a valvular lesion on ventricular function.
- The role of MRI in congenital heart disease is mainly in the postoperative assessment and follow-up of patients.
- MRI and computed tomography (CT) are currently the preferred techniques with which to assess the thoracic great vessels.
- Interventional MR (combined X-radiation and MRI, XMR) is a new and highly promising tool that will soon find its way to clinical use.

Subject Index

List of Contributors

NIDAL AL-SAADI, MD
Institute for Cardiac Magnetic Resonance Tomography, Berlin
Nuernberger Str. 67
10787 Berlin
Germany

JAN BOGAERT, MD, PhD
Professor of Medicine
Department of Radiology
Gasthuisberg University Hospital
Catholic University of Leuven
Herestraat 49
3000 Leuven
Belgium

HILDE BOSMANS, PhD
Department of Radiology
Gasthuisberg University Hospital
Catholic University of Leuven
Herestraat 49
3000 Leuven
Belgium

STEVEN DYMARKOWSKI, MD, PhD
Department of Radiology
Gasthuisberg University Hospital
Catholic University of Leuven
Herestraat 49
3000 Leuven
Belgium

PASCAL HAMAEKERS, RN
Radiological Technician
MR Research Center
Department of Radiology
Gasthuisberg University Hospitals
Catholic University of Leuven
Herestraat 49
3000 Leuven
Belgium

SANJEET R. HEGDE, MD
Research Fellow in Cardiovascular MR
Division of Imaging Science, King's College London
Guy's Hospital Campus
London Bridge
London SE1 9RT
UK

VIVEK MUTHURANGU, BSc, MBChB, MRCPCH
Research Fellow in Cardiovascular MR
Division of Imaging Science, King's College London
Guy's Hospital Campus
London Bridge
London SE1 9RT
UK

YICHENG NI, MD, PhD
Department of Radiology
Gasthuisberg University Hospital
Catholic University of Leuven
Herestraat 49
3000 Leuven
Belgium

REZA RAZAVI, MBBS, MRCP, MRCPCH
Director of Cardiac MRI and
Honorary Consultant Paediatric Cardiologist
Division of Imaging Science, King's College London
Guy's Hospital Campus
London Bridge
London SE1 9RT
UK

ANDREW M. TAYLOR, MD, MRCP, FRCR
Senior Clinical Lecturer and
Honorary Consultant in Cardiovascular MR
Cardiothoracic Unit
Institute of Child Health and
Great Ormond Street Hospital for Children
London WC1N 3JH
UK

MEDICAL RADIOLOGY Diagnostic Imaging and Radiation Oncology

Titles in the series already published

MEDICAL RADIOLOGY Diagnostic Imaging and Radiation Oncology

Titles in the series already published

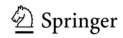

MEDICAL RADIOLOGY Diagnostic Imaging and Radiation Oncology

Titles in the series already published

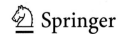 Springer